ROUTLEDGE HANDBOOK OF PHYSICAL ACTIVITY AND MENTAL HEALTH

A growing body of evidence shows that physical activity can be a cost-effective and safe intervention for the prevention and treatment of a wide range of mental health problems. As researchers and clinicians around the world look for evidence-supported alternatives and complements to established forms of therapy (medication and psychotherapy), interest in physical activity mounts.

The *Routledge Handbook of Physical Activity and Mental Health* offers the most comprehensive review of the research evidence on the effects of physical activity on multiple facets of mental health. Written by a team of world-leading international experts, the book covers ten thematic areas:

- physical activity and the 'feel good' effect
- anxiety disorders
- depression and mood disorders
- self-perceptions and self-evaluations
- cognitive function across the lifespan
- psychosocial stress
- pain
- energy and fatigue
- addictions
- quality of life in special populations.

This volume presents a balanced assessment of the research evidence, highlights important directions for future work, and draws clear links between theory, research, and clinical practice. As the most complete and authoritative resource on the topic of physical activity and mental health, this is essential reading for researchers, students and practitioners in a wide range of fields, including clinical and health psychology, psychiatry, neuroscience, behavioural and preventive medicine, gerontology, nursing, public health and primary care.

Panteleimon Ekkekakis is an Associate Professor at the Department of Kinesiology at Iowa State University. His research focuses on the affective responses to physical activity of different levels of intensity, as well as the cognitive and physiological factors that influence these responses. His publications span the areas of affective psychology, psychometrics, personality and individual differences, psychophysiology, health psychology, behavioural and preventive medicine, applied physiology, and exercise science. He is also an elected Fellow of the American College of Sports Medicine.

ROUTLEDGE HANDBOOK OF PHYSICAL ACTIVITY AND MENTAL HEALTH

EDITOR-IN-CHIEF
Panteleimon Ekkekakis

SECTION EDITORS
Dane B. Cook
Lynette L. Craft
S. Nicole Culos-Reed
Panteleimon Ekkekakis
Jennifer L. Etnier
Mark Hamer
Kathleen A. Martin Ginis
Justy Reed
Jasper A.J. Smits
Michael Ussher

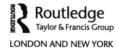

LONDON AND NEW YORK

First published in paperback 2015
First published 2013
by Routledge
2 Park Square, Milton Park, Abingdon, Oxon OX14 4RN

Simultaneously published in the USA and Canada
by Routledge
711 Third Avenue, New York, NY 10017

Routledge is an imprint of the Taylor & Francis Group, an informa business

British Library Cataloguing in Publication Data
A catalogue record for this book is available from the British Library

Library of Congress Cataloging-in-Publication Data
Routledge handbook of physical activity and mental health /
edited by Panteleimon Ekkekakis.
p. cm.
1. Exercise–Physiological aspects. 2. Exercise–Psychological aspects. 3. Cognitive psychology. 4. Mental health. 5. Psychobiology. I. Ekkekakis, Panteleimon, 1968–
QP301.R693 2013
613.7'1–dc23
2012040802

ISBN: 978–0–415–78299–9 (hbk)
ISBN: 978–1–138–92473–4 (pbk)
ISBN: 978–0–203–13267–8 (ebk)

Typeset in Bembo
by Keystroke, Station Road, Codsall, Wolverhampton

Printed and bound in the United States of America by Publishers Graphics, LLC on sustainably sourced paper.

CONTENTS

FIGURES

TABLES

CONTRIBUTORS

Ana M. Abrantes
Assistant Professor (Research)
Alpert Medical School of Brown University
Associate Director of Addictions Research
Butler Hospital
United States of America

Kelly Arbour-Nicitopoulos
Assistant Professor
Faculty of Kinesiology and Physical
Education
University of Toronto
Canada

Lars Arendt-Nielsen
Professor
Laboratory for Musculoskeletal Pain and
Motor Control
Center for Sensory-Motor Interaction (SMI)
Department of Health Science and
Technology
Aalborg University
Denmark

Lisa A. Barella
Assistant Professor
Department of Health, Kinesiology, and
Sport Studies
Coastal Carolina University
United States of America

Deborah Barnes
Associate Professor
Department of Psychiatry
Veterans Affairs Medical Centre
University of California, San Francisco
United States of America

Rebecca Bassett-Gunter
Assistant Professor
School of Kinesiology and Health Science
York University
Canada

Jacqueline L. Beaudry
Graduate Student
School of Kinesiology and Health Science
Muscle Health Research Centre and Physical
Activity and Chronic Disease Unit
York University
Canada

Nicole C. Berchtold
Project Scientist
Institute for Memory Impairments and
Neurological Disorders
University of California, Irvine
United States of America

James A. Blumenthal
Professor of Psychiatry
Department of Psychiatry and Behavioral
Sciences
Division of Behavioral Medicine
Duke University Medical Center
United States of America

Henning Boecker
Professor and Head
Functional Neuroimaging Group
Department of Radiology
University of Bonn
Germany

Richard A. Brown
Professor
Alpert Medical School of Brown University
Director of Addictions Research
Butler Hospital
United States of America

Francis Chaouloff
Researcher
Team Endocannabinoids and
NeuroAdaptation
Neurocentre INSERM U862
University of Bordeaux
France

Michael J. Chen
Assistant Research Professor
Department of Biological Sciences
California State University, Los Angeles
United States of America

Dane B. Cook
Associate Professor
Department of Kinesiology
University of Wisconsin – Madison
United States of America

Carl W. Cotman
Professor
Institute for Memory Impairments and
Neurological Disorders
University of California, Irvine
United States of America

Kerry S. Courneya
Professor, Canada Research Chair in Physical
Activity and Cancer
Faculty of Physical Education and Recreation
University of Alberta
Canada

Lynette L. Craft
Adjunct Assistant Professor
Department of Preventive Medicine
Feinberg School of Medicine
Northwestern University
United States of America

Peter R. E. Crocker
Professor
School of Kinesiology
University of British Columbia
Canada

S. Nicole Culos-Reed
Associate Professor
Faculty of Kinesiology
University of Calgary
Canada

Rod K. Dishman
Professor
Department of Kinesiology
Biomedical Health Sciences Institute,
Neuroscience Division
University of Georgia
United States of America

Anna D'souza
Graduate Student
School of Kinesiology and Health Science
Muscle Health Research Centre and Physical
Activity and Chronic Disease Unit
York University
Canada

Sarah Dubreucq
Graduate Student
Team Endocannabinoids and
NeuroAdaptation
Neurocentre INSERM U862
University of Bordeaux
France

Contributors

Kate M. Edwards
Lecturer
Discipline of Exercise and Sport Science
University of Sydney
Australia

Panteleimon Ekkekakis
Associate Professor
Department of Kinesiology
Iowa State University
United States of America

Steriani Elavsky
Assistant Professor
Department of Kinesiology
Pennsylvania State University
United States of America

Laura D. Ellingson
Post-doctoral Fellow
Department of Kinesiology
University of Wisconsin – Madison
United States of America

Charles F. Emery
Professor
Department of Psychology
Ohio State University
United States of America

Kirk I. Erickson
Assistant Professor
Department of Psychology
Center for the Neural Basis of Cognition
University of Pittsburgh
United States of America

Jennifer L. Etnier
Professor
Department of Kinesiology
University of North Carolina at Greensboro
United States of America

Guy Faulkner
Professor
Faculty of Kinesiology and Physical
Education
University of Toronto
Canada

Monika Fleshner
Professor
Department of Integrative Physiology
Center for Neuroscience
University of Colorado at Boulder
United States of America

Jennifer I. Gapin
Assistant Professor
Department of Kinesiology and Health
Education
Southern Illinois University –
Edwardsville
United States of America

Katharina Gaudlitz
Research Assistant
Department of Psychiatry and
Psychotherapy
Charité – Universitätsmedizin Berlin
Germany

Paul Gorczynski
Post-doctoral Fellow
Centre for Addiction and Mental Health
Canada

Neha Gothe
Graduate Student
Department of Kinesiology and
Community Health
University of Illinois at Urbana-
Champaign
United States of America

Thomas Graven-Nielsen
Professor
Laboratory for Musculoskeletal Pain and
Motor Control
Center for Sensory-Motor Interaction
(SMI)
Department of Health Science and
Technology
Aalborg University
Denmark

Contributors

Benjamin N. Greenwood
Assistant Research Professor
Department of Integrative Physiology
Center for Neuroscience
University of Colorado Boulder
United States of America

Mark Hamer
Principal Research Associate
Psychobiology Group
Department of Epidemiology and Public
Health
University College London
United Kingdom

Matthew P. Herring
Research Associate
Department of Epidemiology
University of Alabama at Birmingham
United States of America

Kelly Ickmans
PhD Researcher
Department of Human Physiology
Faculty of Physical Education and
Physiotherapy
Vrije Universiteit Brussel
Belgium

Lindsay E. Kipp
Lecturer
Department of Kinesiology and Health
Promotion
University of Kentucky
United States of America

Daphne Kos
Post-doctoral Researcher
Division of Occupational Therapy
Department of Health Care Sciences
Artesis University College Antwerp
Belgium
and
Assistant Professor
Katholieke Universiteit Leuven
Belguim

Risa N. Long
Graduate Student
Department of Psychology
The Ohio State University
United States of America

Wendy J. Lynch
Associate Professor
Departments of Psychiatry and
Neurobehavioral Sciences
University of Virginia
United States of America

Michael Mackenzie
Post-doctoral Researcher
Department of Kinesiology and
Community Health
University of Illinois at Urbana-
Champaign
United States of America

Henrik B. Madsen
PhD Fellow
Laboratory for Musculoskeletal Pain and
Motor Control
Center for Sensory-Motor Interaction
(SMI)
Department of Health Science and
Technology
Aalborg University
and
Pain Center South
University Hospital Odense
Denmark

Emily L. Mailey
Assistant Professor
Department of Kinesiology
Kansas State University
United States of America

Petra Majdak
Graduate Student
Neuroscience Program
University of Illinois
United States of America

Giovanni Marsicano
Researcher
Team Endocannabinoids and
NeuroAdaptation
Neurocentre INSERM U862
University of Bordeaux
France

Kathleen A. Martin Ginis
Professor
Department of Kinesiology
McMaster University
Canada

Isabelle Matias
Post-doctoral Researcher
Team Endocannabinoids and
NeuroAdaptation
Neurocentre INSERM U862
University of Bordeaux
France

Stephen Matsko
Graduate Student
University of Rhode Island
Research Associate
Butler Hospital
United States of America

Edward McAuley
Professor
Department of Kinesiology and Community
Health
University of Illinois
United States of America

Carolyn E. McEwen
Graduate Student
School of Kinesiology
University of British Columbia
Canada

Desmond McEwan
Graduate Student
Department of Kinesiology
McMaster University
Canada

Mira Meeus
Post-doctoral Researcher
Department of Human Physiology
Faculty of Physical Education and
Physiotherapy
Vrije Universiteit Brussel
Belgium
and Assistant Professor
Department of Health Care
University College Antwerp
Belgium
and Assistant Professor
Department of Rehabilitation Sciences and
Physiotherapy
Ghent University
Belgium

Jacob D. Meyer
Graduate Student
Department of Kinesiology
University of Wisconsin – Madison
United States of America

Laura E. Middleton
Assistant Professor
Department of Kinesiology
University of Waterloo
Canada

Paul J. Mills
Professor in Residence
Department of Psychiatry
Behavioral Medicine Program
University of California, San Diego
United States of America

Amber D. Mosewich
Graduate Student
School of Kinesiology
University of British Columbia
Canada

Robert W. Motl
Associate Professor
Department of Kinesiology and
Community Health
University of Illinois
United States of America

Jo Nijs
Associate Professor
Department of Human Physiology
Faculty of Physical Education and
Physiotherapy
Vrije Universiteit Brussel
Belgium

KayLoni L. Olson
Graduate Student
Department of Psychology
Ohio State University
United States of America

Michael W. Otto
Professor
Department of Psychology
Boston University
United States of America

Mark B. Powers
Research Assistant Professor
Department of Psychology
Southern Methodist University
United States of America

Timothy W. Puetz
Presidential Management Fellow
Office of the Director
National Institutes of Health
Department of Health and Human Sciences
United States of America

Justy Reed
Professor
Department of Secondary Education,
Professional Studies and Recreation
Chicago State University
United States of America

Justin S. Rhodes
Associate Professor
Department of Psychology
University of Illinois
United States of America

Michael C. Riddell
Associate Professor
School of Kinesiology and Health
Science
Muscle Health Research Centre and
Physical Activity and Chronic Disease
Unit
York University
Canada

Morgan R. Shields
Graduate Student
Department of Kinesiology
University of Wisconsin – Madison
United States of America

Kathleen A. Sluka
Professor
Department of Physical Therapy and
Rehabilitation Science
University of Iowa
United States of America

Mark A. Smith
Professor
Department of Psychology
Davidson College
United States of America

Patrick J. Smith
Assistant Professor of Psychiatry
Department of Psychiatry and Behavioral
Sciences
Division of Behavioral Medicine
Duke University Medical Center
United States of America

Jasper A. J. Smits
Associate Professor
Department of Psychology
Southern Methodist University
United States of America

Aaron J. Stegner
Assistant Scientist
Department of Kinesiology
University of Wisconsin – Madison
United States of America

Andrew Steptoe
British Heart Foundation Professor of
Psychology
Psychobiology Group
Department of Epidemiology and Public
Health
University College London
United Kingdom

Shaelyn M. Strachan
Assistant Professor
Faculty of Kinesiology and Recreation
Management
University of Manitoba
Canada

Andreas Ströhle
Professor, Senior Consultant
Department of Psychiatry and Psychotherapy
Charité – Universitätsmedizin Berlin
Germany

Amanda N. Szabo
Energy Balance Laboratory
University of Kansas
United States of America

Adrian H. Taylor
Professor
School of Sport and Health Sciences
University of Exeter
United Kingdom

Robert S. Thompson
Graduate Student
Department of Integrative Physiology
Center for Neuroscience
University of Colorado Boulder
United States of America

Michael Ussher
Reader in Health Psychology
Division of Population Health Sciences and
Education
St. George's, University of London
United Kingdom

Angela C. Utschig
Research Assistant Professor
Center for Anxiety and Related Disorders
Boston University
United States of America

Jeffrey Vallance
Associate Professor
Faculty of Health Disciplines
Athabasca University
Canada

Inge van Eupen
Post-doctoral Researcher
Division of Occupational Therapy
Department of Health Care Sciences
Artesis University College Antwerp
Belgium

Jessica Van Oosterwijck
Post-doctoral Researcher
Department of Human Physiology
Faculty of Physical Education and
Physiotherapy
Vrije Universiteit Brussel
Belgium

Brigitt-Leila von Lindenberger
Research Assistant
Department of Psychiatry and
Psychotherapy
Charité – Universitätsmedizin Berlin
Germany

Michelle W. Voss
Assistant Professor
Department of Psychology
University of Iowa
United States of America

Maureen R. Weiss
Professor
School of Kinesiology
University of Minnesota
United States of America

Diane E. Whaley
Associate Professor
Curry School of Education
Director, Lifetime Physical Activity
Program
University of Virginia
United States of America

Jessica Wolfe
Research Assistant
Addictions Research
Butler Hospital
United States of America

Kristine Yaffe
Professor
Departments of Psychiatry, Neurology, and
Epidemiology and Biostatistics
Veterans Affairs Medical Centre
University of California, San Francisco
United States of America

Elisabeth Zschucke
Research Assistant
Department of Psychiatry and Psychotherapy
Charité – Universitätsmedizin Berlin
Germany

PHYSICAL ACTIVITY AS A MENTAL HEALTH INTERVENTION IN THE ERA OF MANAGED CARE

A rationale

Panteleimon Ekkekakis

The aim of this introductory chapter is to outline the *raison d'être* of this handbook. This is established by a sequence of arguments substantiating the following points. First, mental health problems are very prevalent in the industrialized world, are of exceptional societal importance, and exact a high cost both in terms of quality of life and in terms of economic impact. Second, a high percentage of individuals suffering from mental health problems do not seek help, and of those who do, many exhibit poor compliance with treatment regimens. Most likely, these phenomena are due to concerns related to the high cost of diagnosis and treatment, questions about the effectiveness of common treatments, and an unwillingness to risk or cope with adverse side-effects. Third, a growing corpus of evidence suggests that physical activity can be an inexpensive, safe, and, most importantly, effective lifestyle intervention that could be used to both prevent and treat a wide range of mental health problems and to improve overall quality of life. However, the effectiveness of physical activity as a mental health intervention is not universally acknowledged. For various reasons, many researchers and practitioners in medicine, psychology, and public health remain either uninformed or unconvinced about the potential of physical activity to promote mental health. Some of these reasons may stem from dualistic and disciplinary rifts and others from legitimate concerns about the methodological rigor of the extant studies. Distinguishing between these, and arriving at an accurate appraisal of the evidence, is becoming increasingly difficult.

This volume was compiled with the goal of offering an encompassing and balanced account of the evidence. World-leading experts from various disciplines review what has been found so far, highlighting notable accomplishments but also pointing out limitations and persistent lacunae that should be addressed in future studies.

Societal importance of public mental health

The prevalence, societal impact, and economic cost of mental disorders are impossible to estimate with accuracy. It is generally acknowledged that published figures most likely represent underestimates. To a large extent, this is attributed to the stigma still attached to mental disorders and the associated unwillingness of many people to undergo a diagnosis for a mental disorder or to disclose information that they perceive as personally embarrassing.

1

Worldwide impact

The World Health Organization (2003) estimates that approximately 450 million people suffer from a mental or behavioral disorder. Worldwide, four of the six leading causes of disability are psychiatric in nature (i.e., depression, alcohol-use disorders, schizophrenia, and bipolar disorder). Collectively, mental disorders (excluding those associated with stroke and brain trauma) account for 12.9% of all disability-adjusted life years lost, compared to 9.3% for cardiovascular disease and 5.2% for all cancers combined (Andlin-Sobocki, Jönsson, Wittchen, & Olesen, 2005). As the prevalence and impact of mental health problems grow, the 14-country World Mental Health Survey shows that 35.5–50.3% of serious cases of mental illness in developed countries and 76.3–85.4% in less-developed countries receive no treatment (WHO World Mental Health Survey Consortium, 2004). Besides social stigmatization, the high cost of therapy and the scarcity of specialized therapeutic resources are believed to contribute to this problem.

In 2000, depression was the fourth leading cause of disease burden according to the Global Burden of Disease (GBD) study, accounting for 4.4% of total disability-adjusted life years. It was also responsible for the largest portion of non-fatal burden, accounting for almost 12% of all years lived with disability (Üstün, Ayuso-Mateos, Chatterji, Mathers, & Murray, 2004). It is estimated that by the year 2020, unipolar major depression will become the second cause of disability worldwide, behind only ischemic heart disease (Murray & Lopez, 1997). By 2030, unipolar depression is projected to be the leading cause of disability in high-income countries (Mathers & Loncar, 2006).

Moreover, dementia, one of the most debilitating mental disorders, is estimated to afflict more than 30 million people worldwide (Ferri et al., 2005; Wimo, Jönsson, & Winblad, 2006). With many countries facing the challenge of an aging population, 4.6 million new cases of dementia are expected every year (one every 7 seconds). At this rate, the number of people affected by this disease is expected to double every 20 years, exceeding 80 million by 2040. In 2009, the total worldwide societal cost of dementia, based on a population of 34.4 million demented persons, was estimated at US$422 billion, including US$142 billion (34%) for informal care. This estimate represents an increase of 34% between 2005 and 2009 (Wimo, Winblad, & Jönsson, 2010).

Across the 27 countries/members of the Europe Union, it is estimated that each year 38.2% of the population suffers from a mental disorder (Wittchen et al., 2011). Even after accounting for comorbidity, this figure corresponds to 164.8 million people. Brain and mental disorders collectively account for 26.6% of the total disability burden. The four most disabling conditions are depression, dementias, alcohol use disorders, and stroke. Very importantly, fewer than one-third of the people affected receive any treatment.

In the United States, according to the replication of the National Comorbidity Survey, about half of Americans meet the criteria for a DSM-IV disorder sometime in their life. Approximately 50% of all lifetime cases of mental illness begin by age 14 and 75% by age 24 (Kessler et al., 2005). Importantly, there are long delays – sometimes decades – between the first onset of symptoms and when people seek treatment (Wang et al., 2005). According to the report by the U.S. Surgeon General on mental health (United States Department of Health and Human Services, 1999), "concerns about the cost of care – concerns made worse by the disparity in insurance coverage for mental disorders in contrast to other illnesses – are among the foremost reasons why people do not seek needed mental health care" (p. 23). Moreover, there are considerable disparities along socioeconomic, geographical, and racial/ethnic lines (González et al., 2010). As a result, according to the data from the National Comorbidity Survey, a nationwide prevalence study based on face-to-face household interviews, only 20.3% of individuals who satisfied diagnostic criteria for a mental disorder received treatment in 1990–1992 and 32.9% in 2001–2003

(Kessler et al., 2005). Interestingly, of those individuals who received treatment, only half met diagnostic criteria for a mental disorder.

Economic cost

The economic cost of mental illness at the societal level is both direct and indirect, the latter being considerably more difficult to estimate. Direct costs include expenses associated with medication use, clinic visits, and hospitalization. The Agency for Healthcare Research and Quality reported that the number of individuals treated for mental disorders nearly doubled from 19.3 million in 1996 to 36.2 million in 2006 (Soni, 2009). The direct cost of their care increased from US$35.2 billion to US$57.5 billion. This made mental disorders the third costliest in terms of direct costs, behind only heart disease (US$78.0 billion) and trauma-related disorders (US$68.1 billion) and at the same level as cancer (US$57.5 billion). However, this estimate does not include several major categories of direct costs, such as drugs. A study conducted by the Substance Abuse and Mental Health Services Administration (Mark et al., 2007) estimated the direct cost of mental health disorders at US$100 billion in 2003, with substance abuse problems costing an additional US$21 billion. These figures exclude costs associated with all types of dementia, tobacco addiction, mental retardation, and mental developmental delays. An estimate subject to the same exclusions puts the annual cost at US$203 billion by 2014 (Levit et al., 2008).

The indirect costs stem from a multitude of sources, including (but not limited to) reduced productivity and increased absenteeism, reduced income and ensuant need for publicly financed assistance (e.g., unemployment compensation, disability benefits, food stamps, public housing), reduced educational attainment, incarceration and other crime-related costs, and homelessness. According to one study (Kessler et al., 2008), after controlling for confounding variables (e.g., age, gender, race, region of the country, as well as alcohol and illicit drug abuse), an individual who had experienced a mental illness in the previous 12 months had an income that was on average US$16,306 less than that of an individual without a mental illness (US$26,435 among men, US$9,302 among women). At the societal level, the cost was astronomical, estimated at US$193.2 billion (US$131.3 billion among men, US$61.9 billion among women). What complicates the estimation of the total societal cost further is the fact that mental disorders exhibit extensive comorbidity with a broad range of physical illnesses, forming a complex web of causal interactions. For example, persons with serious mental illness smoke 44% of all cigarettes in the United States, thus increasing the prevalence of pulmonary disease (Insel, 2008). A study across eight U.S. states documented that clients of public mental health agencies had a risk of death that was 1.2 to 4.9 times higher than that of the average state population. The lives of these individuals were 13.5 to 32.2 years shorter than state averages (Colton & Manderscheid, 2006).

To illustrate the grave economic implications of indirect costs, it is useful to examine two disorders, the impact of which has been analyzed in numerous studies. In 2000, the cost of depression in the United States was estimated at US$83.1 billion. Of this amount, US$26.1 billion (31%) were direct medical costs and US$5.4 billion (7%) were suicide-related mortality costs. On the other hand, the workplace costs were estimated at US$51.5 billion or 62% of the total (Greenberg et al., 2003).

According to the Alzheimer's Association (2010), Alzheimer's disease (AD) is the seventh leading cause of death in the United States, causing approximately as many deaths annually as diabetes. AD is also the fifth leading cause of death among Americans aged 65 and older. Importantly, although the rates of other major causes of death have declined in recent years, the rate due to AD has increased and is projected to continue to increase. For example, between 2000 and 2006, heart disease deaths decreased by 11.1%, stroke deaths decreased by 18.2%, and prostate cancer-related deaths decreased by 8.7%. In contrast, deaths due to AD increased by 46.1%. By 2050, the prevalence of AD in the United States is expected to reach 11 to 16 million people, as the baby boomer generation ages. The Alzheimer's Association estimates that the direct cost of caring for people over 65 with AD and other dementias will reach US$172 billion in 2010, including US$123 billion for Medicare and Medicaid. In 2004, each Medicare beneficiary with AD or another dementia incurred costs (for health care, long-term and hospice) that were three times higher than those of other Medicare beneficiaries of the same age. Likewise, in 2004, each Medicaid beneficiary with AD or another dementia incurred costs (for nursing home and other long-term care for people with very low income and low assets) that were nine times higher than those of other Medicaid beneficiaries of the same age. In addition to these costs, in 2009, approximately 11 million family members and other unpaid caregivers provided an estimated 12.5 billion hours of care to persons with AD and other dementias. This care is valued at nearly US$144 billion. Moreover, caregivers of individuals suffering from AD and other dementias experience increased risk of anxiety, depression, and other mental health problems (Cooper, Balamurali, & Livingston, 2007; Cuijpers, 2005; Etters, Goodall, & Harrison, 2008; Schulz, Boerner, Shear, Zhang, & Gitlin, 2006).

In Canada, Health Canada (2002) estimates that 20% of Canadians will experience a mental illness during their lifetimes. The cost was initially estimated at CA$14.4 billion in 1998 (Stephens & Joubert, 2001). The Canadian Mental Health Association (2004) reported to the House of Commons that mental illnesses account for 50% of physicians' billing and is responsible for more hospital bed days than cancer. After taking into account the costs associated with undiagnosed mental illnesses and the impact on health-related quality of life, a more recent estimate raised the cost for 2003 to CA$51 billion (Lim, Jacobs, Ohinmaa, Schopflocher, & Dewa, 2008).

In England, an extensive study by the King's Fund estimated that 8.65 million people with a mental health problem lived in the country in 2007 (McCrone, Dhanasiri, Patel, Knapp, & Lawton-Smith, 2008). A 14% increase is projected by 2026. The associated costs are expected to increase from £48.6 billion in 2007 to £88.45 billion in 2026. In 2007, almost half of the cost (£22.5 billion) represented money spent on direct NHS and social care services to support people with mental disorders. The rest (£26.1 billion) represented the estimated cost to the economy of earnings lost because of the thousands of people unable to work due to their mental illness. The direct (mental health service) costs were projected to increase by 45% over the next 20 years from £22.5 billion to £47 billion due to more cases of dementia and the projected increase in health care costs. Specifically, due to the aging population, the incidence of dementia is expected to increase by 61%, from 582,827 cases to 937,636 cases. The service costs associated with dementia are far higher than all other conditions put together. In 2007 they accounted for 66% of all mental health service costs, but by 2026 it is estimated that they will make up 73% of all mental health service costs.

Growing skepticism about psycho- and pharmacotherapies

The "formal" methods of treating mental health problems, according to the U.S. Surgeon General's report on mental health (1999), include various types of psychotherapy and pharmacotherapy. Of the two approaches, the use of psychotherapy appears to be steady or declining, whereas the use of pharmacotherapy has increased dramatically in the past several years. The reasons include the scarcity of psychotherapy resources, the relative affordability of pharmacotherapy for most individuals with insurance coverage, and the very aggressive direct-to-consumers advertising of major classes of psychotropic medications (e.g., antidepressants, anxiolytics, mood stabilizers, analgesics, sleep aids).

Psychotherapy

In the United States, the rates of psychotherapy appear to have remained steady, with 3.2% of individuals in 1987, 3.6% in 1997, and 3.18% in 2007 receiving some type of psychotherapy on an outpatient basis (Olfson & Marcus, 2010; Olfson, Marcus, Druss, & Pincus, 2002). In particular, psychotherapy delivered by a psychiatrist declined from 44.4% of all psychotherapy visits in 1996–1997 to 28.9% in 2004–2005 (Mojtabai & Olfson, 2008). Among many academics, the effectiveness of psychotherapy has been in question since Eysenck's (1952) challenge to the field more than 60 years ago. Eysenck argued that the studies that were available until that time "failed to prove that psychotherapy, Freudian or otherwise, facilitates the recovery of neurotic patients. They show that roughly two-thirds of a group of neurotic patients will recover or improve to a marked extent within about two years of the onset of their illness, whether they are treated by means of psychotherapy or not" (p. 322). He added that "definite proof would require a special investigation, carefully planned and methodologically more adequate than these *ad hoc* comparisons" (p. 323). Even after so many years, this kind of "definite proof" remains elusive (Nutt & Sharpe, 2008).

A persistent source of controversy is the fact that meta-analyses generally show no difference between the effect sizes associated with psychotherapy and those associated with placebos. For example, Prioleau, Murdock and Brody (1983) examined 32 studies comparing psychotherapy to a placebo condition and found an average effect size of only .15. Although some subsequent meta-analysts have questioned this finding (Grissom, 1996; Lipsey & Wilson, 1993), a more recent analysis by Baskin, Callen Tierney, Minami, and Wampold (2003) concluded that as long as the placebo interventions are properly designed (i.e., controlling for such structural aspects as number and duration of sessions, training of therapist, format of therapy, etc.), the effect size compared to psychotherapy is indeed very small (.15). The skepticism is fueled by consistent findings that (a) a substantial percentage of patients report an early positive response (Lambert, 2005) and (b) the various types of psychotherapy, despite large differences in their theoretical background and the format of their procedures, seem indistinguishable in terms of therapeutic effectiveness (Smith & Glass, 1977; Wampold et al., 1997). In response to such findings, several psychotherapists have argued that the placebo is not an appropriate control or comparison condition for assessing the effectiveness of psychotherapy (Herbert & Gaudiano, 2005; Kirsch, 2005; Parloff, 1986; Senger, 1987). The main reason in support of this argument is that what is implied by a "placebo" response is in fact an inextricably intertwined component of the psycho-therapeutic process. In essence, the argument is that the so-called "common factors" of all psychotherapeutic modalities (e.g., expectations of benefit, prescription for activity, discussion, attention, compassion, caring, and warmth) may be crucial contributors to the effectiveness of psychotherapy. What this implies, however, is that the therapeutic "active ingredient" in psychotherapy (much less the specific "active ingredient" of different types of psychotherapy) remains unknown. According to a recent authoritative review, "it is remarkable that after decades of psychotherapy research, we cannot provide an evidence-based explanation for how or why even our most well studied interventions produce change" (Kazdin, 2007, p. 23). In other words, if psychotherapy works, no one yet knows why. Moreover, concerns about the safety of psycho-therapy, particularly long-term psychotherapy, are growing (Barlow, 2010; Nutt & Sharpe, 2008).

Pharmacotherapy

The effectiveness and safety of certain types of pharmacotherapy for mental disorders is becoming the subject of intense controversy. In particular, a heated debate has centered around anti-depressants, which, since 2004–2005, have become the most widely prescribed class of drugs in the United States (United States National Center for Health Statistics, 2010). Because of their overwhelming popularity, antidepressants will be used here as an example to illustrate the argument about the growing concerns surrounding the effectiveness and safety of pharmacotherapy for mental disorders.

Across the 27 countries/members of the European Union, 8% of the population overall, and 10% of middle-aged adults, take antidepressants each year (Blanchflower & Oswald, 2011). Antidepressant use exhibits an inverted U-shape relationship with age, being highest for individuals in their late 40s (particularly women) and those who are unemployed, poorly educated, and divorced or separated.

The prescription of antidepressants in the United States nearly doubled in a decade (from 5.84% in 1996 to 10.12% in 2005, or from 13.3 to 27 million users; Olfson & Marcus, 2009). Interestingly, during this period, only 26% of the individuals who received prescriptions for antidepressants were being treated for depression, since these drugs were also commonly prescribed for a wide range of mental health conditions, including back pain and headaches, anxiety, adjustment disorders, sleep disorders, neuropathy, fatigue, and bipolar disorder.

In Canada, antidepressants are the most widely prescribed class of psychotropic medications (Beck et al., 2005), with 5.8% of the population using them. Interestingly, nearly half (47.7%) of antidepressant users have no history of depression (Beck et al., 2005). Antidepressants are even prescribed more frequently than sedatives or hypnotics for individuals with anxiety and more frequently than mood stabilizers for individuals with bipolar disorder. Older tricyclic antidepressants, in particular, are now being prescribed predominantly for diagnoses other than depression (Patten, Esposito, & Carter, 2007). At the same time, 59.6% of individuals with a depression diagnosis in the previous year do not receive a prescription for antidepressants.

In Scotland, the volume of prescribed antidepressants tripled between 1995/1996 and 2006/2007 (Lockhart & Guthrie, 2011). This dramatic increase has been due to a combination of more patients being given prescriptions (from 8% of the population in 1995/1996 to 11.9% in 2000/2001) and increased treatment duration (from 170 days per year to 200). Across the United Kingdom, the number of prescriptions per patient per year increased from 2.8 in 1993 to 5.6 in 2004 (Moore et al., 2009). In England, antidepressant prescriptions increased by 10% per year, on average, over a 13-year period (i.e., 130% overall; Ilyas & Moncrieff, 2012).

The increasing use of antidepressants does not only have economic implications. Two additional problems are receiving increasing attention in the literature. The first deals with questions about their actual effectiveness and the second with their safety profile. On both of these issues, the initial assumptions of clinicians and the positive impressions among the general public must be reevaluated on the basis of emerging evidence.

Meta-analyses on the effectiveness of antidepressants had reached positive conclusions but also included caveats about the fact that the effect sizes were typically small, the methodological quality typically low, the treatment periods short (6–8 weeks), and pharmaceutical companies were providing the funding (Arroll et al., 2009; Arroll et al., 2005). Although the impact of the strong grip of the pharmaceutical industry on the publication of evidence had long been suspected (Healy & Cattell, 2003; McGoey, 2010), the magnitude of this problem was unveiled in a landmark study published in the prestigious *New England Journal of Medicine* (Turner, Matthews, Linardatos, Tell, & Rosenthal, 2008). The researchers compared data from 74 randomized controlled trials (RCTs) that were registered with the U.S. Food and Drug Administration (FDA) with results from the published literature. They found that the findings of 23 of the 74 FDA-registered studies (31%) were unpublished. Of the 74 studies, the FDA deemed 38 (51%) "positive." All but 1 of these 38 "positive" studies were published. The FDA deemed the remaining 36 studies (49%) either "negative" (24 studies) or "questionable" (12 studies). Of these

36 studies, only 3 were published as "non-positive." The remaining 33 either were not published (22 studies) or were published as positive (11 studies). Overall, 48 of 51 published studies were reported as having yielded positive results (94%), although only 38 of the 74 FDA-registered studies actually yielded positive results (51%). Moreover, the mean effect size for published studies was 0.37, whereas the mean effect size for unpublished studies was significantly lower (0.15).

Perhaps the most disconcerting piece of evidence from this analysis was the evaluation of publication practices. First, the effect sizes in published journal articles exceeded the effect size from the FDA reviews of the same studies. The increases in effect sizes ranged from 11% to 69% with a median of 32%. Furthermore, there were instances of (a) presenting data from only one site of a multicenter trial when that site produced positive results but the other sites did not, (b) failing to perform intention-to-treat analyses on the entire original sample, as specified by the approved study protocol, and instead presenting "efficacy" data on a select subsample, and (c) failing to exclude from the analyses "outlier" sites, at which there were significant deviations from the approved study protocol if the exclusion of these sites would have nullified the overall efficacy of the trial.

Another groundbreaking meta-analysis examined the effect of baseline levels of depression on the effectiveness of the six most widely prescribed antidepressants (Kirsch et al., 2008). The investigators retrieved and analyzed data from all the trials that had been submitted by pharmaceutical companies to the FDA for regulatory approval, as well as all studies from the published literature. To evaluate the clinical meaningfulness of the results, the researchers used the commonly employed criteria of either a three-point improvement in Hamilton Rating Scale of Depression (HRSD) scores or an effect size (standardized mean difference) of $d = 0.50$. Overall, the mean improvement among samples who received the drug was 9.60 HRSD points ($d = 1.24$), whereas the mean improvement among placebo samples was 7.80 HRSD points ($d = 0.92$). This 1.80-point difference ($d = 0.32$) was below the established 3-point criterion of clinical meaningfulness.

The relative effectiveness (or lack thereof) of antidepressants did not change as a function of depression severity at baseline. On the other hand, the effectiveness of placebo decreased as the severity of depression at baseline increased. The difference between drug and placebo rose as a linear function of baseline depression severity, reaching the criterion for clinical meaningfulness only for those patients with very high baseline HRSD scores (i.e., 28 or higher, with "very severe" depression defined by the American Psychiatric Association as a score of 23 or higher). However, this difference was due to the decreased effectiveness of placebo when baseline depression was high rather than any increase in the effectiveness of the antidepressants. There was virtually no difference in the improvement scores for drug and placebo for individuals with moderate depression (but note that there was only one study of individuals with moderate depression). The researchers commented that in these trials the placebo accounted for approximately 80% of the effect of the antidepressant drug, when only 50% of the effect of analgesics can be replicated by placebo.

An independent commentator (Ioannidis, 2008) wrote: "Perhaps most people given antidepressants for depressive symptoms would just need some attention from their physician and people to talk to and take some care of them. Antidepressants may be covering largely the lost placebo of human interaction and patient–physician interaction that has become so sparse in modern society" (p. 7). In support of this general assessment, researchers have found that the apparent effectiveness of both antidepressants and placebos increases as a linear function of the number of follow-up visits with the prescribing physician during a trial. In fact, there was a 0.6–0.9-point improvement in the HRSD for each visit that took place during the trial (Posternak & Zimmerman, 2007). Ioannidis (2008) added:

If most of the antidepressant efficacy reflects simply the placebo effect, and if most people just benefit as much as the placebo effect allows, is it unethical to kill a living myth? One might argue that if the general population is informed that antidepressants are not really effective, this might demolish the benefits that we get from the placebo effect when we administer these drugs. However, is it not unethical to lie to patients that an intervention is effective when it is not?

(Ioannidis, 2008, p. 7)

Although the findings of the meta-analysis by Kirsch et al. (2008) are very hard to dismiss, the limitation of having included only one study of individuals with moderate depression (HRSD of 14 to 18) and no studies of individuals with mild (HRSD score of 8 to 13) or severe (HRSD score of 19 to 22) depression was important. To address this limitation, a new meta-analysis pooled together individual data from six large placebo-controlled trials that included patients with a wide range of baseline depression scores (Fournier et al., 2010). In agreement with the findings of Kirsch et al., Fournier et al. found a significant baseline severity by treatment interaction. Specifically, for patients in the mild to moderate range, the effect size was only $d = 0.11$ (with 95% confidence interval from −0.18 to 0.41) and for patients in the severe range the effect size was $d = 0.17$ (with 95% confidence interval from −0.08 to 0.43). Only for patients in the very severe group did the effect size approach the criterion for clinical meaningfulness (i.e., $d = 0.47$, with 95% confidence interval from 0.22 to 0.71). Again supporting the results of the Kirsch et al. meta-analysis, Fournier et al. estimated that antidepressants become more effective than placebo only for patients with very severe baseline depression scores (i.e., HRSD score of 27 or higher).

Besides effectiveness, drugs must also be evaluated for their safety. It is well established that patient adherence to prescriptions for antidepressants is low and the rates of early discontinuation are high (Gartlehner et al., 2005; Goethe, Woolley, Cardoni, Woznicki, & Piez, 2007; Hunot, Horne, Leese, & Churchill, 2007). Specifically, although most prescribing physicians recommend to their patients to stay on antidepressants for at least 6 months (Bull et al., 2002), the majority of patients discontinue antidepressant therapy during the first 30 days (42.4%), whereas only 27.6% continue for more than 90 days (Olfson, Marcus, Tedeschi, & Wan, 2006). Although part of the non-adherence might be due to factors such as misunderstanding the physician's instructions or patient forgetfulness or lack of motivation, the perceived lack of effectiveness and a wide range of adverse side-effects are also responsible. Experiencing one or more "extremely" bothersome side-effects has been found to be associated with more than a doubling of the risk of discontinuation (Goethe et al., 2007).

At the top of the list of the most disconcerting side-effects of modern antidepressants is the increased risk of suicidal ideation and suicide attempts. Accumulating evidence of this risk led the FDA to add a "black box" warning (the strictest type of warning) on the packaging of selective serotonin reuptake inhibitor (SSRIs) antidepressants in 2004. The warning reads in part: "Antidepressants increased the risk of suicidal thinking and behavior (suicidality) in short-term studies in children and adolescents with Major Depressive Disorder (MDD) and other psychiatric disorders." In 2005, the warning was extended to include all antidepressant drugs and in 2007 the warning was extended to young adults (aged 18 to 24 years). Although the absolute number of suicide attempts and suicides is relatively small, the risk associated with the use of antidepressants is significantly elevated compared to placebo (Healy, 2003). For example, a study in the United Kingdom found that, compared with patients who had started taking an antidepressant more than 90 days before developing (nonfatal) suicidal behavior, those who had started taking an antidepressant within 1 to 9 days earlier showed a 4.07-fold higher risk of a suicidal episode, and those who had started taking an antidepressant within 10 to 29 days earlier showed a 2.88-fold higher risk (Jick, Kaye, & Jick, 2004). Similarly, a study in Canada found that SSRI users had a 4.8-fold increased risk of suicide during the first month after receiving their prescription compared to case-matched controls (Juurlink, Mamdani, Kopp, & Redelmeier, 2006).

Second, SSRIs have been found to increase the risk of sexual dysfunction, particularly reducing sexual desire and causing problems in achieving orgasm (Balon, 2006; Kennedy & Rizvi, 2009). A meta-analysis estimated that sexual dysfunction occurs in 25.8% to 80.3% of patients on SSRIs compared to placebo (Serretti & Chiesa, 2009).

Third, SSRIs have been found to increase the risk of bleeding of the upper gastrointestinal tract (Turner, May, Arthur, & Xiong, 2007). The risk has been found to be 3.6 times higher than for non-users but can increase 9.1-fold (de Abajo & García-Rodríguez, 2008) or 12.2-fold (Oksbjerg Dalton et al., 2003) when SSRIs are taken together with aspirin or non-steroidal anti-inflammatory drugs.

Fourth, patients on SSRIs complain of sleep disturbances. In a cohort of 2,853 women over the age of 71 years, the women taking SSRI were 2.15 times more likely than non-users to sleep for 5 hours or less, 2.37 times more likely to experience sleep efficiency of 70% or less, 3.99 times more likely to experience a latency of 1 hour or more before falling asleep, and 1.75 times more likely to experience eight or more long wake episodes (Ensrud et al., 2006). Importantly, in this study sleep variables were assessed objectively by actigraph and analyses were adjusted for a multitude of potential confounders (i.e., age, race, health status, social support, physical activity, alcohol intake, medical conditions, history of depression, functional status, current benzodiazepine use, current use of non-benzodiazepine anxiolytic or hypnotic medications, depressive symptoms, symptoms of anxiety, cognitive function, and BMI).

Fifth, most classes of antidepressants have been known to cause weight gain both acutely and chronically. Weight gain is typically larger with tricyclic antidepressants and monoamine oxidase inhibitors but can also be significant with SSRIs (Deshmukh & Franco, 2003; Schwartz, Nihalani, Jindal, Virk, & Jones, 2004). Furthermore, a population study in Canada (Kisely, Cox, Campbell, Cooke, & Gardner, 2009) showed that older adults (67 years of age or older) had 34% increased risk of developing hypertension as early as 3 months after the initial prescription of SSRIs (after controlling for age, sex, socioeconomic class, schizophrenia, beta blockers, diuretics, anti-psychotics, and other drugs).

Thus, psychotherapy and pharmacotherapy, despite being recognized as the "standard" or "mainstream" approaches for the treatment of mental disorders, may not be as effective or as safe as they are commonly portrayed. Furthermore, it is important to point out that for some mental disorders, neither psychotherapy nor pharmacotherapy can presently offer any plausible preventive or treatment options. For example, in the case of Alzheimer's disease and other dementias, an expert panel convened by the National Institutes of Health in the United States (Daviglus et al., 2010) concluded that "no consistent epidemiologic evidence exists for an association with statins, antihypertensive medications, or anti-inflammatory drugs [while] data are insufficient to comment on cholinesterase inhibitors" (p. 178). Furthermore, "no known medication can be said to reliably delay the onset of Alzheimer disease" (p. 179). To the contrary, "some available evidence shows that certain medications may increase the incidence of Alzheimer disease" (p. 179; also see Plassman, Williams Burke, Holsinger, & Benjamin, 2010).

Physical activity as an underappreciated mental health intervention

The option of physical activity interventions for promoting mental health must be evaluated in the context of the emerging concerns outlined in the previous section. In essence, the growing concerns about the efficacy, safety, and cost of the main forms of therapy have prompted a search for other viable options. It is reasonable to propose that the conditions have now matured for the consideration and acceptance of effective, safe, inexpensive, and widely accessible alternative preventive and therapeutic modalities for a broad spectrum of mental health problems. Of the available options, physical activity seems supremely positioned due to an already-voluminous evidence base, virtual absence of adverse side-effects, minimal cost, limitless global accessibility, and a wide range of collateral benefits, including those on metabolic and cardiovascular health (Phillips, Kiernan, & King, 2003).

Recent advances and emerging challenges

In recent years, some important steps have been taken in bringing exercise and physical activity closer to widespread clinical application in the domain of mental health. For example, the latest (third) edition of the *Practice Guideline for the Treatment of Patients with Major Depressive Disorder*, published by the American Psychiatric Association (Gelenberg et al., 2010), states the following in regard to the role of exercise:

> For most individuals, exercise carries benefits for overall health. Data generally support at least a modest improvement in mood symptoms for patients with major depressive disorder who engage in aerobic exercise or resistance training. Regular exercise may also reduce the prevalence of depressive symptoms in the general population, with specific benefit found in older adults and individuals with co-occurring medical problems . . . If a patient with mild depression wishes to try exercise alone for several weeks as a first intervention, there is little to argue against it, provided the patient is sufficiently monitored for an abrupt worsening of mood or adverse physical effects (e.g., ischemia or musculoskeletal symptoms). The dose of exercise and adherence to an exercise regimen may be particularly important to monitor in the assessment of whether an exercise intervention is useful for major depressive disorder. If mood fails to improve after a few weeks with exercise alone, the psychiatrist should recommend medication or psychotherapy. For patients with depression of any severity and no medical contraindication to exercise, physical activity is a reasonable addition to a treatment plan for major depressive disorder. The optimal regimen is one the patient prefers and will adhere to.
>
> *(Gelenberg et al., 2010, pp. 29–30)*

Likewise, the updated edition of the *Guideline on the Treatment and Management of Depression in Adults*, issued by the National Collaborating Centre for Mental Health and the National Institute for Health and Clinical Excellence (2010) in the United Kingdom, states that "for people with persistent subthreshold depressive symptoms or mild to moderate depression," clinicians should "consider offering one or more of the following interventions, guided by the person's preference: (a) individual guided self-help based on the principles of cognitive behavioral therapy, (b) computerized cognitive behavioral therapy, or (c) a structured group physical activity program" (p. 213). Along similar lines, an evidence-based national clinical guideline for the *Non-pharmaceutical Management of Depression in Adults*, issued by the Scottish Intercollegiate Guidelines Network (2010), states that "structured exercise may be considered as a treatment option for patients with depression" (p. 10).

In other cases, although the evidence is compelling, the response from agencies with authority to issue clinical guidelines or recommendations has been tepid. A case in point is dementia and cognitive decline. An expert panel convened to summarize the conclusions of the state-of-the-science conference on Preventing Alzheimer Disease and Cognitive Decline, organized by the National Institutes of Health (Daviglus et al., 2010), stated the following:

> Some evidence from small interventional studies and selected observational studies suggests that increased physical activity, including walking, may help maintain or improve cognitive function in normal adults. A meta-analysis of several RCTs, many with methodological limitations, concluded that data were insufficient to state that aerobic activity improves or maintains cognitive function. A small, higher-quality randomized trial of physical activity in persons with confirmed memory problems showed modest benefit in reducing cognitive decline; however, these data should be viewed as preliminary. Work is ongoing to further investigate the benefits of physical activity.
>
> *(Daviglus et al., 2010, p. 180)*

Although the language conveys very little enthusiasm, when this statement is juxtaposed to statements regarding other factors whose association to dementia and cognitive decline was also examined at the conference, one gets the impression that physical activity may be among the most promising interventions. For most other potential interventions, the panel found no indication of a beneficial effect. Nevertheless, experts have strongly criticized the conservative tone of this statement, arguing that, by considering solely large clinical trials as sources of evidence, the conclusions of the panel underestimated and misrepresented the strength of the evidence. Flicker, Liu-Ambrose, and Kramer (2011) commented that the evidence for physical activity was "discounted too cursorily for what is now a large and relatively consistent pool of animal and human data" and that "it is difficult to understand why the NIH consensus statement has taken such a cautious approach" (p. 466). Ahlskog, Geda, Graff-Radford, and Petersen (2011) characterized the approach taken by the panel as "nihilistic" (p. 877). Arguably, however, the portrayal of the evidence for physical activity was not only "cautious" and "nihilistic." In a rather remarkable excerpt, the panel clustered together physical activity and "other leisure activities," as if implying that the respective evidence pertaining to these types of "activities" were comparable in size, strength, quality, or consistency: "Preliminary evidence suggests beneficial associations of physical activity and other leisure activities (such as club membership, religious services, painting, or gardening) with preservation of cognitive function" (p. 178).

Over the years, authors from various backgrounds have expressed puzzlement, even frustration, that physical activity, despite its apparent strengths, is not being promoted more actively as a preventive or therapeutic intervention in the domain of public health (Berk, 2007; Callaghan, 2004; Daley, 2002; Donaghy, 2007; Faulkner & Biddle, 2001; Otto et al., 2007; Taylor & Faulkner, 2008; Tkachuk & Martin, 1999). The reality is that, with growing recognition over the years, new challenges have emerged. When physical activity is recommended on a national scale as an effective and safe alternative to established therapies for mild or moderate depression or when physical activity appears to show more promise than any other form of intervention for slowing the progression of cognitive decline, it is natural to stimulate broader interest and, with that, elicit some unintended consequences. These include reactions fueled by dualistic incredulity, opposition stemming from disciplinary territorialism, and, importantly, the wrath of significant financial interests. In combination, these responses raise the risk of bias tingeing the assessments of the evidence that appear in the published literature (MacCoun, 1998). As a result, the literature has been inundated with conflicting, confusing, and misleading conclusions and has become immensely challenging to evaluate, particularly for non-specialists.

The crucial role of paradigms

It would be shortsighted, even outright erroneous, to read the following sections without placing them within a broader epistemological framework. Neither science nor science-driven clinical practice work simply on the basis of what the evidence shows. They work on the basis of paradigms, as defined by Kuhn (1962/1996). Paradigms do not coexist peacefully and do not transition smoothly from one to the next. They battle each other. According to Kuhn, a dominant paradigm imposes "immense restriction of the scientist's vision," to the point that science becomes "increasingly rigid" (p. 64). Consequently, there is always "considerable resistance to paradigm change" (p. 64). Even when scientists "begin to lose faith [and] consider alternatives," they "do not renounce the paradigm that has led them into crisis" (p. 77). The main reason is that "as in manufacture so in science – retooling is an extravagance to be reserved for the occasion that demands it" (p. 76).

Kuhn (1962/1996) emphasized that the transition from an old paradigm to a new one "is far from a cumulative process" (p. 84). Instead, a crisis that forces a field into a search for alternatives essentially induces "a reconstruction of the field from new fundamentals, a reconstruction that changes some of the field's most elementary theoretical generalizations as well as many of its paradigm methods and applications" (p. 85). Because of the radical nature of transitions, such "reconstructions" progress slowly and usually amid considerable tension. Kuhn further suggested that, because the paradigm is such an integral component of the careers of established scientists, researchers who attempt the "reconstruction of the field from new fundamentals" are "almost always . . . either very young or very new to the field whose paradigm they change" (p. 90). These characteristics give them an advantage because they entail that these scientists are "little committed by prior practice to the traditional rules of normal science" and, as a result, they "are particularly likely to see that those rules no longer define a playable game and to conceive another set that can replace them" (p. 90). When a scientific revolution to replace an existing paradigm begins, it is "often restricted to a narrow subdivision of the scientific community" (p. 92).

A relevant example that illustrates the validity of these points is the recognition of the role of exercise in cardiovascular health. Writing in a major medical journal as recently as 1979, Kannel and Sorlie asserted that "it does not seem likely that exercise programs can make as great an impact on incidence of cardiovascular disease as can control of blood pressure, the cigarette habit, obesity, or hyperlipemia" (p. 860). Today, physical activity is widely regarded as one of, if not the most powerful interventions for the promotion of cardiovascular health, and physical activity recommendations are published jointly by the American Heart Association and the American College of Sports Medicine (Haskell et al., 2007). It is therefore doubtful that a similar statement would find its way into a major medical journal.

Simpler times

When the first reviews on the association between physical activity and mental health appeared in the literature, the evidence base consisted only of small-scale correlational and a few quasi-experimental studies. Nevertheless, there was hopeful enthusiasm on the part of exercise scientists that, eventually, the evidence would demonstrate that exercise and physical activity have important roles to play in this domain. With the thin red line separating scientific impartiality from advocacy being somewhat fuzzy, disagreements were bound to emerge. For example, an exercise scientist asserted that "the 'feeling better' sensation that accompanies regular physical activity is so obvious that it is one of the few universally accepted benefits of exercise" (Morgan, 1981, p. 306). At the same time, based on the same limited data, a psychiatrist and a stress physiologist concluded that, although "the psychological benefits of fitness training, especially jogging, have been propagandized by the popular press" (Folkins & Sime, 1981, p. 373), the "status of theorizing about the processes that might explain physical fitness training effects can best be described as a potpourri of speculations" (p. 374) and the "studies of physical fitness effects on psychological health are poorly designed" (p. 386). A little later, another psychiatrist agreed, stating that "the enthusiastic support of exercise to improve mental health has a limited empirical basis and lacks a well tested rationale" (Hughes, 1984, p. 76). These early disagreements can be easily attributed to the fact that one side was basing its statements on belief or intuition whereas the other on a more dispassionate assessment of the scant evidence.

Exercise as analogous to complementary healers

Despite substantial growth in the evidence base during the 1980s and 1990s, views on the role of physical activity in mental health continued to diverge. In 1996, a landmark report of the Surgeon General of the United States on the relationship between physical activity and health included the following statement:

> The literature suggests that physical activity helps improve the mental health of both clinical and nonclinical populations. Physical activity interventions have benefitted persons from the general population who report mood disturbance, including symptoms of anxiety and depression, as well as patients who have been diagnosed with nonbipolar, nonpsychotic depression. These findings are supported by a limited number of intervention studies conducted in community and laboratory settings . . . The psychological benefits of regular physical activity for persons who have relatively good physical and mental health are less clear.
>
> *(United States Department of Health and Human Services, 1996, p. 136)*

In 1999, the 458-page report of the Surgeon General on mental health did not mention physical activity among the recognized methods of treatment for anxiety and depression, which only included psychotherapy and pharmacotherapy. Physical activity was mentioned as one of an "ever-expanding list" of "informal" interventions for coping with stressful life events, alongside "religious and spiritual endeavors" and "complementary healers" (United States Department of Health and Human Services, 1999, p. 232). Citing the earlier report, some possible benefits were acknowledged. However, this was immediately followed by a caveat about the poor methodological quality of the evidence base:

> Physical activities are a means to enhance somatic health as well as to deal with stress. A recent Surgeon General's Report on Physical Activity and Health evaluated the evidence for physical activities serving to enhance mental health. Aerobic physical activities, such as brisk walking and running, were found to improve mental health for people who report symptoms of anxiety and depression and for those who are diagnosed with some forms of depression. The mental health benefits of physical activity for individuals in relatively good physical and mental health were not as evident, but the studies did not have sufficient rigor from which to draw unequivocal conclusions.
>
> *(United States Department of Health and Human Services, 1999, p. 232)*

"There is no evidence"

To date, there is only one empirical study that examined the level of awareness among professionals in clinical psychology of the research literature on physical activity and mental health.

Faulkner and Biddle (2001) conducted interviews with 21 directors of doctoral programs in clinical psychology in the United Kingdom. The interviews showed that physical activity is, for the most part, ignored in clinical psychology curricula. The authors attributed this phenomenon to a certain degree of disciplinary bias, fueled by "a continued adherence to a dualistic notion of mental illness and mental health" (Faulkner & Biddle, 2001, p. 442). What was most relevant to the present review was the finding that the program directors were unaware of research evidence supporting a role of physical activity in the domain of mental health. Faulkner and Biddle (2001) wrote: "Awareness of the exercise and mental health literature was extremely limited, with most participants being unfamiliar with existing research" (p. 439). This conclusion was based on statements by program directors, such as the following:

> There is no evidence. Although you might find the odd paper which says that exercise is effective here and there, as far as treating clinical problems, populations with psychological and psychiatric problems, to my knowledge there is no evidence.
>
> *(Faulkner & Biddle, 2001, p. 439)*

Another program director wondered: "We might want to ask the question, if there's evidence for exercise, why is no one mentioning it?" (p. 439). Other respondents questioned the quality of the extant evidence but were unable to refer to specific problems because this concern was based on suspicion rather than actual first-hand knowledge: "the participants were unable to offer critical insight into the nature of existing research because they were unaware of its existence in the first place" (pp. 439–440).

Perhaps "a bit harsh" but at least a stimulus for improvement

Conflicting assessments continued to appear in the new millennium. A much-discussed issue was depression. Following a systematic review of the evidence on the effects of exercise on depression, commissioned by the Somerset Health Authority in the United Kingdom, a panel of exercise scientists concluded that "overall, the evidence is strong enough for us to conclude that there is support for a causal link between physical activity and reduced clinically defined depression. This is the first time such a statement has been made" (Biddle, Fox, Boutcher, & Faulkner, 2000, p. 155). At the same time, an epidemiologist and a psychiatrist, based on a meta-analysis on the same topic, despite finding that exercise had a substantial positive effect (mean effect size of 1.1) and was no less effective than (much costlier) cognitive therapy, concluded that "the effectiveness of exercise in reducing symptoms of depression cannot be determined because of a lack of good quality research on clinical populations with adequate follow up" (Lawlor & Hopker, 2001, p. 1).

One possible reason for these conflicting evaluations is the scope of the evidence that was considered in each case. Biddle et al. (2000) examined a broad range of sources, spanning the gamut from epidemiologic studies to experiments and neurobiological data. On the other hand, Lawlor and Hopker (2001) considered only RCTs. Furthermore, for Lawlor and Hopker, the evaluation of methodological rigor was based solely on three criteria, namely, "whether allocation was concealed and intention to treat analysis was undertaken, and whether there was blinding" (p. 2). On the basis of these criteria, they judged most studies as being "of poor quality" (p. 3) or "low quality" (p. 5). Closer examination of their criteria, however, reveals a rather peculiar combination of punctiliousness and superficiality. For example, concealment of treatment allocation was judged as "adequate" only if a report specifically mentioned that there was "central randomization at a site remote from the study; computerized allocation in which records are in a locked, unreadable file that can be accessed only after entering patient details; the drawing of sealed and opaque sequentially numbered envelopes" (p. 2). Some of these criteria have been characterized as "arbitrary" (Blumenthal & Ong, 2009, p. 97). At the same time, more consequential threats to internal validity received no attention (Ekkekakis, 2008; Ekkekakis & Backhouse, 2009).

Given the fact that the Lawlor and Hopker (2001) meta-analysis covered studies published until 1999 and the first Consolidated Standards of Reporting Trials (CONSORT) were published in 1996 (Begg et al., 1996), it is unsurprising that methodological details, such as the exact method of randomization and concealment of treatment allocation, were not reported with the greatest degree of specificity. Lawlor and Hopker found that "in no study was treatment allocation described, and contact with authors established that allocation might have been adequately concealed in only three [of 14] studies" (p. 3). In other words, the concealment was judged as inadequate for 79% of the studies. For comparison, prior to the publication of the original CONSORT statement, allocation concealment was judged as "unclear" for 79% of RCTs published in the same highly regarded medical journal in which Lawlor and Hopker published their analysis (Moher, Jones, & Lepage, 2001). Therefore, although highlighting departures from modern reporting guidelines may give a semblance of scientific stringency and provide a basis for summarily dismissing studies as being of low quality, it also overlooks the fact that the standards of this literature were not much different from those of the broader medical literature of the pre-CONSORT era.

The conclusions and critical assessment of the literature by Lawlor and Hopker (2001) prompted a range of responses from researchers working in this field. Defending their approach, Lawlor and Hopker cited an earlier analysis by Schulz, Chalmers, Hayes, and Altman (1995), which found that "trials that reported either inadequate or unclear concealment methods yielded estimates of [odds ratios] that were exaggerated by an average of 41% or 30%, respectively, compared with estimates of [odds ratios] derived from trials that apparently had taken adequate steps to conceal treatment allocation" (p. 411). However, as Callaghan (2004) pointed out, even under the worst-case scenario of inadequate concealment, the exercise effect may be attenuated but remains quite substantial: "on closer scrutiny it would be more accurate to conclude, in my view, that the evidence is weakened but not invalidated. In their review Lawlor and Hopker report an average effect size for exercise . . . of 1.1. Taking the upper end of Schulz et al.'s figure, we can reduce this effect size by 40% to account for methodological weaknesses. This leaves an effect size of 0.66, medium by widely cited estimates" (p. 478).

Other authors criticized the narrow view of the evidence but also conceded that the quality of the evidence was still lacking compared to the strict standards typically expected of RCTs that form the foundation for evidence-based clinical practice:

> It would appear that this assessment is a bit harsh, insofar as there are many studies that, taken together, offer considerable evidence for the benefits of exercise in reducing depression in clinical populations. However, it also is true that there are limited data from well designed clinical trials, which are often considered the gold standard for evaluating the effectiveness of a new therapy . . . Because of the limited data currently available, it could be stated that if the prescription of exercise for [major depressive disorder] required approval from the Food and Drug Administration, it probably would not pass current standards.
>
> *(Brosse, Sheets, Lett, & Blumenthal, 2002, p. 754)*

Despite its arguably inordinate emphasis on technicalities that may be of little practical consequence while missing other crucial problems, the review by Lawlor and Hopker (2001) can be credited with a sensitization of researchers to the need to adhere closely to reporting guidelines and to describe methodological details with greater clarity. For example, using language strongly reminiscent of the Lawlor and Hopker criteria for adequate allocation concealment, Dunn, Trivedi, Kampert, Clark, and Chambliss (2005) wrote that "randomization was implemented with sequentially numbered, opaque, sealed envelopes" (p. 2). Similarly, Blumenthal et al. (2007) wrote that "randomization was performed centrally by computer" and "patients were provided with sealed envelopes containing their group assignment" (Blumenthal et al., 2007, p. 588). As a result, subsequent updates of the meta-analysis have identified more studies that satisfied the quality assessment criteria. The total number, however, remains low. Specifically, out of 25 studies included in the analysis in 2009 (Mead et al., 2009) and 30 that were included in 2012 (Rimer et al., 2012), only three and four, respectively, satisfied all three criteria (i.e., adequate allocation concealment, intention-to-treat analyses, and blinded outcome assessors). Limiting the analysis to such a small group of studies rendered the average effect not statistically significant. Furthermore, although the analysis indicated that "when compared with other established treatments (cognitive behavioral therapy and antidepressants), there was no difference between exercise and the established intervention," the authors insist that "outstanding uncertainties remain about how effective exercise is for depression, mainly because of methodological considerations" (Rimer et al., 2012, p. 17).

Distinguishing findings from their interpretation

Placing emphasis on methodological stringency generally tends to give reviews the semblance of a "strict but fair" impartiality, which is inherently appealing to scientists. However, closely parsing the language of critical reviews can be very revealing. For example, the conclusion of a recent meta-analysis on the effects of exercise on depression among individuals who satisfied diagnostic criteria for depression was:

> The results of this systematic review and meta-analysis suggest that exercise at most has a small benefit in relieving symptoms of depression in patients with clinically diagnosed depression in the short term, based on the [standardized mean difference] of −0.4 which is within the range considered to represent a small effect (0.2 to 0.5).
>
> *(Krogh, Nordentoft, Sterne, & Lawlor, 2011, p. 535)*

First, Cohen (1992) did not define a "small" effect as a range from 0.2 to 0.5 standard deviation but rather as a point estimate of 0.5 standard deviation: "the small, medium, and large [effect sizes] are $d = .20, .50,$ and $.80$. Thus, an operationally defined medium difference between means is half a standard deviation" (Cohen, 1992, p. 157). An effect size of 0.4 is closer to 0.5 (and therefore a "moderate" effect) than it is to 0.2 (or "small").

Second, and more importantly, the non-exercise comparison groups included active treatments, such as pharmacotherapy with regular doses of sertraline hydrochloride, group psychotherapy, and non-aerobic forms of exercise, all of which have been shown effective for reducing depression. By using these comparison groups, studies that showed substantial exercise-induced decreases in symptoms of depression were entered in the analysis as having a null or even a slightly negative effect, lowering the overall pooled standardized mean difference.

Third, the reviewers noted that they found "no evidence that this small effect lasted beyond the duration of the exercise program" (Krogh et al., 2011, pp. 535–536). However, as it has justly been noted, "there is no reason to believe that exercise training would continue to benefit patients after they discontinued exercise any more than patients who stopped taking their antidepressant medication would continue to benefit from medication if they discontinued their medication" (Blumenthal & Ong, 2009, p. 98).

Fourth, the reviewers committed a classic logical fallacy: George has a beard. Goats have beards. Therefore, George is a goat. Now, substitute "George" for "exercise" and "goat" for "placebo effect": "The reduced effect in trials of longer duration might suggest that any effect of exercise is largely placebo in nature, since placebo effects tend to diminish with time" (Krogh et al., 2011, p. 536). There are, of course, numerous other, arguably more likely, scenarios for an effect whose magnitude appears to be reduced over time, before one must arrive at the conclusion that the culprit is the placebo effect.

RCTs as the sole credible source of scientific evidence

Starting with the oft-cited Lawlor and Hopker (2001) review, it has become common practice in systematic reviews dealing with physical activity and various aspects of mental health to limit study selection only to randomized clinical trials, then to reject most of these trials on the basis of various methodological weaknesses, then find a substantial average effect size from the remaining trials, but finally to dismiss this finding because these remaining trials are characterized as too few or too small. On the surface, focusing exclusively on RCTs appears reasonable; after all, this is the standard method used in evaluating the effectiveness of drugs.

On the other hand, this approach essentially sets up an unwinnable game. There are no hard rules for either the number or the size of RCTs that can be thought to constitute an adequate evidentiary basis. So, a reviewer could simply declare, for example, that five RCTs, despite showing strong and consistent positive results, are too few or that their sample sizes are not above a certain arbitrary number that seems large (e.g., 100 participants), regardless of whether the trial was adequately powered. Likewise, a reviewer can always call for even larger and even longer RCTs. Although this may seem hard to refute, there are limits to what can be funded. It should be kept in mind that, unlike trials funded by the pharmaceutical industry, trials of exercise and physical activity are funded mostly by governmental sources and have considerably smaller budgets. Moreover, as the evidence for the benefits of physical activity mounts, governmental funding agencies become increasingly reluctant to approve trials that include the randomization of vulnerable individuals, such as mental health patients or elderly individuals with dementia or cognitive impairment, to control groups (Flicker et al., 2011).

At this point, readers of the literature are confronted with a very confusing situation. Expert panels examine the same evidence base and arrive at conflicting conclusions. For patients and clinicians looking for guidance, it is very difficult to understand how this is possible or what they should do. One apparent cause for the disagreements is that different reviewers apply different study inclusion and exclusion criteria. Some limit their scope to RCTs because this type of design has the potential to provide the most reliable evidence. Others also consider observational and quasi-experimental studies, as well as basic science research, thus drawing information from a much broader and more diverse range of sources. Other possible sources of disagreement are the criteria for evaluating study quality, as well as how consequential each methodological weakness is interpreted to be. Even after taking these different approaches to systematic reviewing into account, however, disagreements are still likely to occur because, ultimately, the process of evaluating the evidence is impossible to disentangle from the element of subjectivity.

As one example, an expert panel, convened under the direction of the Centers for Disease Control and Prevention Healthy Aging Research Network, conducted an extensive review of the evidence on whether exercise and physical activity interventions can maintain or improve the cognitive function of older community-dwelling adults (Snowden et al., 2011). The conclusion of the panel was that "no intervention–outcome pairings had good quality overall" (p. 714) and, therefore, there is "insufficient evidence of cognitive benefits from exercise or physical activity interventions in older adults" (pp. 714–715). As in every other review focusing solely on RCTs, the panel recommended "larger-scale, rigorous clinical trials with longer follow-up periods" (p. 715).

At the same time, another panel of experts (from psychiatry and neurology), after examining evidence that also included neurobiological mechanisms of cognition, concluded that "aerobic exercise is associated with a reduced risk of cognitive impairment and dementia" and "may slow dementing illness." This is because of "two plausible biologic pathways" including attenuating the progression of neurodegenerative processes and reducing vascular risk factors that contribute to dementia risk, particularly via small vessel disease. For these reasons, the authors recommended that "moderate-intensity physical exercise should be considered as a prescription for lowering cognitive risks and slowing cognitive decline across the age spectrum" (Ahlskog et al., 2011, p. 882).

At this point, it should be clear that the process of systematic reviewing is not working as intended. If it did, there would not be as many systematic reviews whose conclusions stand in stark contrast to each other. Therefore, a reasonable proposal is to encourage the standardization of the process and, importantly, increase the transparency by which conclusions are reached and recommendations are made. The practice of summarily rejecting a body of research should be replaced by a specific account of the perceived methodological quality of each study that was considered, the reasons for this judgment, and the weight allocated to each study in reaching a final conclusion. The field of evidence-based medicine has made considerable strides in developing quasi-standardized guidelines, such as the Grading of Recommendations Assessment, Development, and Evaluation (GRADE) protocol. The GRADE approach acknowledges that "the quality of evidence represents a continuum" (Balshem et al., 2011, p. 404) and consistent evidence from observational studies has its rightful place. Furthermore, it appears that, at a minimum, adhering to the GRADE process can reduce some of the arbitrariness and enhance the transparency of systematic reviews in the field of physical activity and mental health:

> There will be cases in which competent reviewers will have honest and legitimate disagreement about the interpretation of evidence. In such cases, the merit of GRADE is that it provides a framework that guides one through the critical components of this assessment and an approach to analysis and communication that encourages transparency and an explicit accounting of the judgments involved.
>
> *(Balshem et al., 2011, p. 405)*

There is pro-exercise bias too, particularly in the exercise literature

Advocacy is seldom a good guide in science and it is true that, over the years, many statements about the mental health benefits of physical activity have tended to "anticipate rather than reflect the accumulation of strong evidence" (Salmon, 2001, p. 36). Therefore, readers would be well served to apply the same degree of scrutiny and skepticism to assessments of the evidence that seem to favor a role for physical activity in mental health as to those that question it.

As an example, one meta-analysis concluded that its results "provide Level 1, Grade A evidence supporting the use of exercise for the alleviation of depressive symptoms" (Rethorst, Wipfli, & Landers, 2009, p. 506) and another that its results represent "Level 1, Grade A evidence for using exercise as a treatment for anxiety disorders" (Wipfli, Rethorst, & Landers, 2008, p. 401). Both meta-analyses were published in highly regarded exercise science journals.

The "Level 1, Grade A" (i.e., top-level) classification refers to a now-obsolete grading system proposed by Guyatt, Cook, Sackett, Eckman, and Pauker (1998) for the evaluation of evidence for different types of antithrombotic medications. According to the logic of this grading system, to achieve the highest level of recommendation, evidence must come from "meta-analysis or a large randomized trial with consistent results" (p. 444S). Thus, for "Grade A," the evidence base must exhibit the following characteristics: "methods strong, results consistent, RCTs, no heterogeneity" (Guyatt et al., 1998, p. 442S, see Table 1). The authors further explained that "one approach to arriving at a best estimate is to conduct rigorous systematic reviews and meta-analyses of RCTs. Another is to employ the results of a single large study if it provides a more accurate estimate of the treatment effect" (p. 442S). Under "Grade A" evidence, there are two levels, 1 and 2. What distinguishes the two levels is whether the effects are clearly beneficial ("Level 1") or equivocal ("Level 2," i.e., it is "uncertain whether the benefits outweigh the risks").

What distinguishes "Grade A" from "Grade B" evidence is the presence (for "Grade A") or absence (for "Grade B") of consistency in the results of the different studies. Thus, for "Grade B" evidence, the criteria are: "methods strong, results inconsistent, RCTs, heterogeneity" (p. 442S, see Table 1). Within "Grade B" evidence, there are again two levels, with "Level 1" evidence requiring "effect clear" (i.e., "that benefits outweigh risks"), and "Level 2" evidence established when the "effect [is] equivocal" (i.e., "uncertainty whether benefits outweigh risks").

In interpreting Guyatt et al.'s (1998) grading system, Wipfli et al. (2008) wrote that, because "large-scale randomized trials are often extremely costly and time consuming to conduct," meta-analysis offers a way to "get around" this problem by "combining results of Level 2 studies, which are smaller randomized, controlled trials" (p. 394). Along the same lines, Rethorst et al. (2009) argued that "Level 1, Grade A evidence can be provided either through one large randomized controlled trial or through a meta-analysis of smaller (Level 2, Grade B) randomized controlled trials" (p. 492). In turn, "Level 2, Grade B studies are similar to Level 1, Grade A studies in that they are randomized controlled trials. However, these studies have smaller sample sizes and thus are susceptible to type II errors" (pp. 492–493).

It seems clear that this interpretation is inconsistent with the logic of Guyatt et al.'s (1998) grading system. For Guyatt et al., the key question was that of consistency. The best case scenario would be to have multiple RCTs yielding consistent results: "Investigators will generate the strongest recommendations when RCTs yielding consistent results (grade A evidence) are available" (p. 442S). If there is only a single RCT, it may still be considered as yielding Grade A evidence ("we classify recommendations as grade A if they are based on even a single RCT"), as long as the RCT is "large," so that its estimate of treatment effect is "accurate." If the single RCT is small, the confidence interval around the point estimate of the treatment effect would be large and, if the lower bound of the confidence interval approaches zero, then there would be more "uncertainty" about the benefits of treatment. Likewise, if multiple RCTs have yielded inconsistent results, especially if some approximate a null effect, there would again be "uncertainty" about the benefit:

> When several RCTs yield widely differing estimates of treatment effect for which there is no explanation (we label this situation "heterogeneity present"), the strength of recommendations from even rigorous RCTs is weaker (grade B evidence) . . . We must acknowledge the heterogeneity of results across studies. In doing so, any recommendation would move from grade A to grade B.
>
> *(Guyatt et al., 1998, p. 442S)*

Furthermore, a crucial point was that for evidence to be classified as either "Grade A" or even "Grade B," the methods must be "strong." It is clear that the random allocation of participants to conditions is not a sufficient condition for a methodology to be labeled "strong." Even if using a randomized design, a methodology would not be characterized as "strong" if treatment allocation was not adequately concealed, assessors were not blinded (particularly when the outcomes are subjective and their assessment is susceptible to bias), when there were large losses to follow-up, when there was no intention-to-treat analysis, when the trial stopped earlier than scheduled, or when there was publication bias (e.g., failure to publish non-significant results).

With this in mind, it is important to point out that one of the aforementioned meta-analyses did not include ratings of quality (Wipfli et al., 2008), whereas the other identified only 5 studies (of 58) with allocation concealment and only 3 studies with intention-to-treat analyses (Rethorst et al., 2009). Moreover, as an indirect indicator of study quality, the authors reported that only 24% (12 of 49) of the studies in one analysis provided adequate information to calculate an exercise dose and approximately half of the effect sizes were derived from studies that did not report the intensity of exercise used (Wipfli et al., p. 403). In the other analysis, only 21% (12 of 58) of the studies provided adequate information to calculate an exercise dose and fewer than half of the studies (24 of 58) reported adequate information about the exercise intensity used (Rethorst et al., 2009). Therefore, it seems that it would not be appropriate to assume that the methods were "strong," which is a requirement for both "Grade A" and "Grade B" evidence.

Research in the era of sloppy journalism and social media

With access to the vast majority of scientific journals still being subscription-based, the privilege of inspecting the "fine print" of published studies is restricted only to those inhabiting the ivory towers of academia. The rest of society is informed via the media. This process is usually mediated by the press offices of universities and research centers. Their role is a crucial one because, unlike scientific journals, which are read by only a few hundred specialists, media pieces are disseminated to millions of people worldwide, including patients in need of treatment options. With more patients becoming active participants in health care decisions, the information reaching them through the media can sway them toward asking their health care providers for one option versus another. It is, therefore, extremely important to provide patients with information that accurately depicts the latest research findings.

Conceivably, however, if the media were provided with inaccurate or misleading information by an ostensibly credible source such as a university press office, it seems fairly clear that most media organizations have neither the technical ability nor the time and inclination to do their own independent fact checking. Therefore, the misinformation would spread at an incredible speed throughout the globe, creating a false impression that would be impossible to contain or ever undo.

As any marketing specialist would attest, "contradictory counter-messaging" can be an extremely powerful tool. For many years, the tobacco industry deliberately used this technique to its advantage (Landman, Cortese, & Glantz, 2008; Smith, 2006) by disseminating a seemingly valid, supposedly science-based, counter-message to the ongoing anti-smoking social marketing campaigns targeting the addictive properties of nicotine. For a smoker who is unwilling or unable to conduct an independent analysis and evaluation of the scientific data, one "science" appears no different from the other "science" and, therefore, the message that nicotine is addictive seems no more valid than the message that it is not. In fact, the "contradictory counter-message" (i.e., that nicotine is non-addictive) does not even have to be believed. Even its mere presence can accomplish the objective, which is to create confusion: many in the public are led to believe that, since there is apparent inconsistency in scientific findings, the addictive properties of nicotine are doubtful. In the end, it really does not matter what the actual research has shown. The battle is fought in the arena of public opinion, following very different rules than the rules of science. For these reasons, the portrayal of research findings in the media can create an additional challenge, a new layer of complexity that readers seeking reliable information have to confront.

On June 6, 2012, a university press office released a statement describing a study that had just been completed. From the opening paragraph, the statement made it clear that the study had been motivated by the clinical practice guidelines for the treatment of depression that have been in place in the United Kingdom (see the earlier subsection entitled "Recent advances and emerging challenges"): "Current clinical guidance recommends physical activity to alleviate the symptoms of depression. However, new research published today in the [*British Medical Journal*], suggests that adding a physical activity intervention to usual care did not reduce symptoms of depression more than usual care alone." Of course, the phrase "physical activity intervention" is understood by most people to mean that, in one experimental condition, people did physical activity, whereas in the other (the control) they did not. Nowhere in the press release is there any specific information about what exactly the "physical activity intervention" consisted of and nowhere is it described as anything other than a "physical activity intervention."

The lead researcher was quoted as saying "Our intervention was not an effective strategy for reducing symptoms. However, it is important to note that increased physical activity is beneficial for people with other medical conditions such as obesity, diabetes and cardiovascular disease." The antithesis created by the use of "however" clearly implies that, unlike the benefits of physical activity for obesity, diabetes, and cardiovascular disease, physical activity is ineffective for reducing symptoms of depression. Another senior researcher further reinforced this interpretation by saying, in no uncertain terms, that "exercise and activity appeared to offer promise as one such treatment, but this carefully designed research study has shown that exercise does not appear to be effective in treating depression."

As was entirely predictable, the British press highlighted the story, as always happens when a new study contradicts what was believed to be established knowledge up to that point. In an interview to the British Broadcast Corporation (BBC), a senior researcher said, "exercise is very good for you, but it's not good for treating people with what was actually quite severe depression." Furthermore, "that buzz we all get from moderate intensity of exercise is certainly acknowledged but it's not sustained and it's not appropriate for treating people with depression."

A professor of public health not associated with the study told the BBC that "this is a huge disappointment because we were hoping exercise would help lift depression." On the same day, *The Guardian*, a major British newspaper, carried the story under the title "Exercise doesn't help depression, study concludes." The opening sentence read: "A study into whether physical activity alleviates the symptoms of depression has found there is no benefit." In another newspaper, *The Telegraph*, under the title "Exercise fails to lift clinical depression," the medical correspondent explained that "exercise should not be 'prescribed' to people with clinical depression, according to a study which found it did nothing to improve their moods."

Only the BBC article hinted at the story behind the story, namely the implications of the study and the associated press release for the role of physical activity in public health policy in the United Kingdom. Reminding readers that the study had been funded by government (i.e., taxpayer) money, the BBC predicted that the findings are "likely to be taken into account when [the National Institute for Health and Clinical Excellence] next reviews its guidelines." A population that paid a substantial sum of money for the study to be carried out and is now convinced by the press release and subsequent media buzz of the ineffectiveness of physical activity is unlikely to accept the continuation of the use of physical activity as a treatment for depression through the national health care system. The National Health Service (NHS) responded a day later, cautioning readers that "despite what several headlines have suggested, new research has not re-examined the effect of exercise on depression" and that "the results do not support the view that exercise is 'useless' for treating depression, as some news sources have suggested." However, it was clearly too little, too late. By that time, the headlines had traveled around the world and reverberated through the social media.

As noted earlier, in a scenario like this, what the actual study showed is ultimately rendered irrelevant. In public opinion, perception is reality and the perception has clearly been formed. Returning to the study to dissect methods and results is likely to strike most people as too technical, too difficult, too confusing, and, after a while, essentially pointless. Depressed patients visiting their primary care physicians are unlikely to accept any advice for physical activity since all major media organizations declared it ineffective. They are also unlikely to have much patience for explanations on what the study did or did not show.

Anyone with the patience to juxtapose the press release and media reports with the actual research publication would be surprised by the extent to which the evidence was distorted. As the NHS pointed out, the study did not investigate the effects of exercise or physical activity on depression. More accurately, although the originally stated aim of the study was, in fact, to "evaluate, in general terms, whether physical activity can be an effective treatment for depression within primary care" (Baxter et al., 2010, p. 6), a series of significant failures in the conceptualization and design of the study precluded the accomplishment of this goal.

The study used a large sample ($N = 361$) of patients who could be characterized as having at least "mild" depression on the basis of scores on the Beck Depression Inventory (i.e., at least a score of 14, on a scale where 0–13 represents minimal depressive symptoms, 14–19 mild, 20–28 moderate, and 29–63 severe depressive symptoms).

Beyond the large sample size, however, most aspects of the study were severely flawed. The patients were randomized to one of two conditions. In one condition, patients received usual care, which within the NHS means the full range of available treatments, including access to antidepressant medications, counseling, referral to exercise on prescription schemes, and secondary care mental health services. In the other condition, in addition to usual care, the patients received an intervention designed to promote physical activity. It should be clear, therefore, that, by design, the study incorporated multiple confounding factors, whose interactions with physical activity were unknown and left uncontrolled. Although recruitment was stratified by the baseline use of antidepressants and an extremely crude measure of physical activity (i.e., self-reported number of days per week of at least 30 minutes of "moderate" or "vigorous" activity), the researchers did not account for the use of other resources, such as counseling.

Furthermore, the researchers admitted initially expecting that only "10% of the sample would have been taking antidepressants at baseline and had intended to exclude them from the main comparative analysis" (p. 4). However, over 50% of the sample was already on antidepressants at baseline, so they "decided to include everyone in the analysis" (p. 4) and, instead, control for antidepressant use statistically, as a covariate. However, the simultaneous exposure of the majority of the intervention group to physical activity and antidepressants represents a confound, and a fatal design flaw, which cannot be remedied by resorting to a statistical control of antidepressant use. First, it is presumed that at least part of the antidepressant effect of physical activity is due to changes in the brain's serotonergic network, the same network targeted by the antidepressant medication. The effects of the interaction of these two parallel interventions on this network remain unclear. Second, it has been found that, when these two treatments are administered in tandem, the antidepressants may undermine the effects of physical activity (Babyak et al., 2000). One possibility is that this interference may be mediated by cognitive processes:

One of the positive psychological benefits of systematic exercise is the development of a sense of personal mastery and positive self-regard, which we believe is likely to play some role in the depression-reducing effects of exercise. It is conceivable that the concurrent use of medication may undermine this benefit by prioritizing an alternative, less self-confirming attribution for one's improved condition. Instead of incorporating the belief "I was dedicated and worked hard with the exercise program; it wasn't easy, but I beat this depression," patients might incorporate the belief that "I took an antidepressant and got better."

(Babyak et al., 2000, p. 636)

The researchers indirectly acknowledged that the statistical control for antidepressant use was only a necessary but imperfect compromise for dealing with the confound, by disclosing that they had originally intended to exclude all participants already on antidepressants. Of course, they should have also done the same with all participants receiving counseling and all those who had opted to use secondary care mental health services. These parallel treatments could also directly confound the effects of physical activity.

The intervention that was used to increase physical activity was also problematic. First, it should be pointed out that the guidelines of the National Institute for Health and Clinical Excellence (2010) specified "a structured group physical activity program" supervised by a physical activity facilitator with a Bachelor's or a Master's degree (the rationale for this was detailed on p. 212 of the guideline document). Instead, the intervention was designed to increase general (lifestyle), unsupervised, physical activity, which is a very different type of intervention.

The intervention to increase physical activity was based on a theory that happens to be in vogue in exercise psychology, namely self-determination theory. Since no specific explanation was offered for why this particular theory was deemed most appropriate for this particular intervention or this particular population, other than that it "seemed particularly relevant" (Haase, Taylor, Fox, Thorp, & Lewis, 2010, p. 86), it is probably safe to assume that a different theory would have been used had the study been designed 5 or 10 years ago, when different theories were in vogue (e.g., the transtheoretical model or social-cognitive theory).

Importantly, this intervention had not been previously tested for its effectiveness or appropriateness in this population. Thus, it is entirely plausible that some of the precepts of self-determination theory might lead to counterproductive effects. For example, it has been found that some participants, due to lack of knowledge and experience with physical activity, feel insecure about making decisions (e.g., selecting an appropriate intensity) and would prefer to relinquish control to a trained professional. Being left with no choice but to decide for themselves, these individuals feel less confident and report reduced pleasure during physical activity (Rose & Parfitt, 2007). However, the promotion of autonomy is a central pillar of self-determination theory and its benefit is considered universal. It was, therefore, one of the main goals of the intervention. This underscores the perils of developing interventions and applying them on a large scale without pilot testing.

Furthermore, the intervention was delivered by non-specialists (mainly graduate students in exercise science, who lacked background in psychology, and students in psychology who lacked background in exercise science), following minimal training (two-day seminar), and through relatively minimal contact (only seven times in 8 months, on average, with only one of these lasting for an hour). As many experts on depression have noted, encouraging depressed adults to exercise is extremely challenging (Salmon, 2001; Seime & Vickers, 2006). Therefore, the decision to use a previously untested intervention and deliver it through non-specialists with minimal qualifications and experience shows that the magnitude of the challenge at hand was clearly underestimated. No one would seriously consider delivering a psychological intervention or prescribing medications to a depressed population through anyone other than a highly trained professional with established credentials. So the assumption that a minimally trained non-specialist, guided only by a 25-page training manual, could conceivably make depressed patients exercise seems to indicate a lack of appreciation for the complexity of exercise motivation in a clinical context. Remarkably, not a single reference in the manual was made to the dysfunctional cognitions that are the hallmarks of depression and nothing in the manual gives any indication that this intervention was specifically developed for a population with this particular psycho-pathology.

As Salmon (2001) aptly described it, convincing a depressed patient to exercise is essentially tantamount to delivering effective psychotherapy, both in terms of difficulty and, to a large extent, in terms of technique: "Exercise in such patients is likely to depend on persuasive or therapeutic maneuvers of the kind that are integral to conventional psychological treatment. That is, the institution of exercise habits could be the *evidence* rather than the basis of successful treat-ment" (p. 38, emphasis in the original). To understand why anyone would think otherwise, one must understand that exercise is not taught in medical or clinical psychological curricula, a situation that often results in the erroneous assumption that exercise is "simple" (Connaughton, Weiler, & Connaughton, 2001; Faulkner & Biddle, 2001; Weiler, Chew, Coombs, Hamer, & Stamatakis, 2012).

The researchers emphasized that the "intervention increased physical activity" (Chalder et al., 2012, p. 5), with the implication being that depression scores were not reduced despite the fact that physical activity was increased. However, from a design standpoint, the intervention was deeply problematic. Because the patients in the "usual case" condition also received encour-agement to join NHS exercise prescription schemes that are available throughout the country, the percentage of those in the usual care group who did at least 1000 MET-minutes per week increased from 26.8% at baseline to 43.4% (by 16.6%) at 4 months. By comparison, the percentage for the intervention group increased from 24.7% to 51.5% (by 26.8%, only about 10% more than usual care). This difference was not statistically significant ($p = 0.08$) and, arguably, clinically negligible. This is crucially important because the "four month follow-up was chosen as the primary outcome endpoint" (p. 2), namely the point at which the outcomes of self-reported depression symptoms and antidepressant use were assessed. It should be clear, however, that at the 4-month time point (i.e., the "primary outcome endpoint"), the intervention had failed to produce a statistically significant (let alone a clinically meaningful) difference in physical activity levels. From an experimental standpoint, since the aim of the study, as stated, was to "evaluate . . . whether physical activity can be an effective treatment for depression" (Baxter et al., 2010, p. 6), once the "manipulation check" indicated that the intervention had failed, carrying on with the analyses makes no sense.

The 4-month time point was chosen because, according to the researchers, it "represented the stage in the intervention period at which [they] expected to observe the largest effect" (p. 2). However, the opposite was the case; not only was physical activity not significantly different between the usual care and the intervention groups at the 4-month time point, but their difference was, in fact, the smallest that was recorded and less than half of the largest difference (at 4 months, 51.5% versus 43.4%, or 8.1%; at 8 months, 63.2% versus 49.4%, or 13.8%; at 12 months, 57.7 versus 40.4, or 17.3%). By opting to compare the groups on the primary outcomes at the 4-month time point, the researchers chose to minimize the strength of the treatment and, by doing so, the statistical power of the analysis.

Furthermore, "there was no evidence that the difference between the groups changed over the duration of the study (time by treatment interaction, $p = 0.71$)" (Chalder et al., 2012, p. 5).

Even at the point of the largest effect of the intervention, which was actually 4 months after the intervention had ended (i.e., at 12 months post-randomization), there was only a 17% difference between the usual care and the intervention group in the percentage of those reaching the criterion of 1000 MET-minutes per week (at 12 months post-randomization). In design terms, there was severe cross-contamination across the experimental groups, since throughout the study 40%–50% of the participants in the usual care group were physically active at levels believed to be sufficient to effect change. Thus, by simultaneously providing encouragement for physical activity to the usual care group, the researchers, once again, chose to minimize the strength of the treatment and, by doing so, reduce the statistical power of the analysis.

Finally, both the measurement of physical activity and the measurement of depression (i.e., the two main variables of interest in the study) were problematic. Physical activity was measured through a 7-day recall diary. This method is known to be prone to a variety of biases and is among the least dependable ways to assess physical activity that are available today. The Beck Depression Inventory II, which was the sole measure of depression, was previously criticized by one of the coauthors of the Chalder et al. (2012) study as a measure that "is difficult to interpret clinically" (Lawlor & Hopker, 2001, p. 6). In spite of its popularity, the Beck Depression Inventory suffers from controversial factorial validity, easy susceptibility of scores to momentary changes in environmental conditions, and relatively poor discriminant validity against anxiety (Richter, Werner, Heerline, Kraus, & Sauer, 1998). For these reasons, sole reliance on the Beck Depression Inventory to operationalize the central outcome variable of the study was a questionable decision. It has become common practice in RCTs to corroborate the data based on this instrument with a different assessment method, namely a standardized clinician interview and rating scale (usually the Hamilton Rating Scale for Depression).

As the previous paragraphs demonstrate, the study by Chalder et al. (2012) had severe methodological flaws that make its findings irrelevant to the originally stated purpose of the study (i.e., to "evaluate . . . whether physical activity can be an effective treatment for depression"). In that sense, the statements in the press release were entirely misleading. However, it is crucial to point out that, by using the criteria for evaluating study quality that Lawlor and Hopker (2001) applied in their meta-analysis, the study by Chalder et al. (2012) would have been judged as being of high quality. Specifically, the authors noted that "treatment allocation, concealed from the study researchers using an automated telephone system, was administered remotely and employed a computer generated code" (p. 2). Furthermore, "the primary comparative analyses were conducted using an intention to treat approach" (p. 3). Finally, even though "owing to the nature of the intervention, none of the participants, general practices, clinicians, or researchers performing the outcome assessments could be blinded to treatment allocation" (p. 2), the use of "a self completion questionnaire" to assess depression was believed to "eliminate any observer bias" (p. 2). There is, therefore, little doubt that this study will appear in future systematic reviews and meta-analyses as being not only relevant to the question of the effect of physical activity on depression but also of high methodological quality. Thus, its null effect will be considered (perhaps with a high weight due to the large sample size) in the calculation of pooled standardized mean differences. This underscores the need for informed, balanced, and critical, as opposed to mechanical and superficial, evaluations of study quality. More broadly, the media coverage of the Chalder et al. study underscores the new challenges that patients and clinicians must face in their quest to make sense of the evidence on physical activity and mental health.

Recapitulation

Mental health problems exact a significant toll on society, both in terms of disability and reduced quality of life and in terms of economic cost. Standard forms of treatment, namely psychotherapy and pharmacotherapy, help a lot of people suffering with mental health challenges. However, they show limited effectiveness for many individuals, they come with a high price for individuals and health care systems, and they do have a range of undesirable side-effects. In this context, physical activity offers a promising alternative form of prevention and treatment. It is safe, inexpensive, and demonstrably effective for a wide range of mental health problems. For these reasons, researchers and clinicians in psychology, psychiatry, primary care, and public health should be informed about the latest research discoveries on the relationship between physical activity and mental health from credible sources. Unfortunately, achieving this goal has been difficult and remains extremely challenging. The literature is plagued by contradictory statements and, due to the technical complexities involved, it is becoming increasingly difficult, especially for non-specialists, to parse the crucial details and make sense of the evidence. As more national clinical practice guidelines recommend the use of physical activity as a treatment option, the potential for bias in the published literature is bound to increase, further obfuscating the evidence. The ambitious goal of this handbook, authored by an international group of experts, is to summarize the current evidence in a comprehensive, balanced, and accessible manner, shedding light on controversial issues, highlighting the progress that has been made, and outlining an agenda for future research.

References

Ahlskog, J.E., Geda, Y.E., Graff-Radford, N.R., & Petersen, R.C. (2011). Physical exercise as a preventive or disease-modifying treatment of dementia and brain aging. *Mayo Clinic Proceedings, 86,* 876–884.

Alzheimer's Association (2010). 2010 Alzheimer's disease facts and figures. *Alzheimer's & Dementia, 6,* 158–194.

Andlin-Sobocki, P., Jonsson, B., Wittchen, H.U., & Olesen, J. (2005). Cost of disorders of the brain in Europe. *European Journal of Neurology, 12* (Suppl 1), 1–27.

Arroll, B., Elley, C.R., Fishman, T., Goodyear-Smith, F.A., Kenealy, T., Blashki, G., & Macgillivray, S. (2009). Antidepressants versus placebo for depression in primary care. *Cochrane Database of Systematic Reviews, 2009* (3), CD007954.

Arroll, B., Macgillivray, S., Ogston, S., Reid, I., Sullivan, F., Williams, B., & Crombie, I. (2005). Efficacy and tolerability of tricyclic antidepressants and SSRIs compared with placebo for treatment of depression in primary care: A meta-analysis. *Annals of Family Medicine, 3,* 449–456.

Babyak, M., Blumenthal, J.A., Herman, S., Khatri, P., Doraiswamy, M., Moore, K., . . . Krishnan, K.R. (2000). Exercise treatment for major depression: Maintenance of therapeutic benefit at 10 months. *Psychosomatic Medicine, 62,* 633–638.

Balon, R. (2006). SSRI-associated sexual dysfunction. *American Journal of Psychiatry, 163,* 1504–1509.

Balshem, H., Helfand, M., Schünemann, H.J., Oxman, A.D., Kunz, R., Brozek, J., . . . Guyatt, G.H. (2011). GRADE guidelines: Rating the quality of evidence. *Journal of Clinical Epidemiology, 64,* 401–406.

Barlow, D.H. (2010). Negative effects from psychological treatments: A perspective. *American Psychologist, 65,* 13–20.

Baskin, T.W., Callen Tierney, S., Minami, T., & Wampold, B.E. (2003). Establishing specificity in psychotherapy: A meta-analysis of structural equivalence of placebo controls. *Journal of Consulting and Clinical Psychology, 71,* 973–979.

Baxter, H., Winder, R., Chalder, M., Wright, C., Sherlock, S., Haase, A., . . . Lewis, G. (2010). Physical activity as a treatment for depression: The TREAD randomised trial protocol. *Trials, 11,* 105.

Beck, C.A., Patten, S.B., Williams, J.V.A., Wang, J.L., Currie, S.R., Maxwell, C.J., & El-Guebaly, N. (2005). Antidepressant utilization in Canada. *Social Psychiatry and Psychiatric Epidemiology, 40,* 799–807.

Beck, C.A., Williams, J.V.A., Wang, J.L., Kassam, A., El-Guebaly, N., Currie, S.R., Maxwell, C.J., & Patten, S.B. (2005). Psychotropic medication use in Canada. *Canadian Journal of Psychiatry, 50,* 605–613.

Begg, C., Cho, M., Eastwood, S., Horton, R., Moher, D., Olkin, I., . . . Stroup, D.F. (1996). Improving the quality of reporting of randomized controlled trials: The CONSORT statement. *Journal of the American Medical Association, 276*, 637–639.

Berk, M. (2007). Should we be targeting exercise as a routine mental health intervention? *Acta Neuropsychiatrica, 19*, 217–218.

Biddle, S.J.H., Fox, K.R., Boutcher, S.H., & Faulkner, G.E. (2000). The way forward for physical activity and the promotion of psychological well-being. In S.J.H. Biddle, K.R. Fox, & S.H. Boutcher (Eds.), *Physical activity and psychological well-being* (pp. 154–168). London: Routledge.

Blanchflower, B.G., & Oswald, A.J. (2011). *Antidepressants and age*. Bonn, Germany: Institute for the Study of Labor.

Blumenthal, J.A., Babyak, M.A., Doraiswamy, P.M., Watkins, L., Hoffman, B.M., Barbour, K.A., . . . Sherwood, A. (2007). Exercise and pharmacotherapy in the treatment of major depressive disorder. *Psychosomatic Medicine, 69*, 587–596.

Blumenthal, J.A., & Ong, L. (2009). Commentary on "Exercise and depression" (Mead et al., 2009): And the verdict is . . . *Mental Health and Physical Activity, 2*, 97–99.

Brosse, A.L., Sheets, E.S., Lett, H.S., & Blumenthal, J.A. (2002). Exercise and the treatment of clinical depression in adults: Recent findings and future directions. *Sports Medicine, 32*, 741-760.

Bull, S.A., Hu, X.H., Hunkeler, E.M., Lee, J.Y., Ming, E.E., Markson, L.E., & Fireman, B. (2002). Discontinuation of use and switching of antidepressants: Influence of patient–physician communication. *Journal of the American Medical Association, 288*, 1403–1409.

Callaghan, P. (2004). Exercise: A neglected intervention in mental health care? *Journal of Psychiatric and Mental Health Nursing, 11*, 476–483.

Canadian Mental Health Association (2004). *Meeting the mental health needs of the people of Canada: A submission to the House of Commons Standing Committee on Finance*. Ottawa, ON: Author.

Chalder, M., Wiles, N.J., Campbell, J., Hollinghurst, S.P., Haase, A.M., Taylor, A.H., . . . Lewis, G. (2012). Facilitated physical activity as a treatment for depressed adults: Randomised controlled trial. *British Medical Journal, 344*, e2758.

Cohen, J. (1992). A power primer. *Psychological Bulletin, 112*, 155–159.

Colton, C.W., & Manderscheid, R.W. (2006). Congruencies in increased mortality rates, years of potential life lost, and causes of death among public mental health clients in eight states. *Preventing Chronic Disease, 3* (2), 1–14.

Connaughton, A.V., Weiler, R.M., & Connaughton, D.P. (2001). Graduating medical students' exercise prescription competence as perceived by deans and directors of medical education in the United States: Implications for healthy people 2010. *Public Health Reports, 116*, 226–234.

Cooper, C., Balamurali, T.B., & Livingston, G. (2007). A systematic review of the prevalence and covariates of anxiety in caregivers of people with dementia. *International Psychogeriatrics, 19*, 175–195.

Cuijpers, P. (2005). Depressive disorders in caregivers of dementia patients: A systematic review. *Aging & Mental Health, 9*, 325–330.

Daley, A.J. (2002). Exercise therapy and mental health in clinical populations: Is exercise therapy a worthwhile intervention? *Advances in Psychiatric Treatment, 8*, 262–270.

Daviglus, M.L., Bell, C.C., Berrettini, W., Bowen, P.E., Connolly, E.S. Jr., Cox, N.J. . . . Maurizio Trevisan (2010). National Institutes of Health state-of-the-science conference statement: Preventing Alzheimer disease and cognitive decline. *Annals of Internal Medicine, 153*, 176–181.

de Abajo, F.J., & García-Rodríguez, L.A. (2008). Risk of upper gastrointestinal tract bleeding associated with selective serotonin reuptake inhibitors and venlafaxine therapy: Interaction with nonsteroidal anti-inflammatory drugs and effect of acid-suppressing agents. *Archives of General Psychiatry, 65*, 795–803.

Deshmukh, R., & Franco, K. (2003). Managing weight gain as a side effect of antidepressant therapy. *Cleveland Clinic Journal of Medicine, 70*, 614–623.

Donaghy, M.E. (2007). Exercise can seriously improve your mental health: Fact or fiction? *Advances in Physiotherapy, 9*, 76–88.

Dunn, A.L., Trivedi, M.H., Kampert, J.B., Clark, G.G., & Chambliss, H.O. (2005). Exercise treatment for depression efficacy and dose response. *American Journal of Preventive Medicine, 28*, 1–8.

Ekkekakis, P. (2008). The genetic tidal wave finally reached our shores: Will it be the catalyst for a critical overhaul of the way we think and do science? *Mental Health and Physical Activity, 1*, 47–52.

Ekkekakis, P., & Backhouse, S.H. (2009). Exercise and psychological well-being. In R. Maughan (Ed.), *Olympic textbook of science in sport* (pp. 251–271). Hoboken, NJ: Wiley-Blackwell.

Ensrud, K.E., Blackwell, T.L., Ancoli-Israel, S., Redline, S., Yaffe, K., Diem, S., . . . Stone, K.L. (2006). Use of selective serotonin reuptake inhibitors and sleep disturbances in community-dwelling older women. *Journal of the American Geriatrics Society, 54*, 1508–1515.

Etters, L., Goodall, D., & Harrison, B.E. (2008). Caregiver burden among dementia patient caregivers: A review of the literature. *Journal of the American Academy of Nurse Practitioners, 20*, 423–428.

Eysenck, H.J. (1952). The effects of psychotherapy: An evaluation. *Journal of Consulting Psychology, 16*, 319–324.

Faulkner, G., & Biddle, S. (2001). Exercise and mental health: It's just not psychology! *Journal of Sports Sciences, 19*, 433–444.

Ferri, C.P., Prince, M., Brayne, C., Brodaty, H., Fratiglioni, L., Ganguli, M., . . . Alzheimer's Disease International (2005). Global prevalence of dementia: A Delphi consensus study. *Lancet, 366*, 2112–2117.

Flicker, L., Liu-Ambrose, T., & Kramer, A.F. (2011). Why so negative about preventing cognitive decline and dementia? The jury has already come to the verdict for physical activity and smoking cessation. *British Journal of Sports Medicine, 45*, 465–467.

Folkins, C.H., & Sime, W.E. (1981). Physical fitness training and mental health. *American Psychologist, 36*, 373–389.

Fournier, J.C., DeRubeis, R.J., Hollon, S.D., Dimidjian, S., Amsterdam, J.D., Shelton, R.C., & Fawcett, J. (2010). Antidepressant drug effects and depression severity: A patient-level meta-analysis. *Journal of the American Medical Association, 303*, 47–53.

Gartlehner, G., Hansen, R.A., Carey, T.S., Lohr, K.N., Gaynes, B.N., & Randolph, L.C. (2005). Discontinuation rates for selective serotonin reuptake inhibitors and other second-generation antidepressants in outpatients with major depressive disorder: A systematic review and meta-analysis. *International Clinical Psychopharmacology, 20*, 59–69.

Gelenberg, A.J., Freeman, M.P., Markowitz, J.C., Rosenbaum, J.F., Thase, M.E., Trivedi, M.H., & Van Rhoads, R.S. (2010). *Practice guideline for the treatment of patients with major depressive disorder* (3rd ed.). Arlington, VA: American Psychiatric Association.

Goethe, J.W., Woolley, S.B., Cardoni, A.A., Woznicki, B.A., & Piez, D.A. (2007). Selective serotonin reuptake inhibitor discontinuation: Side effects and other factors that influence medication adherence. *Journal of Clinical Psychopharmacology, 27*, 451–458.

González, H.M., Vega, W.A., Williams, D.R., Tarraf, W., West, B.T., & Neighbors, H.W. (2010). Depression care in the United States: Too little for too few. *Archives of General Psychiatry, 67*, 37–46.

Greenberg, P.E., Kessler, R.C., Birnbaum, H.G., Leong, S.A., Lowe, S.W., Berglund, P.A., & Corey-Lisle, P.K. (2003). The economic burden of depression in the United States: How did it change between 1990 and 2000? *Journal of Clinical Psychiatry, 64*, 1465–1475.

Grissom, R.J. (1996). The magical number .7 ± .2: Meta-meta-analysis of the probability of superior outcome in comparisons involving therapy, placebo, and control. *Journal of Consulting and Clinical Psychology, 64*, 973–982.

Guyatt, G.H., Cook, D.J., Sackett, D.L., Eckman, M., & Pauker, S. (1998). Grades of recommendation for antithrombotic agents. *Chest, 114*, 441S–444S.

Haase, A.M., Taylor, A.H., Fox, K.R., Thorp, H., & Lewis, G. (2010). Rationale and development of the physical activity counselling intervention for a pragmatic TRial of Exercise and Depression in the UK (TREAD-UK). *Mental Health and Physical Activity, 3*, 85–91.

Haskell, W.L., Lee, I.M., Pate, R.R., Powell, K.E., Blair, S.N., Franklin, B.A., . . . Bauman, A. (2007). Physical activity and public health: Updated recommendation for adults from the American College of Sports Medicine and the American Heart Association. *Medicine and Science in Sports and Exercise, 39*, 1423–1434.

Health Canada (2002). *A report on mental illnesses in Canada*. Ottawa, ON: Author.

Healy, D. (2003). Lines of evidence on the risks of suicide with selective serotonin reuptake inhibitors. *Psychotherapy and Psychosomatics, 72*, 71–79.

Healy, D., & Cattell, D. (2003). Interface between authorship, industry and science in the domain of therapeutics. *British Journal of Psychiatry, 183*, 22–27.

Herbert, J.D., & Gaudiano, B.A. (2005). Moving from empirically supported treatment lists to practice guidelines in psychotherapy: The role of the placebo concept. *Journal of Clinical Psychology, 61*, 893–908.

Hughes, J.R. (1984). Psychological effects of habitual aerobic exercise: A critical review. *Preventive Medicine, 13*, 66–78.

Hunot, V.M., Horne, R., Leese, M.N., & Churchill, R.C. (2007). A cohort study of adherence to antidepressants in primary care: The influence of antidepressant concerns and treatment preferences. *Primary Care Companion to the Journal of Clinical Psychiatry, 9*, 91–99.

Ilyas, S., & Moncrieff, J. (2012). Trends in prescriptions and costs of drugs for mental disorders in England, 1998–2010. *British Journal of Psychiatry, 200*, 393–398.

Insel, K.R. (2008). Assessing the economic costs of serious mental illness. *American Journal of Psychiatry, 165*, 663–665.

Ioannidis, J.P.A. (2008). Effectiveness of antidepressants: An evidence myth constructed from a thousand randomized trials? *Philosophy, Ethics, and Humanities in Medicine, 3*, 14.

Jick, H., Kaye, J.A., & Jick, S.S. (2004). Antidepressants and the risk of suicidal behaviors. *Journal of the American Medical Association, 292*, 338–343.

Juurlink, D.N., Mamdani, M.M., Kopp, A., & Redelmeier, D.A. (2006). The risk of suicide with selective serotonin reuptake inhibitors in the elderly. *American Journal of Psychiatry, 163*, 813–821.

Kannel, W.B., & Sorlie, P. (1979). Some health benefits of physical activity: The Framingham study. *Archives of Internal Medicine, 139*, 857–861.

Kazdin, A.E. (2007). Mediators and mechanisms of change in psychotherapy research. *Annual Review of Clinical Psychology, 3*, 1–27.

Kennedy, S.H., & Rizvi, S. (2009). Sexual dysfunction, depression, and the impact of antidepressants. *Journal of Clinical Psychopharmacology, 29*, 157–164.

Kessler, R.C., Berglund, P., Demler, O., Jin, R., Merikangas, K.R., & Walters, E.E. (2005). Lifetime prevalence and age-of-onset distributions of DSM-IV disorders in the National Comorbidity Survey Replication. *Archives of General Psychiatry, 62*, 593–602.

Kessler, R.C., Heeringa, S., Lakoma, M.D., Petukhova, M., Rupp, A.E., Schoenbaum, M., . . . Zaslavsky, A.M. (2008). Individual and societal effects of mental disorders on earnings in the United States: Results from the National Comorbidity Survey Replication. *American Journal of Psychiatry, 165*, 703–711.

Kirsch, I. (2005). Placebo psychotherapy: Synonym or oxymoron? *Journal of Clinical Psychology, 61*, 791–803.

Kirsch, I., Deacon, B.J., Huedo-Medina, T.B., Scoboria, A., Moore, T.J., & Johnson, B.T. (2008). Initial severity and antidepressant benefits: A meta-analysis of data submitted to the Food and Drug Administration. *PLoS Medicine, 5*, e45.

Kisely, S., Cox, M., Campbell, L.A., Cooke, C., & Gardner, D. (2009). An epidemiologic study of psychotropic medication and obesity-related chronic illnesses in older psychiatric patients. *Canadian Journal of Psychiatry, 54*, 269–274.

Krogh, J., Nordentoft, M., Sterne, J.A.C., & Lawlor, D.A. (2011). The effect of exercise in clinically depressed adults: Systematic review and meta-analysis of randomized controlled trials. *Journal of Clinical Psychiatry, 72*, 529–538.

Kuhn, T.S. (1962/1996). *The structure of scientific revolutions* (3rd ed.). Chicago: University of Chicago Press.

Lambert, M.J. (2005). Early response in psychotherapy: Further evidence for the importance of common factors rather than "placebo effects." *Journal of Clinical Psychology, 61*, 855–869.

Landman, A., Cortese, D.K., & Glantz, S. (2008). Tobacco industry sociological programs to influence public beliefs about smoking. *Social Science & Medicine, 66*, 970–981.

Lawlor, D.A., & Hopker, S.W. (2001). The effectiveness of exercise as an intervention in the management of depression: Systematic review and meta-regression analysis of randomised control trials. *British Medical Journal, 322*, 1–8.

Levit, K.R., Kassed, C.A., Coffey, R.M., Mark, T.L., McKusick, D.R., King, E., . . . Stranges, E. (2008). *Projections of national expenditures for mental health services and substance abuse treatment, 2004–2014* (SAMHSA Publication No. SMA 08-4326). Rockville, MD: Substance Abuse and Mental Health Services Administration.

Lim, K.-L., Jacobs, P., Ohinmaa, A., Schopflocher, D., & Dewa, C.S. (2008). A new population-based measure of the economic burden of mental illness in Canada. *Chronic Diseases in Canada, 28*, 92–98.

Lipsey, M.W., & Wilson, D.B. (1993). The efficacy of psychological, educational, and behavioral treatment: Confirmation from meta-analysis. *American Psychologist, 48*, 1181–1209.

Lockhart, P., & Guthrie, B. (2011). Trends in primary care antidepressant prescribing 1995–2007: A longitudinal population database analysis. *British Journal of General Practice, 61*, e565–e572.

MacCoun, R.J. (1998). Biases in the interpretation and use of research results. *Annual Review of Psychology, 49*, 259–287.

Mark, T.L., Levit, K.R., Coffey, R.M., McKusick, D.R., Harwood, H.J., King, E.C., . . . Ryan, K. (2007). *National expenditures for mental health services and substance abuse treatment, 1993–2003* (SAMHSA Publication No. SMA 07–4227). Rockville, MD: Substance Abuse and Mental Health Services Administration.

Mathers, C.D., & Loncar, D. (2006). Projections of global mortality and burden of disease from 2002 to 2030. *PLoS Medicine, 3* (11), e442.

McCrone, P., Dhanasiri, S., Patel, A., Knapp, M., & Lawton–Smith, S. (2008). *Paying the price: The cost of mental health care in England to 2026.* London: King's Fund.

McGoey, L. (2010). Profitable failure: Antidepressant drugs and the triumph of flawed experiments. *History of the Human Sciences, 23,* 58–78.

Mead, G.E., Morley, W., Campbell, P., Greig, C.A., McMurdo, M., & Lawlor, D.A. (2009). Exercise for depression. *Cochrane Database of Systematic Reviews, 2009* (3), CD004366.

Moher, D., Jones, A., & Lepage, L. (2001). Use of the CONSORT statement and quality of reports of randomized trials: A comparative before-and-after evaluation. *Journal of the American Medical Association, 285,* 1992–1995.

Mojtabai, R., & Olfson, M. (2008). National trends in psychotherapy by office-based psychiatrists. *Archives of General Psychiatry, 65,* 962–970.

Moore, M., Yuen, H.M., Dunn, N., Mullee, M.A., Maskell, J., & Kendrick, T. (2009). Explaining the rise in antidepressant prescribing: A descriptive study using the general practice research database. *British Medical Journal, 339,* b3999.

Morgan, W.P. (1981). Psychological benefits of physical activity. In F.J. Nagle & H.J. Montoye (Eds.), *Exercise in health and disease* (pp. 299–314). Springfield, IL: Charles C. Thomas.

Murray, C.J., & Lopez, A.D. (1997). Alternative projections of mortality and disability by cause 1990–2020: Global Burden of Disease Study. *Lancet, 349,* 1498–1504.

National Collaborating Centre for Mental Health and National Institute for Health and Clinical Excellence (2010). *Depression: The treatment and management of depression in adults* (updated edition). Leicester and London: British Psychological Society and Royal College of Psychiatrists.

Nutt, D.J., & Sharpe, M. (2008). Uncritical positive regard? Issues in the efficacy and safety of psychotherapy. *Journal of Psychopharmacology, 22,* 3–6.

Oksbjerg Dalton, S., Johansen, C., Mellemkjær, L., Nørgård, B., Toft Sørensen, H., & Olsen, J.H. (2003). Use of selective serotonin reuptake inhibitors and risk of upper gastrointestinal tract bleeding: A population-based cohort study. *Archives of Internal Medicine, 163,* 59–64.

Olfson, M., & Marcus, S.C. (2009). National patterns in antidepressant medication treatment. *Archives of General Psychiatry, 66,* 848–856.

Olfson, M., & Marcus, S.C. (2010). National trends in outpatient psychotherapy. *American Journal of Psychiatry, 167,* 1456–1463.

Olfson, M., Marcus, S.C., Druss, B., & Pincus, H.A. (2002). National trends in the use of outpatient psychotherapy. *American Journal of Psychiatry, 159,* 1914–1920.

Olfson, M., Marcus, S.C., Tedeschi, M., & Wan, G.J. (2006). Continuity of antidepressant treatment for adults with depression in the United States. *American Journal of Psychiatry, 163,* 101–108.

Otto, M.W., Church, T.S., Craft, L.L., Greer, T.L., Smits, J.A.J., & Trivedi, M.H. (2007). Exercise for mood and anxiety disorders. *Journal of Clinical Psychiatry, 68,* 669–676.

Parloff, M.B. (1986). Placebo controls in psychotherapy research: A sine qua non or a placebo for research problems? *Journal of Consulting and Clinical Psychology, 54,* 79–87.

Patten, S.B., Esposito, E., & Carter, B. (2007). Reasons for antidepressant prescriptions in Canada. *Pharmacoepidemiology and Drug Safety, 16,* 746–752.

Phillips, W.T., Kiernan, M., & King, A.C. (2003). Physical activity as a nonpharmacological treatment for depression: A review. *Complementary Health Practice Review, 8,* 139–152.

Plassman, B.L., Williams, J.W. Jr., Burke, J.R., Holsinger, T., & Benjamin, S. (2010). Systematic review: Factors associated with risk for and possible prevention of cognitive decline in later life. *Annals of Internal Medicine, 153,* 182–193.

Posternak, M.A., & Zimmerman, M. (2007). Therapeutic effect of follow-up assessments on antidepressant and placebo response rates in antidepressant efficacy trials: Meta-analysis. *British Journal of Psychiatry, 190,* 287–292.

Prioleau, L., Murdock, M., & Brody, N. (1983). An analysis of psychotherapy versus placebo studies. *Behavioral and Brain Sciences, 6,* 275–310.

Rethorst, C.D., Wipfli B.M., & Landers, D.M. (2009). The antidepressive effects of exercise: A meta-analysis of randomized trials. *Sports Medicine, 39,* 491–511.

Richter, P., Werner, J., Heerlein, A., Kraus, A., & Sauer, H. (1998). On the validity of the Beck Depression Inventory: A review. *Psychopathology, 31,* 160–168.

Rimer, J., Dwan, K., Lawlor, D.A., Greig, C.A., McMurdo, M., Morley, W., & Mead, G.E. (2012). Exercise for depression. *Cochrane Database of Systematic Reviews, 2012* (7), CD004366.

Rose, E.A., & Parfitt, G. (2007). A quantitative analysis and qualitative explanation of the individual differences in affective responses to prescribed and self-selected exercise intensities. *Journal of Sport & Exercise Psychology, 29,* 281–309.

Salmon, P. (2001). Effects of physical exercise on anxiety, depression, and sensitivity to stress: A unifying theory. *Clinical Psychology Review, 21,* 33–61.

Schulz, K.F., Chalmers, I., Hayes, R.J., & Altman, D.G. (1995). Empirical evidence of bias: Dimensions of methodological quality associated with estimates of treatment effects in controlled trials. *Journal of the American Medical Association, 273,* 408–412.

Schulz, R., Boerner, K., Shear, K., Zhang, S., & Gitlin, L.N. (2006). Predictors of complicated grief among dementia caregivers: A prospective study of bereavement. *American Journal of Geriatric Psychiatry, 14,* 650–658.

Schwartz, T.L., Nihalani, N., Jindal, S., Virk, S., & Jones, N. (2004). Psychiatric medication-induced obesity: A review. *Obesity Reviews, 5,* 115–121.

Scottish Intercollegiate Guidelines Network (2010). *Non-pharmaceutical management of depression in adults: A national clinical guideline.* Edinburgh: Author.

Seime, R.J., & Vickers, K.S. (2006). The challenges of treating depression with exercise: From evidence to practice. *Clinical Psychology: Science and Practice, 13,* 194–197.

Senger, H.L. (1987). The "placebo" effect of psychotherapy: A moose in the rabbit stew. *American Journal of Psychotherapy, 41,* 68–81.

Serretti, A., & Chiesa, A. (2009). Treatment-emergent sexual dysfunction related to antidepressants: A meta-analysis. *Journal of Clinical Psychopharmacology, 29,* 259–266.

Smith, E.A. (2006). "It's interesting how few people die from smoking": Tobacco industry efforts to minimize risk and discredit health promotion. *European Journal of Public Health, 17,* 162–170.

Smith, M.L., & Glass, G.V. (1977). Meta-analysis of psychotherapy outcome studies. *American Psychologist, 32,* 752–760.

Snowden, M., Steinman, L., Mochan, K., Grodstein, F., Prohaska, T.R., Thurman, D.J., . . . Anderson, L.A. (2011). Effect of exercise on cognitive performance in community-dwelling older adults: Review of intervention trials and recommendations for public health practice and research. *Journal of the American Geriatrics Society, 59,* 704–716.

Soni, A. (2009). *The five most costly conditions, 1996 and 2006: Estimates for the U.S. civilian noninstitutionalized population* (Statistical Brief 248). Rockville, MD: Agency for Healthcare Research and Quality.

Stephens, T., & Joubert, N. (2001). The economic burden of mental health problems in Canada. *Chronic Diseases in Canada, 22,* 18–23.

Taylor, A.H., & Faulkner, G. (2008). Inaugural editorial. *Mental Health and Physical Activity, 1,* 1–8.

Tkachuk, G.A., & Martin, G.L. (1999). Exercise therapy for patients with psychiatric disorders: Research and clinical implications. *Professional Psychology: Research and Practice, 30,* 275–282.

Turner, E.H., Matthews, A.M., Linardatos, E., Tell, R.A., & Rosenthal, R. (2008). Selective publication of antidepressant trials and its influence on apparent efficacy. *New England Journal of Medicine, 358,* 252–260.

Turner, M.S., May, D.B., Arthur, R.R., & Xiong, G.L. (2007). Clinical impact of selective serotonin reuptake inhibitors therapy with bleeding risks. *Journal of Internal Medicine, 261,* 205–213.

United States Department of Health and Human Services (1996). *Physical activity and health: A report of the Surgeon General.* Atlanta, GA: Author, Centers for Disease Control and Prevention, National Center for Chronic Disease Prevention and Health Promotion.

United States Department of Health and Human Services (1999). *Mental health: A report of the Surgeon General.* Rockville, MD: Author, Substance Abuse and Mental Health Services Administration, Center for Mental Health Services, National Institutes of Health, National Institute of Mental Health.

United States National Center for Health Statistics (2010). *Health, United States, 2009: With special feature on medical technology.* Hyattsville, MD: United States Department of Health and Human Services, Centers for Disease Control and Prevention, National Center for Health Statistics.

Üstün, T.B., Ayuso-Mateos, J.L., Chatterji, S., Mathers, C., & Murray, C.J. (2004). Global burden of depressive disorders in the year 2000. *British Journal of Psychiatry, 184,* 386–392.

Wampold, B.E., Mondin, G.W., Moody, M., Stich, F., Benson, K., & Ahn, H. (1997). A meta-analysis of outcome studies comparing bona fide psychotherapies: Empirically, "all must have prizes." *Psychological Bulletin, 122,* 203–215.

Wang, P.S., Berglund, P., Olfson, M., Pincus, H.A., Wells, K.B., & Kessler, R.C. (2005). Failure and delay in initial treatment contact after first onset of mental disorders in the National Comorbidity Survey Replication. *Archives of General Psychiatry, 62,* 603–613.

Weiler, R., Chew, S., Coombs, N., Hamer, M., & Stamatakis, E. (2012). Physical activity education in the undergraduate curricula of all UK medical schools: Are tomorrow's doctors equipped to follow clinical guidelines? *British Journal of Sports Medicine, 46,* 1024–1026.

WHO World Mental Health Survey Consortium (2004). Prevalence, severity, and unmet need for treatment of mental disorders in the World Health Organization World Mental Health Surveys. *Journal of the American Medical Association, 291,* 2581–2590.

Wimo, A., Jönsson, L., & Winblad, B. (2006). An estimate of the worldwide prevalence and direct costs of dementia in 2003. *Dementia and Geriatric Cognitive Disorders, 21,* 175–181.

Wimo, A., Winblad, B., & Jönsson, L. (2010). The worldwide societal costs of dementia: Estimates for 2009. *Alzheimer's & Dementia, 6,* 98–103.

Wipfli, B.M., Rethorst, C.D., & Landers, D.M. (2008). The anxiolytic effects of exercise: A meta-analysis of randomized trials and dose-response analysis. *Journal of Sport & Exercise Psychology, 30,* 392–410.

Wittchen, H.U., Jacobi, F., Rehm, J., Gustavsson, A., Svensson, M., Jönsson, B., . . . Steinhausen, H.C. (2011). The size and burden of mental disorders and other disorders of the brain in Europe 2010. *European Neuropsychopharmacology, 21,* 655–679.

World Health Organization (2003). *Investing in mental health.* Geneva, Switzerland: Author.

PART 1

The physical activity "feel-good" effect

Edited by
Panteleimon Ekkekakis

1

PLEASURE FROM THE EXERCISING BODY

Two centuries of changing outlooks in psychological thought

Panteleimon Ekkekakis

The mere exertion of the muscles after long rest or confinement is in itself a pleasure, as we ourselves feel, and as we see in the play of young animals.

(Darwin, 1872, p. 77)

Researchers working on the effects of physical activity on mental health often express puzzlement, even frustration, that physical activity is not recognized more widely as a *bona fide* mental health intervention in spite of mounting evidence. Attempts to probe the causes of this phenomenon typically reveal two contributing factors, namely a hypercritical treatment of the evidence (e.g., Mead et al., 2009) and, perhaps surprisingly, a lack of awareness of the evidence. For example, when Faulkner and Biddle (2001) asked directors of doctoral training programs in clinical psychology in England about their perceptions of the role of exercise in mental health, one striking finding was their "extremely limited" (p. 439) awareness of relevant studies. One program director remarked: "We might want to ask the question, if there's evidence for exercise, why is noone mentioning it? That would be a more interesting question to us, to be honest" (p. 439). Critiquing a research literature on conceptual and methodological grounds, and choosing to accept or reject its findings on that basis, is perfectly reasonable. In fact, it is the basis of responsible evidence-based practice. So, of the two contributing factors, the former is scientifically warranted and potentially fruitful, in that it can stimulate efforts to further improve the quality of the evidence base (Ekkekakis, 2008). The latter, however, is a different issue altogether. Choosing to ignore an entire literature, or claiming that it does not exist, cannot be construed as either helpful or healthy (Ekkekakis & Backhouse, 2009). Therefore, a contemplation of the historical processes that led to the current situation may prove enlightening.

Like most scientific disciplines, psychology is not immune to the problem of faltering memory (Watson, 1960). The frame of reference for past research and theorizing typically extends over a period of a few years, not decades or centuries. What probably drives this phenomenon is the assumption that the size of the evidence base and the sophistication of theories grow following a monotonic and more-or-less linear trajectory. In other words, there is a belief that there is no backtracking or looping in how scientific knowledge evolves over time. If this were so, being aware of only the latest empirical and theoretical literature would suffice, as that would encapsulate the accumulated experience of the past. In reality, however, the topics, the methods, and the interpretive frameworks that science utilizes at a particular historical juncture are dictated by Kuhnian paradigms, which are ephemeral and often non–cumulative (Kuhn, 1962/1996). Psychology is no exception (Robins, Gosling, & Craik, 1999).

This chapter traces the history of references to the exercise–pleasure relationship in psychological works since the mid-1800s. The goal of this review is to answer the intriguing question posed by the anonymous director of the clinical psychology program, namely "why is noone mentioning [exercise]"? The crucial role of shifting paradigmatic perspectives in shaping the attitudes toward exercise within the field of psychology should become apparent. In particular, readers should recognize the non-cumulative, even regressive and cyclical, nature of the knowledge development process, a phenomenon that can be attributed directly to the changing paradigms. Finally, a synopsis of what is presently known about the exercise–pleasure relationship is provided.

Alexander Bain (1818–1903)

In the second half of the nineteenth and the early part of the twentieth century, the nascent field of psychology fully embraced the idea of a close relationship between exercise and pleasure. Scottish philosopher Alexander Bain (1855), in his opus entitled "Senses and the Intellect," published a remarkably detailed and insightful analysis of the "feelings of muscular exercise." For Bain, a logician considered one of the forefathers of the scientific psychology of the twentieth century, this interest in exercise was not merely a fortuitous occurrence. He believed that demonstrating a close link between a physical act, such as bodily movement, and a sensory perception or an emotional response would safeguard psychology against critics eager to accuse it of dealing solely with immaterial or metaphysical phenomena.

According to Bain (1855), provided that someone is healthy and adequately rested, exercise induces "a feeling of vigor, strength, or intense vitality" (p. 92). Along with the overall state of good health that ensues from exercise, these feelings account "for a considerable portion of the sum of human pleasure" (p. 92). Echoing the hedonistic ideas of the British Utilitarians, such as Jeremy Bentham (1748–1832) and John Stuart Mill (1806–1873), Bain believed strongly in the "deep-seated bond which connects feeling with action" (p. 102): "When we descend into the gymnastic arena to convert surplus energy into pleasure, the conscious state [the pleasure] is then the spur and guide of our action. We continue our exercise while the pleasure lasts, and cease when it ceases" (p. 98). In fact, Bain believed that human beings have an inherent propensity for exercise: "without any conscious end, in other words, without our willing it, action commences when the body is refreshed and invigorated" (p. 250). Moreover, if this spontaneous tendency is resisted, as in the case of a child not allowed to play or a person imprisoned in a cell, "intense uneasiness or craving is felt" (p. 251). Thus, Bain wrote of a "necessity of bodily exercise [which is] felt by everyone, and most of all by the young" (p. 78).

At the same time, Bain recognized that the pleasure of exercise is not universal but rather conditional. This feeling is at its highest when there is "concurrence of youth with high muscular energy, or the athletic constitution at its prime" (p. 99). Under these conditions, "the pleasure will be very great indeed, and the volitional promptings to keep it up equally great" (p. 99). On the other hand, "with the generality of men, however, the same strong terms cannot be applied to describe this species of emotion, which in them sinks down to a second or third-rate pleasure" (p. 99). In turn, this may explain "the utter neglect of physical exercise as a habitual element of life" (p. 95).

Furthermore, Bain pointed out that the nature of the feelings may change depending on the intensity of the activity. Under most circumstances, "we may derive the greatest amount of pleasurable sensibility, at the least cost of exertion, through the means of well-concerted slow movements"; this is because "the emotional state is not overwhelmed by the expenditure of active power, and hence the enjoyment is keen" (p. 101). The benefits of slow activity include "soothing down a morbid excitement," "preparing the way for absolute repose," and restoring tranquility after a bustling day (p. 102). However, "slow movements are entirely out of keeping with a fresh and active bodily tone"; they may even be "repugnant and intolerable in such a situation" (p. 102).

Fast or high-intensity movements, on the other hand, have the "tendency to excite and inflame the system into a still more intense condition, such as we term elation, animal spirits, with boisterous manifestations" (p. 103). For example, "in a rapid walk, still more in a run, the consciousness is excited, the gesticulations and speech are rapid, the features betray a high tension. The increase of emotional fervor must be attributed to an exalted condition of the nervous system, of the kind produced by intoxicating stimulants in general" (p. 104). A similar example is "the gleesome and joyous excitement of the young in the midst of their active sports" (p. 98); in this case, "the pleasurable stimulus of exertion diffuses itself over the whole system, lighting up the features with gaiety and mirth, and prompting the vocal organs to cries of delight" (p. 98).

Importantly, Bain, showing his sensitivity to "differences of individual character" (p. 95), pointed out that it is "easier in some temperaments than in others, to perform rapid movements with coolness" (p. 104). He noted that "it is one of the peculiarities of what is called the nervous temperament, or a nervous system naturally prone to vigorous exertion [. . .] to expend itself copiously in all its efforts" (p. 328). Although he recognized that physiological differences in the muscles can explain some of this proneness to vigorous exertion, he insisted that "the power of continuing the exercise without fatigue" (p. 328) is ultimately due to the nervous system: "I must account the quality of the muscle of far inferior importance, and indeed quite trifling in comparison with the quality of the nervous framework" (p. 329).

If intense effort is continued for too long, the pleasure "changes into pain" (p. 97), the "pain of fatigue" (p. 108). In contradistinction to "ordinary fatigue" which Bain considered pleasant, this "over-fatigue" produces "acute pains of various degrees of intensity, from the easily endurable up to severe suffering" (p. 91). As the function of pleasure was to encourage and sustain movement, the function of fatigue is to force its termination: "The peculiarity of the state being exhaustion consequent on exercise, it naturally follows that a cessation of activity should be one of the accompanying circumstances of the feeling. As a mere physical fact, fatigue would lead to inaction. Thus there would be a discouragement to new effort" (p. 93).

James Mark Baldwin (1861–1934)

Baldwin was one of the most prominent psychologists in North America around the turn of the twentieth century. He was a key figure in the establishment of the American Psychological Association (and its sixth president), co-founder (with James McKeen Cattell) of the *Psychological Review*, and the founding editor of the *Psychological Bulletin* (later passing the editorship to John B. Watson).

In the second volume of his highly acclaimed *Handbook of Psychology*, subtitled "Feeling and Will," Baldwin (1891) addressed the relationship between exercise and pleasure, noting that "muscular sensations are pleasurable within the range of easy effort" (p. 120). This is based on the general principle that, when an activity is of moderate intensity and well matched to the properties of the muscles involved, it tends to be pleasant. If the intensity or duration of exercise exceeds the moderate range, then we experience "the pains of fatigue" (p. 121). Agreeing with Bain, Baldwin considered the pleasure associated with exercise among the most enthralling elements in human experience: "these pleasures of activity, such as pleasures of the chase, of sports, of general vigor, are more positive apparently than any other sensuous pleasures" (p. 120). Also in agreement with Bain, Baldwin accepted the notion of an inherent propensity for exercise:

> After confining myself to my writing-table all the morning, my attention loses its elasticity and readiness of concentration: but my muscular system begins to feel an overabundance of energy, a pressing readiness for exercise. And when I give up my intellectual task and indulge my craving for exercise, I have a peculiar feeling of throwing off the mental weight, of getting rid of the thraldom of ideas, in the easy enjoyment of muscular activity.
>
> *(p. 287)*

As was the case with most intellectuals of his time, Baldwin's thinking was greatly affected by the theory of evolution. His *Mental Development in the Child and the Race*, first published in 1894, reflects influences from Darwin's *On the Origin of Species* (published in 1859) and *The Expression of the Emotions in Man and Animals* (published in 1872), as well as the elaboration of the implications of evolutionary ideas for psychology in the revised edition of Herbert Spencer's *Principles of Psychology* (published in 1873). The framework of the theory of evolution enabled Baldwin to explore the broader significance of the effects of exercise on pleasure, in essence providing, for the first time, an answer to the "why" question: why is exercise pleasurable?

According to Baldwin (1894), organisms exhibit an innate "susceptibility to certain organic stimulations, such as food, oxygen, etc." (p. 191). When the need for these "stimulations" is satisfied, pleasure occurs. Pleasure brings forth a "heightened central vitality" which, in turn, results in a "motor excess discharge," manifested in "abundant and varied movements" (p. 191). Of those movements, however, there is a tendency to select those "which bring more of these vital stimulations again; and these finally keep up the vitality of the organism" (p. 191). Exercise, according to Baldwin, is pleasant because it is vitally beneficial for the organism: "In as far as the exercise of muscle in high organisms, or the mere fact of contractility itself in the lower, is vitally good, in so far as it also gives pleasure, and this pleasure serves to issue in excess discharge to the same regions again" (p. 191). Along the same line, Baldwin (1891) wrote in *Feeling and Will*: "Nature's design is that the heart should beat regular and strong. She secures this by my enjoyment of physical exercise" (p. 232). Therefore, exercise is pleasant because it is useful; the function of the pleasure exercise produces is to encourage more exercise.

William James (1842–1910)

In 1890, William James published his *Principles of Psychology*, which he had begun writing in 1878. The two-volume textbook became one of the most widely read psychological texts of all time. In 1892, James was encouraged by the administration of Harvard to organize seminars for teachers, highlighting the connection between psychology and education. Not surprisingly for someone of James' charisma and intellectual renown, the lectures were hugely popular. The transcriptions were published as magazine articles and finally in book form in 1899 under the title *Talks to Teachers on Psychology and to Students on Some of Life's Ideals*.

In one lecture to students, entitled "The Gospel of Relaxation," James (1899) addressed the role of exercise in improving how people feel. What is unique in James' treatment of the subject is that he placed his remarks within the context of his famous theory of emotion. Challenging the conventional view, James had proposed that the experience of emotion consists of the perception of the physiological and behavioral changes that occur upon exposure to a relevant stimulus: "our emotions are mainly due to those organic stirrings that are aroused in us in a reflex way by the stimulus of the exciting object or situation" (p. 199). For James, this meant that, if the theory is true (and, for him, "it is certain that the main core of it is true," p. 200), there are clear implications for the regulation of emotional reactions: "were this bodily commotion suppressed, we should not so much feel fear as call the situation fearful; we should not feel surprise, but coldly recognize that the object was indeed astonishing" (pp. 199–200). The therapeutic potential of this approach is considerable because what one does is under direct volitional control: "by regulating the action, which is under the more direct control of the will, we can indirectly regulate the feeling, which is not" (p. 201).

Although the role that James saw for exercise as a therapeutic modality was becoming apparent at this point of his lecture, he took his reasoning a step further by making a surprising reference to psychoanalytic theory (at a time when Freud and his ideas were still unknown in North America). He endorsed the view that "bodily discomforts . . . breed a general self-mistrust and sense that things are not as they should be" (p. 203) and these, in turn, form the causal basis of an unhealthy mind. With this, he was ready to begin laying out his views on exercise: "Consider, for example, the effects of a well-toned motor-apparatus, nervous and muscular, on our general personal self-consciousness, the sense of elasticity and efficiency that results" (p. 204). He presented several interesting examples. Because of skiing, Norwegian women, who used to be "sedentary fireside tabby-cats," were transformed into "lithe and audacious creatures, for whom no night is too dark or height too giddy, and who are not only saying good-bye to the traditional feminine pallor and delicacy of constitution, but actually taking the lead in every educational and social reform" (pp. 204–205). Similarly, "the strength of the British Empire . . . is perennially nourished and kept up by nothing so much as by the national worship, in which all classes meet, of athletic outdoor life and sport" (p. 205).

Finally, concerned about the prospect of a technological future that "will more and more require mental power from us, and less and less will ask for bare brute strength" (p. 206), James (1899) said the following about the importance of exercise and physical fitness:

> I cannot believe that our muscular vigor will ever be a superfluity. Even if the day ever dawns in which it will not be needed for fighting the old heavy battles against Nature, it will still always be needed to furnish the background of sanity, serenity, and cheerfulness to life, to give moral elasticity to our disposition, to round off the wiry edge of our fretfulness, and make us good-humored and easy of approach. Weakness is too apt to be what the doctors call irritable weakness. And that blessed internal peace and confidence, that *acquiescentia in seipso*, as Spinoza used to call it, that wells up from every part of the body of a muscularly well-trained human being, and soaks the indwelling soul of him with satisfaction, is, quite apart from every consideration of its mechanical utility, an element of spiritual hygiene of supreme significance.
>
> (p. 207)

The personal significance of these strong words is better understood by taking into account two facts about James' own life. First, he had been having recurring bouts of severe and debilitating depression since the late 1860s. Second, he had started having problems with his heart a year earlier, in 1898. These problems eventually led to his death of cardiac failure in 1910, at the age of 68.

The era of behaviorism

Since the early 1890s, William James had been looking for a way out of academic psychology. The reason was that North American psychology was changing in a direction that left him uninspired. The "reflexology" pioneered by Ivan Pavlov and the experimental approach of Wilhelm Wundt were proving enormously influential, as they were seen as offering psychology, only recently divorced from philosophy, a path toward scientific legitimacy. At the dawn of the twentieth century, behaviorism, spearheaded by Edward Thorndike and John B. Watson, became the dominant paradigm. This meant the eradication of subjective constructs, such as pleasure, from the range of topics considered acceptable for scientific study. Exercise, mostly in the form of runway and maze running in animal learning experiments, was treated almost exclusively as an observable dependent variable. In the few cases in which it was used as an independent variable, exercise was presumed to represent a means of inducing arousal.

What is astonishing in the studies published during the early part of the twentieth century is how complete the disregard for the introspection-based theorizing of the late nineteenth century was. The slate was wiped clean and psychologists started "discovering" behavioral phenomena and speculating about their causes entirely anew, as if nothing had been said about them before. For example, it was not long after the systematic observation of rodent behavior began that investigators noticed that animals would run "spontaneously," without being coerced by an extrinsic factor such as food. This was an anomalous observation for the behaviorist paradigm; movement without a readily apparent objective, such as the approach of food or the avoidance of shock, did not make sense. While searching for the "internal stimulus" of this inexplicable behavior, attention was initially directed to such factors as "age, hunger and diet, and hormones" (Shirley, 1929, p. 342).

It was not until the 1950s (Kagan & Berkun, 1954) and 1960s (Hundt & Premack, 1963) that running was openly characterized as "rewarding" or "reinforcing," essentially (though not directly) recognizing once again the ability of exercise to produce pleasure. Several authors (e.g., Hill, 1956) also suggested that there may be an inherent drive for "activity." On one hand, this was an acknowledgment that there is an intrinsic propensity for physical activity, but, on the other, by invoking the concept of "drive," researchers were able to avoid the question of the processes that mediate this propensity and thus any direct reference to subjective factors (i.e., pleasure).

The era of cognitivism

Between the 1960s and the 1980s, psychology witnessed the advent of the cognitive revolution and the shift to a new dominant paradigm. Although this new paradigm was more accepting of subjective states, its attitude toward the body reflected varying degrees of neglect.

Two related trends are evident during the period of cognitivism with respect to how bodily activation, including activation induced by exercise, was viewed. According to one of these perspectives, information from the body has no inherent affective meaning; it only acquires meaning following a process of cognitive appraisal. Thus, afferent information generated from the exercising body is viewed as undifferentiated, diffuse, and highly malleable, such that the same physiological condition can be experienced as pleasant or unpleasant, depending on the outcome of the cognitive appraisal. According to the second perspective, pleasant and unpleasant affective responses emanating from the body are so automated and reflex-like that they are of little or no interest as psychological phenomena.

The origins of these ideas can be traced to Walter Cannon's (1915, 1927) critique of the theory of emotion proposed by William James. Cannon's critique was five-fold: (a) separation of the viscera from the central nervous system does not alter emotional behavior in experimental animals, (b) the same visceral changes occur in very different emotional, as well as non-emotional, states, (c) the viscera are relatively insensitive structures, (d) visceral changes are too slow to be a source of emotional feelings, and (e) artificial induction of visceral changes typical of certain emotions does not produce these emotions in a manner felt as experientially identical.

Based on these points, Stanley Schachter and Jerome Singer (1962) conducted a now-famous study showing that physiological arousal, induced by infusions of epinephrine, could be associated with diverse emotions such as euphoria and anger, following an appropriate cognitive manipulation. The results of this experiment, which was, of course, delimited to specific emotions, epinephrine dosages, experimental manipulations, and participants, led Schachter (1964) to draw some rather grand generalizations: "Cognitions arising from the immediate situation as interpreted by past experience provide the framework within which one understands and labels his feelings. It is the cognition which determines whether the state of physiological arousal will be labeled 'anger,' 'joy,' or whatever" (p. 51). Despite the limitations of the study itself, the idea that physiological arousal provides nothing but an amorphous substrate that can be readily manipulated by cognitive "labeling" became very popular. The timing of the study, in 1962, as the cognitive revolution was gaining momentum, probably played a crucial role in this regard.

Thus, in the 1970s, the same essential idea found expression in Dolf Zillmann's notion of "excitation transfer." Since physiological arousal was seen as devoid of inherent affective meaning, Zillmann, Katcher, and Milavsky (1972) proposed that high "excitation" generated by exercise (cycling) could be "transferred" to intensify subsequent retaliatory aggressive behavior following a provocation scenario. Exercise-induced "excitation" was "conceived of as [nothing more than] general drive or energy" (p. 249). Zillmann and Bryant (1974) found that the intensification of aggressive behavior is still observable if the exercise-induced "excitation" has subsided by the time the opportunity for retaliatory aggression is given, as long as it was present during the provocation. In subsequent refinements of the "excitation transfer" idea, however, it was emphasized that the transfer effect does not appear as long as the individual can still consciously perceive the exercise-induced excitation and correctly attribute it to the preceding exercise (Cantor, Zillmann, & Bryant, 1975; Zillmann, Johnson, & Day, 1974). Furthermore, because highly physically fit individuals recover quickly from exercise, they are unlikely to manifest a transfer effect (Zillmann et al., 1974). Nevertheless, echoing Cannon, Zillmann hastened to clarify that the absence of a transfer effect immediately post-exercise "is not to say that [the participant] receives highly specific, reliable feedback [from the body]" (p. 504). Instead, the explanations that were offered were that "the subjects may have been preoccupied with 'catching their breath' [or] the intense arousal they experienced distracted them" (p. 513). Likewise, the finding that "the physically most fit persons proved to be the least susceptible to behavior-modifying transfer effects" was attributed to the fact that "they had best recovered from the induced state of sympathetic arousal" (p. 514). Nevertheless, Zillmann et al. did recognize that "provoked subjects enjoying excellent fitness displayed the least aggressive behavior, and those showing the poorest fitness displayed the most," noting that the possibility that "persons of superior fitness are emotionally more secure . . . cannot be ruled out at present" (p. 514).

By the 1980s, cognitivism was reinforced by the parallel rise of other movements with which it shared a strong skepticism toward physicalism, namely postmodernism and social constructionism. With their emphasis on social and cultural environments, these movements had grown increasingly disembodied (Cromby, 2004), extending the distance between the physical body and lived experience: "Such movements [of the body] surely cannot in themselves be our thoughts, the content of our inner lives? Whereas our bodily reactions and responses constitute the indeterminate beginnings of our thoughts and intentions, our perceptions and understandings, they become determinate only in our voicing of them in relation to a form of life" (Shotter, 1997, p. 19). As soon as social constructionism gained a footing in psychology (Gergen, 1985), it found proponents in the study of emotion. As the balance of interest tilted heavily toward culturally framed social emotions, the importance attributed to bodily processes diminished, installing a cognitive homunculus to a commanding position as monitor, data analyst, and executive officer. According to Averill (1980), "[bodily] feedback is subject to second-order monitoring . . . and it is the monitoring that determines the quality of experience, not the feedback per se" (p. 317).

In certain theories of emotion developed during the period of cognitivism, pleasant and unpleasant states emanating from the body in response to such stimuli as heat or warmth, coldness or coolness, starvation, dehydration, pain, or exercise were recognized as evolutionary forerunners to social emotions. However, these states were either theorized to occur only following a cognitive analysis and interpretation, even a rudimentary one, or they were considered of limited or no interest from a psychological perspective. For example, Scherer (1984) recognized that "even internally generated sensations" can be "emotion producing stimuli" but, for this to happen, they must be subjected to an appraisal process consisting of "a very rapidly occurring sequence of hierarchically organized stimulus processing steps" (p. 306). Following a first check for the novelty or unexpectedness of the stimulus, the second check "consists of the evaluation of the intrinsic pleasantness or unpleasantness of a stimulus which causes the organism to experience pleasure or distress" (p. 307).

Because Scherer (1984) noted that "this check has to do with the inherent pleasantness or unpleasantness of a stimulus, and is not dependent on its relevance to the goals of an organism at that particular moment" (p. 307), Lazarus rejected the characterization of this type of check as part of the "appraisal" process. Lazarus opted instead to classify "inherent pleasantness and unpleasantness" as mere perceptions: "pleasant and unpleasant sensations (e.g., being touched in a particular way or muscle fatigue) . . . should be regarded as perceptual information" (Lazarus & Smith, 1988, p. 287). Furthermore,

> Pleasure and pain are sensory states, not emotions; they lead to emotions when their significance is evaluated and the quality of the resulting emotion depends on the outcome of this evaluation. Muscle fatigue and pain, for example, are often appraised positively and lead to positive emotions for the athlete who believes this is a desirable goal of exercise or practice (as in the expression, "go for the burn") but are appraised quite negatively and lead to negative emotions when some other goal is involved, as when one is struggling to finish a contest in the best position possible, or when pain or distress signifies physical impairment or illness to the person.
>
> *(p. 287)*

By disqualifying sensory pleasure and pain from the domain of emotions, Lazarus essentially questions whether these states are of veritable interest as topics of psychological investigation. He describes them by such adjectives as "universal," "automatic," "hard–wired," "built–in," "innate," "rigid," and "inflexible," to arrive at the suggestion that these phenomena constitute nothing more than neural loops, designed to serve "particular internal homeostatic needs" (Smith & Lazarus, 1990, p. 613) or correct "internal tissue deficits" (p. 612):

> We are built so that sensorimotor pleasure, such as a sweet taste, physical rest, stroking the body, or certain kinds of full stomachs, is almost always elicited by definable physical stimuli in a neurologically intact and receptive person. So, too, with pain.
>
> *(Lazarus, 1991a, p. 55)*

Although Lazarus accepted that sensory "perceptions" of pleasure and displeasure can ultimately lead to emotions following an appropriate appraisal, he agreed with Schachter and Singer that the power of this appraisal in determining the nature of the emotion is absolute. According to Lazarus (1991a), "we do not experience an emotion merely in response to . . . exercising even though homeostatic processes essential to survival are set in motion and coordinated in these situations" (p. 197). "Exercising vigorously," Lazarus (1984) wrote, produces "arousal." This will become an emotion "only if we appraise the encounter (e.g., the physical and social conditions and the bodily state it produces) as having a bearing on our well-being" (p. 124). The appraisal process is theorized to be so omnipotent that even inherently "painful fatigue" can be transformed to an experience of "satisfaction":

> Pain and pleasure are transformed into emotional distress or satisfaction only as a result of appraisals of their significance. For example, competitive runners in a close race who are experiencing painful fatigue on the way to the finish line will probably react with distress because the pain signifies that they are running out of steam and that the race may be lost. However, when the same runners are seeking to condition themselves in training, they are apt to feel satisfaction when they experience the same painful fatigue, because it now signifies that their bodies are being strengthened for future races without much being at stake.
>
> *(Lazarus, 1991b, p. 821)*

In concluding this overview of the references to exercise and pleasure in the psychological literature during the era of cognitivism, it is important to emphasize that the various assertions reviewed here were made in the absence of empirical evidence. Neither Zillmann nor Lazarus, for example, conducted an experiment in which participants were asked to provide self-reports of pleasure–displeasure in response to exercise. Their assertions, therefore, were based entirely on assumptions derived from the cognitivist framework.

Exercise in psychological experiments, 1970s to present

Such was the impact of Zillmann's idea of "excitation transfer" that, by the 1980s, psychology laboratories were teeming with studies involving running, stepping, and cycling (e.g., Clark, Milberg, & Ross, 1983; Hansen, Hansen, & Crano, 1989; Isen, Daubman, & Nowicki, 1987; McDonald, Harris, & Maher, 1983; Sanbonmatsu & Kardes, 1988; Wegner & Giuliano, 1980, 1983; White, Fishbein, & Rutstein, 1981; White & Kight, 1984). Without exception, exercise was used as a means of raising arousal and, in each case, the studies by Zillmann from the 1970s were cited as the basis for this usage. Without testing to ensure that this assumption is true, exercise was chosen because researchers were convinced that it represents a "neutral source of arousal" (White & Kight, 1984, p. 56) or the best method to avoid "confounding the effects of arousal with the effects of valence" (Pham, 1996, p. 375). This usage of exercise, based on the same rationale, continued during the 1990s (e.g., Martin, Harlow, & Strack, 1992; Sinclair, Hoffman, Mark, Martin, & Pickering, 1994) and 2000s (e.g., Lange & Fleming, 2005; Nakajima & Fleming, 2008).

As one example, citing Zillmann's work, Isen et al. (1987) used exercise to induce "affectless arousal" (p. 1122) or "arousal devoid of any particular affective tone" (p. 1128). So convinced were the authors that exercise produces "affectless arousal" that they did not consider it necessary to compare the participants' "affective tone" before and after the exercise; they only asked after exercise. In fact, they even questioned the wisdom of asking participants any affect-related questions in conjunction with an exercise treatment. They criticized their own measure (feel "positive" versus "negative") for being "inappropriate . . . for treatments such as the exercise condition, in which . . . there is no apparent reason for the question and it is therefore too reactive" (p. 1125).

In another example, Anderson, Deuser, and DeNeve (1995) conducted a study to investigate the effects of hot temperatures on state hostility and positive/negative affect. Exercise was included to provide an opportunity to test the validity of a self-report measure of arousal. Reportedly, the measure was found to be "sensitive to changes in perceived arousal created by brief exercise" (p. 441), as the mean score increased from before to after exercise, and subsequently decreased during the recovery period. One important attribute of the measure of arousal, however, was that the item pool represented a nearly perfect confound of arousal and pleasure–displeasure. Almost all high-arousal items denoted some degree of pleasure (e.g., energetic, lively, vigorous, excited, sharp, alert, powerful) and, conversely, almost all low-arousal items denoted some degree of displeasure (e.g., depressed, weak, drowsy, exhausted, sluggish, weary, dull, tired, worn-out, fatigued, sleepy). Therefore, although it was just as likely that exercise induced pleasure, the researchers interpreted their findings as indicative only of arousal.

What is particularly noteworthy in this body of research is the strong reliance on the assumption that the arousal induced by exercise is "affectless." With very few exceptions (Kim & Baron, 1988; Stangor, 1990), researchers accepted this assumption without making any attempt at empirical verification, despite the fact that Zillmann also had not provided any such evidence. Even in the few cases in which the assumption was put to a test, the methods were generally inadequate, as if they were aimed primarily to appease readers rather than provide a rigorous assessment. For example, Kim and Baron (1988) used a purpose-made questionnaire inquiring about very specific emotional states of no relevance to the experimental situation (anger, relaxation, anxiety, friendliness) and only compared a "high" to a "low" exercise condition rather than a no-exercise control. In another case, when a reviewer suggested that the assumption should be tested, the researchers questioned whether exercise could have affect-altering effects, arguing instead that any such findings would probably be artifactual (Sinclair et al., 1994, see Note 3).

Erber and Erber (2000) also used exercise but their intention was not to induce "affectless" arousal. They theorized that any activity requiring effort would "take the mind off" a previously induced happy or sad mood and, in effect, "attenuate" that mood. They found that 10 minutes of step exercise, much like working on difficult math problems, could produce the hypothesized "attenuation" effect. As noted by Thayer (2000), in putting forth their "attenuation" interpretation, the researchers did not consider alternative explanations: "exercise is a powerful mood regulator, and easily could become the overriding influence on mood measurements with weak film manipulations having little effect by comparison" (p. 203).

Beyond assumptions: evidence for the exercise-induced "feel-better" effect

It took a century for research to begin to put Alexander Bain's introspective observations to the test. Starting in the 1960s, reviewers from medicine (e.g., Hammett, 1967) and sport science (e.g., Morgan, 1969) began piecing together fragments of rudimentary evidence from correlational studies linking physical fitness to emotional stability. The first quasi-experimental and experimental designs appeared in the 1970s. While most of the emphasis continued to be on personality traits and self-perceptions, the first studies examining the effects of chronic exercise training (e.g., Greist et al., 1978; Morgan, Roberts, Brand, & Feinerman, 1970; Schwartz, Davidson, & Goleman, 1978) and acute exercise bouts (e.g., Bahrke & Morgan, 1978; Morgan, Roberts, & Feinerman, 1971; Nowlis & Greenberg, 1979) on variables from the affective domain also started to emerge.

A considerable boost to the study of the phenomenon that came to be known as the exercise-induced "feel-better" effect was given with the publication of state measures of affective variables, including the state version of the State-Trait Anxiety Inventory (Spielberger, Gorsuch, & Lushene, 1970) and the Profile of Mood States (McNair, Lorr, & Droppleman, 1971). These measures were the first standardized questionnaires appropriate for operationalizing this phenomenon. Thus, essentially by necessity, the "feel-better" effect was operationally defined as (and treated as tantamount to) post-exercise anxiety reduction and mood enhancement. As the availability and popularity of these measures grew during the 1980s, the studies demonstrating post-exercise anxiolysis (e.g., Boutcher & Landers, 1988; Raglin & Morgan, 1987; Wilson, Berger, & Bird, 1981) and positive mood shifts (e.g., Berger & Owen, 1983; Lichtman & Poser, 1983; Roth, 1989; Steptoe & Bolton, 1988; Steptoe & Cox, 1988) increased in number. Furthermore, over time, their methodological quality improved substantially.

It is important to note that, although most of these studies were conducted by researchers with academic backgrounds in exercise science, a significant number were published in journals from the broader field of psychology, including psychotherapy, psychosomatic medicine, health psychology, and psychophysiology. Evidently, these studies did not go unnoticed by psychologists specializing in the study of affective phenomena. Starting in the 1980s, both Robert Thayer (1987a, 1987b), developer of the Activation Deactivation Adjective Check List (Thayer, 1986), and David Watson (1988; McIntyre, Watson, & Cunningham, 1990), co-developer of the Positive and Negative Affect Schedule (Watson, Clark, & Tellegen, 1988), conducted studies examining the link between physical activity and mood using their own measures. Thus, during the 1980s, research on the exercise-induced "feel-better" effect broke the confines of specialty journals, appearing for the first time in "mainstream" psychological publications, such as the *Journal of Personality and Social Psychology* (e.g., Thayer, 1987a; Watson, 1988), in addition to several other journals published by the American Psychological Association.

Perhaps an important part of the answer to the question posed at the beginning of this chapter (i.e., "why is noone mentioning [exercise]?") can be found in the following observation. In the January 1987 issue of the *Journal of Personality and Social Psychology*, Thayer (1987a), based on research evidence, reported an "unexpectedly strong effect associated with the 10-min brisk walk—up to 2 hr of reduced tension and increased energy" (p. 124). This article has 126 entries in the Citation Index (as of June 2012). Six months later, in the same journal, as noted earlier, Isen et al. (1987), based solely on assumptions, used exercise to induce "affectless arousal" (p. 1122) or "arousal devoid of any particular affective tone" (p. 1128). However, this article is cited at approximately five times the rate (617 times), according to the Citation Index.

By the end of the 1990s, the database on the "feel-better" phenomenon included hundreds of studies (for reviews, see Ekkekakis & Petruzzello, 1999; Tuson & Sinyor, 1993; Yeung, 1996). This led one reviewer to conclude that "both survey and experimental research . . . provide support to the well publicized statement that 'exercise makes you feel good'" (Fox, 1999, p. 413) and another to state that "there is no need for further research or reviews dealing with the question of whether or not physical activity results in improved mood" (Morgan, 1997, p. 230).

Coming full circle: nineteenth-century ideas in twenty-first-century laboratories

In the early part of the twenty-first century, research on the exercise–pleasure relationship entered a new phase, characterized by an updated methodological and conceptual approach. What is remarkable about the findings from this contemporary line of research, however, is the similarity of the themes that are emerging and the conclusions that are drawn to the observations of

Alexander Bain and James Mark Baldwin, stated well over a century ago. It could be argued that modern laboratory experimentation is now, finally, testing their seminal hypotheses and providing empirical support for their pioneering insights. In essence, contrary to any assumptions about the supposedly linear pattern of growth of scientific knowledge, research is only now, after a long, paradigm-imposed embargo, continuing the work that they started in the 1800s.

First, affective responses are examined from a more global perspective, now extending beyond state anxiety and the six distinct mood states tapped by the Profile of Mood States. In newer studies, affect is conceptualized as a dimensional domain, defined by two orthogonal and bipolar dimensions, namely affective valence (ranging from pleasure to displeasure) and perceived activation or arousal. The advantage afforded by this model, named the affect circumplex, is that, at least theoretically, it allows for comprehensive coverage of the content domain of interest in a very efficient manner (requiring the measurement of only two constructs).

Second, instead of limiting assessment to only the pre- and post-exercise time points, newer studies use repeated measurements to track changes in valence and activation throughout the exercise bout and recovery period. Because affect responds dynamically and often instantaneously to changing conditions, such as the progressively intensifying physical strain of exercise or the termination of strenuous effort, examination of pre-to-post changes may misrepresent the true shape of the response trajectory as it unfolds over time.

Third, instead of focusing solely on analyses of change at the level of the entire sample, recent studies also include examinations of change at the level of subgroups and individual participants. The reason for this is that not all individuals respond to the same exercise stimulus in the same direction; some may report increases but others decreases in pleasure. Consequently, analyses of change at the level of the sample mean may conceal disparate and divergent patterns of change at the level of individuals.

Fourth, instead of defining exercise intensity as percentages of maximal capacity (e.g., maximal heart rate of oxygen consumption), several recent studies use metabolic markers, such as the ventilatory (or "gas exchange") threshold and the respiratory compensation point. The ventilatory threshold occurs when relatively more carbon dioxide is produced than the oxygen that is consumed. The respiratory compensation point is the intensity at which pulmonary ventilation begins to rise disproportionately to the amount of carbon dioxide that is produced (see Figure 1.1).

These are adaptationally important benchmarks because of what they mean for the ability of the person to continue exercise. Below the ventilatory threshold, in the so-called "moderate" domain of intensity, an individual can exercise for a long time while physiological indices, such as heart rate, oxygen uptake, and blood lactate, can remain stable. When the intensity exceeds the ventilatory threshold, in what is called the "heavy" domain of intensity, physiological steady-state is disrupted (i.e., even when the workload remains constant, physiological indices begin to rise) and an organism-wide stress response begins (e.g., lactate accumulation rises, accompanied by increases in catecholamine and cortisol concentrations, and a sympathetic shift in autonomic activity). Provided that the distance from the ventilatory threshold is not too large, if a person continues to exercise, a physiological steady-state may be re-established after several minutes. However, judging by most physiological indicators, the organism would be exhibiting a full-blown stress response. Finally, when the intensity exceeds the respiratory compensation point, the maintenance of physiological steady-state is no longer possible; physiological indices rise continuously until the person reaches the limits of tolerance and has to stop. This domain of intensity is termed "severe."

According to the dual-mode theory (Ekkekakis, 2003), affective responses are matched to these domains of intensity in a manner that corresponds to their adaptational implications (see

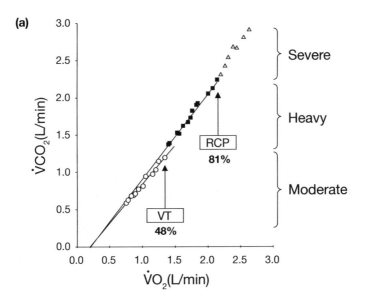

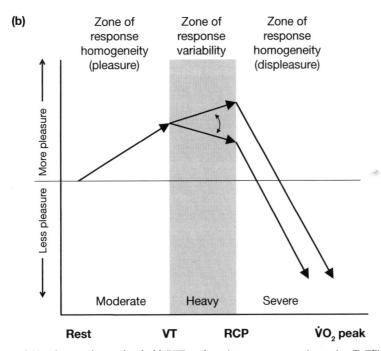

Figure 1.1 Panel (a): The ventilatory threshold (VT) and respiratory compensation point (RCP) represent distinct changes in the slope of the gas-exchange relationship and demarcate the domains of moderate, heavy, and severe exercise intensity. In this example, the first change in slope (VT, beginning of the *heavy* domain) occurs at 48% and the second change in slope (RCP, beginning of the *severe* domain) occurs at 81% of peak oxygen uptake ($\dot{V}O_2$peak). Panel (b): According to the dual-mode theory (Ekkekakis, 2003), there is (1) homogeneity of affective responses in the moderate domain, with the predominant response being pleasure, (2) variability in the heavy domain, with some individuals reporting increases and others decreases in pleasure, and (3) homogeneity in the severe domain, with the predominant response being displeasure.

Figures 1.1 and 1.2; also see Ekkekakis, Parfitt, & Petruzzello, 2011, for a review). Specifically, within the moderate domain, most healthy individuals report stable or increasing levels of pleasure during exercise, typically followed by further improvements during the post–exercise period (also see Reed, Chapter 8, this volume). For example, during and after self-paced walks, most participants report higher pleasure, activation, and perceived energy (Ekkekakis, Backhouse, Gray, & Lind, 2008; Ekkekakis, Hall, Van Landuyt, & Petruzzello, 2000). From an evolutionary perspective, it has been suggested that this positive response was selected to reward and encourage the vitally important subsistence activities (hunting, gathering) that occupied a substantial portion of daily life in the Pleistocene environment (Ekkekakis, Hall, & Petruzzello, 2005a; Raichlen, Foster, Gerdeman, Seillier, & Giuffrida, 2012; Sher, 1998). These speculations are, of course, highly reminiscent of Baldwin's (1891) thoughts on the evolutionary significance of exercise-induced pleasure, which were, in turn, inspired by the writings of Darwin and Spencer.

In the domain of heavy intensity, as the exerciser begins to experience a challenging barrage of interoceptive cues generated by the perturbation of the physiological state, affective responses begin to exhibit interindividual variability. Some individuals continue to report increases in pleasure, while others report decreases (Ekkekakis et al., 2005a; Van Landuyt, Ekkekakis, Hall, & Petruzzello, 2000). This is again consistent with Bain's (1855) observation that it is "easier in some temperaments than in others, to perform rapid movements with coolness" (p. 104). From an evolutionary standpoint, while strong adaptational pressures tend to produce response homogeneity, such variability is interpreted as a response that has ambiguous adaptational implications. Put differently, continuing to experience pleasure while the body is exhibiting symptoms of stress foretelling of an impending metabolic crisis is like a double-edged sword. On one hand, this trait may provide an adaptational advantage by enabling someone to persist and gain the competitive edge in a physical effort (e.g., while fighting or hunting). On the other hand, challenging one's biological limits raises the level of risk (e.g., for exhaustion, heatstroke, skeletal or muscular injury, cardiac arrest). Thus, on balance, neither those individuals who continue to experience pleasure at this level of intensity nor those who begin to experience displeasure will have an unambiguous adaptational advantage. Evidence shows that people differ in their preference for different levels of exercise intensity and exhibit different levels of tolerance to high-intensity exercise. These individual differences account for significant portions of the variability in affective responses in this domain of intensity, beyond what is accounted for by such factors as sex, age, and maximal aerobic capacity (Ekkekakis, Hall, & Petruzzello, 2005b).

Within the domain of severe intensity, there is no chance of re-establishing physiological stability and the risk of a potentially fatal metabolic crisis grows with every step. Therefore, the body must issue an unambiguous directive to consciousness that the activity must be stopped or

Figure 1.2 Panel (a): Affective responses to exercise, plotted in a two-dimensional space, where the horizontal axis represents affective valence (pleasure vs displeasure) and the vertical axis represents perceived activation. The solid line shows the trajectory of change during a graded treadmill test to volitional fatigue (average duration 11.3 minutes). The dotted line shows the change in response to a 15-minute self-paced treadmill walk. Panel (b): The two lines represent the responses of 44.4% of a sample ($N = 63$) who reported gradual improvements (rightward shift) and 41.3% who reported gradual declines (leftward shift) in affective valence during a 30-minute session of cycle-ergometry at 60% of maximal aerobic capacity. These results illustrate (1) the predominantly positive affective response below the ventilatory threshold (walk), (2) the predominantly negative affective response above the ventilatory threshold (graded test to fatigue), and (3) the variable affective response at intensities proximal to the ventilatory threshold (cycling at 60%) (data drawn from Ekkekakis, Hall, Van Landuyt, & Petruzzello (2000), Hall et al. (2002), and Van Landuyt, Ekkekekis, Hall, & Petruzzello (2000), respectively).

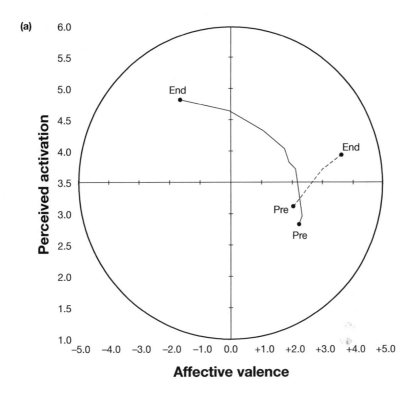

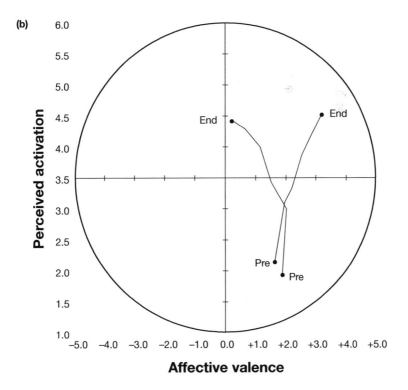

its intensity reduced immediately, in order to prevent collapse and irreparable damage. This directive comes in the form of a universal, automatic, and cognitively unmanageable negative affective response that quickly and effectively diminishes any desire to continue. This irrepressible negative affective response appears to be driven by two factors acting jointly, as redundant safeguards (Ekkekakis & Acevedo, 2006). First, there is an overwhelming intensification of afferent cues from the strained body. Physiological variables, such as ventilation, oxygen uptake, lactate concentration, and core temperature, account for most of the reliable variance in reports of affective valence within the domain of severe intensity (Ekkekakis, 2003). Second, there is significant reduction in the oxygenation and, therefore, presumably the activity of the dorsolateral prefrontal cortex, an area known to be involved in the cognitive control of negative affect (Ekkekakis, 2009).

Finally, once the strenuous activity is stopped, there is a rapid (among physically fit individuals, instantaneous) affective rebound from negativity to positivity (see Figure 1.3), consistent with the "affective or hedonic contrast" phenomenon described by Solomon (1980, 1991). The magnitude of the rebound is proportional to the extent of the negative shift during a strenuous bout of exercise, but typically somewhat larger in absolute terms (Ekkekakis, Hall, & Petruzzello, 2008). Thus, as a result of this rebound, within seconds or minutes, the post-exercise affective state may become more positive than the pre-exercise state. Although such pre- to post-improvements in affect were interpreted in the past as additional evidence for the exercise-induced "feel-better" effect, this interpretation is debatable. A more appropriate interpretation is that the positivity is not a response to the exercise itself but rather to the cessation of exercise (Backhouse, Ekkekakis, Biddle, Foskett, & Williams, 2007).

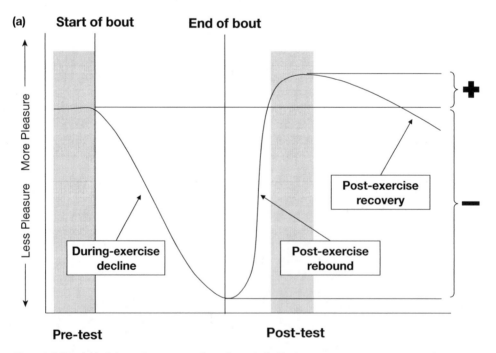

Figure 1.3, Panel (a): Schematic representation of a typical affective response to strenuous exercise (e.g., at intensity exceeding the ventilatory threshold), illustrating the affective decline during the bout (-) and the affective rebound after the bout, leading to a post-exercise state that is more positive than the pre-exercise one (+).

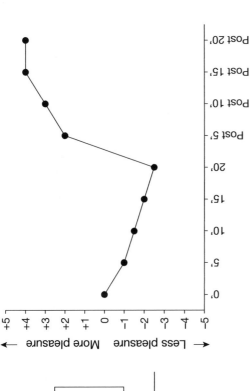

Figure 1.3, Panel (b): This type of response is consistent with Solomon's (1980, 1991) opponent-process model. According to Solomon and Corbit (1974), the "exhilaration following . . . endurance-challenging exercise" (p. 143) is an example of the operation of an opponent process. Solomon postulated that, for each stimulus charged with negative affect (termed a-process), an opponent-process (or b-process), charged with positive affect, is aroused. The function of the opponent-process is to return the organism to a state of affective equilibrium. Solomon (1980) proposed that the a-process "closely tracks the stimulus intensity" (p. 710) and, once it "reaches a critical intensity" (Solomon, 1991, p. 339), it "trips" the opponent-process into action. In turn, the opponent-process "has a long latency, a sluggish course of increase, and a sluggish course of decay" (Solomon, 1980, p. 710) after the a-process is terminated. Solomon (1980) speculated that the b-process might reflect the function of endogenous opioids (see Chapter 2 by Boecker and Dishman, this volume). Assuming a progressive homeostatic perturbation (a-process) during exercise (top-left graph), an opponent-process with the characteristics described by Solomon might be aroused (bottom-left graph). Through the function of an affect summator computing |a-b|, the resultant affect (right graph) would closely resemble the response pattern shown in panel (a).

Supporting another of the observations of Bain and Baldwin, recent studies have provided empirical evidence for a link between affective responses to exercise and exercise behavior. The more pleasant the exercise is, the more physical activity a person is likely to do (Schneider, Dunn, & Cooper, 2009; Williams et al., 2008; Williams, Dunsiger, Jennings, & Marcus, 2012). However, skeptics might argue that, if exercise can be pleasant, what accounts for the persistently low rates of public physical activity participation or what Bain (1855) called "the utter neglect of physical exercise as a habitual element of life" (p. 95)? The answer to this challenging question may lie, at least in part, in what is essentially an evolutionary aberration, namely the extremely poor physical condition of many contemporary humans.

To illustrate, consider the example of a participant from a study conducted by the author. A 41-year-old woman weighed 61 kg and had a Body Mass Index of 25 kg/m^2, on the cusp between being considered normal weight or overweight. She was apparently healthy, as she had not been diagnosed with a chronic cardiorespiratory, circulatory, or metabolic condition and was not receiving any medication. However, as a result of sedentary living over a period of decades, her maximal aerobic capacity was very poor. Her peak aerobic capacity was only 17 ml of oxygen per kilogram of body weight per minute (bottom 1% according to normative data). Her ventilatory threshold was at 60% of that, or at approximately 10 ml per kg per min (2.86 times the basal metabolic rate, or MET). Examples of physical activities rated at 2.5 METs and, therefore, within her "moderate" range of intensity include slow walking (less than 4 miles per hour) without carrying any extra weight, mild stretching, fishing from a seated position, dusting, washing dishes, watering flowers, playing the piano, and sewing. In contrast, physical activities rated at 3.0 METs, and therefore within her "heavy" domain of intensity, include such common everyday tasks as slow walking while carrying an external load (e.g., bags of groceries weighing under 20 lbs or 9 kg), fishing from a standing position, cleaning windows, sweeping the floor, washing the car, painting the walls, picking fruit from a tree, bowling, or golfing. Because these activities would require her to enter the domain of heavy intensity, they would probably suffice to induce a reduction in pleasure. To make matters worse, being overweight or obese (conditions now shared by over 60% of the population in industrialized countries) is associated with significantly reduced levels of pleasure over most of the range of exercise intensity compared to being normal weight (Ekkekakis & Lind, 2006; Ekkekakis, Lind, & Vazou, 2010).

Conclusion

Although the exercise-induced "feel-better" effect is not universal, it is now a reliably established phenomenon. It is typically associated with moderate levels of exercise intensity (i.e., below the ventilatory threshold) and, for some individuals, even with intensities that are slightly higher. However, as the rate of obesity rises and the average level of aerobic capacity falls, the phenomenon may become increasingly harder to detect in modern humans. Therein lies the challenge for public health, including public mental health. To keep people physically active and thus enable them to benefit from the effects of exercise, the exercise must be pleasant. When it is not, dropout is likely to ensue, leading to an even poorer state of physical conditioning, and a perpetuation of the vicious cycle.

As to the question posed at the beginning of this chapter, namely why so many colleagues in psychology appear unaware of evidence linking exercise to pleasure, a critical reading of the literature indicates that the reason is not the absence of evidence. Rather, the culprit must be sought among the list of usual suspects: artificial disciplinary chasms, dualistic rifts, paradigm-induced tunnel vision, uncritical adoption of assumptions, and a faltering historical memory.

References

Anderson, C.A., Deuser, W.E., & DeNeve, K.M. (1995). Hot temperatures, hostile affect, hostile cognition, and arousal: Tests of a general model of affective aggression. *Personality and Social Psychology Bulletin, 21*, 434–448.

Averill, J.R. (1980). A constructivist view of emotion. In R. Plutchik & H. Kellerman (Eds.), *Emotion: Theory, research, and experience* (Vol. 1, pp. 305–339). New York: Academic Press.

Backhouse, S.H., Ekkekakis, P., Biddle, S.J.H., Foskett, A., & Williams, C. (2007). Exercise makes people feel better but people are inactive: Paradox or artifact? *Journal of Sport and Exercise Psychology, 29*, 498–517.

Bahrke, M.S., & Morgan, W.P. (1978). Anxiety reduction following exercise and meditation. *Cognitive Therapy and Research, 2*, 323–333.

Bain, A. (1855). *The senses and the intellect.* London: John W. Parker & Son.

Baldwin, J.M. (1891). *Handbook of psychology: Feeling and will.* New York: Henry Holt & Company.

Baldwin, J.M. (1894). *Mental development in the child and the race: Methods and processes.* New York: Macmillan.

Berger, B.G., & Owen, D.R. (1983). Mood alteration with swimming: Swimmers really do "feel better." *Psychosomatic Medicine, 45*, 425–433.

Boutcher, S.H., & Landers, D.M. (1988). The effects of vigorous exercise on anxiety, heart rate, and alpha activity of runners and nonrunners. *Psychophysiology, 25*, 696–702.

Cannon, W.B. (1915). *Bodily changes in pain, hunger, fear and rage: An account of recent researches into the function of emotional excitement.* New York: D. Appleton & Company.

Cannon, W.B. (1927). The James-Lange theory of emotions: A critical examination and an alternative theory. *American Journal of Psychology, 39*, 106–124.

Cantor, J.R., Zillmann, D., & Bryant, J. (1975). Enhancement of experienced sexual arousal in response to erotic stimuli through misattribution of unrelated residual excitation. *Journal of Personality and Social Psychology, 32*, 69–75.

Clark, M.S., Milberg, S., & Ross, J. (1983). Arousal cues arousal-related material in memory: Implications for understanding effects of mood on memory. *Journal of Verbal Learning and Verbal Behavior, 22*, 633–649.

Cromby, J. (2004). Between constructionism and neuroscience: The societal co-constitution of embodied subjectivity. *Theory and Psychology, 14*, 797–821.

Darwin, C. (1872). *The expression of the emotions in man and animals.* London: John Murray.

Ekkekakis, P. (2003). Pleasure and displeasure from the body: Perspectives from exercise. *Cognition and Emotion, 17*, 213–239.

Ekkekakis, P. (2008). The genetic tidal wave finally reached our shores: Will it be the catalyst for a critical overhaul of the way we think and do science? *Mental Health and Physical Activity, 1*, 47–52.

Ekkekakis, P. (2009). Illuminating the black box: Investigating prefrontal cortical hemodynamics during exercise with near-infrared spectroscopy. *Journal of Sport and Exercise Psychology, 31*, 505–553.

Ekkekakis, P., & Acevedo, E.O. (2006). Affective responses to acute exercise: Toward a psychobiological dose-response model. In E.O. Acevedo & P. Ekkekakis (Eds.), *Psychobiology of physical activity* (pp. 91–109). Champaign, IL: Human Kinetics.

Ekkekakis, P., & Backhouse, S.H. (2009). Exercise and psychological well-being. In R. Maughan (Ed.), *Olympic textbook of science in sport* (pp. 251–271). Hoboken, NJ: Wiley-Blackwell.

Ekkekakis, P., Backhouse, S.H., Gray, C., & Lind, E. (2008). Walking is popular among adults but is it pleasant? A framework for clarifying the link between walking and affect as illustrated in two studies. *Psychology of Sport and Exercise, 9*, 246–264.

Ekkekakis, P., Hall, E.E., & Petruzzello, S.J. (2005a). Variation and homogeneity in affective responses to physical activity of varying intensities: An alternative perspective on dose-response based on evolutionary considerations. *Journal of Sports Sciences, 23*, 477–500.

Ekkekakis, P., Hall, E.E., & Petruzzello, S.J. (2005b). Some like it vigorous: Individual differences in the preference for and tolerance of exercise intensity. *Journal of Sport and Exercise Psychology, 27*, 350–374.

Ekkekakis, P., Hall, E.E., & Petruzzello, S.J. (2008). The relationship between exercise intensity and affective responses demystified: To crack the forty-year-old nut, replace the forty-year-old nutcracker! *Annals of Behavioral Medicine, 35*, 136–149.

Ekkekakis, P., Hall, E.E., Van Landuyt, L.M., & Petruzzello, S.J. (2000). Walking in (affective) circles: Can short walks enhance affect? *Journal of Behavioral Medicine, 23*, 245–275.

Ekkekakis, P., & Lind, E. (2006). Exercise does not feel the same when you are overweight: The impact of self-selected and imposed intensity on affect and exertion. *International Journal of Obesity, 30*, 652–660.

Ekkekakis, P., Lind, E., & Vazou, S. (2010). Affective responses to increasing levels of exercise intensity in normal-weight, overweight, and obese middle-aged women. *Obesity, 18*, 79–85.

Ekkekakis, P., Parfitt, G., & Petruzzello, S.J. (2011). The pleasure and displeasure people feel when they exercise at different intensities: Decennial update and progress towards a tripartite rationale for exercise intensity prescription. *Sports Medicine, 41,* 641–671.

Ekkekakis, P., & Petruzzello, S.J. (1999). Acute aerobic exercise and affect: Current status, problems, and prospects regarding dose-response. *Sports Medicine, 28,* 337–374.

Erber, R., & Erber, M.W. (2000). The self-regulation of moods: Second thoughts on the importance of happiness in everyday life. *Psychological Inquiry, 11,* 142–148.

Faulkner, G., & Biddle, S. (2001). Exercise and mental health: It's just not psychology! *Journal of Sports Sciences, 19,* 433–444.

Fox, K.R. (1999). The influence of physical activity on mental well-being. *Public Health Nutrition, 2,* 411–418.

Gergen, K.J. (1985). The social constructionist movement in modern psychology. *American Psychologist, 40,* 266–275.

Greist, J.H., Klein, M.H., Eischens, R.R., Faris, J., Gurman, A.S., & Morgan, W.P. (1978). Running through your mind. *Journal of Psychosomatic Research, 22,* 259–294.

Hall, E.E., Ekkekakis, P., & Petruzzello, S.J. (2002). The affective beneficence of vigorous exercise revisited. *British Journal of Health Psychology, 7,* 47–66.

Hammett, V.B.O. (1967). Psychological changes with physical fitness training. *Canadian Medical Association Journal, 96,* 764–768.

Hansen, R.D., Hansen, C.H., & Crano, W.D. (1989). Sympathetic arousal and self-attention: The accessibility of interoceptive and exteroceptive arousal cues. *Journal of Experimental Social Psychology, 25,* 437–449.

Hill, W.F. (1956). Activity as an autonomous drive. *Journal of Comparative and Physiological Psychology, 49,* 15–19.

Hundt, A.G., & Premack, D. (1963). Running as both a positive and negative reinforcer. *Science, 142,* 1087–1088.

Isen, A.M., Daubman, K.A., & Nowicki, G.P., (1987). Positive affect facilitates creative problem solving. *Journal of Personality and Social Psychology, 52,* 1122–1131.

James, W. (1890). *The principles of psychology.* New York: Henry Holt.

James, W. (1899). *Talks to teachers on psychology and to students on some of life's ideals.* New York: Henry Holt & Company.

Kagan, J., & Berkun, M. (1954). The reward value of running activity. *Journal of Comparative and Physiological Psychology, 47,* 108.

Kim, H.-S., & Baron, R.S. (1988). Exercise and the illusory correlation: Does arousal heighten stereotypic processing? *Journal of Experimental Social Psychology, 24,* 366–380.

Kuhn, T.S. (1962/1996). *The structure of scientific revolutions* (3rd ed.). Chicago: University of Chicago Press.

Lange, L.J., & Fleming, R. (2005). Cognitive influences on the perception of somatic change during a feigned chemical release. *Journal of Applied Social Psychology, 35,* 463–486.

Lazarus, R.S. (1984). On the primacy of cognition. *American Psychologist, 39,* 124–129.

Lazarus, R.S. (1991a). *Emotion and adaptation.* New York: Oxford University Press.

Lazarus, R.S. (1991b). Progress on a cognitive-motivational-relational theory of emotion. *American Psychologist, 46,* 819–834.

Lazarus, R.S., & Smith, C.A. (1988). Knowledge and appraisal in the cognition-emotion relationship. *Cognition and Emotion, 2,* 281–300.

Lichtman, S., & Poser, E.G. (1983). The effects of exercise on mood and cognitive functioning. *Journal of Psychosomatic Research, 27,* 43–52.

Martin, L.L., Harlow, T.F., & Strack, F. (1992). The role of bodily sensations in the evaluation of social events. *Personality and Social Psychology Bulletin, 18,* 412–419.

McDonald, P.J., Harris, S.G., & Maher, J.E. (1983). Arousal-induced self-awareness: An artifactual relationship? *Journal of Personality and Social Psychology, 44,* 285–289.

McIntyre, C.W., Watson, D., & Cunningham, A.C. (1990). The effects of social interaction, exercise, and test stress on positive and negative affect. *Bulletin of the Psychonomic Society, 28,* 141–143.

McNair, D.M., Lorr, M., & Droppleman, L.F. (1971). *Manual for the Profile of Mood States.* San Diego, CA: Educational and Industrial Testing Service.

Mead, G.E., Morley, W., Campbell, P., Greig, C.A., McMurdo, M.E.T., & Lawlor, D.A. (2009). Exercise for depression. *Mental Health and Physical Activity, 2,* 95–96.

Morgan, W.P. (1969). Physical fitness and emotional health: A review. *American Corrective Therapy Journal, 23,* 124–127.

Morgan, W.P. (1997). Conclusion: State of the field and future research. In W.P. Morgan (Ed.), *Physical activity and mental health* (pp. 227–232). Washington, DC: Taylor & Francis.

Morgan, W.P., Roberts, J.A., Brand, F.R., & Feinerman, A.D. (1970). Psychological effect of chronic physical activity. *Medicine and Science in Sports, 2,* 213–217.

Morgan, W.P., Roberts, J.A., & Feinerman, A.D. (1971). Psychologic effect of acute physical activity. *Archives of Physical Medicine and Rehabilitation, 52,* 422–425.

Nakajima, M., & Fleming, R. (2008). Cognitive and physiological determinants of symptom perception and interpretation. *Journal of Applied Biobehavioral Research, 13,* 42–66.

Nowlis, D.P., & Greenberg, N. (1979). Empirical description of effects of exercise on mood. *Perceptual and Motor Skills, 49,* 1001–1002.

Pham, M.T. (1996). Cue representation and selection effects of arousal on persuasion. *Journal of Consumer Research, 22,* 373–387.

Raglin, J.S., & Morgan, W.P. (1987). Influence of exercise and quiet rest on state anxiety and blood pressure. *Medicine and Science in Sports and Exercise, 19,* 456–463.

Raichlen, D.A., Foster, A.D., Gerdeman, G.L., Seillier, A., & Giuffrida, A. (2012). Wired to run: Exercise-induced endocannabinoid signaling in humans and cursorial mammals with implications for the "runner's high." *Journal of Experimental Biology, 215,* 1331–1336.

Robins, R.W., Gosling, S.D., & Craik, K.H. (1999). An empirical analysis of trends in psychology. *American Psychologist, 54,* 117–128.

Roth, D.L. (1989). Acute emotional and psychophysiological effects of aerobic exercise. *Psychophysiology, 26,* 593–602.

Sanbonmatsu, D.M., & Kardes, F.R. (1988). The effects of physiological arousal on information processing and persuasion. *Journal of Consumer Research, 15,* 379–385.

Schachter, S. (1964). The interaction of cognitive and physiological determinants of emotional state. *Advances in Experimental Social Psychology, 1,* 49–80.

Schachter, S., & Singer, J.E. (1962). Cognitive, social, and physiological determinants of emotional state. *Psychological Review, 69,* 379–399.

Scherer, K.H. (1984). On the nature and function of emotion: A component process approach. In K.R. Scherer & P. Ekman (Eds.), *Approaches to emotion* (pp. 293–317). Hillsdale, NJ: Lawrence Erlbaum.

Schneider, M., Dunn, A., & Cooper, D. (2009). Affect, exercise, and physical activity among healthy adolescents. *Journal of Sport and Exercise Psychology, 31,* 706–723.

Schwartz, G.E., Davidson, R.J., & Goleman, D.J. (1978). Patterning of cognitive and somatic processes in the self-regulation of anxiety: Effects of meditation versus exercise. *Psychosomatic Medicine, 40,* 321–328.

Sher, L. (1998). The endogenous euphoric reward system that reinforces physical training: A mechanism for mankind's survival. *Medical Hypotheses, 51,* 449–450.

Shirley, M. (1929). Spontaneous activity. *Psychological Bulletin, 26,* 341–365.

Shotter, J. (1997). The social construction of our inner selves. *Journal of Constructivist Psychology, 10,* 7–24.

Sinclair, R.C., Hoffman, C., Mark, M.M., Martin, L.L., & Pickering, T.L. (1994). Construct accessibility and the misattribution of arousal: Schachter and Singer revisited. *Psychological Science, 5,* 15–19.

Smith, C.A., & Lazarus, R.S. (1990). Emotion and adaptation. In L.A. Pervin (Ed.), *Handbook of personality: Theory and research* (pp. 609–637). New York: Guilford.

Solomon, R.L. (1980). The opponent-process theory of acquired motivation: The costs of pleasure and the benefits of pain. *American Psychologist, 35,* 691–712.

Solomon, R.L. (1991). Acquired motivation and affective opponent-processes. In J. Madden (Ed.), *Neurobiology of learning, emotion, and affect* (pp. 307–347). New York: Raven.

Solomon, R.L., & Corbit, J.D. (1974). An opponent-process theory of motivation: Temporal dynamics of affect. *Psychological Review, 81,* 119–145.

Spielberger, C.D., Gorsuch, R.L., & Lushene, R.E. (1970). *Manual for the State-Trait Anxiety Inventory.* Palo Alto, CA: Consulting Psychologists Press.

Stangor, C. (1990). Arousal, accessibility of trait constructs, and person perception. *Journal of Experimental Social Psychology, 26,* 305–321.

Steptoe, A., & Bolton, J. (1988). The short-term influence of high and low intensity physical exercise on mood. *Psychology and Health, 2,* 91–106.

Steptoe, A., & Cox, S. (1988). Acute effects of aerobic exercise on mood. *Health Psychology, 7,* 329–340.

Thayer, R.E. (1986). Activation-Deactivation Adjective Check List: Current overview and structural analysis. *Psychological Reports, 58,* 607–614.

Thayer, R.E. (1987a). Energy, tiredness, and tension effects of a sugar snack versus moderate exercise. *Journal of Personality and Social Psychology, 52,* 119–125.

Thayer, R.E. (1987b). Problem perception, optimism, and related states as a function of time of day (diurnal rhythm) and moderate exercise: Two arousal systems in interaction. *Motivation and Emotion, 11*, 19–36.

Thayer, R.E. (2000). Mood regulation and general arousal systems. *Psychological Inquiry, 11*, 202–204.

Tuson, K.M., & Sinyor, D. (1993). On the affective benefits of acute aerobic exercise: Taking stock after twenty years of research. In P. Seraganian (Ed.), *Exercise psychology: The influence of physical exercise on psychological processes* (pp. 80–121). New York: Wiley.

Van Landuyt, L.M., Ekkekakis, P., Hall, E.E., & Petruzzello, S.J. (2000). Throwing the mountains into the lakes: On the perils of nomothetic conceptions of the exercise–affect relationship. *Journal of Sport and Exercise Psychology, 22*, 208–234.

Watson, D. (1988). Intraindividual and interindividual analyses of positive and negative affect: Their relation to health complaints, perceived stress, and daily activities. *Journal of Personality and Social Psychology, 54*, 1020–1030.

Watson, D., Clark, L.A., & Tellegen, A. (1988). Development and validation of brief measures of positive and negative affect: The PANAS scales. *Journal of Personality and Social Psychology, 54*, 1063–1070.

Watson, R.I. (1960). The history of psychology: A neglected area. *American Psychologist, 15*, 251–255.

Wegner, D.M., & Giuliano, T. (1980). Arousal-induced attention to self. *Journal of Personality and Social Psychology, 38*, 719–726.

Wegner, D.M., & Giuliano, T. (1983). On sending artifact in search of artifact: Reply to McDonald, Harris, and Maher. *Journal of Personality and Social Psychology, 44*, 290–293.

White, G.L., Fishbein, S., & Rutstein, J. (1981). Passionate love and the misattribution of arousal. *Journal of Personality and Social Psychology, 41*, 56–62.

White, G.L., & Kight, T.D. (1984). Misattribution of arousal and attraction: Effects of salience of explanations for arousal. *Journal of Experimental Social Psychology, 20*, 55–64.

Williams, D.M., Dunsiger, S., Ciccolo, J.T., Lewis, B.A., Albrecht, A.E., & Marcus, B.H. (2008). Acute affective response to a moderate-intensity exercise stimulus predicts physical activity participation 6 and 12 months later. *Psychology of Sport and Exercise, 9*, 231–245.

Williams, D.M., Dunsiger, S., Jennings, E.G., & Marcus, B.H. (2012). Does affective valence during and immediately following a 10-min walk predict concurrent and future physical activity? *Annals of Behavioral Medicine, 44*, 43–51.

Wilson, V.E., Berger, B.G., & Bird, E.I. (1981). Effects of running and of an exercise class on anxiety. *Perceptual and Motor Skills, 53*, 472–474.

Yeung. R.R. (1996). The acute effects of exercise on mood state. *Journal of Psychosomatic Research, 40*, 123–141.

Zillmann, D., & Bryant, J. (1974). Effect of residual excitation on the emotional response to provocation and delayed aggressive behavior. *Journal of Personality and Social Psychology, 30*, 782–791.

Zillmann, D., Johnson, R.C., & Day, K.D. (1974). Attribution of apparent arousal and proficiency of recovery from sympathetic activation affecting excitation transfer to aggressive behavior. *Journal of Experimental Social Psychology, 10*, 503–515.

Zillmann, D., Katcher, A.H., & Milavsky, B. (1972). Excitation transfer from physical exercise to subsequent aggressive behavior. *Journal of Experimental Social Psychology, 8*, 247–259.

2

PHYSICAL ACTIVITY AND REWARD

The role of endogenous opioids

Henning Boecker and Rod K. Dishman

In humans, regular physical activity has been associated with a wide range of positive mental health outcomes in various affect-related domains beyond well-established effects on specific aspects of cognition (Hillman, Erickson, & Kramer, 2008). These include reduced symptoms of depression and anxiety (Byrne & Byrne, 1993; De Moor, Boomsma, Stubbe, Willemsen, & de Geus, 2008; Herring, O'Connor, & Dishman, 2010; Herring, Puetz, O'Connor, & Dishman, 2012; Krogh, Nordentoft, Sterne, & Lawlor, 2011; Mead, Morley, Campbell, Greig, McMurdo, & Lawlor, 2009; Morgan, 1985; Ströhle, 2009), lowered odds of developing depressive disorders or feelings of distress (Physical Activity Guidelines Advisory Committee, 2008), and elevated mood (Janal, Colt, Clark, & Glusman, 1984; Wildmann, Kruger, Schmole, Niemann, & Matthaei, 1986). Mood effects range from feelings of general well-being (Knechtle, 2004; Sher, 1996) and accomplishment (Conroy, Smith, & Felthous, 1982) to ecstatic affective states, referred to as "runner's high" (Partin, 1983; Wagemaker & Goldstein, 1980). Deprivation from regular exercise can be associated with mood disturbances, notably increased state anxiety, tension, depression, and confusion (Mondin et al., 1996). Beyond mood, there are indications that exercise training influences pain perception (Koltyn, 2000) and studies in humans (Droste, Greenlee, Schreck, & Roskamm, 1991; Janal et al., 1984; Koltyn, 2000) and animals (Shyu, Andersson, & Thoren, 1982) have demonstrated elevated pain detection thresholds as a consequence of exercise, although muscle pain during intense exercise may not depend on opiodergic influences on nociception (Cook, O'Connor, & Ray, 2000).

Despite considerable research efforts, up to now the neurobiological mechanisms underlying the benefits of being physically active remain poorly understood (Dishman et al., 2006) and also the circumstances (e.g., exercise duration and intensity, associated factors, etc.) causing positive aspects of exercise on mental health remain unclear (De Moor et al., 2008). While there is considerable progress in unveiling neurobiological mechanisms that may mediate cognitive improvement by exercise (Hillman et al., 2008), including neurotrophic factor release (Gomez-Pinilla, 2008; Vaynman & Gomez-Pinilla, 2005, 2006; Vaynman, Ying, & Gomez-Pinilla, 2004), neurogenesis/angiogenesis (van Praag, 2008), and neuroplasticity (Cotman & Berchtold, 2002), the central mechanisms mediating reward and pleasure in athletes remain far less well understood. Moreover, the understanding of the motivation to initiate and maintain a physically active lifestyle is still in its infancy, despite evidence that physical activity is strongly heritable (Bray et al., 2009; Stubbe et al., 2006).

There are different theories how exercise affects mood. Dietrich has proposed the "transient hypofrontality hypothesis" claiming an exercise-induced state of frontal hypofunction to account for effects of exercise on emotion and cognition (Dietrich, 2006). This theory has found support by ^{18}F-fluorodeoxyglucose (FDG) PET data of decreased prefrontal cortex metabolism during exercise (Tashiro et al., 2008), along with EEG changes in frontal brain areas (Schneider et al., 2009). However, the results of a recent systematic review and meta-analysis of 21 studies of exercise on brain hemodynamics measured by near-infrared spectroscopy (NIRS) in healthy adults are inconsistent with the "transient hypofrontality hypothesis" when it is applied to sub-maximal exercise (Rooks, Thom, McCully, & Dishman, 2010). The pattern of cerebral oxygenation, deoxygenation, and blood volume in the studies reviewed suggested responses opposite to the hypothesis. Only during highly intense, exhaustive exercise were cerebral oxygen values lowered. In contrast, moderate to hard sub-maximal exercise, the intensities that people select for their exercise and that elicit favorable moods, was accompanied by increases in cerebral oxygen and blood volume (Rooks et al., 2010). Related to this, Ekkekakis brought up the "dual-mode theory" (Ekkekakis, 2009), postulating that cognitive processing in prefrontal cortex shifts toward interoceptive processing in an exercise-intensity dependent manner. Other theories have focused on central neurotransmission, claiming effects of exercise on mood to be linked to biogenic amines (Chaouloff, 1989) and endorphinergic neurotransmission (Francis, 1983; Harber & Sutton, 1984).

This review will focus on the role of endorphins in exercise and how they affect pleasure and reward processing in athletes. The influential "endorphin hypothesis" (for a review, see Hoffmann, 1997) claims that endogenous opioid peptides are released in the human brain where they modulate affective processing and pain perception. However, after more than 30 years of human exercise research, the "endorphin hypothesis" is still under critical debate (Dishman, 1985; Dishman & O'Connor, 2009; Hinton & Taylor, 1986) as, for various reasons including methodological constraints, there has as yet been no direct proof in humans that exercise-induced mood changes are directly induced by endorphins in the central nervous system (CNS). Although opiate antagonists like Naloxone or Naltrexone have evoked positive associations of opioid actions and mood effects in most studies (Daniel, Martin, & Carter, 1992; Janal et al., 1984; Jarvekulg & Viru, 2002), although not unequivocally (Markoff, Ryan, & Young, 1982), the human findings generated so far were in essence indirect measures; for example, the demonstration of elevated beta-endorphin levels in plasma after exercise challenges does not inform about changes in central opioidergic neurotransmission because peripheral endorphins can only marginally reenter the brain through the blood–brain barrier (Dearman & Francis, 1983) and, thus, the relation between the peripheral and central opioidergic compartments remains unknown.

Only recently, PET ligand studies have been introduced as a more direct approach for studying opioidergic mechanisms in human exercise research (Boecker, Henriksen, et al., 2008; Boecker et al., 2010; Boecker, Sprenger, et al., 2008). Thereby, it has become possible to image opioidergic receptor binding within the entire human CNS *in vivo* and to assess binding changes related to exercise challenges. From a first application of this imaging method in athletes, evidence emerged to support that endogenous opioids are released in human brains after prolonged exercise (Boecker, Sprenger, et al., 2008). This technique may in future help resolve some of the unknown links between exercise, the central opioidergic compartment, and affective modulation in human athletes. Thus, future applications of behavioral and neuroimaging neuroscience to physical activity studies are necessary to elucidate, or eliminate, plausible opioidergic mechanisms, thereby advancing our understanding of the choice to be physically active and whether physical activity truly benefits mental health.

In the following, we will summarize the current state of research on the opioidergic system in exercise studies: first, we will describe the opioidergic system at the level of transmitters and receptors; second, we will summarize models of reward, hedonics, and motivation; third, we will summarize animal studies, and, finally, human studies examining the role of the central opioidergic system in mediating affective states through exercise.

The opioidergic system

Endogenous opioids have pharmacological actions similar to exogenous opiates like morphine. They act by binding to mu, kappa, or delta opioid receptors, and all three major representatives of the endogenous opioids carry variable affinities for mu, kappa, or delta opioid receptors. Due to their widespread distribution throughout the peripheral and central nervous system, endogenous opioids influence various bodily functions, from hedonics to pain regulation, but also cardiovascular, appetite, thirst, and temperature regulation (Akil et al., 1998; Evans, Hammond, & Fredrickson, 1988).

There are three major types of endogenous opioids: the beta-endorphins found primarily in the anterior and intermediate regions of the pituitary and released into the bloodstream, as well as the enkephalins and dynorphin, both distributed throughout many different CNS structures. More recently, another group of endogenous substances termed endomorphins (endomorphin-1 and endomorphin-2) have been discovered (Fichna, Janecka, Costentin, & Do Rego, 2007); through their particular affinity to the mu-receptor they can mimic their effects (Fichna et al., 2007). Whereas generation of euphoria has been linked to mu-receptor activation, dysphoric mood states have been associated with kappa-receptor activation (Bodnar, 2007).

In exercise research, studies on opioids have focused on beta-endorphins. They interact with mu- and delta-opioid receptors (Raynor et al., 1994). Peripherally, they are found in multiple organs like the eyes, the heart, the kidneys, the gastrointestinal tract, and the adrenal glands. Centrally, they are found in the spinal cord and in the brain (Imura & Nakai, 1981), the highest concentration being in the hypothalamus, but also in the limbic system, the periaqueductal gray (PAG), and the brainstem (Hegadoren, O'Donnell, Lanius, Coupland, & Lacaze-Masmonteil, 2009). The PAG is a key area of the descending anti-nociceptive pathway that mediates opioidergic anti-nociceptive effects (Sandkuhler, 1996). Neurons expressing the precursor protein proopiomelanocortin (POMC) are also found in the ventral tegmental area (VTA) and the nucleus accumbens (Leriche, Cote-Velez, & Mendez, 2007), whereby beta-endorphins are thought to modulate hedonics and appetitively motivated behaviors. Beta-endorphins produce hypoalgesia, respiratory depression, bradycardia, miosis, and hypothermia.

The enkephalins (leu-ENK and met-ENK) bind preferentially to delta-opioid receptors (Akil et al., 1998) and influence nociception, reward, and stress responses. Enkaphalins are thought to maintain normal affective tone through their interaction with delta receptors (Perrine, Sheikh, Nwaneshiudu, Schroeder, & Unterwald, 2008; Torregrossa et al., 2006) and ENK desensitization of delta opioid receptors in the ventral striatum, a critical neural circuit for affective modulation of endogenous opioids (Smith & Berridge, 2007), induces anxiety and depression-like effects. Furthermore, ENK influence stress, and nociception via the amygdala, the PAG, and the dorsal horn of the spinal cord (Akil et al., 1998; Jonsdottir, 2000a).

The distribution of dynorphin (DYN A, DYN B) generally overlaps with that of ENK but the behavioral functions are often opposite. DYN binds primarily to kappa-opioid receptors, thereby mediating stress-induced dysphoria (Land et al., 2008) and aversion via projections from the dorsal raphe nuclei to the nucleus accumbens (Land et al., 2009). Within the striatum, DYN is found particularly in medium spiny neurons that express the dopamine D-1 receptor subtype

(Jonsdottir, 2000b). DYN effects on the kappa-opioid receptor inhibit dopamine release in the VTA and nucleus accumbens (Mansour, Fox, Akil, & Watson, 1995; Nestler & Carlezon, 2006; Shippenberg & Rea, 1997).

Models of reward, hedonics, and motivation

It is important to consider that neurobiological theories of mechanisms mediating motivational and hedonic behavioral processes are not focused on the opioidergic system alone. Functional interactions exist between the opioidergic and the dopaminergic system and both transmitter systems are implicated in partly overlapping aspects of behavioral regulation. Beyond their involvement in central pain control (Bencherif et al., 2002; Casey et al., 2000; Zubieta, Heitzeg, et al., 2003; Zubieta et al., 2001), endogenous opioids mediate affective (Carr, 1984; Kehoe & Boylan, 1994; Zubieta, Ketter, et al., 2003), motivational (Carr, 1984), and stress responses (Drolet et al., 2001). Dopamine, on the other hand, is the principal neurotransmitter for central motor control (Brooks, 2001), but is also involved in cognitive processing (Kaasinen & Rinne, 2002; Pillon, Czernecki, & Dubois, 2003; Rinne et al., 2000), motivation (Volkow et al., 2002), and reward-associated behavior (Hakyemez, Dagher, Smith, & Zald, 2008; Martin-Soelch et al., 2001; Pappata et al., 2002; Zald et al., 2004). Finally, both, the opioidergic (DiChiara, Acquas, & Tanda, 1996; Herz, 1996, 1997) and dopaminergic (Volkow, Fowler, & Wang, 2004; Volkow et al., 2003) systems are "key players" in the development and maintenance of addictive behavior.

Dopamine and opioid receptors are G-protein coupled metabotropic receptors. Anatomically, there is widespread overlap in the expression of the opioidergic and the dopaminergic system in many parts of the CNS, which have been characterized best in the basal ganglia and midbrain circuits. In the rat VTA, approximately 50–60% of enkephalin-immunoreactive terminals that have synaptic contacts show association with tyrosine hydroxylase (TH) -labeled dendrites (Sesack & Pickel, 1992). Fluorescent micrographs suggest that high-affinity opiate binding sites are located primarily on dopaminergic presynaptic terminals (Stefano, Zukin, & Kream, 1982); however, enkephalin immunoreactivity has also been described in small unmyelinated axons (Garzon & Pickel, 2002). Dopaminergic neurons in the substantia nigra (SN) express kappa-opioid receptors on the terminal regions of their perikaria (Yamada, Groshan, Phung, Hisamitsu, & Richelson, 1997) and mu-opioid receptors are expressed in the retrorubral field, the substantia nigra (SN), and the VTA. The opioidergic receptor expression in these nuclei is region specific (German, Speciale, Manaye, & Sadeq, 1993). For instance, whereas the ventral pars compacta of the SN, which contains numerous DA neurons, has prominent mu-opioid receptor binding, lower receptor densities were observed in rostral portions of the VTA (German et al., 1993).

Hence, in order to understand the relative roles of motivational and hedonic processes in the antecedents and consequences of exercise, one must consider mutual interactions between opioid peptides and dopamine. The mesolimbic dopamine system has been associated with mediating behavioral responses to natural rewards, including food intake, reproductive behavior, play, etc. (Berridge & Robinson, 1998; Lutter & Nestler, 2009; Robbins & Everitt, 1996; Wise, 2004). Although dopamine was traditionally conceived as mediating hedonic aspects of reward (Koob & Le Moal, 1997; Wise, 2008), there is now accumulating evidence that it is more involved in motivational aspects of reward, rather than "pleasure" per se (Berridge & Robinson, 1998; Flagel et al., 2011; Smith & Berridge, 2007).

There are two important models related to dopamine-opioid interactions and their implications for addictive behavior: the "incentive salience hypothesis" which emphasizes the importance of dopamine as a motivator, driving the "wanting" aspect triggered by conditioned stimuli.

According to the "incentive salience hypothesis," the "liking" or "pleasure" associated with reward is mediated by other hedonic-based systems like GABA and opioid peptides (Smith & Berridge, 2007). On the other hand, models centered on the role of hedonics rather than motivational processes, such as the "hedonic allostasis theory," conceptualize addictive behaviors as a response to hypoactivity in dopamine systems (Koob & Le Moal, 1997). This hypo-dopaminergic state is postulated to induce compensatory behavioral activation (e.g., sensation-seeking, drug-seeking, compulsive exercise, etc.) to restore normal hedonic tone. Compulsive exercise or "addiction" to exercise thus would depend on correcting a dysphoric state caused by low dopaminergic (and presumably also opioidergic) tone. This is in contrast to the "incentive salience hypothesis," which predicts that higher dopaminergic transmission would lead to appetitively motivated behaviors such as exercise.

The opioid system in animal exercise studies

Elevated serum opioid activity has been demonstrated after exercise challenges in animals (Debruille et al., 1999), but it is unique to animal work that opioid receptor distributions can be directly studied in the CNS. Early ligand-binding studies showed altered opiate receptor occupancy in the rat brain following acute exercise (Pert & Bowie, 1979; Wardlaw & Frantz, 1980). However, subsequent studies produced conflicting results: chronic treadmill running did not alter basal levels of brain opioid peptides (Houghten, Pratt, Young, Brown, & Spann, 1986); upon acute exercise challenges, either beta-endorphin levels were higher in the nucleus accumbens after 2 hours of forced treadmill running (Blake, Stein, & Vomachka, 1984), or exercise was associated with lower levels of endorphins (Sforzo, Seeger, Pert, Pert, & Dotson, 1986), as evidenced by increased [^{3}H]diprenorphine binding in target brain regions after 2 hours of forced swimming. As those studies used forced exercise paradigms – which may be problematic as stress hormones can cause opioid release (Nikolarakis, Pfeiffer, Stalla, & Herz, 1987) – and did not measure behavioral responses representative of euphoria, hypoalgesia, or anxiolysis, these results neither supported nor refuted the "endorphin hypothesis" of exercise on mood and/or pain. It has been shown, however, that voluntary exercise increases DYN-converting enzyme activity in rat CSF, thereby converting DYN to leu-enkephalin (Persson et al., 1993). DYN is also released in the paraventricular nucleus (PVN), together with leu-ENK in the caudate-putamen after high-intensity aerobic exercise (Chen, Zhao, Yue, & Wang, 2007).

The role of the dopaminergic system will be further elucidated in other chapters of this book. It should be briefly noted here that treadmill running also increases dopamine release (Meeusen, Piacentini, & De Meirleir, 2001). Exercise also increases dopamine turnover (Hattori, Naoi, & Nishino, 1994) and chronically up-regulates D2 receptors (MacRae, Spirduso, Walters, Farrar, & Wilcox, 1987) in the striatum of rats. In contrast to acute effects of treadmill running, striatal DA activity has been reduced after chronic exposure to wheel running in highly fit rats (Swallow et al., 2008), whereas gene expression for D2 receptors in the nucleus accumbens was unchanged (Knab, Bowen, Hamilton, Gulledge, & Lightfoot, 2009) or decreased after chronic wheel running (Greenwood et al., 2011).

Another approach to determine whether an experimental challenge activates a specific endogenous neurotransmitter is to test whether repeated exposure to that manipulation produces tolerance to drugs that mimic the neurotransmitter. For the opioidergic system, the anti-nociceptive effects of exogenous opiates are attenuated by exercise. This is referred to as "cross-tolerance" (Mathes & Kanarek, 2001) and it was shown that exercise produces a cross-tolerance to the analgesic effects of morphine (Smith & Lyle, 2006). Similar effects can also be elicited directly by local morphine administration into the PAG (Mathes & Kanarek, 2006). Naloxone-precipitated withdrawal is also exaggerated following chronic wheel running (Kanarek, D'Anci, Jurdak, & Mathes, 2009).

Exercise genetics have become another line of investigation, as there is evidence that physical activity impacts gene expression of beta-endorphin, ENK, and DYN (Jonsdottir, Hoffmann, & Thoren, 1997; Mathe, Bjornebekk, & Brene, 2006). Running increases DYN mRNA levels in the caudate putamen of rats bred for running and drug preference (Werme, Thoren, Olson, & Brene, 2000). Additionally, the effect is blocked by the opioid receptor antagonist naloxone, indicating not only up-regulation of mRNA, but also mu-receptor activation (Werme et al., 2000). As opioid modulation of brain dopamine is a core feature in models of motivated behavior and addiction (see above), it is interesting to notice that the transcription factor DeltaFosB is overexpressed in the nucleus accumbens of rats exhibiting spontaneous wheel running (Werme et al., 2002). DeltaFosB could facilitate wheel running by inhibiting the release by GABA neurons of co-localized dynorphin, which otherwise binds with kappa-opioid receptors to inhibit DA release in the VTA or accumbens (Werme et al., 2002). In short, it is plausible that central opioids modulate dopamine and/or other neurotransmitter systems that control metabolic or hedonic drives regulating physical activity (Nestler & Carlezon, 2006; Werme et al., 2002).

Human plasma beta-endorphin studies in exercise

Mood and affect can be investigated most informatively in humans, as the use of affective self-evaluations and neuropsychological scales for mood and hedonics provide a major advantage compared to animal studies. Indeed, a general problem in animal research is that operational measures of hedonics are difficult to validate (Holmes, 2003). Up to now, human research has focused on endorphin levels in the peripheral compartment, as direct investigations of the CNS in athletes have been prohibited due to ethical constraints.

During vigorous exercise, beta-endorphin release from the pituitary is usually accompanied by increases in ACTH, which is derived along with beta-endorphin and melanocortin from the common precursor POMC. Hence, peripheral levels of beta-endorphins during and shortly after acute exercise may be viewed as an indication of the stress response to the exercise. Opioid peptides are reliably elevated in the plasma of humans during intense exercise (Carr et al., 1981; Farrell, Gates, Maksud, & Morgan, 1982; Gambert et al., 1981), but they show a considerable intra- (Sheps, Koch, Bragdon, Ballenger, & McMurray, 1988) and inter-individual (Farrell et al., 1982; Goldfarb & Jamurtas, 1997) variability. According to a recent review (Boecker et al., 2010), a large majority (59 of 65) of studies (from 1982 to 2008) showed significant increases of peripheral beta-endorphin concentrations, despite highly heterogeneous exercise challenges. It remains unclear whether plasma beta-endorphins, and their precursor molecule POMC, show a clear dose-gradient response to exercise (Goldfarb & Jamurtas, 1997; Harbach & Hempelmann, 2005; Nybo & Secher, 2004). Although several studies (Bullen et al., 1984; de Vries, Bernards, de Rooij, & Koppeschaar, 2000; Farrell, Kjaer, Bach, & Galbo, 1987; Goldfarb, Hatfield, Armstrong, & Potts, 1990; Goldfarb, Hatfield, Potts, & Armstrong, 1991; Goldfarb et al., 1998; McMurray, Forsythe, Mar, & Hardy, 1987; McMurray, Hardy, Roberts, Forsythe, & Mar, 1989; Rahkila, Hakala, Alen, Salminen, & Laatikainen, 1988; Viru & Tendzegolskis, 1995; Viswanathan, Vandijk, Graham, Bonen, & George, 1987) have demonstrated that strenuous exercise regimes are associated with higher magnitudes of peripheral endorphins than low-intensity exercise challenges, research suggests that these peripheral changes are not reflective of beta-endorphin concentrations in the brain (Boecker et al., 2010). After strenuous exercise, raised beta-endorphins in plasma tend to wash out slowly over a time-span of several hours and this wash-out was slower during recovery from a marathon race than after an exhausting incremental graded treadmill exercise (Heitkamp, Schmid, & Scheib, 1993). In humans, protracted miosis up to 6 hours has been demonstrated after more than 30 minutes of exercise, an effect that is very likely due to opioidergic mechanisms, as it can be blocked by naloxone eye drops (Allen, Thierman, & Hamilton, 1983). This review (Boecker et al., 2010) revealed that the endorphin literature up to now has not been able to establish consistent links between (peripheral) opioid peptides in plasma and (central) behavioral effects on mood and pain perception. The association between peripheral beta-endorphin values and mood is highly inconsistent, with only two out of seven reviewed studies showing a positive relationship between both factors (Harte, Eifert, & Smith, 1995; Janal et al., 1984). Hence, levels of opioid peptides in plasma following exercise challenges do not allow extrapolating upon central opioidergic transmitters or upon central transmitter actions at the opioid receptor level. It has been claimed, therefore, that the brain during exercise is affected by opioids other than those derived from POMC in the pituitary (Fallon & Leslie, 1986), whereas peripheral opioid peptides help regulate physiological responses that support energy expenditure and modulate nociception during exercise (Dishman, 1985; Nybo & Secher, 2004; Rossier et al., 1977).

Human opioid receptor PET studies in exercise

Recent developments in functional neuroimaging have provided alternative and promising approaches for unveiling opioidergic effects in human exercise research: the applicability of PET with suitable opioidergic tracers allows non-invasive *in vivo* monitoring of both acute opioidergic transmitter trafficking and chronic changes of opioid receptor expression in human athletes. Available are PET tracers with either non-specific ([^{11}C]diprenorphine, [^{18}F]diprenorphine, non-selective antagonist) or subtype-specific binding properties ([^{11}C]carfentanil, mu-opioid receptor agonist; [^{18}F]fluoro-cyclofoxy, mu/kappa-opioid receptor antagonist). As studies in humans have the advantage, as compared to animals, that mood effects can be captured using appropriate rating scales, acute opioid trafficking and long-term opioid receptor binding changes associated with exercise can be linked to individual affective states. In the following, we will summarize the findings of a first published opioid PET ligand study using endurance exercise training as experimental challenge (Boecker, Sprenger, et al., 2008).

The tracer 6-O-(2-[^{18}F]fluoroethyl)-6-O-desmethyldiprenorphine ([^{18}F]FDPN), which has similar selectivity to mu, delta, and kappa opioid receptors (Wester et al., 2000), was applied in 10 trained male athletes (mean age 36.9 years ± 2.6) to test the effect of 2 hours' endurance running as exercise challenge. Each participant received two PET scans on separate days in random order: rest (no sport 24 hours prior to PET), post-exercise (directly after 2 hours of running). During exercise, the average pace was of 11.0 ± 2.3 km/h, the average heart rate 144±7 min^{-1}. The euphoria ratings on visual analog scales increased significantly from 37.6 ± 19.6/100 (prior to exercise) to 73.3 ± 13.2/100. This was associated with a significant reduction of [^{18}F]FDPN binding after exercise, confirming the study hypothesis of elevated endogenous opioid tone induced by running. For the first time it was possible to study the localization of these ligand binding changes after acute exercise bouts *in vivo*. Interestingly, the most preponderant effects were encountered in prefrontal/orbitofrontal cortices, and also extensively in limbic structures (anterior cingulate cortex, insula).

The opioid PET data are indicative of elevated endogenous opioid levels post-exercise in areas of the brain (anterior cingulate cortex, and insula/parainsular cortex) implicated in affective processing (Dalgleish, 2004). More specifically, the location of these effects is well in accord with current theories of opioid-generated pleasure (Kringelbach & Berridge, 2010).

Summary

How exercise influences mood states is an important experimental question; however, after more than 30 years of research, the role of opioids in exercise-related hedonics is still unclear. While exogenously administered opiates induce euphoric states, it is rather unusual that athletes have comparably strong mood changes simply by engaging in physical activity, as this would not make "biological sense" in the absence of severe physical stress or trauma. Although a great deal of research data argue for the participation of endogenous opioids in mood regulation during and after exercise, most of the evidence is "indirect," and up to now causal effects of opioids on mood processing remain to be determined.

Animal studies show increased levels of endorphins or altered enkephalin receptor binding in the brain after acute exercise, but emotional effects are difficult to study in animals. In humans, the current state of knowledge is also still in a premature stage: studies using opioid receptor blocking approaches have revealed equivocal results regarding exercise effects on mood. The relation between endorphins in the peripheral blood and the CNS is still unknown, so it is questionable whether conventional blood-based methods yield relevant information on central neurotransmitter effects. It is expected for the future that ligand PET applications in athletes may help uncover some of the hitherto unknown links between opioidergic neurotransmission and psychophysiological effects in exercise. The authors of this chapter, therefore, make the claim that future studies should synergize human brain imaging with behavioral neuroscience approaches based on animal models.

References

Akil, H., Owens, C., Gutstein, H., Taylor, L., Curran, E., & Watson, S. (1998). Endogenous opioids: Overview and current issues. *Drug and Alcohol Dependence, 51*(1–2), 127–140.

Allen, M., Thierman, J., & Hamilton, D. (1983). Naloxone eye drops reverse the miosis in runners: Implications for an endogenous opiate test. *Canadian Journal of Applied Sport Sciences, 8*(2), 98–103.

Bencherif, B., Fuchs, P. N., Sheth, R., Dannals, R. F., Campbell, J. N., & Frost, J. J. (2002). Pain activation of human supraspinal opioid pathways as demonstrated by [^{11}C]-carfentanil and positron emission tomography (PET). *Pain, 99*(3), 589–598.

Berridge, K. C., & Robinson, T. E. (1998). What is the role of dopamine in reward: Hedonic impact, reward learning, or incentive salience? *Brain Research Reviews, 28*(3), 309–369.

Blake, M. J., Stein, E. A., & Vomachka, A. J. (1984). Effects of exercise training on brain opioid peptides and serum LH in female rats. *Peptides, 5*(5), 953–958.

Bodnar, R. J. (2007). Endogenous opiates and behavior: 2006. *Peptides, 28*(12), 2435–2513.

Boecker, H., Henriksen, G., Sprenger, T., Miederer, I., Willoch, F., Valet, M., et al. (2008). Positron emission tomography ligand activation studies in the sports sciences: Measuring neurochemistry in vivo. *Methods, 45*(4), 307–318.

Boecker, H., Othman, A., Mueckter, S., Scheef, L., Pensel, M., Daamen M., et al. (2010). Advocating neuroimaging studies of transmitter release in human physical exercise challenges studies. *Open Access Journal of Sports Medicine, 1*, 167–175.

Boecker, H., Sprenger, T., Spilker, M. E., Henriksen, G., Koppenhoefer, M., Wagner, K. J., . . . Tolle, T. R. (2008). The runner's high: Opioidergic mechanisms in the human brain. *Cerebral Cortex, 18*(11), 2523–2531.

Bray, M. S., Hagberg, J. M., Perusse, L., Rankinen, T., Roth, S. M., Wolfarth, B., . . . Bouchard, C. (2009). The human gene map for performance and health-related fitness phenotypes: The 2006–2007 update. *Medicine & Science in Sports & Exercise, 41*(1), 35–73.

Brooks, D. J. (2001). Functional imaging studies on dopamine and motor control. *Journal of Neural Transmission, 108*(11), 1283–1298.

Bullen, B. A., Skrinar, G. S., Beitins, I. Z., Carr, D. B., Reppert, S. M., Dotson, C. O., . . . McArthur, J. W. (1984). Endurance training effects on plasma hormonal responsiveness and sex hormone excretion. *Journal of Applied Physiology, 56*(6), 1453–1463.

Byrne, A., & Byrne, D. G. (1993). The effect of exercise on depression, anxiety and other mood states: A review. *Journal of Psychosomatic Research*, *37*(6), 565–574.

Carr, D. B., Bullen, B. A., Skrinar, G. S., Arnold, M. A., Rosenblatt, M., Beitins, I. Z., . . . McArthur, J. W. (1981). Physical conditioning facilitates the exercise-induced secretion of beta-endorphin and beta-lipotropin in women. *New England Journal of Medicine*, *305*(10), 560–563.

Carr, K. D. (1984). The physiology of opiate hedonic effects and the role of opioids in motivated behavior. *Advances in Alcohol & Substance Abuse*, *3*(3), 5–18.

Casey, K. L., Svensson, P., Morrow, T. J., Raz, J., Jone, C., & Minoshima, S. (2000). Selective opiate modulation of nociceptive processing in the human brain. *Journal of Neurophysiology*, *84*(1), 525–533.

Chaouloff, F. (1989). Physical exercise and brain monoamines: A review. *Acta Physiologica Scandinavica*, *137*(1), 1–13.

Chen, J. X., Zhao, X., Yue, G. X., & Wang, Z. F. (2007). Influence of acute and chronic treadmill exercise on rat plasma lactate and brain NPY, L-ENK, DYN A1-13. *Cellular and Molecular Neurobiology*, *27*(1), 1–10.

Conroy, R. W., Smith, K., & Felthous, A. R. (1982). The value of exercise on a psychiatric hospital unit. *Hospital & Community Psychiatry*, *33*(8), 641–645.

Cook, D. B., O'Connor, P. J., & Ray, C. A. (2000). Muscle pain perception and sympathetic nerve activity to exercise during opioid modulation. *American Journal of Physiology – Regulatory, Integrative, and Comparative Physiology*, *279*(5), R1565–1573.

Cotman, C. W., & Berchtold, N. C. (2002). Exercise: A behavioral intervention to enhance brain health and plasticity. *Trends in Neurosciences*, *25*(6), 295–301.

Dalgleish, T. (2004). The emotional brain. *Nature Reviews Neurosciences*, *5*(7), 583–589.

Daniel, M., Martin, A. D., & Carter, J. (1992). Opiate receptor blockade by naltrexone and mood state after acute physical activity. *British Journal of Sports Medicine*, *26*(2), 111–115.

De Moor, M. H., Boomsma, D. I., Stubbe, J. H., Willemsen, G., & de Geus, E. J. (2008). Testing causality in the association between regular exercise and symptoms of anxiety and depression. *Archives of General Psychiatry*, *65*(8), 897–905.

de Vries, W. R., Bernards, N. T., de Rooij, M. H., & Koppeschaar, H. P. (2000). Dynamic exercise discloses different time-related responses in stress hormones. *Psychosomatic Medicine*, *62*(6), 866–872.

Dearman, J., & Francis, K. T. (1983). Plasma levels of catecholamines, cortisol, and beta-endorphins in male athletes after running 26.2, 6, and 2 miles. *Journal of Sports Medicine and Physical Fitness*, *23*(1), 30–38.

Debruille, C., Luyckx, M., Ballester, L., Brunet, C., Odou, P., Dine, T., . . . Cazin, J.C. (1999). Serum opioid activity after physical exercise in rats. *Physiological Research*, *48*(2), 129–133.

DiChiara, G., Acquas, E., & Tanda, G. (1996). Ethanol as a neurochemical surrogate of conventional reinforcers: The dopamine–opioid link. *Alcohol*, *13*(1), 13–17.

Dietrich, A. (2006). Transient hypofrontality as a mechanism for the psychological effects of exercise. *Psychiatry Research*, *145*(1), 79–83.

Dishman, R. K. (1985). Medical psychology in exercise and sport. *Medical Clinics of North America*, *69*(1), 123–143.

Dishman, R. K., Berthoud, H. R., Booth, F. W., Cotman, C. W., Edgerton, V. R., Fleshner, M. R., et al. (2006). Neurobiology of exercise. *Obesity (Silver Spring)*, *14*(3), 345–356.

Dishman, R. K., & O'Connor, P. J. (2009). Lessons in exercise neurobiology: The case of endorphins. *Mental Health and Physical Activity*, *2*, 4–9.

Drolet, G., Dumont, E. C., Gosselin, I., Kinkead, R., Laforest, S., & Trottier, J. F. (2001). Role of endogenous opioid system in the regulation of the stress response. *Progress in Neuropsychopharmacology and Biological Psychiatry*, *25*(4), 729–741.

Droste, C., Greenlee, M. W., Schreck, M., & Roskamm, H. (1991). Experimental pain thresholds and plasma beta-endorphin levels during exercise. *Medicine & Science in Sports & Exercise*, *23*(3), 334–342.

Ekkekakis, P. (2009). Illuminating the black box: Investigating prefrontal cortical hemodynamics during exercise with near-infrared spectroscopy. *Journal of Sport & Exercise Psychology*, *31*(4), 505–553.

Evans, C. J. H., Hammond, D. L., & Fredrickson, R. C. A. (1988). The opioid peptides. In G. W. Pasternak (Ed.), *The opiate receptors* (pp. 23–74). Clifton, NJ: Humana Press.

Fallon, J. H., & Leslie, F. M. (1986). Distribution of dynorphin and enkephalin peptides in the rat brain. *Journal of Comparative Neurology*, *249*(3), 293–336.

Farrell, P. A., Gates, W. K., Maksud, M. G., & Morgan, W. P. (1982). Increases in plasma beta-endorphin/beta-lipotropin immunoreactivity after treadmill running in humans. *Journal of Applied Physiology*, *52*(5), 1245–1249.

Farrell, P. A., Kjaer, M., Bach, F. W., & Galbo, H. (1987). Beta-endorphin and adrenocorticotropin response to supramaximal treadmill exercise in trained and untrained males. *Acta Physiologica Scandinavica, 130*(4), 619–625.

Fichna, J., Janecka, A., Costentin, J., & Do Rego, J. C. (2007). The endomorphin system and its evolving neurophysiological role. *Pharmacological Reviews, 59*(1), 88–123.

Flagel, S. B., Clark, J. J., Robinson, T. E., Mayo, L., Czuj, A., Willuhn, I., . . . Akil, H. (2011). A selective role for dopamine in stimulus-reward learning. *Nature, 469*(7328), 53–57.

Francis, K. (1983). The role of endorphins in exercise: A review of current knowledge. *Journal of Orthopaedic & Sports Physical Therapy, 4*(3), 169–173.

Gambert, S. R., Garthwaite, T. L., Pontzer, C. H., Cook, E. E., Tristani, F. E., Duthie, E. H., et al. (1981). Running elevates plasma beta-endorphin immunoreactivity and ACTH in untrained human subjects. *Proceedings of the Society for Expimental Biology and Medicine, 168*(1), 1–4.

Garzon, M., & Pickel, V. M. (2002). Ultrastructural localization of enkephalin and mu-opioid receptors in the rat ventral tegmental area. *Neuroscience, 114*(2), 461–474.

German, D. C., Speciale, S. G., Manaye, K. F., & Sadeq, M. (1993). Opioid receptors in midbrain dopaminergic regions of the rat. I. Mu receptor autoradiography. *Journal of Neural Transmission – General Section, 91*(1), 39–52.

Goldfarb, A. H., Hatfield, B. D., Armstrong, D., & Potts, J. (1990). Plasma beta-endorphin concentration: Response to intensity and duration of exercise. *Medicine & Science in Sports & Exercise, 22*(2), 241–244.

Goldfarb, A. H., Hatfield, B. D., Potts, J., & Armstrong, D. (1991). Beta-endorphin time course response to intensity of exercise: Effect of training status. *International Journal of Sports Medicine, 12*(3), 264–268.

Goldfarb, A. H., & Jamurtas, A. Z. (1997). Beta-endorphin response to exercise. An update. *Sports Medicine, 24*(1), 8–16.

Goldfarb, A. H., Jamurtas, A. Z., Kamimori, G. H., Hegde, S., Otterstetter, R., & Brown, D. A. (1998). Gender effect on beta-endorphin response to exercise. *Medicine & Science in Sports & Exercise, 30*(12), 1672–1676.

Gomez-Pinilla, F. (2008). The influences of diet and exercise on mental health through hormesis. *Ageing Ressearch and Reviews, 7*(1), 49–62.

Greenwood, B. N., Foley, T. E., Le, T. V., Strong, P. V., Loughridge, A. B., Day, H. E. W., et al. (2011). Long-term voluntary wheel running is rewarding and produces plasticity in the mesolimbic reward pathway. *Behavioural Brain Research, 217*(2), 354–362.

Hakyemez, H. S., Dagher, A., Smith, S. D., & Zald, D. H. (2008). Striatal dopamine transmission in healthy humans during a passive monetary reward task. *Neuroimage, 39*(4), 2058–2065.

Harbach, H. W., & Hempelmann, G. (2005). Proopiomelanocortin and exercise. In W. J. Kraemer & A. D. Rogol (Ed.), *The endocrine system and exercise* (pp. 134–155). Malden, MA: Blackwell Publishing.

Harber, V. J., & Sutton, J. R. (1984). Endorphins and exercise. *Sports Medicine, 1*(2), 154–171.

Harte, J. L., Eifert, G. H., & Smith, R. (1995). The effects of running and meditation on beta-endorphin, corticotropin-releasing hormone and cortisol in plasma, and on mood. *Biological Psychology, 40*(3), 251–265.

Hattori, S., Naoi, M., & Nishino, H. (1994). Striatal dopamine turnover during treadmill running in the rat: Relation to the speed of running. *Brain Research Bulletin, 35*(1), 41–49.

Hegadoren, K. M., O'Donnell, T., Lanius, R., Coupland, N. J., & Lacaze-Masmonteil, N. (2009). The role of beta-endorphin in the pathophysiology of major depression. *Neuropeptides, 43*(5), 341–353.

Heitkamp, H. C., Schmid, K., & Scheib, K. (1993). Beta-endorphin and adrenocorticotropic hormone production during marathon and incremental exercise. *European Journal of Applied Physiology and Occupational Physiology, 66*(3), 269–274.

Herring, M. P., O'Connor, P. J., & Dishman, R. K. (2010). The effect of exercise training on anxiety symptoms among patients: A systematic review. *Archives of Internal Medicine, 170*(4), 321–331.

Herring, M. P., Puetz, T. W., O'Connor, P. J., & Dishman, R. K. (2012). Effect of exercise training on depressive symptoms among patients with a chronic illness: A systematic review and meta-analysis of randomized controlled trials. *Archives of Internal Medicine, 172*, 101–111.

Herz, A. (1996). Biological bases of addiction: Bidirectional modulation by opioids. *Nervenheilkunde, 15*(8), 466–468.

Herz, A. (1997). Endogenous opioid systems and alcohol addiction. *Psychopharmacology, 129*(2), 99–111.

Hillman, C. H., Erickson, K. I., & Kramer, A. F. (2008). Be smart, exercise your heart: Exercise effects on brain and cognition. *Nature Reviews Neuroscience, 9*(1), 58–65.

Hinton, E. R., & Taylor, S. (1986). Does placebo response mediate runner's high? *Perceptual and Motor Skills, 62*(3), 789–790.

Hoffmann, P. (1997). The endorphin hypothesis. In W. P. Morgan (Ed.), *Physical activity and mental health* (pp. 163–177). Washington, DC: Taylor & Francis.

Holmes, P. V. (2003). Rodent models of depression: Reexamining validity without anthropomorphic inference. *Critical Reviews in Neurobiology, 15*(2), 143–174.

Houghten, R. A., Pratt, S. M., Young, E. A., Brown, H., & Spann, D. R. (1986). Effect of chronic exercise on beta-endorphin receptor levels in rats. *NIDA Research Monographs, 75*, 505–508.

Imura, H., & Nakai, Y. (1981). "Endorphins" in pituitary and other tissues. *Annual Review of Physiology, 43*, 265–278.

Janal, M. N., Colt, E. W., Clark, W. C., & Glusman, M. (1984). Pain sensitivity, mood and plasma endocrine levels in man following long-distance running: Effects of naloxone. *Pain, 19*(1), 13–25.

Jarvekulg, A., & Viru, A. (2002). Opioid receptor blockade eliminates mood effects of aerobic gymnastics. *International Journal of Sports Medicine, 23*(3), 155–157.

Jonsdottir, I. H. (2000a). Neuropeptides and their interaction with exercise and immune function. *Immunology & Cell Biology, 78*(5), 562–570.

Jonsdottir, I. H. (2000b). Effects of exercise on the immune system: Neuropeptides and their interaction with exercise and immune function. *Immunology & Cell Biology, 78*(5), 562–570.

Jonsdottir, I. H., Hoffmann, P., & Thoren, P. (1997). Physical exercise, endogenous opioids and immune function. *Acta Physiologica Scandinavica Supplement, 640*, 47–50.

Kaasinen, V., & Rinne, J. O. (2002). Functional imaging studies of dopamine system and cognition in normal aging and Parkinson's disease. *Neuroscience and Biobehavioral Reviews, 26*(7), 785–793.

Kanarek, R. B., D'Anci, K. E., Jurdak, N., & Mathes, W. F. (2009). Running and addiction: Precipitated withdrawal in a rat model of activity-based anorexia. *Behavioral Neuroscience, 123*(4), 905–912.

Kehoe, P., & Boylan, C. B. (1994). Behavioral effects of kappa-opioid-receptor stimulation on neonatal rats. *Behavioral Neuroscience, 108*(2), 418–423.

Knab, A. M., Bowen, R. S., Hamilton, A. T., Gulledge, A. A., & Lightfoot, J. T. (2009). Altered dopaminergic profiles: Implications for the regulation of voluntary physical activity. *Behavioural Brain Research, 204*(1), 147–152.

Knechtle, B. (2004). Influence of physical activity on mental well-being and psychiatric disorders. *Praxis (Bern), 93*(35), 1403–1411.

Koltyn, K. F. (2000). Analgesia following exercise: A review. *Sports Medicine, 29*(2), 85–98.

Koob, G. F., & Le Moal, M. (1997). Drug abuse: Hedonic homeostatic dysregulation. *Science, 278*(5335), 52–58.

Kringelbach, M. L., & Berridge, K. C. (2010). The functional neuroanatomy of pleasure and happiness. *Discovery Medicine, 9*(49), 579–587.

Krogh, J., Nordentoft, M., Sterne, J. A., & Lawlor, D. A. (2011). The effect of exercise in clinically depressed adults: Systematic review and meta-analysis of randomized controlled trials. *Journal of Clinical Psychiatry, 72*(4), 529–538.

Land, B. B., Bruchas, M. R., Lemos, J. C., Xu, M., Melief, E. J., & Chavkin, C. (2008). The dysphoric component of stress is encoded by activation of the dynorphin kappa-opioid system. *Journal of Neuroscience, 28*(2), 407–414.

Land, B. B., Bruchas, M. R., Schattauer, S., Giardino, W. J., Aita, M., Messinger, D., et al. (2009). Activation of the kappa opioid receptor in the dorsal raphe nucleus mediates the aversive effects of stress and reinstates drug seeking. *Proceedings of the National Academy of Science of the United States of America, 106*(45), 19168–19173.

Leriche, M., Cote-Velez, A., & Mendez, M. (2007). Presence of pro-opiomelanocortin mRNA in the rat medial prefrontal cortex, nucleus accumbens and ventral tegmental area: Studies by RT-PCR and in situ hybridization techniques. *Neuropeptides, 41*(6), 421–431.

Lutter, M., & Nestler, E. J. (2009). Homeostatic and hedonic signals interact in the regulation of food intake. *Journal of Nutrition, 139*(3), 629–632.

MacRae, P. G., Spirduso, W. W., Walters, T. J., Farrar, R. P., & Wilcox, R. E. (1987). Endurance training effects on striatal D2 dopamine receptor binding and striatal dopamine metabolites in presenescent older rats. *Psychopharmacology (Berlin), 92*(2), 236–240.

Mansour, A., Fox, C. A., Akil, H., & Watson, S. J. (1995). Opioid-receptor mRNA expression in the rat CNS: Anatomical and functional implications. *Trends in Neurosciences, 18*(1), 22–29.

Markoff, R. A., Ryan, P., & Young, T. (1982). Endorphins and mood changes in long-distance running. *Medicine & Science in Sports & Exercise, 14*(1), 11–15.

Martin-Soelch, C., Leenders, K. L., Chevalley, A. F., Missimer, J., Kunig, G., Magyar, S., et al. (2001). Reward mechanisms in the brain and their role in dependence: Evidence from neurophysiological and neuroimaging studies. *Brain Research Reviews, 36*(2–3), 139–149.

Mathe, A. A., Bjornebekk, A., & Brene, S. (2006). Running has differential effects on NPY, opiates, and cell proliferation in an animal model of depression and controls. *Neuropsychopharmacology, 31*(2), 256–264.

Mathes, W. F., & Kanarek, R. B. (2001). Wheel running attenuates the antinociceptive properties of morphine and its metabolite, morphine-6-glucuronide, in rats. *Physiology & Behavior, 74*(1–2), 245–251.

Mathes, W. F., & Kanarek, R. B. (2006). Chronic running wheel activity attenuates the antinociceptive actions of morphine and morphine-6-glucouronide administration into the periaqueductal gray in rats. *Pharmacology and Biochemistry of Behavior, 83*(4), 578–584.

McMurray, R. G., Forsythe, W. A., Mar, M. H., & Hardy, C. J. (1987). Exercise intensity-related responses of beta-endorphin and catecholamines. *Medicine & Science in Sports & Exercise, 19*(6), 570–574.

McMurray, R. G., Hardy, C. J., Roberts, S., Forsythe, W. A., & Mar, M. H. (1989). Neuroendocrine responses of type A individuals to exercise. *Behavioral Medicine, 15*(2), 84–92.

Mead, G. E., Morley, W., Campbell, P., Greig, C. A., McMurdo, M., & Lawlor, D. A. (2009). Exercise for depression. *Cochrane Database of Systematic Reviews, 2009*, (3), CD004366.

Meeusen, R., Piacentini, M. F., & De Meirleir, K. (2001). Brain microdialysis in exercise research. *Sports Medicine, 31*(14), 965–983.

Mondin, G. W., Morgan, W. P., Piering, P. N., Stegner, A. J., Stotesbery, C. L., Trine, M. R., et al. (1996). Psychological consequences of exercise deprivation in habitual exercisers. *Medicine & Science in Sports & Exercise, 28*(9), 1199–1203.

Morgan, W. P. (1985). Affective beneficence of vigorous physical activity. *Medicine & Science in Sports & Exercise, 17*(1), 94–100.

Nestler, E. J., & Carlezon, W. A., Jr. (2006). The mesolimbic dopamine reward circuit in depression. *Biological Psychiatry, 59*(12), 1151–1159.

Nikolarakis, K., Pfeiffer, A., Stalla, G. K., & Herz, A. (1987). The role of CRF in the release of ACTH by opiate agonists and antagonists in rats. *Brain Research, 421*(1–2), 373–376.

Nybo, L., & Secher, N. H. (2004). Cerebral perturbations provoked by prolonged exercise. *Progress in Neurobiology, 72*(4), 223–261.

Pappata, S., Dehaene, S., Poline, J. B., Gregoire, M. C., Jobert, A., Delforge, J., et al. (2002). In vivo detection of striatal dopamine release during reward: A PET study with [C-11]raclopride and a single dynamic scan approach. *Neuroimage, 16*(4), 1015–1027.

Partin, C. (1983). Runner's "high." *Journal of American Medical Association, 249*(1), 21.

Perrine, S. A., Sheikh, I. S., Nwaneshiudu, C. A., Schroeder, J. A., & Unterwald, E. M. (2008). Withdrawal from chronic administration of cocaine decreases delta opioid receptor signaling and increases anxiety- and depression-like behaviors in the rat. *Neuropharmacology, 54*(2), 355–364.

Persson, S., Jonsdottir, I., Thoren, P., Post, C., Nyberg, F., & Hoffmann, P. (1993). Cerebrospinal fluid dynorphin-converting enzyme activity is increased by voluntary exercise in the spontaneously hypertensive rat. *Life Sciences, 53*(8), 643–652.

Pert, C. B., & Bowie, D. L. (1979). Behavioral manipulations of rats causes alterations in opiate receptor occupancy. In E. Usdin, W. E. Bunney, & N. S. Kline (Ed.), *Endorphins in mental health research* (pp. 93–104). New York: Oxford University Press.

Physical Activity Guidelines Advisory Committee. (2008). *Physical activity guidelines advisory committee report.* Washington, DC: U.S. Department of Health and Human Services.

Pillon, B., Czernecki, V., & Dubois, B. (2003). Dopamine and cognitive function. *Current Opinion in Neurology, 16* (Suppl. 2), S17–22.

Rahkila, P., Hakala, E., Alen, M., Salminen, K., & Laatikainen, T. (1988). Beta-endorphin and corticotropin release is dependent on a threshold intensity of running exercise in male endurance athletes. *Life Sciences, 43*(6), 551–558.

Raynor, K., Kong, H., Chen, Y., Yasuda, K., Yu, L., Bell, G. I., et al. (1994). Pharmacological characterization of the cloned kappa-, delta-, and mu-opioid receptors. *Molecular Pharmacology, 45*(2), 330–334.

Rinne, J. O., Portin, R., Ruottinen, H., Nurmi, E., Bergman, J., Haaparanta, M., et al. (2000). Cognitive impairment and the brain dopaminergic system in Parkinson disease: [18F]fluorodopa positron emission tomographic study. *Archives of Neurology, 57*(4), 470–475.

Robbins, T. W., & Everitt, B. J. (1996). Neurobehavioural mechanisms of reward and motivation. *Current Opinion in Neurobiology, 6*(2), 228–236.

Rooks, C. R., Thom, N. J., McCully, K. K., & Dishman, R. K. (2010). Effects of incremental exercise on cerebral oxygenation measured by near-infrared spectroscopy: A systematic review. *Progress in Neurobiology, 92*(2), 134–150.

Rossier, J., Bayon, A., Vargo, T. M., Ling, N., Guillemin, R., & Bloom, F. (1977). Radioimmunoassay of brain peptides: Evaluation of a methodology for the assay of beta-endorphin and enkephalin. *Life Sciences, 21*(6), 847–852.

Sandkuhler, J. (1996). The organization and function of endogenous antinociceptive systems. *Progress in Neurobiology, 50*(1), 49–81.

Schneider, S., Askew, C. D., Diehl, J., Mierau, A., Kleinert, J., Abel, T., et al. (2009). EEG activity and mood in health orientated runners after different exercise intensities. *Physiology & Behavior, 96*(4–5), 709–716.

Sesack, S. R., & Pickel, V. M. (1992). Dual ultrastructural localization of enkephalin and tyrosine hydroxylase immunoreactivity in the rat ventral tegmental area: Multiple substrates for opiate–dopamine interactions. *Journal of Neuroscience, 12*(4), 1335–1350.

Sforzo, G. A., Seeger, T. F., Pert, C. B., Pert, A., & Dotson, C. O. (1986). In vivo opioid receptor occupation in the rat-brain following exercise. *Medicine & Science in Sports & Exercise, 18*(4), 380–384.

Sheps, D. S., Koch, G., Bragdon, E. E., Ballenger, M. N., & McMurray, R. G. (1988). The reproducibility of resting and post exercise plasma beta-endorphins. *Life Sciences, 43*(9), 787–791.

Sher, L. (1996). Exercise, wellbeing, and endogenous molecules of mood. *Lancet, 348*(9025), 477.

Shippenberg, T. S., & Rea, W. (1997). Sensitization to the behavioral effects of cocaine: Modulation by dynorphin and kappa-opioid receptor agonists. *Pharmacology and Biochemistry of Behavior, 57*(3), 449–455.

Shyu, B. C., Andersson, S. A., & Thoren, P. (1982). Endorphin mediated increase in pain threshold induced by long-lasting exercise in rats. *Life Sciences, 30*(10), 833–840.

Smith, K. S., & Berridge, K. C. (2007). Opioid limbic circuit for reward: Interaction between hedonic hotspots of nucleus accumbens and ventral pallidum. *Journal of Neuroscience, 27*(7), 1594–1605.

Smith, M. A., & Lyle, M. A. (2006). Chronic exercise decreases sensitivity to mu opioids in female rats: Correlation with exercise output. *Pharmacology and Biochemistry of Behavior, 85*(1), 12–22.

Stefano, G. B., Zukin, R. S., & Kream, R. M. (1982). Evidence for the presynaptic localization of a high affinity opiate binding site on dopamine neurons in the pedal ganglia of Mytilus edulis (Bivalvia). *Journal of Pharmacology and Experimental Therapeutics, 222*(3), 759–764.

Ströhle, A. (2009). Physical activity, exercise, depression and anxiety disorders. *Journal of Neural Transmission, 116*(6), 777–784.

Stubbe, J. H., Boomsma, D. I., Vink, J. M., Cornes, B. K., Martin, N. G., Skytthe, A., et al. (2006). Genetic influences on exercise participation in 37,051 twin pairs from seven countries. *PLoS One, 1*, e22.

Swallow, J. G., Waters, R. P., Renner, K. J., Pringle, R. B., Summers, C. H., Britton, S. L., et al. (2008). Selection for aerobic capacity affects corticosterone, monoamines and wheel-running activity. *Physiology & Behavior, 93*(4–5), 1044–1054.

Tashiro, M., Itoh, M., Fujimoto, T., Masud, M. M., Watanuki, S., & Yanai, K. (2008). Application of positron emission tomography to neuroimaging in sports sciences. *Methods, 45*(4), 300–306.

Torregrossa, M. M., Jutkiewicz, E. M., Mosberg, H. I., Balboni, G., Watson, S. J., & Woods, J. H. (2006). Peptidic delta opioid receptor agonists produce antidepressant-like effects in the forced swim test and regulate BDNF mRNA expression in rats. *Brain Research, 1069*(1), 172–181.

van Praag, H. (2008). Neurogenesis and exercise: Past and future directions. *Neuromolecular Medicine, 10*(2), 128–140.

Vaynman, S., & Gomez-Pinilla, F. (2005). License to run: Exercise impacts functional plasticity in the intact and injured central nervous system by using neurotrophins. *Neurorehabilitation and Neural Repair, 19*(4), 283–295.

Vaynman, S., & Gomez-Pinilla, F. (2006). Revenge of the "sit": How lifestyle impacts neuronal and cognitive health through molecular systems that interface energy metabolism with neuronal plasticity. *Journal of Neuroscience Research, 84*(4), 699–715.

Vaynman, S., Ying, Z., & Gomez-Pinilla, F. (2004). Hippocampal BDNF mediates the efficacy of exercise on synaptic plasticity and cognition. *European Journal of Neuroscience, 20*(10), 2580–2590.

Viru, A., & Tendzegolskis, Z. (1995). Plasma endorphin species during dynamic exercise in humans. *Clinical Physiology, 15*(1), 73–79.

Viswanathan, M., Vandijk, J. P., Graham, T. E., Bonen, A., & George, J. C. (1987). Exercise-induced and cold-induced changes in plasma beta-endorphin and beta-lipotropin in men and women. *Journal of Applied Physiology, 62*(2), 622–627.

Volkow, N. D., Fowler, J. S., & Wang, G. J. (2004). The addicted human brain viewed in the light of imaging studies: Brain circuits and treatment strategies. *Neuropharmacology, 47*, 3–13.

Volkow, N. D., Wang, G. J., Fowler, J. S., Logan, J., Jayne, M., Franceschi, D., et al. (2002). "Nonhedonic" food motivation in humans involves dopamine in the dorsal striatum and methylphenidate amplifies this effect. *Synapse, 44*(3), 175–180.

Volkow, N. D., Wang, G. J., Maynard, L., Jayne, M., Fowler, J. S., Zhu, W., et al. (2003). Brain dopamine is associated with eating behaviors in humans. *International Journal of Eating Disorders, 33*(2), 136–142.

Wagemaker, H., & Goldstein, L. (1980). The runner's high. *Journal of Sports Medicine and Physical Fitness, 20*(2), 227–229.

Wardlaw, S. L., & Frantz, A. G. (1980). Effect of swimming stress on brain β-endorphin and ACTS (abstract). *Clinical Research (London) 28*, 482.

Werme, M., Messer, C., Olson, L., Gilden, L., Thoren, P., Nestler, E. J., et al. (2002). Delta FosB regulates wheel running. *Journal of Neuroscience, 22*(18), 8133–8138.

Werme, M., Thoren, P., Olson, L., & Brene, S. (2000). Running and cocaine both upregulate dynorphin mRNA in medial caudate putamen. *European Journal of Neuroscience, 12*(8), 2967–2974.

Wester, H. J., Willoch, F., Tolle, T. R., Munz, F., Herz, M., Oye, I., et al. (2000). 6-O-(2-[18F]fluoroethyl)-6-O-desmethyldiprenorphine ([18F]DPN): Synthesis, biologic evaluation, and comparison with [11C]DPN in humans. *Journal of Nuclear Medicine, 41*(7), 1279–1286.

Wildmann, J., Kruger, A., Schmole, M., Niemann, J., & Matthaei, H. (1986). Increase of circulating beta-endorphin-like immunoreactivity correlates with the change in feeling of pleasantness after running. *Life Sciences, 38*(11), 997–1003.

Wise, R. A. (2004). Dopamine, learning and motivation. *Nat Rev Neurosci, 5*(6), 483–494.

Wise, R. A. (2008). Dopamine and reward: The anhedonia hypothesis 30 years on. *Neurotoxicity Research, 14*(2–3), 169–183.

Yamada, M., Groshan, K., Phung, C. T., Hisamitsu, T., & Richelson, E. (1997). The expression of mRNA for a kappa opioid receptor in the substantia nigra of Parkinson's disease brain. *Brain Research – Molecular Brain Research, 44*(1), 12–20.

Zald, D. H., Boileau, I., El-Dearedy, W., Gunn, R., McGlone, F., Dichter, G. S., et al. (2004). Dopamine transmission in the human striatum during monetary reward tasks. *Journal of Neuroscience, 24*(17), 4105–4112.

Zubieta, J. K., Heitzeg, M. M., Smith, Y. R., Bueller, J. A., Xu, K., Xu, Y., et al. (2003). COMT val158met genotype affects mu-opioid neurotransmitter responses to a pain stressor. *Science, 299*(5610), 1240–1243.

Zubieta, J. K., Ketter, T. A., Bueller, J. A., Xu, Y., Kilbourn, M. R., Young, E. A., et al. (2003). Regulation of human affective responses by anterior cingulate and limbic mu-opioid neurotransmission. *Archives of General Psychiatry, 60*(11), 1145–1153.

Zubieta, J. K., Smith, Y. R., Bueller, J. A., Xu, Y., Kilbourn, M. R., Jewett, D. M., et al. (2001). Regional mu opioid receptor regulation of sensory and affective dimensions of pain. *Science, 293*(5528), 311–315.

3

PHYSICAL ACTIVITY FEEL-GOOD EFFECT

The role of endocannabinoids

Francis Chaouloff, Sarah Dubreucq, Isabelle Matias,
and Giovanni Marsicano

It is recognized worldwide that physical exertion provides health benefits. This positive effect is linked to the improvement of numerous functions, including cardiovascular, immunological, metabolic, osteoarticular, and brain functions. The identification of the mechanisms through which physical exercise exerts these health-protective effects is considered essential as it paves the way for future fundamental and therapeutic knowledge (Powell & Paffenbarger, 1985). Among health benefits provided by exercise, those related to central functions have been well documented. In particular, the observations of positive consequences of acute and chronic exercise on emotional behaviors in humans, including through anti-stress properties (Salmon, 2001), have led clinicians to use exercise as a therapeutic tool against several psychopathologies, especially mild depression and anxiety (Martinsen & Morgan, 1997; Raglin, 1997; Salmon, 2001; Ströhle, 2009). Thus, exercise alone, or in combination with subeffective antidepressant/anxiolytic medications, is reported to trigger mood and emotional improvements similar to those elicited by classical antidepressants and anxiolytics (Martinsen & Morgan, 1997; Raglin, 1997).

In keeping with these psychological effects of physical exercise, it is now more than 30 years since scientists have tried to uncover the neurobiological bases for these positive effects of physical exercise. For obvious reasons, much of the work has been performed in laboratory animals using models of forced (treadmill running) and voluntary (wheel running) exercise. The first model requires a period of conditioning. During that phase, animals placed on a shock grid that is located at one end of the treadmill belt learn rapidly that running on that belt is the only means to escape from footshocks. Although the need for such a conditioning step is one disadvantage, the ability to modify the speed and the slope of the treadmill and the possibility to perform experiments during the inactive (i.e., light) phase of the diurnal cycle of the animals explain the success of this running paradigm. On the other hand, wheel running is a spontaneous and voluntary behavior which, as such, does not require conditioning. Plateau levels of endurance are generally reached after 1 week and animals can be provided limited or unlimited access to the wheels. As opposed to the treadmill, one limit of wheels is the lack of spontaneous running behavior during the inactive phase of the diurnal cycle, thereby requiring phase shifts in the diurnal cycle so as to allow a coincidence between the active (i.e., dark) phase of that cycle and the daily working period of the experimenters. Another limit is related to the most appropriate sedentary control to which the runners need to be compared. Thus, control animals are usually hosted either in standard cages or in cages with a locked wheel. As we will see below, choosing between either control conditions is not easy as each of these conditions suffers its own limits, especially when dealing with the emotional impacts of running activity.

Works aimed at deciphering the neurobiological impacts of physical exercise have initially focused on brain monoamine neurochemistry (see reviews from Chaouloff, 1989, 1997; Dunn & Dishman, 1991; Meeusen, Piacentini, & De Meirleir, 2001). Indeed, such a deliberate choice was dictated by the growing interest scientists showed at that time for the monoaminergic theory of depression (Ransford, 1982). Exercise in treadmill-trained animals was reported to stimulate monoamine synthesis, turnover, and/or release rates in brain regions associated with the control of mood (e.g., frontal cortex, hippocampus, striatum, hypothalamus). Although these results brought some support for the "monoamine hypothesis" of the antidepressant effects of physical exercise, this direct link suffered a lack of compelling evidence for (1) functional changes in monoamine transmission, and (2) a causal relationship between these changes in monoamine synthesis/metabolism and the mood-elevating effects of exercise. Besides the monoaminergic systems, the opioidergic systems have also received much attention (see review by Hoffmann, 1997). This interest surged with the observation that exercise increased circulating endorphin levels while a pretreatment with the opioid receptor antagonist naloxone prevented the mood-elevating effects of acute exercise. These results led to the well-known "endorphin hypothesis." However, both the inability to reproduce these data in several laboratories and methodological issues have hampered that hypothesis (Dietrich & McDaniel, 2004). Among other neurobiological candidates for the positive effects of exercise on emotionality, much interest has been devoted to neurotrophins (Hillman, Ericksson, & Kramer, 2008; van Praag, 2009). Thus, exercise increases peripheral and central levels of trophic factors (such as brain-derived neurotrophic factor; BDNF), which are involved in both the mood-elevating properties of antidepressants – possibly through their regulation of hippocampal synaptic plasticity and neurogenesis – and in the exercise-induced facilitation of learning and memory processes. However, the mechanisms leading to the release of trophic factors during exercise are still under investigation.

Physical exercise and the endocannabinoid system

In 2003, it was reported that 50 minutes of moderate exercise through treadmill running or ergometer cycling increased the circulating levels of the endogenous cannabinoid (endocannabinoid) anandamide (AEA) in trained male college students (Sparling, Giuffrida, Piomelli, Rosskopf, & Dietrich, 2003). As AEA is one of the main peripheral and central endocannabinoids (Piomelli, 2003), this seminal observation suggested that exercise may indeed stimulate the endocannabinoid system (ECS). Because the ECS is one key modulator of numerous brain functions/processes including food intake, energy balance, pain sensitivity, emotionality, learning and memory, thermoregulation, and neuroinflammation (Freund, Katona, & Piomelli, 2003; Marsicano & Lutz, 2006; Pacher, Bàtkai, & Kunos, 2006; Piomelli, 2003), the observation of increased circulating AEA levels after exercise opened the promising hypothesis that some physiological effects of physical exercise might indeed be mediated by the ECS (Dietrich & McDaniel, 2004). Furthermore, because the ECS is the target of Δ^9-tetrahydrocannabinol (THC, the main psychoactive component of marijuana; Mechoulam & Hanus, 2000), the observation that several psychological effects of acute exercise – the so-called "runner's high" (well-being, happiness, elation, inner harmony, time distortion) – are similar to those often observed after marijuana consumption has led to the proposal that the ECS may play a crucial role in the feel-good properties of exercise (Dietrich & McDaniel, 2004).

The endocannabinoid system

The ECS is composed of endocannabinoids, the machinery for their synthesis/degradation, and the receptors, namely CB1 and CB2 receptors, through which endocannabinoids exert their functions (Freund et al., 2003; Marsicano & Lutz, 2006; Pacher et al., 2006; Piomelli, 2003). Endocannabinoids, which are lipid messengers synthesized "on demand" from membrane precursors, comprise numerous members. Among these, AEA and 2-arachidonoylglycerol (2-AG) are the best-studied molecules. In the brain, activation of voltage-gated Ca^{2+} channels with/without the concomitant activation of Gq/11-coupled receptors (such as the group 1 metabotropic glutamate receptors or the muscarinic 1/3 receptors) leads to AEA and/or 2-AG synthesis (Alger, 2002; Chevaleyre, Takahashi, & Castillo, 2006; Ohno-Shosaku, Tanimura, Hashimotodani, & Kano, 2011; Piomelli, 2003). Following their transport into the cells, the degradation of AEA and 2-AG is thought to occur respectively at the postsynapse and at the presynapse (Figure 3.1A). The effects of endocannabinoids are mainly mediated by their retrograde action at CB1 receptors located on presynaptic neuronal terminals and on glial cells. Besides CB1 receptors, endocannabinoids may also act on CB2 receptors, which are mainly located on microglial cells in the CNS. As the activation of CB1 receptors by endocannabinoids leads to an inhibition of cyclic AMP levels, an inhibition of voltage-gated Ca^{2+} channels, and an activation of K^+ channels, the result of the retrograde action of endocannabinoids on neurons is a net decrease in presynaptic excitability and thus neurotransmitter release (Figure 3.1B). Stimulation of CB1 receptors is thus a means to control for excessive presynaptic activity (Alger, 2002; Chevaleyre et al., 2006; Ohno-Shosaku et al., 2011). At GABAergic and glutamatergic synapses, such an inhibitory influence of endocannabinoids on transmitter release will bear consequences on synaptic plasticity, whether this plasticity is short lasting (as illustrated by the so-called depolarization-induced suppression of inhibition or suppression of excitation) or long lasting (Alger, 2002; Chevaleyre et al., 2006; Ohno-Shosaku et al., 2011). Recent results have indicated that 2-AG, rather than AEA, is the lipid-derived molecule involved in the inhibitory effects of endocannabinoids on short-lasting synaptic plasticity (Gao et al., 2010; Tanimura et al., 2010). In addition to the brain, the ECS is also present in the periphery, as illustrated by the presence of CB1 receptors in the heart, the liver, the muscles, the gastrointestinal tract, the endocrine pancreas, and the adipose tissue (Pacher et al., 2006; Pagotto, Marsicano, Cota, Lutz, & Pasquali, 2006). However, as opposed to the brain ECS (see below), there is still no information as to the specific relationships that may link physical exercise and peripheral CB1 receptors.

As indicated above, the ECS regulates many brain functions. Such a property is accounted for by the key inhibitory role of CB1 receptors on the release of different neurotransmitters (including the main inhibitory and excitatory neurotransmitters, namely GABA and glutamate), and by the location of this receptor in numerous brain regions (Herkenham et al., 1990; Marsicano & Lutz, 1999). This is illustrated by the observation of CB1 gene/protein expression in the cerebral cortex, the amygdala, the hippocampus, the ventral and dorsal striata, the basal ganglia, the nucleus accumbens, the midbrain (including the dorsal raphe nuclei and the ventral tegmental area), and the hypothalamus. Therein, CB1 receptors are involved in the control of essential brain functions, of which several are documented to be engaged or affected by physical exercise. For example, motor activity, food intake, energy expenditure, anxiety, learning/memory, and hedonia/motivation processes are all found to be controlled by CB1 receptors (El Manira & Kyriakatos, 2010; Lafenêtre, Chaouloff, & Marsicano, 2007; Maldonado, Valverde, & Berrendero, 2006; Pagotto et al., 2006).

(a)

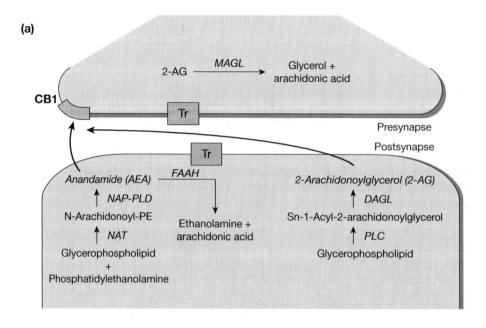

(b)

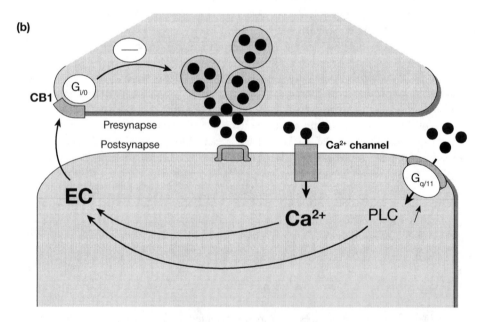

Figure 3.1 The endocannabinoid system. (a) Synthesis and degradation of the principal endocannabinoids, anandamide (AEA) and 2-arachidonoylglycerol (2-AG), in neurons. (b) Mechanisms underlying the retrograde action of endocannabinoids on transmitter release. DAGL: diacylglycerol lipase; FAAH: fatty acid amide hydrolase; MAGL: monoacylglycerol lipase; NAP-PLD: N-acylphosphatidylethanolamine-hydrolyzing phospholipase D; NAT: N-acyltransferase; PLC: phospholipase C; Tr: endocannabinoid transporter.

Wheel running activity and the endocannabinoid system

Except for the seminal study by Sparling et al. (2003) and for two recent studies confirming that exercise increases circulating AEA levels, albeit in an intensity-dependent manner (Heyman et al., 2012; Raichlen, Foster, Seillier, Giuffrida & Gerdeman, in press), all studies aimed at examining the relationships between physical exercise and the ECS have been conducted in laboratory animals provided with running wheels. The first issue that has been the focus of investigation relates to the impacts of wheel running on the synthesis/release of endocannabinoids. In rats housed with unlimited access to running wheels for 8 days, hippocampal, but not frontocortical, AEA was found to be increased in the morning of the ninth day (Hill et al., 2010). On the other hand, analyses of the other major endocannabinoid, namely 2-AG, revealed a lack of influence of wheel running in either brain region. It is worthy of mention that in this study control animals were housed with PVC tubing as a means to enrich the environment, thus leaving open the possibility that the results would have been different if controls were housed with locked wheels (see below). We have also recently addressed the question of wheel running effects on brain, but also blood, endocannabinoid levels. Besides the animal species (mice were used in the present study), our study differed from the former in several ways. Thus, our mice were allowed to run for 3h/day during 8 days and endocannabinoid levels were estimated after 30 minutes of running. These estimations were compared to those conducted in controls that were housed with locked wheels for a similar duration. As shown in Figure 3.2A, neither circulating levels of AEA nor brain concentrations of this endocannabinoid displayed changes with running activity. The former observation contrasts with that obtained in the blood samples from exercising human subjects, this contrast being likely accounted for by species differences in the physiological and psychological salience of each exercise paradigm. The analysis of 2-AG levels led to a similar picture to that observed for AEA levels, except for a significant decrease in the hippocampus of mice allowed to run that was associated with a similar trend in the frontal cortex (Figure 3.2B). Although the real significance of these observations is unknown, it is interesting to note that mice exposed for 7 days to a daily episode of social stress displayed an opposite pattern to that measured in exercising mice. Thus, 2-AG levels were found to be increased in the hippocampus and the frontal cortex when measured 40 minutes after the last stress episode (Dubreucq et al., 2012). Interestingly, such a brain region–dependent pattern of reactivity of 2-AG has been observed in rats submitted repeatedly to another type of stress, namely restraint (Patel & Hillard, 2008). These results raise the hypothesis that the respective patterns of reactivity of 2-AG after running and stress are indicative of the psychological salience of each experimental condition. Other issues that merit consideration are the possibilities that wheel running triggers major changes on rat and mouse endocannabinoid levels in discrete brain regions and/or the need for different timings than those used in our study.

In addition to endocannabinoid levels, several studies have explored the effects of wheel running on CB1 receptors. These analyses have focused on the protein itself (number and affinity of the receptor protein) and/or on its functional characteristics. In the above-mentioned study aimed at exploring the impact of wheel running on rat brain endocannabinoid levels, CB1 receptor binding capacities in controls and exercising animals were also investigated. It was found that the number of binding sites for a CB1 receptor agonist increased in the hippocampus, but not in the frontal cortex (Hill et al., 2010). However, such an increase was counterbalanced by a reduction in receptor affinity for the ligand (as revealed by an increased dissociation constant). Besides, one study reported that 10 days of wheel running increased the gene expression of the CB1 receptor in the hippocampus of female mice (Wolf et al., 2010). Concerning CB1 receptor function, 8 days of wheel running hypersensitized the activation of hippocampal

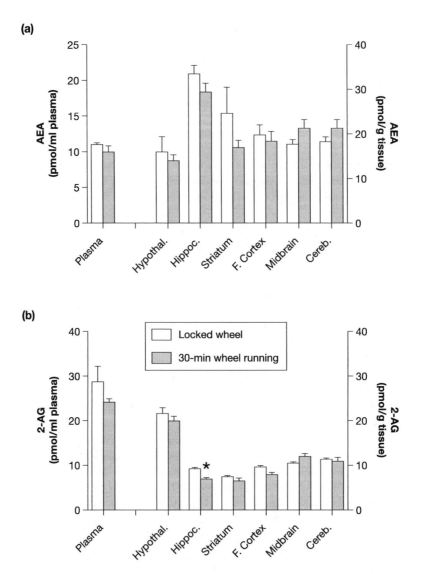

Figure 3.2 Endocannabinoids and wheel running. (a) Plasma and brain tissue anandamide (AEA), and (b) 2-arachidonoylglycerol (2-AG) levels 30 minutes after the initiation of wheel running in animals housed for 8 days with free wheels or with locked wheels. Values are the mean ± S.E.M. of 3 (blood) and 8 (brain regions) samples/group. ★ $P < 0.05$ for the difference between sedentary and running subjects.

CB1 receptor-associated G proteins by a CB1 receptor agonist, thus suggesting that wheel running bears stimulatory consequences on hippocampal CB1 receptor function (Hill et al., 2010). Indeed, such a conclusion may extend to another brain region, namely the striatum. Thus, the ability of a CB1 receptor agonist to decrease striatal GABA neurotransmission, as assessed by the reduction in the frequency of spontaneous and miniature inhibitory postsynaptic currents (IPSCs), was reinforced after 15 days (but not 7 days) of wheel running activity (de Chiara et al., 2010). Such a sensitizing effect of wheel running was selective for GABAergic neurons as the CB1 receptor-mediated decrease in striatal glutamatergic transmission was of similar amplitude in control mice and in running mice. It is important to note here that providing control mice with a sweetened drinking solution led also to increased sensitivity of CB1 receptors on striatal GABAergic neurons (de Chiara et al., 2010). On the basis of this parallel, it has been proposed that it is the hedonic impact of running that may account for the above-mentioned electro-physiological results. It should be noted, however, that in this study the controls were housed in standard cages, leaving unaddressed the possibility that in addition to the hedonic impact of running, the enrichment of the environment contributed to the increased sensitivity of striatal CB1 receptors. This issue is particularly important in view of the promising observation that the desensitization of the inhibitory control exerted by CB1 receptors on striatal GABAergic transmission that is observed in animals exposed to three daily stress episodes was reported to be reversed by 1 day of housing with running wheels (Rossi et al., 2008).

Role of the endocannabinoid system during physical exercise

As illustrated above, the available data gathered so far strongly suggest that physical exercise impacts on the ECS in humans and possibly in laboratory rodents. However, it should be acknowledged that this relationship has been poorly documented, which is in keeping with the very recent surge of interest in this area of research. As shown in the present section, this paucity of results actually extends to the quest for the role exerted by the ECS during or immediately after exercise.

The tools to study the role of the endocannabinoid system in exercising subjects

The study of the functional role of any transmitter system involves classically the characterization of the responses elicited by direct agonists for the receptors of that transmitter. This strategy is often completed by the use of indirect receptor agonists, i.e., drugs acting respectively on the membrane transporters for that transmitter or on the synthesis/release of that transmitter. Such studies bring information on the potential impact of that transmitter system on a vast array of functions but do not inform on the tonic and permissive role that transmitter system may exert during particular situations. Pharmacological and genetic assays based respectively on the administration of antagonists or on the use of constitutive/conditional mutants for these targets are nowadays the routine procedures to gather that information. Studies on the relationships between the ECS and exercise have all focused on the tonic role the ECS may be endowed with during exercise, doing so by means of CB1 receptor antagonists, such as SR141716 (Rinaldi-Carmona et al., 1994) and AM251 (Gatley, Gifford, Volkow, Lan, & Makriyannis, 1996), or using constitutive mutants for the CB1 receptor wherein this receptor is absent from the whole body (Ledent et al., 1999; Marsicano et al., 2002; Zimmer, Zimmer, Hohmann, Herkenham, & Bonner, 1999). Because CB1 receptors are located on different neuronal (and glial) populations and expressed in numerous brain regions (see above), it is useful, however, to further define the population of CB1 receptors through which the ECS may play a role. This can be achieved using conditional mutants for CB1 receptors, and we will illustrate below the potential use of this strategy. The generation of these conditional mutations is based on the so-called "Cre/lox P" technique (Morozov, Kellendonk, Simpson, & Tronche, 2003). This technique is based on the ability of a recombinase protein (Cre) to excise any sequence of DNA flanked by short sequences called "loxP" sites. Given their small dimensions (34 base pairs), the introduction of loxP sites into the genome of mice flanking a given gene to generate "floxed" mutant mice does not change its expression. Therefore, "floxed" mice can be considered phenotypically wild-type mice. However, the presence of the Cre recombinase in specific cell types or tissues will lead to the specific excision of the "floxed" gene, generating conditional (i.e., spatially and/or temporally restricted) mutant mice. Thus, crossing mice bearing a Cre recombinase specific for a given cell population with mice hosting a CB1 gene sequence flanked by loxP sites ("floxed CB1") generates two types of subjects in the progeny: (a) those bearing just the floxed CB1 gene sequence (phenotypically wild-type animals) and (b) those lacking the CB1 sequence in the cell populations expressing the Cre recombinase (conditional CB1 mutant animals). As an illustration, crossing mice that either carry or do not carry the Cre recombinase Nex with mice hosting a floxed CB1 gene generates wild-type controls (termed below Glu-CB1$^{+/+}$) and mice lacking CB1 receptors from glutamatergic neurons (termed below Glu-CB1$^{-/-}$; Monory et al., 2006). Using other mutant mice expressing a Cre recombinase specific to a cell population (Monory et al., 2007) allows further dissecting the functional role of CB1 receptors with respect to the cell population where these receptors are expressed. For example, the respective roles of CB1 receptors located on GABAergic neurons (the brain cells in which CB1 receptors are the most abundantly expressed; Marsicano & Lutz, 1999; Monory et al., 2006) and on glutamatergic cells (where CB1 are expressed to a low level; Marsicano & Lutz, 1999; Monory et al., 2006) have been recently documented with respect to the control of fasting-induced food intake (Bellochio et al., 2010) and long-term memory deficits triggered by THC (Puighermanal et al., 2009). As indicated above, investigations on the relationships between the ECS and exercise have used CB1 receptor antagonists and constitutive/conditional CB1 receptor mutants (see below). Undoubtedly, the use of conditional mutants for the CB1 receptor will expand in the near future to further define the role of the ECS during exercise. This is also true for other promising tools that have been generated recently, among which (a) selective inhibitors of the enzymes degrading the endocannabinoids or of the transporter that allows the cellular uptake of these lipids (Long et al., 2009; Piomelli, 2003; Schlosburg et al., 2010), and (b) mouse mutants for FAAH (Cravatt et al., 2001), DAGL (Gao et al., 2010; Tanimura et al., 2010), and MAGL (Chanda et al., 2010).

The endocannabinoid system and running performance

In 2004, it was reported that an acute pretreatment with the CB1 receptor antagonist AM251 before the active phase of the diurnal cycle increased in a dose-dependent manner the wheel running distance covered overnight by lean mice while decreasing that distance for the highest doses in obese mice (Zhou & Shearman, 2004). However, several years later, a study using the same antagonist reported that this drug, even if provided repeatedly, did not influence wheel running in rats (Hill et al., 2010). It should be noted here, however, that the latter study relied on the administration of the CB1 receptor antagonist at the beginning of the inactive phase of the diurnal cycle, i.e., 10 hours before the normal onset of the running episode. This opens the possibility that the antagonist was devoid of activity when the animals started their running activities. In a third work, it was documented that the administration of the CB1 receptor antagonist SR141716 2 hours after the onset of wheel running activity decreased the running distances in a dose-dependent manner (Keeney et al., 2008). This decrease, which was observed both in a control mouse line and in a mouse line selected for high wheel running activity, was accounted for by sex-dependent decreases in running duration and/or speed (Keeney et al., 2008). These three pharmacological studies thus lead to different conclusions, that heterogeneity being accounted for by their respective experimental settings (acute/repeated treatment, delay between treatment and running activity). Besides these experimental differences, one additional variable that differed between the studies was the duration of time provided to the animals to habituate to the wheels before pharmacological treatments. In the first and third studies, mice were provided with a 5- to 7-day training period beforehand, whereas in the second study rats received their daily antagonist administration on the first day of housing with wheels. In our hands, pretreatment with the CB1 receptor antagonist SR 141716 30 minutes before a 3-hour daily wheel running episode that started at the onset of the dark phase of the diurnal cycle actually decreased running activity in 7-day trained mice, a finding extended to mice given the opportunity to run for the first time (Dubreucq et al., 2013). Taken together with the data from the study from Keeney et al. (2008), our data strongly suggest that the ECS acts as a tonic stimulatory control of running activity, including when running activity has already been engaged. The use of CB1 mutant mice provides definitive evidence for this suggestion. Thus, in a study in which mice were given unrestricted access to running wheels, constitutive CB1 mutant mice displayed a 30–40% decrease in wheel running activity compared to their wild-type littermates (Dubreucq, Koehl, Abrous, Marsicano, & Chaouloff, 2010). A detailed analysis of the behaviors of CB1 mutant mice revealed that the negative consequence of CB1 receptor deletion on running activity was accounted for by decreased time spent running and decreased maximal velocity. Furthermore, wheel running differences between CB1 receptor mutants and wild-type littermates were already observed when mice began to engage in their running activity, i.e., during the dark phase of the diurnal cycle (Chaouloff, Dubreucq, Bellocchio, & Marsicano, 2011). In the present context, the following observations are noteworthy. First, this inhibitory consequence of CB1 receptor deletion on running performance is unlikely to be accounted for by an intrinsic impact on locomotor activity as CB1 receptor knock-out mice do not differ from their wild-type littermates when housed for 1 week in cages provided with horizontal and vertical actimeters (Chaouloff et al., 2011). Second, the inhibitory impact of CB1 receptor deletion on wheel running activity was also observed in mice provided with a restricted (3-h) daily access to the running wheels (Dubreucq et al., 2013).

Whenever a reduction in wheel running activity in SR141716-pretreated/treated animals is observed (see above), the amplitude of that reduction ranges between 30 and 60% of the activity measured in vehicle-injected animals. As already mentioned above, CB1 knock-out mice display a 30 to 40% decrease in wheel running activity, compared to wild-type animals. Taken together, these observations suggest that the ECS exerts only a partial tonic stimulatory control of wheel running activity. Where and how such a control is exerted is a question we have recently tried to address although (1) wheel running is a complex behavior (Sherwin, 1998), and (2) the ECS controls many functions in the CNS as well as in the periphery. Thus, in the CNS, the ECS exerts a tight stimulatory control of motoric behavior through the CB1 receptor-dependent modulation of the excitability of neuronal networks in the neocortex, the striatum, the cerebellum, and the spinal cord (El Manira & Kyriakatos, 2010). Accordingly, pharmacological antagonism or genetic silencing of CB1 receptors in either of these networks could have inhibitory consequences on running activity. The same holds true for the impact that the ECS exerts over metabolism through actions on food intake and energy expenditure (Pacher et al., 2006; Pagotto et al., 2006). Another hypothesis, which does not exclude the former ones, lies in the observation that rodents will lever-press to get access to running wheels (Belke & Wagner, 2005) and display conditioned place preference for brief and sustained wheel access (Greenwood et al., 2011; Lett, Grant, & Koh, 2001). These results are in keeping with the proposal that although wheel running is an extremely complex behavior, it can be considered a natural reward with high motivation roots (Sherwin, 1998). Because the ECS, through CB1 receptors, modulates in a positive manner rewarding and motivational processes (Maldonado et al., 2006), we recently suggested that the ECS might control running activity by acting on the naturally rewarding properties of running. Indeed, our most recent experiments using conditional CB1 mutant lines wherein CB1 receptors are deleted from selective neuronal or glial populations indicated that (1) the tonic control exerted by CB1 receptors on running performance is fully accounted for by CB1 receptors located on GABAergic neurons, (2) these receptors are located on GABAergic nerve terminals lying in the ventral tegmental area (VTA), a key area involved in reward-based motivation processes, and (3) the presence of CB1 receptors on GABAergic neurons prevents the negative after-effects of exercise on VTA dopaminergic activity (Dubreucq et al., 2013).

The endocannabinoid system and the emotional consequences of running

We have indicated above the importance of laboratory animal studies in the quest for the neurobiological mechanisms underlying the positive emotional effects of physical exercise in humans. However, this quest lies on a prerequisite, which is that these animal models of human physical activity have positive emotional effects. The literature on that particular aspect of exercise has yielded numerous, albeit contradictory, data. Indeed, part of that heterogeneity is accounted for by the respective experimental settings among which the conditions under which the sedentary/control animals are housed (see below).

Tools to measure anxiety and fear memory in laboratory animals

Emotionality is the behavioral repertoire that any individual expresses when confronted by novel situations. Accordingly, it is made of different dimensions, including anxiety, fear, curiosity, joy, sadness, . . . etc. (Lazarus, 1991), several of which may be modeled in laboratory rodents (File, 1987; Ramos & Mormède, 1998). Among these dimensions, anxiety and fear memory have received a great deal of attention, including in studies aimed at measuring the impact of voluntary/forced exercise.

Anxiety tests are classically divided into two categories, the first one grouping unconditioned tests where the innate behavioral reactions of the animal are measured when placed in a novel environment (File, 1987; Treit, 1985). Anxiety is measured as the conflict between the curiosity for that novel environment and the reticence for the same environment due to its potential danger. Typically, this conflict is assessed by, e.g., measuring the number of transits from the closed/protected arms to the open/unprotected arms of an elevated plus-maze, the number of visits from the dark compartment to the highly lit compartment of a light/dark box, or the exploration of the highly illuminated center, as opposed to the less illuminated periphery, of an open field. In the second group of tests, conditioned anxiety, which is also based on conflict, is assessed by measuring vital behaviors, such as feeding or drinking, under conditions wherein these consumptions are punished by mild footshocks.

Another dimension that has received some particular attention is conditioned fear memory. In the classical fear conditioning protocol, a neutral cue (conditioned stimulus), which can be an environmental context – a light, a sound, or an odor – is associated with an aversive stimulus (unconditioned stimulus), usually an electric footshock. The pairing between both stimuli elicits a fear response to the presentation of the conditioned stimulus alone (Davis & Whalen, 2001; LeDoux, 2000). Such a fear response is assessed by means of the so-called "freezing" behavior, characterized by the absence of movements except those necessary for breathing (Blanchard & Blanchard, 1969).

The key role of the housing conditions when assessing the effects of wheel running on unconditioned anxiety and fear memory

As indicated above, the literature on the consequences of voluntary running on unconditioned anxiety and, to a lesser extent, on fear memory is somewhat contradictory. Thus, several studies have reported that wheel running exerts anxiolytic effects while others reported that such an activity either had no effect on anxiety or proved to be anxiogenic (Binder, Droste, Ohl, & Reul,

2004; Burghardt, Fulk, Hand, & Wilson, 2004; Duman, Schlesinger, Russell, & Duman, 2008; Fuss et al., 2010). Among the issues that have been highlighted to explain such discrepancies, we have recently focused on the housing condition of the control animals to which the exercising subjects are compared (Dubreucq, Marsicano, & Chaouloff, 2011). Thus, several studies used control animals housed under standard conditions while others used control animals housed with a locked wheel. The main argument for housing animals under the former condition stems from the observation that a wheel, even if locked, may promote behavioral activities (e.g., wheel hanging) that may bias the results. However, besides the fact that a locked wheel may enrich the environment, and thus bear important consequences (e.g., on hippocampal neurogenesis and neuroplasticity; Lledo, Alonso, & Grubb, 2006), such an argument is contradicted by the observation of lid hanging in animals housed in standard cages as well as the importance of wheel hanging in animals housed with free wheels (Koteja, Garland, Sax, Swallow, & Carter, 1999). To explore the intrinsic impacts of the two aforementioned control housing conditions (standard housing without any wheel, housing with a locked wheel) when compared with housing with a free wheel, we have recently used mice housed under any of these three conditions for more than 3 weeks. Thereafter, all the mice were tested for several emotional behaviors, including anxiety in a light/dark box and contextual fear memory expression. The results show that the effects of wheel running on anxiety and fear memory depend on the experimental condition under which the controls are housed (Dubreucq et al., 2011). As an illustration, wheel running proved anxiolytic in the light/dark box when compared with the standard housing condition but not when compared with housing with a locked wheel.

Role of the endocannabinoid system in the emotional profile displayed by wheel running subjects

To our knowledge, only one study has explored the respective influences of wheel running and CB1 receptors on some aspects of emotionality (Dubreucq et al., 2010). In that study, male CB1 mutant mice were compared with their wild-type littermates for their behavioral responses in an open field and their cued fear memory after a 6-week housing with locked or free wheels. It was observed that neither the exploration of the center of the open field, an index of anxiety (see above), nor the peripheral locomotion in that test were sensitive to wheel running in the two genotypes (Dubreucq et al., 2010). This result confirms the above-mentioned difficulty of revealing the anxiolytic impact of wheel running, if any. On the other hand, examination of cued fear memory expression, which is an amygdala-dependent process (as opposed to contextual fear memory, which is hippocampus-dependent; Maren & Quirk, 2004), revealed a significant interaction between wheel running and CB1 receptor expression. Confirming previous observations, CB1 receptor deletion *per se* increased cued fear expression and delayed fear extinction during recall sessions, as assessed from freezing reactions to a tone previously associated with a shock during the conditioning session (Marsicano et al., 2002). Interestingly, wheel running, which was ineffective in wild-type animals, counteracted both the increased fear expression and the delayed extinction that are observed in sedentary CB1 mutant mice (Dubreucq et al., 2010). The observation that wheel running was ineffective on cued fear memory in wild-type animals contrasts with previous findings showing that wheel running increases contextual fear memory (Burghardt, Pasumarthi, Wilson, & Fadel, 2006; Greenwood, Strong, Foley, & Fleshner, 2009). This may indicate that wheel running bears differential effects on hippocampal- and amygdala-dependent fear memories. In keeping with the inhibitory impact of wheel running on the hypersensitized fear expression displayed by CB1 receptor mutants, we recently wondered whether such an interaction between wheel running and CB1 receptor deletion would still be observed if CB1 receptors were selectively deleted from selective neuronal populations. As indicated above, the Cre/lox P technique has allowed the generation of CB1 receptor mutants wherein CB1 receptors are missing from selected neuronal populations, including cortical glutamatergic neurons (Bellocchio et al., 2010; Monory et al., 2006, 2007; Puighermanal et al., 2009). We thus housed male Glu–CB1$^{-/-}$ and male Glu–CB1$^{+/+}$ mice for 3 weeks with either locked or free wheels, and then examined in both genotypes anxiety-related behaviors using the elevated plus-maze (see above), and cued fear memory expression and extinction during fear recall tests. In the elevated plus-maze, wheel running was found to exert hypolocomotor influences, as assessed by the number of visits to the closed (i.e., protected) arms of the maze (Figure 3.3A). On the other hand, wheel running counteracted the decrease in the percent time spent in the open (i.e., unprotected) arms of the maze that was displayed by the mutant mice (Figure 3.3B). Taken with the data mentioned above, this set of observations thus suggests that wheel running in mice does not bear intrinsic anxiolytic effects but may be able to reverse innate anxiety. Whether this counteracting effect of wheel running extends to environmental situations that further raise anxiety levels is an issue that surely deserves future investigation. When Glu–CB1$^{-/-}$ and male Glu–CB1$^{+/+}$ mice were cued fear conditioned by a tone-shock pairing, fear expression responses to single tone exposure 1 to 3 days later revealed that wheel running had an influence in mutant, but not in wild-type mice (Figures 3.3C and 3.3D). Thus, wheel running

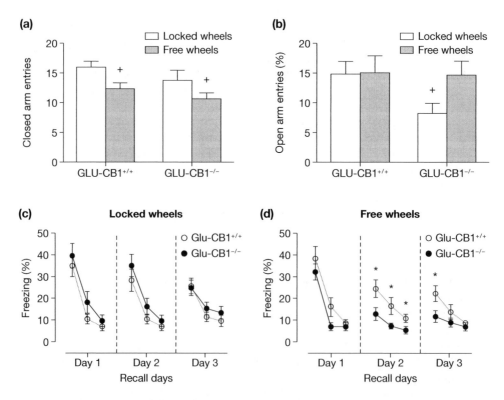

Figure 3.3 CB1 receptors and behavioral consequences of wheel running. (a) Activity and (b) anxiety-related behavior in the elevated plus-maze of Glu–CB1$^{+/+}$ and Glu–CB1$^{-/-}$ mice housed for 3 weeks with either locked or free wheels. Cued fear memory during recall sessions in Glu–CB1$^{+/+}$ and Glu–CB1$^{-/-}$ mice housed for 3 weeks with locked wheels (c) or with free wheels (d). Values are the mean ± S.E.M. of 13–15 mice/group. $^+$ P < 0.05 for the main influence of the housing condition in the two genotypes. ⋆ at least P < 0.05 for the difference between sedentary and running subjects.

decreased fear expression and accelerated fear extinction on recall sessions 2 and 3 in Glu-CB1$^{-/-}$, but not in Glu-CB1$^{+/+}$, mice. Such a differential effect of wheel running in the two genotypes closely resembles that measured in constitutive CB1 mutants, as opposed to their wild-type littermates (see above). This indicates that (1) wheel running controls in a tonic manner cued fear memory expression/extinction and (2) that such a control involves CB1 receptors located on cortical glutamatergic neurons. In turn, the former finding opens the promising hypothesis that physical exercise in humans may set back to normal levels abnormally high fear expression and/or delayed extinction (as observed, e.g., in patients suffering post-traumatic stress disorder). Our finding reinforces former evidence for a tight control of fear memory by the ECS (Marsicano et al., 2002); however, how such a control is exerted in exercising subjects remains to be explored.

The endocannabinoid system and the neurogenic impact of wheel running

Adult neurogenesis, i.e., the formation of new neurons, occurs in the hippocampus where it is highly sensitive to wheel running (Ernst, Olson, Pinel, Lam, & Christie, 2006; van Praag, 2009). Thus, housing with running wheels increases neurogenesis in the dentate gyrus, an effect already observed after 1 week of wheel running. However, such a stimulatory impact of exercise is not specific to running as environmental enrichments also share that capacity (Kempermann, Kuhn, & Gage, 1997). As already underlined above with regard to the emotional effects of wheel running, the neurogenic impact of an enrichment in the environment raises the question of the intrinsic consequence of the presence of the wheel. Indeed, a recent study wherein mice were housed in standard cages or in cages complemented with either locked wheels or free wheels revealed the following. Housing with wheels, whether locked or unlocked, stimulated the proliferative phase of the neurogenic process, compared with standard housing (Bednarczyk et al., 2010). However, when focusing on later stages of the neurogenic process (i.e., survival, differentiation, maturation), mice housed with free wheels displayed increased neurogenesis, as compared to the two other mouse groups. This indicates that exercise has an intrinsic stimulatory influence on the last phases of the neurogenic process only.

Several studies have analyzed whether the ECS contributes to the stimulatory effects of wheel running on neurogenesis. In the aforementioned study in which a CB1 receptor antagonist was administered daily for 8 days to male rats, it was observed that such a treatment prevented the stimulatory influence of wheel running on hippocampal cell proliferation (Hill et al., 2010). Supporting this, one study using female mice reported that wheel running elicited cell proliferation in the dentate gyrus, as compared to standard housing, a change that was absent in CB1 mutant mice (Wolf et al., 2010). On the other hand, another study using male CB1 mutant and wild-type mice reported that although CB1 receptor mutation decreased neurogenesis, in line with past results (Aguado et al., 2006; Jin et al., 2004) and running performance (see above), the percent stimulatory influence of wheel running on neurogenesis was independent from the mouse genotype (Dubreucq et al., 2010). Taken together, these results indicate the need for future experiments to delineate the role of CB1 receptors on exercise-induced neurogenesis. In keeping with the contradictory data that have emerged on that subject, these experiments will need to detail the respective roles of CB1 receptors at each stage of the neurogenic process and compare the effects of wheel running to standard housing and housing with locked wheels.

Conclusions

The ECS plays a major role in the regulation of central functions, including well-being. This chapter has tried to provide arguments in favor of a role for that key modulatory system during exercise. The data reviewed above highlight the likelihood that the ECS is involved in the control of exercise performance, but much remains to be done before identifying the mechanisms underlying such a control. Besides, there is experimental support for a role of the ECS in the modulation of fear memory and neurogenic processes in exercising subjects, but again much work is needed to detail such a relationship. We have seen that the main experimental evidence for a role of the ECS during exercise stems from animal studies. In turn, this indicates the need for a real appreciation of the limits of animal models of exercise. This chapter has tried to raise several of them, including the need to compare exercising animals to appropriate controls. However, besides these issues, other ones that were not covered in the present chapter need to be taken into account before translating animal studies to the clinics. These include the difficulty of building the most appropriate animal models of human psychopathologies such as depression, and the awareness that laboratory animals live in impoverished environments. Accordingly, wheel running activity, even if compared with that related to the simple presence of a wheel, may bear a valence that largely exceeds that usually measured in human beings offered a vast array of occupational activities.

References

Aguado, T., Palazuelos, J., Monory, K., Stella, N., Cravatt, B., Lutz, B., Marsicano, G., Kokaia, Z., Guzmán, M., & Galve-Roperh, I. (2006). The endocannabinoid system promotes astroglial differentiation by acting on neural progenitor cells. *Journal of Neuroscience, 26*, 1551–1561.

Alger, E. (2002). Retrograde signaling in the regulation of synaptic transmission: Focus on endocannabinoids. *Progress in Neurobiology, 68*, 247–286.

Bednarczyk, M.R., Hacker, L.C., Fortin-Nunez, S., Aumont, A., Bergeron, R., & Fernandes, K.J. (2010). Distinct stages of adult hippocampal neurogenesis are regulated by running and the running environment. *Hippocampus, 21*, 1334–1347.

Belke, T.W., & Wagner, J.P. (2005). The reinforcing property and the rewarding aftereffect of wheel running in rats: A combination of two paradigms. *Behavioral Processes, 68*, 165–172.

Bellocchio, L., Lafenêtre, P., Cannich, A., Cota, D., Puente, N., Grandes, P., Chaouloff, F., Piazza, P.V., & Marsicano, G. (2010). Bimodal control of stimulated food intake by the endocannabinoid system. *Nature Neuroscience, 13*, 281–283.

Binder, E., Droste, S.K., Ohl, F., & Reul, J.M.H.M. (2004). Regular voluntary exercise reduces anxiety-related behavior and impulsiveness in mice. *Behavioral Brain Research, 155*, 197–206.

Blanchard, R.J., & Blanchard, D.C. (1969). Passive and active reactions to fear-eliciting stimuli. *Journal of Comparative and Physiological Psychology, 68*, 129–135.

Burghardt, P.R., Fulk, L.J., Hand, G.A., & Wilson, M.A. (2004). The effects of chronic treadmill and wheel running on behavior in rats. *Brain Research, 1019*, 84–96.

Burghardt, P.R., Pasumarthi, R.K., Wilson, M.A., & Fadel, J. (2006). Alterations in fear conditioning and amygdalar activation following chronic wheel running. *Pharmacology Biochemistry and Behavior, 84*, 306–312.

Chanda, P.K., Gao, Y., Mark, L., Btesh, J., Strassle, B.W., Lu, P., . . . Samad, T.A. (2010). Monoacylglycerol lipase activity is a critical modulator of the tone and integrity of the endocannabinoid system. *Molecular Pharmacology, 78*, 996–1003.

Chaouloff, F. (1989). Physical exercise and brain monoamines: A review. *Acta Physiologica Scandinavica, 137*, 1–13.

Chaouloff, F. (1997). Effects of acute physical exercise on central serotonergic systems. *Medicine and Science in Sports and Exercise, 29*, 58–62.

Chaouloff, F., Dubreucq, S., Bellocchio, L., & Marsicano, G. (2011). Endocannabinoids and motor behavior: CB1 receptors also control running activity. *Physiology, 26*, 76–77.

Chevaleyre, V., Takahashi, K.A., & Castillo, P.E. (2006). Endocannabinoid-mediated synaptic plasticity in the CNS. *Annual Review of Neuroscience, 29*, 37–76.

Cravatt, B.F., Demarest, K., Patricelli, M.P., Bracey, M.H., Giang, D.K., Martin, B.R., & Lichtman, A.H. (2001). Supersensitivity to anandamide and enhanced endogenous cannabinoid signaling in mice lacking fatty acid amide hydrolase. *Proceedings of the National Academy of Sciences USA, 98*, 9371–9376.

Davis, M., & Whalen, P.J. (2001). The amygdala: Vigilance and emotion. *Molecular Psychiatry, 6*, 13–34.

De Chiara, V., Errico, F., Musella, A., Rossi, S., Mataluni, G., Sacchetti, L., . . . Centonze, D. (2010). Voluntary exercise and sucrose consumption enhance cannabinoid CB1 receptor sensitivity in the striatum. *Neuropsychopharmacology, 35*, 374–387.

Dietrich, A., & McDaniel, W.F. (2004). Endocannabinoids and exercise. *British Journal of Sports Medicine, 38*, 536–541.

Dubreucq, S., Durand, A., Matias, I., Bénard, G., Richard, E., Soria-Gomez, E., . . . Chaouloff, F. (2013). Ventral tegmental area cannabinoid type-1 receptors control voluntary exercise performance. *Biological Psychiatry,* in press.

Dubreucq, S., Koehl, M., Abrous, D.N., Marsicano, G., & Chaouloff, F. (2010). CB1 receptor deficiency decreases wheel-running activity: Consequences on emotional behaviors and hippocampal neurogenesis. *Experimental Neurology, 224*, 106–113.

Dubreucq, S., Marsicano, G., & Chaouloff, F. (2011). Emotional consequences of wheel running in mice: Which is the appropriate control? *Hippocampus, 21*, 239–242.

Dubreucq, S., Matias, I., Cardinal, P., Häring, M., Lutz, B., Marsicano, G., & Chaouloff, F. (2012). Genetic dissection of the role of cannabinoid type-1 receptors in the emotional consequences of repeated social stress in mice. *Neuropsychopharmacology, 37*, 1885–1900.

Duman, C., Schlesinger, L., Russell, D.S., & Duman, R.S. (2008). Voluntary exercise produces antidepressant and anxiolytic behavioral effects in mice. *Brain Research, 199*, 148–158.

Dunn, A.L., & Dishman, R.K. (1991). Exercise and the neurobiology of depression. *Exercise and Sport Sciences Reviews, 19*, 41–98.

El Manira, A., & Kyriakatos, A. (2010). The role of endocannabinoid signaling in motor control. *Physiology, 25*, 230–238.

Ernst, C., Olson, A.K., Pinel, J.P., Lam, R.W., & Christie, B.R. (2006). Antidepressant effects of exercise: Evidence for an adult-neurogenesis hypothesis? *Journal of Psychiatry and Neuroscience, 31*, 84–92.

File, S.E. (1987). The contribution of behavioral studies to the neuropharmacology of anxiety. *Neuropharmacology, 26*, 877–886.

Freund, T.F., Katona, I., & Piomelli, D. (2003). Role of endogenous cannabinoids in synaptic signaling. *Physiological Reviews, 83*, 1017–1066.

Fuss, J., Ben Abdallah, N.M.B., Vogt, M.A., Touma, C., Pacifici, P.G., Palme, R., . . . Gass, P. (2010). Voluntary exercise induces anxiety-like behavior in adult C57BL/6J mice correlating with hippocampal neurogenesis. *Hippocampus, 20*, 364–376.

Gao, Y., Vasilyev, D.V., Goncalves, M.B., Howell, F.V., Hobbs, C., Reisenberg, M., . . . Doherty, P. (2010). Loss of retrograde endocannabinoid signaling and reduced adult neurogenesis in diacylglycerol lipase knock-out mice. *Journal of Neuroscience, 30*, 2017–2024.

Gatley, S.J., Gifford, A.N., Volkow, N.D., Lan, R., & Makriyannis, A. (1996). ^{123}I-labeled AM251: A radioiodinated ligand which binds in vivo to mouse brain cannabinoid CB1 receptors. *European Journal of Pharmacology, 307*, 331–338.

Greenwood, B.N., Foley, T.E., Le, T.V., Strong, P.V., Loughridge, A.B., Day, H.E., & Fleshner, M. (2011). Long-term voluntary wheel running is rewarding and produces plasticity in the mesolimbic reward pathway. *Behavioral Brain Research, 217*, 354–362.

Greenwood, B.N., Strong, P.V., Foley, T.E., & Fleshner, M. (2009). A behavioral analysis of the impact of voluntary physical activity on hippocampus-dependent contextual conditioning. *Hippocampus, 19*, 988–1001.

Herkenham, M., Lynn, A.B., Little, M.D., Johnson, M.R., Melvin, L.S., de Costa, B.R., & Rice, K.C. (1990). Cannabinoid receptor localization in brain. *Proceedings of the National Academy of Sciences USA, 87*, 1932–1936.

Heyman, E., Gamelin, F.X., Goekint, M., Piscitelli, F., Roelands, B., Leclair, E., . . . Meeusen, R. (2012). Intense exercise increases circulating endocannabinoid and BDNF levels in humans: Possible implications for reward and depression. *Psychoneuroendocrinology, 37*, 844–851.

Hill, M.N., Titterness, A.K., Morrish, A.C., Carrier, E.J., Lee, T.T., Gil-Mohapel, J., . . . Christie, B.R. (2010). Endogenous cannabinoid signaling is required for voluntary exercise-induced enhancement of progenitor cell proliferation in the hippocampus. *Hippocampus, 20*, 513–523.

Hillman, C.H., Erickson, K.I., & Kramer, A.F. (2008). Be smart, exercise your heart: Exercise effects on brain and cognition. *Nature Reviews Neuroscience, 9*, 58–65.

Hoffmann, P. (1997). The endorphin hypothesis. In W.P. Morgan (Ed.), *Physical activity and mental health* (pp. 163–177). Washington, DC: Taylor & Francis.

Jin, K., Xie, L., Kim, S.H., Parmentier-Batteur, S., Sun, Y., Mao, X.O., Childs, J., & Greenberg, D.A. (2004). Defective adult neurogenesis in CB1 cannabinoid receptor knockout mice. *Molecular Pharmacology, 66*, 204–208.

Keeney, B.K., Raichlen, D.A., Meek, T.H., Wijeratne, R.S., Middleton, K.M., Gerdeman, G.L., & Garland Jr., T. (2008). Differential response to a selective cannabinoid receptor antagonist (SR141716: rimonabant) in female mice from lines selectively bred for high voluntary wheel-running behavior. *Behavioral Pharmacology, 19*, 812–820.

Kempermann, G., Kuhn, H.G., & Gage, F.H. (1997). More hippocampal neurons in adult mice living in an enriched environment. *Nature, 386*, 493–495.

Koteja, P., Garland Jr., T., Sax, J.K., Swallow, J.G., & Carter, P.A. (1999). Behavior of house mice artificially selected for high levels of voluntary wheel running. *Animal Behavior, 58*, 1307–1318.

Lafenêtre, P., Chaouloff, F., & Marsicano, G. (2007). The endocannabinoid system in the processing of anxiety and fear and how CB1 receptors may modulate fear extinction. *Pharmacological Research, 56*, 367–381.

Lazarus, R.S. (1991). Progress on a cognitive-motivational-relational theory of emotion. *American Psychologist, 46*, 819–834.

Ledent, C., Valverde, O., Cossu, G., Petitet, F., Aubert, J.F., Beslot, F., . . . Parmentier, M. (1999). Unresponsiveness to cannabinoids and reduced addictive effects of opiates in CB1 receptor knockout mice. *Science, 283*, 401–404.

LeDoux, J.E. (2000). Emotion circuits in the brain. *Annual Review of Neuroscience, 23*, 155–184.

Lett, B.T., Grant, V.L., & Koh, M.T. (2001). Naloxone attenuates the conditioned place preference induced by wheel running in rats. *Physiology and Behavior, 72*, 355–358.

Lledo, P.M., Alonso, M., & Grubb, M.S. (2006). Adult neurogenesis and functional plasticity in neuronal circuits. *Nature Reviews Neuroscience, 7*, 179–193.

Long, J.Z., Nomura, D.K., Vann, R.E., Walentiny, D.M., Booker, L., Jin, X., . . . Cravatt, B.F. (2009). Dual blockade of FAAH and MAGL identifies behavioral processes regulated by endocannabinoid crosstalk in vivo. *Proceedings of the National Academy of Sciences USA, 106*, 20270–20275.

Maldonado, R., Valverde, O., & Berrendero, F. (2006). Involvement of the endocannabinoid system in drug addiction. *Trends in Neurosciences, 29*, 225–232.

Maren, S., & Quirk, G.J. (2004). Neuronal signalling of fear memory. *Nature Reviews Neuroscience, 5*, 844–852.

Marsicano, G., & Lutz, B. (1999). Expression of the cannabinoid receptor CB1 in distinct neuronal subpopulations in the adult mouse forebrain. *European Journal of Neuroscience, 11*, 4213–4225.

Marsicano, G., & Lutz, B. (2006). Neuromodulatory functions of the endocannabinoid system. *Journal of Endocrinological Investigation, 29*, 27–46.

Marsicano, G., Wotjak, C.T., Azad, S., Bisogno, T., Rammes, G., Cascio, M.G., . . . Lutz, B. (2002). The endogenous cannabinoid system controls extinction of aversive memories. *Nature, 418*, 530–534.

Martinsen, E.W., & Morgan, W.P. (1997). Antidepressant effects of physical activity. In W.P. Morgan (Ed.), *Physical activity and mental health* (pp. 93–106). Washington, DC: Taylor & Francis.

Mechoulam, R., & Hanus, L. (2000). A historical overview of chemical research on cannabinoids. *Chemistry and Physics of Lipids, 108*, 1–13.

Meeusen, R., Piacentini, M.F., & De Meirleir, K. (2001). Brain microdialysis in exercise research. *Sports Medicine, 31*, 965–983.

Monory, K., Blaudzun, H., Massa, F., Kaiser, N., Lemberger, T., Schütz, G., . . . Marsicano, G. (2007). Genetic dissection of behavioral and autonomic effects of delta^9-tetrahydrocannabinol in mice. *PloS Biology, 5*, e269.

Monory, K., Massa, F., Egertová, M., Eder, M., Blaudzun, H., Westenbroek, R., . . . Marsicano, G. (2006). The endocannabinoid system controls key epileptogenic circuits in the hippocampus. *Neuron, 51*, 455–466.

Morozov, A., Kellendonk, C., Simpson, E., & Tronche, F. (2003). Using conditional mutagenesis to study the brain. *Biological Psychiatry, 54*, 1125–1133.

Ohno-Shosaku, T., Tanimura, A., Hashimotodani, Y., & Kano, M. (2011). Endocannabinoids and retrograde modulation of synaptic transmission. *Neuroscientist, 18*, 119–132.

Pacher, P., Bátkai, S., & Kunos, G. (2006). The endocannabinoid system as an emerging target of pharmacotherapy. *Pharmacological Reviews, 58*, 389–462.

Pagotto, U., Marsicano, G., Cota, D., Lutz, B., & Pasquali, R. (2006). The emerging role of the endocannabinoid system in endocrine regulation and energy balance. *Endocrine Reviews, 27*, 73–100.

Patel, S., & Hillard, C.J. (2008). Adaptations in endocannabinoid signaling in response to repeated homotypic stress: A novel mechanism for stress habituation. *European Journal of Neuroscience, 27*, 2821–2829.

Piomelli, D. (2003). The molecular logic of endocannabinoid signalling. *Nature Reviews Neuroscience, 4*, 873–884.

Powell, K.E., & Paffenbarger Jr., R.S. (1985). Workshop on epidemiologic and public health aspects of physical activity and exercise: A summary. *Public Health Reports, 100*, 118–126.

Puighermanal, E., Marsicano, G., Busquets-Garcia, A., Lutz, B., Maldonado, R., & Ozaita, A. (2009). Cannabinoid modulation of hippocampal long-term memory is mediated by mTOR signaling. *Nature Neuroscience, 12*, 1152–1158.

Raglin, J.S. (1997). Anxiolytic effects of physical activity. In W.P. Morgan (Ed.), *Physical Activity and Mental Health* (pp. 107–126). Washington, DC: Taylor & Francis.

Raichlen, D.A., Foster, A.D., Seillier, A., Giuffrida, A., & Gerdeman, G.L. (in press). Exercise-induced endocannabinoid signalling is modulated by intensity. *European Journal of Applied Physiology*.

Ramos, A., & Mormède, P. (1998). Stress and emotionality: A multidimensional and genetic approach. *Neuroscience and Biobehavioral Reviews, 22*, 33–57.

Ransford, C.P. (1982). A role for amines in the antidepressant effect of exercise: A review. *Medicine and Science in Sports and Exercise, 14*, 1–10.

Rinaldi-Carmona, M., Barth, F., Héaulme, M., Shire, D., Calandra, B., Congy, C., . . . Le Fur, G. (1994). SR141716A, a potent and selective antagonist of the brain cannabinoid receptor. *FEBS Letters, 350*, 240–244.

Rossi, S., De Chiara, V., Musella, A., Kusayanagi, H., Mataluni, G., Bernardi, G., . . . Centonze, D. (2008). Chronic psychoemotional stress impairs cannabinoid-receptor-mediated control of GABA transmission in the striatum. *Journal of Neuroscience, 28*, 7284–7292.

Salmon, P. (2001). Effects of physical exercise on anxiety, depression, and sensitivity to stress: A unifying theory. *Clinical Psychology Review, 21*, 33–61.

Schlosburg, J.E., Blankman, J.L., Long, J.Z., Nomura, D.K., Pan, B., Kinsey, S.G., . . . Cravatt, B.F. (2010). Chronic monoacylglycerol lipase blockade causes functional antagonism of the endocannabinoid system. *Nature Neuroscience, 13*, 1113–1119.

Sherwin, C.M. (1998). Voluntary wheel running: A review and novel interpretation. *Animal Behavior, 56*, 11–27.

Sparling, P.B., Giuffrida, A., Piomelli, D., Rosskopf, L., & Dietrich, A. (2003). Exercise activates the endocannabinoid system. *Neuroreport, 14*, 2209–2211.

Ströhle, A. (2009). Physical activity, exercise, depression and anxiety disorders. *Journal of Neural Transmission, 116*, 777–784.

Tanimura, A., Yamazaki, M., Hashimotodani, Y., Uchigashima, M., Kawata, S., Abe, M., . . . Kano, M. (2010). The endocannabinoid 2-arachidonoylglycerol produced by diacylglycerol lipase alpha mediates retrograde suppression of synaptic transmission. *Neuron, 65*, 320–327.

Treit, D. (1985). Animal models for the study of anti-anxiety agents: A review. *Neuroscience and Biobehavioral Reviews, 9*, 203–222.

van Praag, H. (2009). Exercise and the brain: Something to chew on. *Trends in Neurosciences, 32*, 283–290.

Wolf, S.A., Bick-Sander, A., Fabel, K., Leal-Galicia, P., Tauber, S., Ramirez-Rodriguez, G., . . . Kempermann, G. (2010). Cannabinoid receptor CB1 mediates baseline and activity-induced survival of new neurons in adult hippocampal neurogenesis. *Cell Communication and Signaling, 8*, 12.

Zhou, D., & Shearman, L.P. (2004). Voluntary exercise augments acute effects of CB1-receptor inverse agonist on body weight loss in obese and lean mice. *Pharmacology Biochemistry and Behavior, 77*, 117–125.

Zimmer, A., Zimmer, A.M., Hohmann, A.G., Herkenham, M., & Bonner, T.I. (1999). Increased mortality, hypoactivity, and hypoalgesia in cannabinoid CB1 receptor knockout mice. *Proceedings of the National Academy of Sciences USA, 96*, 5780–5785.

4

PHYSICAL ACTIVITY AND REWARD

The role of dopamine

Justin S. Rhodes and Petra Majdak

The idea that physical activity could be rewarding may seem counter-intuitive because many people find exercise aversive and would prefer to be inactive. Arguably one of the greatest health problems facing the United States today is inactivity, which is associated with obesity and metabolic syndrome, e.g., diabetes, heart disease, and stroke (Must et al., 1999). On the other hand, clearly, certain individual humans find at least some types of physical activity rewarding, as they choose to exercise multiple times per week and even report that they feel euphoria from exercise, as in the case of the runner's high (Boecker et al., 2008). Moreover, many people who regularly exercise report withdrawal symptoms if they are unable to exercise, including irritability, anxiety, difficult time focusing, and bad mood (Mondin et al., 1996). Hence, in certain predisposed humans, it seems that physical activity can be rewarding and reinforcing to the extent that individuals choose to engage in the activities and show withdrawal when prevented from an exercise routine.

In industrialized nations such as the United States where physical activity is typically low, individuals who find exercise rewarding and reinforcing have a health advantage because regular bouts of aerobic physical exercise maintain cardiovascular, immune, and mental health, and delay aging. Exercise reverses many of the causes and symptoms of metabolic syndrome by reducing body fat, increasing sensitivity of insulin receptors, and decreasing blood pressure (when not exercising) (Helmrich, Ragland, Leung, & Paffenbarger, 1991). Exercise also appears to enhance brain health. For example, in humans and rodent models, exercise improves performance on cognitive tasks and can reduce stress and aging-induced cognitive deficits (Colcombe & Kramer, 2003; Greenwood & Fleshner, 2011). Therefore, understanding the mechanisms underlying reward and motivation for physical activity has broad implications for improving health and longevity.

Behavioral evidence that physical activity can be rewarding in animals

Cumulative evidence from the animal literature supports the contention that physical activity can be rewarding. First, many animals will work for access to physical activity in an operant conditioning task (Iversen, 1993). In addition, studies have established that rats prefer to spend time in environments paired with the aftereffects of wheel running using the conditioned place preference (CPP) assay (Belke & Wagner, 2005; Lett, Grant, Byrne, & Koh, 2000). One limitation is that it is not clear whether physical activity per se was rewarding or whether access to the running wheel served as a form of enrichment for the animals. In other words, animals housed in standard laboratory cages could have been relatively deprived of stimuli, and the wheel provides a novel stimulus for the animals. Seeking a more enriched experience could explain why animals chose to press levers to obtain access to a running wheel and showed preference for contexts paired with a wheel.

On the other hand, a large body of literature has established that many animals choose to run long distances when presented with the opportunity even when there is no clear goal or objective (e.g., to obtain food, water, or mates). Moreover, animals will engage in the physical activity repeatedly over weeks and months, long after the stimulus or experience could have been perceived as novel. For example, standard inbred strains of mice run between 2 and 10 km/day, depending on the genotype, when running wheels are available (Clark, Kohman et al., 2011). Hence, combined with the operant and classical conditioning data, the cumulative evidence favors the hypothesis that physical activity itself can be rewarding and reinforcing in animals.

Neurobiological indicators of physical activity reward

A number of rodent animal studies have discovered neurobiological changes induced from chronic voluntary wheel running that are analogous to changes that take place in the brain in response to drugs of abuse (Greenwood et al., 2011; Rhodes, Garland, & Gammie, 2003; Werme, Thoren, Olson, & Brene, 2000). If one assumes that the molecular changes induced from chronic drugs reflect the rewarding properties of the drugs, then these data provide additional evidence that physical activity can be rewarding and reinforcing, similar to drugs of abuse. However, despite the massive drug abuse literature, it is difficult to prove that a specific molecule is involved in rewarding as opposed to aversive properties of drugs, their side effects, or compensatory mechanisms associated with chronic drug administration not directly related to reward (Rhodes & Crabbe, 2005). Most proposed causal molecular mechanisms for addiction and reward remain contentious in the field. However, in one group of relatively convincing studies, Werme et al. (2002) found that rats that ran for 30 days at approximately 10 km/day displayed increased levels of ΔFosB in the nucleus accumbens compared to rats exposed to locked running wheels. Similar increases in ΔFosB occurred in rats exposed to chronic drugs of abuse (Perrotti et al., 2008). Moreover, mice that overexpressed ΔFosB selectively in striatal dynorphin-containing neurons increased their daily running compared with control littermates, consistent with previous work showing ΔFosB overexpression within this same neuronal population increases the rewarding properties of drugs of abuse (Werme et al., 2002). Based on the observations that ΔFosB accumulates in the nucleus accumbens and striatum with repeated drug use and is sufficient to induce drug-seeking behavior, ΔFosB has been suggested to be a molecular switch for addiction (Nestler, Barrot, & Self, 2001). It is known that ΔFosB is a transcription factor, i.e., it binds to protein complexes that bind to DNA to cause the expression of genes (Nestler, Kelz, & Chen, 1999). However, how exactly ΔFosB contributes to reward or addiction, and the specificity of ΔFosB in reward as compared to aversion is not known and remains an active area of research. For example, ΔFosB is induced from a variety of stimuli in addition to drugs of abuse and wheel running, including electroconvulsive seizures, brain lesions, and chronic stress (Chen, Kelz, Hope, Nakabeppu, & Nestler, 1997; Vialou et al., 2010). Taken together, the available data suggest that ΔFosB may be an important molecule involved in the reinforcing effects of physical activity and drugs of abuse, but how ΔFosB contributes to the perception of reward or reinforcement and the specificity of the ΔFosB response to reward has not been established.

Replicate lines of mice selectively bred for increased voluntary wheel running behavior

Additional neurobiological evidence that physical activity can be rewarding and reinforcing comes from a long-term selective breeding experiment for increased voluntary wheel running behavior in mice (Swallow, Carter, & Garland, 1998). The experiment began in 1993 and is still ongoing. Mice generated from this experiment represent an invaluable resource for discovering common mechanisms underlying physical activity reward. One of the great strengths of the model is the replication of the lines. An unprecedented four replicate high-runner lines and four replicate control lines are maintained. The replication of the lines combined with the large divergence in levels of voluntary wheel running produced over 18 years and 60+ generations of breeding provides a unique and statistically powerful genetic animal model to identify neurobiological mechanisms underlying the increase in the running behavior (Rhodes, Gammie, & Garland, 2005).

Note that there is no a priori reason why increased voluntary running induced from selection would have to involve changes in brain reward circuits. For example, changes in exercise-physiological traits such as increases in mitochondria in muscles or size of the heart could have changed to allow the animals to run farther. In fact, the original rationale for conducting the experiment was to identify correlated changes in exercise-physiological traits (such as heart mass or aerobic capacity) – not brain reward – that were hypothesized to support the high activity levels (Swallow, Garland, Carter, Zhan, & Sieck, 1998). A number of exercise-physiological changes have been documented in the lines including a small muscle phenotype with high concentration of enzymes involved in aerobic metabolism (Guderley, Joanisse, Mokas, Bilodeau, & Garland, 2008). Moreover, aerobic capacity, the maximum amount of oxygen an animal can consume during forced exercise, has increased in the high-runner lines (Rezende, Garland, Chappell, Malisch, & Gomes, 2006). Nonetheless, a number of pieces of evidence that will be reviewed in this chapter also suggest that the brain reward circuit has undergone substantial evolution to cause increased motivation for running in the high-runner lines. In retrospect, it is intuitive that selection on a voluntary behavior would have to involve changes in brain reward circuits given that at the start of the experiment most of the animals probably did not choose to run at maximum physiological capacity, and therefore individual differences in levels of running were most likely attributed to differences in perceptions of reward or motivation for the activity.

Over the years of selection, voluntary levels of running increased in the high-runner lines from an average of approximately 4 km/day at the start of the experiment, up to an average of 15 km/day by generation 15. After generation 15, levels of running reached a plateau and have remained at approximately a 15-km/day average through the current generations. A pivotal experiment was conducted in generation 29 that identified brain regions in the high-runner mice putatively involved in motivation for running (Rhodes et al., 2003). Animals were placed on wheels for 6 days. On day 7, during the daytime when the animals were resting, a tile was placed between the wheel access tunnel and the cage so that the animals would not be able to run during their normal active period. The other half of the animals remained undisturbed and freely able to run. All animals were euthanized at a time when they would normally be running at peak levels and their brains were removed and processed to measure patterns of neuronal activation in 25 different brain regions using a standard technique described below. The idea behind the blocked running group was to examine brain activity when animals were expecting and wanting to run but were unable to do so. Because running itself activates neuronal systems, we reasoned that if the animals were running at the time of euthanasia (as they were in the free-runner group), we would not be able to differentiate brain regions involved in motivation from brain regions merely reflecting the sensory stimulation of running itself. Hence, the animals prevented from running were considered to be in a state of withdrawal from running, potentially involving many emotions, including frustration, anxiety, expectation, and craving, among others, most of which we argued would reflect wanting or desire to run (Rhodes et al., 2003).

Immediately after euthanasia, the brains of all the animals were removed, sectioned, and stained for immunohistochemical detection of c-Fos. c-Fos is another transcription factor like ΔFosB discussed in the preceding section, except unlike ΔFosB, c-Fos is transiently expressed in response to a stimulus, reaching peak concentrations approximately 2 hours after a stimulus and then rapidly degrading to undetectable levels rather than accumulating with repeated exposures as does ΔFosB (Nestler et al., 2001). The technique of immunohistochemical detection of c-Fos is widely used to capture and quantify neuronal activation occurring up to 2 hours in the brain before animals are euthanized (Clark, Bhattacharya, Miller, & Rhodes, 2011). Neurons that were stimulated or firing action potentials to a large enough degree to induce a transcriptional response within the cells during this period will express high levels of c-Fos and appear darkly stained under the microscope (Clayton, 2000) (see Figure 4.1).

We observed a striking and surprising result. Many brain regions that are classically considered components of the natural reward circuit (see below) displayed high numbers of c-Fos-positive cells in the animals prevented from running (Rhodes et al., 2003). An example is shown in Figure 4.1 for the dorsal striatum. Similar patterns of c-Fos were observed when animals were exposed to contexts paired with drugs of abuse (Johnson, Revis, Burdick, & Rhodes, 2010; Rhodes, Ryabinin, & Crabbe, 2005; Zombeck et al., 2008). Perhaps even more striking was that animals from the selected high-runner lines displayed significantly greater c-Fos responses in these reward regions as compared to control unselected animals. Although high-runner animals are more active than controls in cages without running wheels (Malisch et al., 2009; Rhodes et al., 2001), we concluded that differences in physical activity were unlikely to account for the c-Fos responses in reward regions when animals were prevented from running. This is because the complementary group of animals that were freely able to run up to the point of euthanasia displayed low c-Fos levels in these regions and the c-Fos levels were uncorrelated with individual differences in running behavior. Hence, we concluded that components of the natural reward circuit in the brain had undergone evolutionary changes in the high-runner lines to predispose high motivation for running (Rhodes et al., 2003).

The natural reward circuit and the role of dopamine in the brain

The natural reward circuit (see Figure 4.2) can be defined as the set of brain regions involved in the perception of pleasure from rewarding experiences leading to reinforcement of behaviors involved in seeking the experience. Such a circuit is hypothesized to have evolved to enable animals to behave in ways that increase survival and reproductive success. The identity of some of the key brain regions comprising the natural reward circuit was originally discovered by Olds and Milner in 1954 (Olds & Milner, 1954) using electrodes placed in the brains of rats performing an operant task to deliver mild electric shocks in the region where the electrode was placed. They discovered that a rat would repeatedly press the lever to self-administer shocks when the electrode was placed at many different regions throughout the brain. However, when the electrode was placed anywhere near the medial forebrain bundle, a group of axons connecting the septal area, lateral hypothalamus, nucleus accumbens, and ventral tegmental area (VTA) of the brain, the effect was particularly pronounced, oftentimes resulting in the animals forgoing food and water in order to continue lever-pressing. The interpretation was that electrical activation of the medial forebrain bundle results in perception of pleasure similar to but on a much larger scale compared to physiological activation produced by natural rewards such as food and sex.

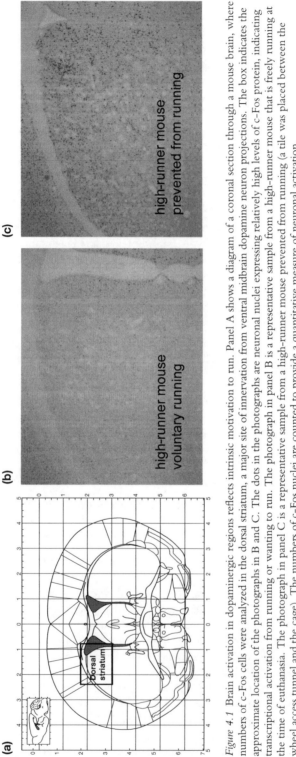

Figure 4.1 Brain activation in dopaminergic regions reflects intrinsic motivation to run. Panel A shows a diagram of a coronal section through a mouse brain, where numbers of c-Fos cells were analyzed in the dorsal striatum, a major site of innervation from ventral midbrain dopamine neuron projections. The box indicates the approximate location of the photographs in B and C. The dots in the photographs are neuronal nuclei expressing relatively high levels of c-Fos protein, indicating transcriptional activation from running or wanting to run. The photograph in panel B is a representative sample from a high-runner mouse that is freely running at the time of euthanasia. The photograph in panel C is a representative sample from a high-runner mouse prevented from running (a tile was placed between the wheel access tunnel and the cage). The numbers of c-Fos nuclei are counted to provide a quantitative measure of neuronal activation.

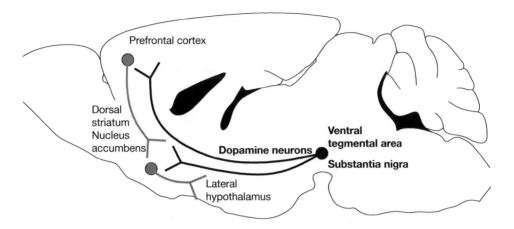

Figure 4.2 The natural reward circuit. A sagittal section of a mouse brain illustrating the location of the ventral midbrain dopamine neuron cell bodies and major projections to the dorsal striatum, nucleus accumbens, and prefrontal cortex. Interconnections with the lateral hypothalamus are shown for reference with the text. Many other brain regions contribute to the natural reward circuit. The full collection is arguably most of the brain. This is not surprising given the importance of the circuit for motivating animals to behave in ways that increase survival and reproductive success.

The VTA is one of the two main locations in the brain where neurons are located that synthesize and release dopamine, and the projection of dopamine neurons from the VTA to the nucleus accumbens is considered a key component, or final common pathway, involved in the perception of reward and reinforcement. All drugs of abuse with diverse mechanisms of action, including ethanol, cocaine, heroin, nicotine, and marijuana, and natural rewards such as food and sex increase dopamine in extracellular spaces in the nucleus accumbens (Damsma, Pfaus, Wenkstern, Phillips, & Fibiger, 1992; Doyon et al., 2003; Hernandez & Hoebel, 1988; Nisell, Nomikos, & Svensson, 1994; Tanda, Pontieri, & Di Chiara, 1997). For a long time, these findings, among many others, led to the belief that dopamine was the neurochemical substrate for reward. However, it is now established and well appreciated that dopamine plays a much more complicated role in the brain than simply acting as the reward substrate (Salamone, Correa, Mingote, & Weber, 2005). Many other stimuli that produce strong aversion or the opposite of pleasure, such as pain or stress, also induce dopamine release into the nucleus accumbens (Scott, Heitzeg, Koeppe, Stohler, & Zubieta, 2006). Moreover, dopamine has diverse functions in the brain depending on the environmental context and neuroanatomical region.

As mentioned above, dopamine projections from the VTA to the nucleus accumbens are thought to play an important role in reward and reinforcement. The VTA also makes more diffuse projections to the prefrontal and cingulate cortices and these connections, together with the accumbens, are referred to as the mesolimbic dopamine reward pathway. It is rather unfortunate that the pathway is referred to as the reward pathway because it could just as well be referred to as the aversion pathway. Rather than playing a specific role in reward, the current understanding is that dopamine in the mesolimbic circuit acts as a salience detector (Horvitz, 2000). In other words, dopamine is important for the animal to evaluate the relative importance of the stimulus for survival or reproductive success. A sudden approach of a predator that threatens the animal's life is a salient event, even more salient than finding a large meal after going hungry for several days, and both will involve dopamine release and reinforcement learning.

By acting as a salience detector, dopamine plays a pivotal role in reinforcement. This is most easily illustrated with an example. In a series of pioneering studies, Wolfram Schultz recorded the discharge of dopamine cells located in the VTA while a monkey was performing a task to obtain a juice reward (as reviewed in Schultz, 2007). What Shultz discovered is that initially, before the monkey learned the task, dopamine discharges occurred during the receipt of the unpredicted rewards. But as the monkey learned the task, the dopamine discharges began to occur in response to the cues that predicted the reward rather than from the reward itself. Moreover, if the reward was not received as expected, then depressions in discharges were observed (Fiorillo, Tobler, & Schultz, 2003). These observations are consistent with a role for dopamine in learning appropriate behaviors and associations in response to salient stimuli, in this case a juice reward.

The other main location in the brain, besides the VTA, where dopamine cell bodies reside is the substantia nigra pars compacta. The projection of dopamine neurons to the dorsal striatum, known as the nigrostriatal pathway, is part of the basal ganglia circuit that mediates the coordination of locomotor function. Loss of dopamine neurons in the nigrostriatal pathway causes Parkinson's disease and erratic, uncoordinated motor behavior. The nigrostriatal pathway is also thought to play a key role in the natural reward circuit, specifically integrating information about rewarding or aversive experiences, making decisions, and coordinating goal-directed movement toward or away from salient experiences (Wise, 2009).

A very important unresolved question is how the reward circuit is modified by experiences to produce strong reinforcement learning and compulsive behavior, as in the case of addiction or dependence. Another important unresolved question is how the reward circuit develops or functions differently to predispose individuals to engage in specific behaviors caused by genetic and/or environmental factors. The same brain regions and neurochemicals implicated in addiction are thought to be components of the natural reward circuit, and the specific differences in the circuit (e.g., more or fewer dopamine receptors of one or several types, neuroanatomical distribution, differences in numerous second messengers involved in dopamine signaling cascade, etc.) that make an animal motivated for one behavior (e.g., physical activity) versus another (e.g., drug abuse) are not known. Discovering the specificity in the neural circuits involved in drug abuse and addiction versus motivation for natural rewards is an important area for future research because it will help define the neurobiology of compulsive maladaptive behavior as compared to healthy behavior, and potentially identify useful targets for pharmacotherapy.

Dopamine signaling in physical activity reward

Given that physical activity can be inherently rewarding in animals and humans, and given the extensive literature on the role of the dopamine neurotransmitter system in reward, reinforcement, and the voluntary control of movement, it is not surprising that dopamine signaling appears to play a role in physical activity reward. Microdialysis studies, where extracellular fluid from the nucleus accumbens and dorsal striatum was sampled and analyzed for dopamine and dopamine metabolite concentrations during forced treadmill running at a variety of speeds, have been conducted in rats (for a review see Table II in Meeusen, Piacentini, & De Meirleir, 2001). The extracellular fluid was analyzed using high-performance liquid chromatography to quantify concentrations of dopamine and metabolites. It appears that a threshold speed is needed somewhere between 3 and 7 m/min for rats, but at or above this speed, dopamine concentrations in extracellular spaces increase above resting levels. Moreover, dopamine turnover, as measured by accumulation of dopamine metabolites (DOPAC and HVA) in extracellular spaces, increases linearly with the speed of running (Hattori, Naoi, & Nishino, 1994). As discussed in the previous sections, increased extracellular dopamine does not necessarily imply reward. Dopamine signaling in the nucleus accumbens or dorsal striatum could reflect voluntary control of movement. Moreover, the dopamine signaling could simply reflect the salient experience of forced running that would occur regardless of whether the experience was perceived as aversive or rewarding.

Although the rodent animal literature consistently reports increased extracellular dopamine from treadmill running, the human literature is less consistent. A recent study conducted in humans using positron emission tomography (PET) to non-invasively quantify extracellular dopamine in the striatum found no evidence that synaptic dopamine concentrations changed in response to 30 minutes of treadmill running at a moderate intensity (approximately 10 km/hr) (Wang et al., 2000). However, the PET technique to quantify dopamine and other molecules in the rat studies is very different from microdialysis. Rather than directly measuring dopamine and metabolites from extracellular fluid in the brain, the PET method uses non-invasive imaging of radio-labeled raclopride, a dopamine D2-receptor antagonist, which is injected intravenously into the subject to estimate the magnitude of binding to D2 receptors. The theory is that raclopride will compete with endogenous dopamine for D2 receptors, and hence, if extracellular dopamine increases after exercise, it can be detected by measuring proportional decreases in binding of raclopride. A major limitation of the PET method is that receptor binding could also be influenced by changes in dopamine receptors on cellular membranes, which can be transported to and from the cytoplasm in response to local concentrations of extracellular dopamine (Dumartin et al., 2000). However, the evidence suggests that the method works for detecting large changes in extracellular dopamine such as that induced from stimulant drugs that block dopamine uptake. Simultaneous microdialysis and PET imaging studies in nonhuman primates have shown a linear relation between the changes in dopamine induced from stimulant drugs as assessed with microdialysis and those obtained using imaging (Breier et al., 1997; Laruelle et al., 1997). Therefore, the method appears to work for detecting large dopamine fluctuations, but it may be limited for detecting smaller changes such as those induced from running on a treadmill.

Additional evidence that the dopamine neurotransmitter system is involved with motivation for physical activity comes from a study using mice deficient in expression of the Nurr1 gene, a gene involved in the development of midbrain dopamine neurons (Werme et al., 2003). Mice were engineered to carry a null mutation that prevents transcription of Nurr1. Heterozygous mice, deficient in Nurr1 because they carry one copy of the mutation and one copy of an intact Nurr1 gene, were compared to "wild-type" littermates carrying two intact Nurr1 copies in levels of voluntary wheel running displayed over 21 days. The heterozygous Nurr1 deficient mice displayed reduced dopamine levels in the striatum and low levels of wheel running (approximately 2 km/day) compared to their wild-type littermates (approximately 10 km/day). Hence, the authors concluded that dopamine plays a role in motivation for voluntary wheel running behavior because the dopamine deficient mice displayed low levels of running. However, another interpretation is that the dopamine deficiency impaired voluntary control of movement rather than affecting physical activity reward. Given that dopamine is required to control voluntary movement, it is possible that the dopamine deficient mice ran less not because they found physical activity less rewarding than wild-type mice but rather because they were unable to control their movement sufficiently to produce high levels of running. The authors favored the reward hypothesis because the dopamine deficient mice also drank less ethanol than wild-type mice, suggesting that they were less motivated for both natural and drug rewards. They ruled out the possibility that a mild motor impairment could affect ethanol drinking by showing that the dopamine deficiency did not affect intake of a sweetened or bitter solution (see Figure 2A, B in Werme et al., 2003). However, it is possible that drinking is not as difficult a motor task as running on a wheel, and that the mild motor impairment could still have caused the reduced wheel running.

The specificity of dopamine involvement in physical activity reward as compared to a more general role in processing salient experiences or voluntary control of movement is difficult to establish. However, the lines of mice selectively bred for increased voluntary wheel running described above provide additional evidence that seems to tip the balance in favor of the reward hypothesis. In a series of studies, it was demonstrated that the high runners respond very differently to drugs that increase dopamine in extracellular spaces (including methylphenidate, cocaine, and GBR12909). In high-runner lines, these drugs tend to reduce running, whereas at similar doses in control unselected mice, these drugs either had no effect or increased running (Rhodes & Garland, 2003; Rhodes et al., 2001). The difference is particularly striking because the increased distances run in high-runner lines are primarily due to increased speeds of running rather than increased duration of running, and the drugs mainly reduced running speed, not duration. Both control and high-runner mice spend most of the dark cycle running; the high runners just run faster during these running bouts (Girard, McAleer, Rhodes, & Garland, 2001). Hence, by artificially increasing dopamine in extracellular spaces using drugs, it is possible to turn a high runner into an animal that appears more like a mouse from a control unselected line. Methylphenidate data are shown in Figure 4.3A and B to illustrate the general result.

Additional experiments examining the effects of dopamine agonists and antagonists on wheel running behavior in the replicate high-runner and control lines suggest that dopamine signaling via D1-like receptors has likely been altered by selection. Specifically, high-runner mice were significantly less sensitive to the locomotor-reducing effects of dopamine D1-like but not D2-like antagonists. Figure 4.3C and D illustrate the result for the dopamine D1-like antagonist drug SCH23390. At a dose of 0.05 mg/kg, SCH23390 severely reduces wheel running in control unselected mice, whereas it barely has any effect in mice from high-runner lines. No differences were observed between high-runner and control mice in response to the serotonin reuptake inhibitor fluoxetine and the mu-opioid receptor antagonists naloxone and naltrexone. All these drugs dose dependently decreased wheel running to a similar extent in all the lines (Li, Rhodes, Girard, Gammie, & Garland, 2004; Rhodes et al., 2001). Hence, the behavioral pharmacology data specifically identify the dopamine neurotransmitter system as being changed in some way from selection and not the other candidates examined including opioid and serotonin systems.

Our current hypothesis is that specific molecules downstream of dopamine D1-receptors are altered in high-runner mice and that these molecular differences contribute to the altered sensitivity to dopamine drugs and increased motivation for physical activity. We first considered the possibility that dopamine levels or dopamine turnover or metabolism could explain the pharmacology results. However, high runners and controls showed no detectable differences in total dopamine concentrations or dopamine metabolites in the striatum under resting conditions or when forced to run on a treadmill at varying speeds (Rhodes, Gammie, & Garland, 2005). We also considered the possibility that dopamine D1 or D2 receptors were differentially expressed in the striatum. However, no significant differences were detectable using standard radio–ligand binding assays (unpublished data). Therefore, our current hypothesis is that intracellular molecules

Figure 4.3 Dopamine D1-like receptor signaling implicated in high voluntary wheel running behavior. Mean wheel running (revolutions) ± SEM is plotted in 10-min increments 1 h before and 2 h after an injection of either saline or methylphenidate (Ritalin) (30 mg/kg) (n = 24 per data point). Panel A shows data for unselected control lines and panel B for high-runner lines. Methylphenidate increased wheel running in control lines and decreased running in high-runner lines. Panels B and C show the same graphs as A and B except in response to a dopamine D1-like receptor antagonist, SCH 23390. High-runner mice were less sensitive than controls to the behavioral effects of SCH 23390. Panels A–D are redrawn from Rhodes & Garland (2003).

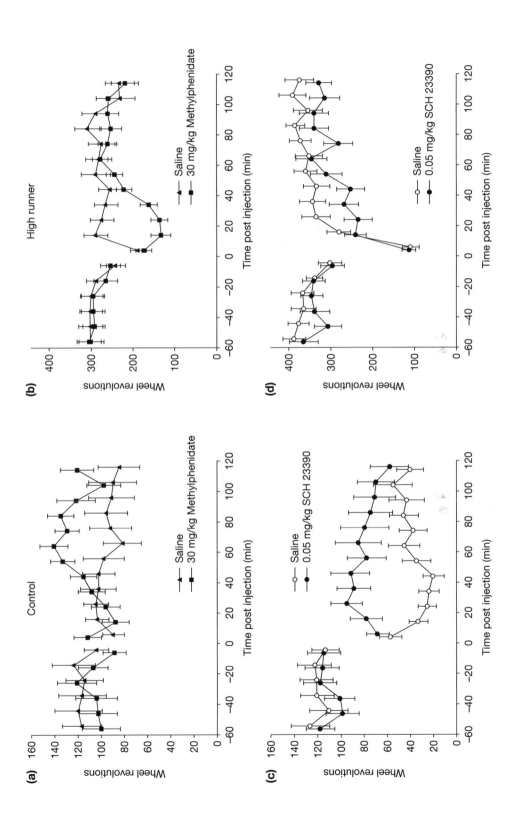

in the dopamine signaling cascade, besides dopamine and its receptors, were the direct targets of selection. The identity of these molecules is currently unknown and is the topic of future investigation. The dopamine signaling system is extraordinarily complex, with numerous molecules including those in the DARPP-32/protein phosphatase-1 cascade (Greengard, Allen, & Nairn, 1999). Many of these molecules are also influenced by receptor signaling from other neurotransmitter systems besides dopamine, such as glutamate, GABA, serotonin, and neuropeptides, thus making them attractive candidates for integrative regulation of brain function.

Future directions

The cumulative evidence that dopamine plays a role in the motivation for physical activity is convincing, but which molecules in the dopamine signaling cascade are critical regulators of physical activity reward remains presently unknown. One of the biggest challenges is identifying specificity of dopamine involvement in behavior. Dopamine is a neuromodulator in the brain with diverse functions. It regulates neuronal activation and signaling between many different types of neurons throughout the brain. Given the complexity of the system, i.e., numerous molecules with different expression patterns in different brain regions, it is not surprising that dopamine signaling serves diverse functions. Discovering which components change to increase voluntary wheel running seems a tractable goal, but will be challenging. A large literature on brain reward circuits implicated in drug abuse has yet to agree on clear molecular mechanisms leading to craving for drugs and addiction. Moreover, the specificity in the neural circuits or molecular components involved in motivation for drugs versus natural rewards and aversive stimuli is not established and will be difficult to determine (Johnson et al., 2010; Zombeck et al., 2008).

One advantage for the physical activity phenotype as compared to the drug models is the availability of the statistically powerful replicated selective breeding experiment for increased voluntary wheel running behavior. It seems plausible to use genomic approaches to identify common patterns of gene expression in brain reward regions under different conditions of voluntary wheel access in the replicate selected and unselected lines. Discovering the molecules and structural changes that are different in animals highly motivated for physical activity could provide new insight into mechanisms of behavior and motivation. Knowledge of how a brain functions to motivate physical activity has broad therapeutic applications in a modern culture where inactivity threatens health and longevity.

References

Belke, T. W., & Wagner, J. P. (2005). The reinforcing property and the rewarding aftereffect of wheel running in rats: A combination of two paradigms. *Behavioural Processes, 68*(2), 165–172.

Boecker, H., Sprenger, T., Spilker, M. E., Henriksen, G., Koppenhoefer, M., Wagner, K. J., . . . Tolle, T. R. (2008). The runner's high: Opioidergic mechanisms in the human brain. *Cerebral Cortex, 18*(11), 2523–2531.

Breier, A., Su, T. P., Saunders, R., Carson, R. E., Kolachana, B. S., de Bartolomeis, A., . . . Pickar, D. (1997). Schizophrenia is associated with elevated amphetamine-induced synaptic dopamine concentrations: Evidence from a novel positron emission tomography method. *Proceedings of the National Academy of Sciences of the United States of America, 94*(6), 2569–2574.

Chen, J., Kelz, M. B., Hope, B. T., Nakabeppu, Y., & Nestler, E. J. (1997). Chronic Fos-related antigens: Stable variants of deltaFosB induced in brain by chronic treatments. *Journal of Neuroscience, 17*(13), 4933–4941.

Clark, P. J., Bhattacharya, T. K., Miller, D. S., & Rhodes, J. S. (2011). Induction of c-Fos, Zif268, and Arc from acute bouts of voluntary wheel running in new and pre-existing adult mouse hippocampal granule neurons. *Neuroscience, 184*, 16–27.

Clark, P. J., Kohman, R. A., Miller, D. S., Bhattacharya, T. K., Brzezinska, W. J., & Rhodes, J. S. (2011). Genetic influences on exercise-induced adult hippocampal neurogenesis across 12 divergent mouse strains. *Genes, Brain and Behavior, 10*(3), 345–353.

Clayton, D. F. (2000). The genomic action potential. *Neurobiology of Learning and Memory, 74*(3), 185–216.

Colcombe, S., & Kramer, A. F. (2003). Fitness effects on the cognitive function of older adults: A meta-analytic study. *Psychological Science, 14*(2), 125–130.

Damsma, G., Pfaus, J. G., Wenkstern, D., Phillips, A. G., & Fibiger, H. C. (1992). Sexual behavior increases dopamine transmission in the nucleus accumbens and striatum of male rats: Comparison with novelty and locomotion. *Behavioral Neuroscience, 106*(1), 181–191.

Doyon, W. M., York, J. L., Diaz, L. M., Samson, H. H., Czachowski, C. L., & Gonzales, R. A. (2003). Dopamine activity in the nucleus accumbens during consummatory phases of oral ethanol self-administration. *Alcoholism: Clinical and Experimental Research, 27*(10), 1573–1582.

Dumartin, B., Jaber, M., Gonon, F., Caron, M. G., Giros, B., & Bloch, B. (2000). Dopamine tone regulates D1 receptor trafficking and delivery in striatal neurons in dopamine transporter-deficient mice. *Proceedings of the National Academy of Science of the United States of America, 97*(4), 1879–1884.

Fiorillo, C. D., Tobler, P. N., & Schultz, W. (2003). Discrete coding of reward probability and uncertainty by dopamine neurons. *Science, 299*(5614), 1898–1902.

Girard, I., McAleer, M. W., Rhodes, J. S., & Garland, T., Jr. (2001). Selection for high voluntary wheel-running increases speed and intermittency in house mice (Mus domesticus). *Journal of Experimental Biology, 204*(Pt 24), 4311–4320.

Greengard, P., Allen, P. B., & Nairn, A. C. (1999). Beyond the dopamine receptor: The DARPP-32/protein phosphatase-1 cascade. *Neuron, 23*(3), 435–447.

Greenwood, B. N., & Fleshner, M. (2011). Exercise, stress resistance, and central serotonergic systems. *Exercise and Sport Sciences Reviews, 39*(3), 140–149.

Greenwood, B. N., Foley, T. E., Le, T. V., Strong, P. V., Loughridge, A. B., Day, H. E., . . . Fleshner, M. (2011). Long-term voluntary wheel running is rewarding and produces plasticity in the mesolimbic reward pathway. *Behavioural Brain Research, 217*(2), 354–362.

Guderley, H., Joanisse, D. R., Mokas, S., Bilodeau, G. M., & Garland, T., Jr. (2008). Altered fibre types in gastrocnemius muscle of high wheel-running selected mice with mini-muscle phenotypes. *Comparative Biochemistry and Physiology – Part B: Biochemistry & Molecular Biology, 149*(3), 490–500.

Hattori, S., Naoi, M., & Nishino, H. (1994). Striatal dopamine turnover during treadmill running in the rat: Relation to the speed of running. *Brain Research Bulletin, 35*(1), 41–49.

Helmrich, S. P., Ragland, D. R., Leung, R. W., & Paffenbarger, R. S., Jr. (1991). Physical activity and reduced occurrence of non-insulin-dependent diabetes mellitus. *New England Journal of Medicine, 325*(3), 147–152.

Hernandez, L., & Hoebel, B. G. (1988). Food reward and cocaine increase extracellular dopamine in the nucleus accumbens as measured by microdialysis. *Life Sciences, 42*(18), 1705–1712.

Horvitz, J. C. (2000). Mesolimbocortical and nigrostriatal dopamine responses to salient non-reward events. *Neuroscience, 96*(4), 651–656.

Iversen, I. H. (1993). Techniques for establishing schedules with wheel running as reinforcement in rats. *Journal of the Experimental Analysis of Behavior, 60*(1), 219–238.

Johnson, Z. V., Revis, A. A., Burdick, M. A., & Rhodes, J. S. (2010). A similar pattern of neuronal Fos activation in 10 brain regions following exposure to reward- or aversion-associated contextual cues in mice. *Physiology & Behavior, 99*(3), 412–418.

Laruelle, M., Iyer, R. N., al-Tikriti, M. S., Zea-Ponce, Y., Malison, R., Zoghbi, S. S., . . . Bradberry, C. W. (1997). Microdialysis and SPECT measurements of amphetamine-induced dopamine release in nonhuman primates. *Synapse, 25*(1), 1–14.

Lett, B. T., Grant, V. L., Byrne, M. J., & Koh, M. T. (2000). Pairings of a distinctive chamber with the aftereffect of wheel running produce conditioned place preference. *Appetite, 34*(1), 87–94.

Li, G., Rhodes, J. S., Girard, I., Gammie, S. C., & Garland, T., Jr. (2004). Opioid-mediated pain sensitivity in mice bred for high voluntary wheel running. *Physiology & Behavior, 83*(3), 515–524.

Malisch, J. L., Breuner, C. W., Kolb, E. M., Wada, H., Hannon, R. M., Chappell, M. A., . . . Garland, T., Jr. (2009). Behavioral despair and home-cage activity in mice with chronically elevated baseline corticosterone concentrations. *Behavior Genetics, 39*(2), 192–201.

Meeusen, R., Piacentini, M. F., & De Meirleir, K. (2001). Brain microdialysis in exercise research. *Sports Medicine, 31*(14), 965–983.

Mondin, G. W., Morgan, W. P., Piering, P. N., Stegner, A. J., Stotesbery, C. L., Trine, M. R., . . . Wu, M. Y. (1996). Psychological consequences of exercise deprivation in habitual exercisers. *Medicine & Science in Sports & Exercise, 28*(9), 1199–1203.

Must, A., Spadano, J., Coakley, E. H., Field, A. E., Colditz, G., & Dietz, W. H. (1999). The disease burden associated with overweight and obesity. *Journal of the American Medical Association, 282*(16), 1523–1529.

Nestler, E. J., Barrot, M., & Self, D. W. (2001). DeltaFosB: A sustained molecular switch for addiction. *Proceedings of the National Academy of Sciences of the United States of America, 98*(20), 11042–11046.

Nestler, E. J., Kelz, M. B., & Chen, J. (1999). DeltaFosB: A molecular mediator of long-term neural and behavioral plasticity. *Brain Research, 835*(1), 10–17.

Nisell, M., Nomikos, G. G., & Svensson, T. H. (1994). Systemic nicotine-induced dopamine release in the rat nucleus accumbens is regulated by nicotinic receptors in the ventral tegmental area. *Synapse, 16*(1), 36–44.

Olds, J., & Milner, P. (1954). Positive reinforcement produced by electrical stimulation of septal area and other regions of rat brain. *Journal of Comparative and Physiological Psychology, 47*(6), 419–427.

Perrotti, L. I., Weaver, R. R., Robison, B., Renthal, W., Maze, I., Yazdani, S., . . . Nestler, E. J. (2008). Distinct patterns of DeltaFosB induction in brain by drugs of abuse. *Synapse, 62*(5), 358–369.

Rezende, E. L., Garland, T., Jr., Chappell, M. A., Malisch, J. L., & Gomes, F. R. (2006). Maximum aerobic performance in lines of Mus selected for high wheel-running activity: Effects of selection, oxygen availability and the mini-muscle phenotype. *Journal of Experimental Biology, 209*(Pt 1), 115–127.

Rhodes, J. S., & Crabbe, J. C. (2005). Gene expression induced by drugs of abuse. *Current Opinion in Pharmacology, 5*(1), 26–33.

Rhodes, J. S., Gammie, S. C., & Garland, T., Jr. (2005). Neurobiology of mice selected for high voluntary wheel running activity. *Integrative and Comparative Biology, 45*, 438–455.

Rhodes, J. S., & Garland, T. (2003). Differential sensitivity to acute administration of Ritalin, apomorphine, SCH 23390, but not raclopride in mice selectively bred for hyperactive wheel-running behavior. *Psychopharmacology (Berlin), 167*(3), 242–250.

Rhodes, J. S., Garland, T., Jr., & Gammie, S. C. (2003). Patterns of brain activity associated with variation in voluntary wheel-running behavior. *Behavioral Neuroscience, 117*(6), 1243–1256.

Rhodes, J. S., Hosack, G. R., Girard, I., Kelley, A. E., Mitchell, G. S., & Garland, T., Jr. (2001). Differential sensitivity to acute administration of cocaine, GBR 12909, and fluoxetine in mice selectively bred for hyperactive wheel-running behavior. *Psychopharmacology (Berlin), 158*(2), 120–131.

Rhodes, J. S., Ryabinin, A. E., & Crabbe, J. C. (2005). Patterns of brain activation associated with contextual conditioning to methamphetamine in mice. *Behavioral Neuroscience, 119*(3), 759–771.

Salamone, J. D., Correa, M., Mingote, S. M., & Weber, S. M. (2005). Beyond the reward hypothesis: Alternative functions of nucleus accumbens dopamine. *Current Opinion in Pharmacology, 5*(1), 34–41.

Schultz, W. (2007). Behavioral dopamine signals. *Trends in Neurosciences, 30*(5), 203–210.

Scott, D. J., Heitzeg, M. M., Koeppe, R. A., Stohler, C. S., & Zubieta, J. K. (2006). Variations in the human pain stress experience mediated by ventral and dorsal basal ganglia dopamine activity. *Journal of Neuroscience, 26*(42), 10789–10795.

Swallow, J. G., Carter, P. A., & Garland, T., Jr. (1998). Artificial selection for increased wheel-running behavior in house mice. *Behavior Genetics, 28*(3), 227–237.

Swallow, J. G., Garland, T., Jr., Carter, P. A., Zhan, W. Z., & Sieck, G. C. (1998). Effects of voluntary activity and genetic selection on aerobic capacity in house mice (Mus domesticus). *Journal of Applied Physiology, 84*(1), 69–76.

Tanda, G., Pontieri, F. E., & Di Chiara, G. (1997). Cannabinoid and heroin activation of mesolimbic dopamine transmission by a common mu1 opioid receptor mechanism. *Science, 276*(5321), 2048–2050.

Vialou, V., Robison, A. J., Laplant, Q. C., Covington, H. E., 3rd, Dietz, D. M., Ohnishi, Y. N., . . . Nestler, E. J. (2010). DeltaFosB in brain reward circuits mediates resilience to stress and antidepressant responses. *Nature Neuroscience, 13*(6), 745–752.

Wang, G. J., Volkow, N. D., Fowler, J. S., Franceschi, D., Logan, J., Pappas, N. R., . . . Netusil, N. (2000). PET studies of the effects of aerobic exercise on human striatal dopamine release. *Journal of Nuclear Medicine, 41*(8), 1352–1356.

Werme, M., Hermanson, E., Carmine, A., Buervenich, S., Zetterstrom, R. H., Thoren, P., . . . Brené, S. (2003). Decreased ethanol preference and wheel running in Nurr1-deficient mice. *European Journal of Neuroscience, 17*(11), 2418–2424.

Werme, M., Messer, C., Olson, L., Gilden, L., Thoren, P., Nestler, E. J., . . . Brené, S. (2002). Delta FosB regulates wheel running. *Journal of Neuroscience, 22*(18), 8133–8138.

Werme, M., Thoren, P., Olson, L., & Brené, S. (2000). Running and cocaine both upregulate dynorphin mRNA in medial caudate putamen. *European Journal of Neuroscience, 12*(8), 2967–2974.

Wise, R. A. (2009). Roles for nigrostriatal—not just mesocorticolimbic—dopamine in reward and addiction. *Trends in Neurosciences, 32*(10), 517–524.

Zombeck, J. A., Chen, G. T., Johnson, Z. V., Rosenberg, D. M., Craig, A. B., & Rhodes, J. S. (2008). Neuroanatomical specificity of conditioned responses to cocaine versus food in mice. *Physiology & Behavior, 93*(3), 637–650.

PART 2

Anxiety disorders

Edited by
Jasper A. J. Smits

5

THE RELATIONSHIP BETWEEN PHYSICAL ACTIVITY AND ANXIETY AND ITS DISORDERS

*Angela C. Utschig, Michael W. Otto, Mark B. Powers,
and Jasper A. J. Smits*

Regular physical activity (PA) is associated with fewer symptoms of anxiety and depression, lower levels of stress, anger, and cynical distrust, as well as better social functioning and vitality among persons with anxiety disorders. In this chapter, we review cross-sectional, longitudinal, and randomized studies that highlight the interplay between PA and anxiety and its disorders. Our aim is to summarize what is known about the PA–anxiety relation with the intent to guide future directions for research in this area.

Physical activity is associated with reduced anxiety in population-based studies

A number of population-based studies support the association between PA and reduced levels of mood and anxiety symptoms (Goodwin, 2003; Hassmen, Koivula, & Uutela, 2000; Stephens, 1988). In a pooled, representative sample of U.S. and Canadian individuals aged 10 to 74 ($N = 55,979$), PA was associated with improved mental health, including fewer symptoms of depression and anxiety, even after controlling for education, social economic status, and physical illness. The link between PA and mental health was strongest among those who were over 40 and female (Stephens, 1988). In another study, Goodwin (2003) examined data from approximately 6,000 individuals (aged 15–54) in the National Comorbidity Survey. The study compared the 12-month prevalence of DSM diagnoses among persons who indicated that they exercised "regularly" (60.3%) to those who exercised occasionally, rarely, or never. Individuals who reported regular PA were significantly less likely to be diagnosed with panic, agoraphobia, social phobia, generalized anxiety disorder (GAD), or specific phobias. These associations did not vary by gender or age and remained significant after controlling for comorbid physical illness and demographic variables.

Ströhle and colleagues (2007) found evidence suggesting that PA may offer protective effects against the onset of anxiety disorders. They assessed a cohort of 2,458 individuals (aged 14–24) for DSM-IV anxiety disorders over a span of four years. Cross-sectional results indicated that those individuals who engaged in regular PA were less likely to meet criteria for DSM-IV psychiatric disorders (particularly anxiety disorders) and less likely to have comorbid conditions compared to those who were inactive (OR = 0.70). Similarly, the longitudinal data showed that participants engaging in regular PA had a lower incidence rate of anxiety disorders compared to those who were inactive (OR = 0.52). This study provides correlational evidence indicating that PA may prospectively reduce the incidence of anxiety disorders.

The hypothesis that PA directly confers protective effects against anxiety disorders was challenged in a population-based study from the Netherlands. De Moor and colleagues (2008) examined leisure time PA and levels of anxiety and depression in a sample of twins (N = 5,952), additional siblings (N =1,249), and parents (N = 1,249). Cross-sectional and longitudinal results revealed a negative association between PA and anxiety in twins. However, when examining the relationship in the context of genetic and environmental factors, genetic correlations were significant, whereas environmental correlations were not, thus suggesting that the association between PA and anxiety disorders may be best explained by overlapping genetic factors. Indeed, heritable tendencies toward avoidance appear to play a role in the onset of anxiety disorders (Arnold, Zai, & Richter, 2004) and may also reduce the likelihood of voluntary leisure time PA (see our discussion of these factors below). Hence, lower rates of PA among those with anxiety disorders may be the result of genetically linked avoidance tendencies. Despite the role of genetics in both lower PA and anxiety, there is good evidence to suggest that programmed exercise can reduce both risk factors for the development of anxiety disorders and anxiety severity once these disorders are developed. Nonetheless, prior to reviewing this evidence, it is important to note that genetic influences may moderate the degree of benefit of these interventions. For example, in a longitudinal study of adolescent girls, PA was protective against depression only for those girls with a genetic variation in brain-derived neurotrophic factor (BDNF; Mata, Thompson, & Gotlib, 2010). More specifically, this genetic variation (Val66Met polymorphism in the BDNF gene) is associated with lower BDNF, and exercise is known to increase BDNF levels (Egan et al., 2003). BDNF is important for brain plasticity, neurogenesis, neuronal survival, and hippocampal function (Egan et al., 2003). Moreover, reduced levels of BDNF are associated with depressed mood, reduced response to CBT, and disturbances in memory (Egan et al., 2003; Lu, 2003). Hence, the Met allele may identify those individuals most likely to achieve affective benefits from PA-related BDNF stimulation (Mata et al., 2010). As such, the role of genetic variants in the effects of exercise on anxiety and mood requires additional study.

Physical activity reduces anxiety reactivity to stressors

Stress has been implicated in the development and maintenance of anxiety disorders (Last, Barlow, & O'Brien, 1984; Kessler, Davis, & Kendler, 1997). Many studies indicate that PA may prepare the body to handle stressors by improving its ability to adapt to such demands (e.g., Brownley et al., 2003; Sothman et al., 1996; Steptoe, Kimbell, & Basford, 1998). For example, Throne and colleagues (2000) randomly assigned firefighters to either a 16-week exercise program (rowing machine for 40 minutes four times per week) or their own continued PA routine (control condition) following initial measurements of heart rate, blood pressure, anxiety, and mood in a simulated fire drill. Following the intervention, the firefighters repeated the simulated fire drill. Those who completed the rowing program showed significantly lower heart rate, blood pressure, state anxiety, and negative affect compared to those in the control condition.

With respect to reducing reactivity to anxiety disorder-relevant stressors, growing evidence suggests that PA offers protective effects (Esquivel, Schruers, Kuipers, & Griez, 2002; Esquivel et al., 2008; Rejeski, Thompson, Brubaker, & Miller, 1992; Smits et al., 2009, 2011; Strohle et al., 2005, 2009). For example, Rejeski and colleagues (1992) compared the effects of a 40-minute bout of aerobic exercise to 40 minutes of quiet rest on responses to psychosocial stress (i.e., interpersonal threat) in low to moderately physically fit women. Participants were counter-balanced to experience both conditions and results suggested that both blood pressure and self-reported anxiety were significantly lower following the psychosocial stressor when participants had engaged in exercise prior to the stressor (Rejeski et al., 1992). Similarly, Esquivel and colleagues (2002) examined the effects of exercise compared to minimal activity prior to a single vital capacity inhalation of 35% CO_2 in healthy adults. Participants who exercised reported significantly fewer panic symptoms compared to those in the minimal activity condition. Consistent with these findings, Smits and colleagues (2009) found less anxious responding among participants who exercised prior to a single vital capacity inhalation of 35% CO_2 compared to those in a quiet rest control condition. Importantly, these effects remained significant after controlling for negative affect and anxiety sensitivity (AS), an established cognitive risk factor for panic and related disorders, as well as fearful responding to CO_2 challenge (McNally, 2002). In a recent follow-up study, these findings were extended to show that the relation between regular exercise and reduced fearful responding to CO_2-enriched air is stronger among individuals with elevated AS than among individuals with normative AS levels, suggesting that the protective effects of regular PA with respect to anxiety vulnerability may be particularly applicable to persons at risk – i.e., those who have elevated AS (Smits et al., 2011).

More relevant to PA as a treatment for anxiety are studies that demonstrate the effects of PA as a buffer to stress in individuals diagnosed with anxiety disorders (Esquivel et al., 2008; Strohle et al., 2009). For example, Strohle and colleagues (2009) examined the effects of 30 minutes of aerobic exercise compared to 30 minutes of rest on panic attacks induced by cholecystokinin tetrapeptide (CCK_4) in individuals with panic disorder and healthy controls. Panic disordered individuals showed increases in somatic symptoms following exercise, but no increases in anxiety compared to control participants. Additionally, those participants with panic disorder who underwent exercise before the CCK_4 challenge were significantly less likely to have a panic attack compared to those who did not exercise (Strohle et al., 2009).

Additional evidence for the anti-panic effects of PA comes from the study of exercise as an intervention for reducing (instead of modulating the effects of) AS (Smits, Berry, Tart, & Powers, 2008b). Specifically, Broman-Fulks and colleagues (2004) randomly assigned participants with high levels of AS (measured with the Anxiety Sensitivity Index; Reiss, Peterson, Gursky, & McNally, 1986) to either six 20-minute high-intensity (60–90% max HR) or six 20-minute low-intensity (below 60% of max HR) exercise sessions. Results revealed that the high-intensity intervention was associated with significantly greater reductions in AS compared to the low-intensity intervention. In a follow-up study, Broman-Fulks and Storey (2008) observed significant reductions in AS following six sessions of aerobic exercise compared to a no-exercise control in participants with high AS. Later work used a similar protocol comparing six 20-minute high-intensity exercise sessions to six sessions of exercise plus cognitive restructuring and a waitlist control in participants with high AS (Smits et al., 2008a). Both exercise conditions were equally efficacious in reducing AS compared to the waitlist condition, suggesting that guiding participants through threat reappraisal may not add to the efficacy of aerobic exercise.

Acute physical activity is followed by reduced anxiety

Research on the effects of acute bouts of PA on anxiety indicates differential effects for aerobic compared to anaerobic (i.e., resistance training) activity. Reductions in state anxiety appear evident immediately and up to 120 minutes following aerobic activity (Bahrke & Morgan, 1978; Hale & Raglin, 2002; Raglin & Wilson, 1996). However, anaerobic activity, especially at high intensities, appears to temporarily increase state anxiety during or immediately following the activity, followed by a slow return to baseline (or lower) over a period of 20 to 60 minutes (Bibeau, Moore, Mitchell, Vargas-Tonsing, & Bartholomew, 2010; Raglin, Turner, & Eksten, 1993).

More recently, research on the acute anxiolytic affects of PA has expanded to include examination of the effect of prescribed versus self-selected intensities for aerobic and anaerobic activity (Focht, 2002; Knapen et al., 2009). Overall, self-selected PA intensity appears as efficacious in reducing anxiety as prescribed intensities; in a qualitative review, Ekkekakis and colleagues (2011) found that acute bouts of exercise, particularly at intensities chosen by participants, are associated with significant reductions in state anxiety (Ekkekakis, Parfitt, & Petruzello, 2011). Knapen and colleagues (2009) examined the effects of 20 minutes of prescribed versus self-selected aerobic exercise in individuals with anxiety and depressive disorders (Knapen et al., 2009). Participants completed three exercise conditions: (1) 50% of maximum heart rate; (2) self-selected intensity with heart rate feedback; and (3) self-selected intensity without heart rate feedback. All three conditions showed pre- to post-exercise reductions in state anxiety and negative affect; heart rate feedback did not influence the response. Additionally, self-selected intensity exercise, regardless of heart rate feedback, resulted in significant increases in well-being and decreases in fatigue. A similar study examining the effects of prescribed versus self-selected resistance exercise or resting condition found comparable results (Focht, 2002). State anxiety was reduced in both the prescribed and self-selected conditions at 5, 20, 60, and 120 minutes following acute exercise in those participants classified as high-state anxiety individuals, while reductions in state anxiety were only seen at 60 and 120 minutes following exercise in the low-state anxiety group (Focht, 2002). Additionally, all participants had significantly higher ratings of perceived exertion in the prescribed exercise condition, compared to the self-selected condition. These findings parallel other work suggesting that exercise (particularly self-selected compared to prescribed intensities) is associated with positive affect (Ekkekakis & Petruzello, 1999) and also extend the literature by providing some insight into the timing of anxiety reduction in high versus low anxious individuals during self-selected intensities. Specifically, the anxiolytic effects of anaerobic PA are greater for persons with higher levels of baseline anxiety compared to those with low levels (Hale & Raglin, 2002); however, individuals with low baseline anxiety show significant anxiety reduction following acute anaerobic activity when the exercise is self-selected and after a considerable post-exercise period (60–120 minutes; Focht, 2002).

Together, these findings suggest that acute bouts of PA are associated with reductions in anxiety, if not immediately, very shortly following the conclusion of activity. However, control groups were not employed in all studies, limiting causal conclusions. Additionally, it remains unclear whether these effects vary as a function of other person variables such as age or gender, or different types of anxiety.

Anxiety symptoms decrease with physical activity training programs

Several recent meta-analyses suggest medium effect sizes for PA interventions in the reduction of anxiety (Conn, 2010; Long & van Stavel, 1995; Petruzzello, Landers, Hatfield, Kubitz, & Salazar, 1991; Wipfli, Rethorst & Landers, 2008). For example, Wipfli and colleagues (2008) found that PA outperformed other active treatments (e.g., CBT, pharmacotherapy) and no-treatment control groups in the treatment of anxiety ($d = .48$ and $d = .19$ respectively). Additionally, Long and van Stavel (1995) found that several factors influenced the relationship between PA and anxiety reduction. First, interventions focusing only on PA were significantly more effective in anxiety reduction ($d = .45$) than those attempting to change other behaviors as well ($d = .01$). Second, supervised PA ($d = .47$) outperformed non-supervised ($d = .09$) interventions. Finally, effect sizes for studies using high-stressed samples (e.g., work, school, social) were significantly larger than those using low-stressed samples ($d =.51$ and .28, respectively; Long & van Stavel, 1995).

With regard to the influence of specific PA parameters, longer duration of the intervention is generally associated with greater reductions in trait anxiety, with the largest effects for those programs that are at least 16 weeks in length ($d = .90$; Petruzzello et al., 1991). Similarly, sessions lasting 21 to 30 minutes provide the most anxiety reduction ($d = .41$; Petruzzello et al., 1991). Analysis of the effect of frequency of PA on anxiety reductions indicates that engaging in PA three to four times per week elicits significantly larger effects than one to two or more than five times per week (Wipfli et al., 2008). Moreover, as indicated in the previous section, the intensity of PA is associated with changes in *positive* affect during and immediately following acute activity, where higher intensities are associated with reduced positive affect (Ekkekakis & Petruzzello, 1999). In non-clinical samples, higher intensity activity relates to greater anxiety reduction in fit compared to unfit individuals, indicating that degree of benefit from high-intensity programs may be moderated by fitness (Ekkekakis & Petruzzello, 1999).

In contrast to findings for acute PA, aerobic and anaerobic training programs appear to yield comparable patterns of anxiety reduction immediately following intervention. Specifically, in healthy adults, both aerobic and anaerobic programs elicit changes in state and trait anxiety immediately following long-term programs, which often range from 10 to 24 weeks in length (Blumenthal, Williams, Needles, & Wallace, 1982; DiLorenzo et al., 1999; Tsutsumi, Don, Zaichowsky, & Delizonna, 1997; Cassilhas, Antunes, Tufik, & de Mello, 2010). Additionally, aerobic programs demonstrate maintenance of anxiety reductions up to 12 months following the intervention (DiLorenzo et al., 1999). Interestingly, a longer-term program (12 weeks) of yoga/tai chi, characterized as an aerobic activity, was associated with significant reductions in trait anxiety and exhaustion and greater improvements in tranquility and revitalization compared to a metabolically matched walking program (Streeter et al., 2010). Thus, both longer-term aerobic and anaerobic programs invoke change in anxiety immediately following the intervention in non-clinical populations, while aerobic programs demonstrate their efficacy up to a year post-program. Importantly, more research is needed to determine the long-term effects of anaerobic activity in clinical and non-clinical populations. Additionally, the beneficial impact of yoga on anxiety and mood symptoms is important for the continued development of PA interventions, as it offers an alternative for individuals who may not be willing or capable of more vigorous or high-impact aerobic exercise.

Clinical trials of physical activity for anxiety disorders are limited in number

Overall, the evidence base for PA as an intervention for anxiety is less developed than that for depression (Stathopoulou, Powers, Berry, Smits, & Otto, 2006). To date, randomized controlled trials investigating the effects of PA interventions in patients with anxiety disorders have included panic disorder, social phobia, and generalized anxiety disorder (GAD; Broocks et al., 1998; Herring, Jacob, Suveg, Dishman, & O'Connor, 2012; Martinsen, Raglin, Hoffart, & Friis, 1998). Open trials have examined PA for obsessive-compulsive disorder (OCD) and post-traumatic stress disorder (PTSD; Brown et al., 2007; Manger & Motta, 2005). In general, evidence suggests that PA is associated with significant reductions in specific anxiety disorder symptoms, as well as more general anxiety. For example, Broocks and colleagues (1998) examined the efficacy of aerobic exercise relative to clomipramine and pill placebo in patients with panic disorder. Patients randomized to the exercise condition engaged in a 10-week aerobic endurance-training program. Results suggested that clomipramine was significantly more effective at reducing anxiety symptoms after four weeks of treatment compared to placebo, while exercise was significantly more effective than placebo after 10 weeks. Both treatments resulted in equal reductions in anxiety and outperformed placebo at post-treatment; however, clomipramine yielded greater changes in global improvement ratings compared to exercise.

Examining a broader range of disorders, Martinsen and colleagues (1998) compared an aerobic exercise condition to an anaerobic exercise condition among in-patient participants with panic disorder with agoraphobia, social phobia, or GAD. Both eight-week exercise conditions showed similar post-treatment improvements in anxiety, while only aerobic exercise was associated with greater improvements in physical fitness (Martinsen et al., 1998). This indicates that cardio-respiratory fitness may not account for the effectiveness of exercise programs in reducing pathological anxiety. Similarly, exercise (150 minutes of moderate intensity per week), in combination with group CBT, resulted in significantly reduced symptoms of depression, stress, and anxiety among patients with panic disorder, social phobia, and GAD, compared to group CBT alone (Merom et al., 2008). Likewise, in a small feasibility study, patients with GAD achieved significantly greater reductions in worry symptoms following six weeks of resistance or aerobic exercise training as compared to a wait list control (Herring et al., 2012).

PA interventions have also gained some support for their beneficial impact on symptoms of OCD and PTSD. For example, patients with OCD who engaged in a 12-week moderate-intensity aerobic group program in conjunction with regular care showed significant reductions in Y-BOCS scores from pre- to post-treatment and at a 6-month follow-up (Brown et al., 2007). Moreover, clinically meaningful changes were observed for 69% and 50% of patients at post-treatment and six-month follow up, respectively. Patients also reported improvement in overall sense of well-being after the 12-week intervention (Brown et al., 2007). Additional analyses to determine the acute effects of exercise on symptoms of anxiety, obsessions, and compulsions suggested medium to large effects for reductions in pre- to post-exercise on all three variables at week one and small effects for all three factors at week 12 (Abrantes et al., 2009). These findings suggest that exercise provided the greatest reductions in symptoms earlier in treatment, offering initial support for the utility of exercise as an inexpensive and effective brief treatment for anxiety.

Similarly, exercise interventions may be useful for reduction of PTSD symptoms (Diaz & Motta, 2008; Manger & Motta, 2005; Newman & Motta, 2007). A study investigating the effects of five weeks of speed walking on symptoms of anxiety and PTSD in a sample of adolescents suggested that over 90% of participants reported significant reductions in PTSD immediately following the intervention and at one month follow-up (Diaz & Motta, 2008). Additionally, over 50% of participants reported significant reductions in general anxiety. Although these early findings are promising, the lack of a control group makes solid conclusions difficult to draw.

Further investigation is needed to determine the level of benefit for specific anxiety disorders, including PTSD and OCD. This additional research may also help to clarify the mechanisms through which PA reduces anxiety. Additionally, more work needs to be done to clarify potential moderators of the relationship between PA and anxiety reduction. That is, does the efficacy of PA for anxiety disorders vary as a function of certain dispositional variables such as genetic factors, as discussed earlier, or dispositional variables such as cardiorespiratory fitness, gender, and age? Similarly, future work investigating the timing of treatment effects (i.e., when changes actually occur) will lend insight into development of interventions that provide optimal effects in the most efficient manner.

There also remains a paucity of research on the dose-response relationship of PA and anxiety reduction. One criticism of PA research is that no studies have examined the *combined* effect of varying intensity, duration, and frequency of exercise (Dunn, Trivedi, & O'Neal, 2001). Most research comes from quantitative analyses of numerous studies providing some information, yet a clear picture of a dose-response relationship is still lacking. When looking at the available research, it seems that consistent exercise, in line with current public health recommendations

(USDHHS, 2008), seems to be a good starting point. This type of long-term exercise will likely be beneficial for reductions in overall stress and anxiety over time, while more intense interventions, using PA as an interoceptive technique (e.g., Smits et al., 2008a), may be necessary to drive changes in more specific symptoms, such as those associated with panic disorder (i.e., AS). Ekkekakis and colleagues (2011) further highlighted that intensity of exercise was inversely related to affective response, such that higher intensity produces more negative affect. Given the promising findings on the use of self-selected intensity activity, additional research on this topic will likely provide useful information on whether a dose–response relationship is indeed present, or whether reductions in anxiety are moderated by other variables (e.g., level of anxiety, fitness level, health-related factors such as body mass index (BMI)). Together, such research will help determine the clinical utility of PA interventions for the anxiety disorders.

Anxiety may result in physical *in*activity

Thus far, we have reviewed data suggesting that PA may prevent or reduce symptoms of anxiety. We now turn to work indicating that anxiety may reduce PA. Anxiety may contribute to physical inactivity through several proposed mechanisms. First, individuals with significant anxiety, particularly AS, generally find PA aversive. One theory attempting to explain variability in affective responses to PA is the dual-mode theory, which posits that two factors, cognitive appraisals and interoceptive cues, interact to generate an affective response (Ekkekakis, 2003). Specifically, when individuals exercise at intensities at or around their ventilatory threshold (VT) or lactate threshold (LT), the affective response is thought to be driven mainly by cognitive appraisals of the exercise experience, whereas exercise that exceeds one's VT/LT, by definition being much more strenuous, will be driven more by interoceptive cues (e.g., racing heart, trouble breathing), resulting in more negative affect, especially for individuals with heightened sensitivity to these cues (e.g., high AS). Research examining affective states during exercise supports these hypotheses (Lind, Joens-Matre, & Ekkekakis, 2005; Parfitt, Rose, & Burgess, 2006; Rose & Parfitt, 2007, 2008). For example, in a study comparing affective responses to exercise at intensities below LT, above LT, and self-selected intensity, affect was least positive in the above LT condition and most positive in the low LT and self-selected conditions (Rose & Parfitt, 2007). Moreover, perceptions of exercise ability, interpretation of exercise intensity, and perceptions of control influenced positive affective responses (Rose & Parfitt, 2007).

Additional research suggests that individuals choose to exercise at intensities around or at their VT/LT, and the intensity is increased over the duration of the exercise session, while affective responses remain stable and positive (Lind et al., 2005; Rose & Parfitt, 2007, 2008). Data also support a decline in affect during exercise above VT, which may be related to the experience of intense interoceptive cues, creating a negative affective message from the body (Ekkekakis, 2003; Rose & Parfitt, 2007). This decline in affect over VT threshold seems to be especially true among overweight/obese individuals (Ekkekakis, Lind, & Vazou, 2010). Interestingly, overweight individuals report more negative affect when exercise intensity is prescribed, rather than self-imposed, compared to normal-weight individuals. Obese individuals also tend to rate both perceived exertion and breathlessness intensity higher than those who are normal weight (Ekkekakis & Lind, 2006; Ofir et al., 2007). Thus, PA interventions, especially in individuals with intolerance for physiological sensations (i.e., high AS and panic disorder) as well as overweight/obese individuals, should work to reduce this intolerance during the early phase of exercise to improve the likelihood of positive affect during and immediately following exercise and ultimately facilitate the maintenance of a long-term PA program, similar to those interventions targeting anxiety sensitivity (Smits et al., 2008b).

Research examining physical inactivity and AS has expanded to determine whether other factors, such as BMI, may play a role in this relationship. Specifically, when examining the relationship between AS, BMI, and exercise following randomization to either a 20-minute bout of aerobic exercise or 20 minutes of quiet rest, results indicated that fear was highest among individuals with high BMIs, but only when they also had elevated AS (Smits, Tart, Presnell, Rosenfield, & Otto, 2010). Moreover, the relationship between BMI and AS did not predict levels of fear in those individuals in the quiet rest condition (Smits et al., 2010). Overall, these findings suggest that elevated AS may play an essential role in physical inactivity in those who are more likely to experience exertion-related symptoms as a result of excessive weight.

In addition to AS, social physique anxiety (SPA), described as an individual's anxiety regarding others' evaluation of physical appearance (Hart, Leary, Rejeski, 1989), may influence the relationship between PA and anxiety. High SPA is associated with reduced PA (e.g., Atalay & Gençöz, 2008; Lantz, Hardy, & Ainsworth, 1997), is more common among adolescent and young adult females (Hayes, Crocker & Kowalski, 1999; Hart et al., 1989), and correlates directly with body weight, such that overweight/obese individuals report higher levels of SPA (Spink, 1992). In a study examining the affective responses to increasing levels of exercise intensity in normal-weight, overweight, and obese women, Ekkekakis and colleagues (2010) found that SPA was negatively related to pleasure during exercise for obese women, but not for normal-weight or overweight women. Interestingly, this association was only significant at intensities near VT, not at low or maximal intensities. Given that individuals with high SPA may avoid exercise to avoid negative evaluation of their physical appearance, at low intensities, overweight/obese individuals may not have been concerned with evaluation from others because they were likely able to maintain their composure and pace, and at maximal intensity they may have been more concerned with the interoceptive cues of exercise, making SPA less salient. In an attempt to reduce SPA, Lindwall and Lindgren (2005) investigated changes in SPA over the course of a six-month exercise intervention compared to waitlist control among sedentary adolescent females. Following the intervention, those girls in the exercise condition demonstrated significant reductions in SPA compared to those in the control condition (Lindwall & Lindgren, 2005). Interestingly, SPA levels increased among those in the waitlist condition after the six-month timeframe.

Conclusions and future directions

The literature examining the relationship between PA and anxiety and its disorders continues to expand. Overall, the findings are that PA is beneficial for most anxiety, most of the time. More specifically, PA reduces existing anxiety and appears to be associated with lower risk of developing an anxiety disorder. Conversely, anxiety disorders are associated with reduced PA, indicating that the PA–anxiety relation may be bidirectional.

There is still a relative dearth of research examining PA (aerobic or anaerobic) as an intervention for individuals with anxiety disorders. More research is also needed on the dose-response relationship between PA and anxiety. Here, it is important that the influence of exercise dose parameters (intensity, duration, frequency) or exercise modality on anxiety may very well vary by individual difference variables such as AS, SPA, and BMI (Ekkekakis & Lind, 2006; Ekkekakis et al., 2010; Smits et al., 2010).

Research also suggests there may be benefits of self-selected over prescribed exercise intensities in both anxiety reduction and PA adoption and maintenance. Recent work demonstrates that individuals typically pick intensities at or around their VT when given the opportunity to self-select and generally see higher levels of positive affect than those who are prescribed the same intensities (Rose & Parfitt, 2007, 2008). One course for additional research is to examine how self-selected intensities endure in longer-term interventions, rather than acute exercise bouts. Moreover, work investigating the role of self-selected intensity in clinical anxiety populations needs to be established. Combining self-selected intensity research with research on frequency and duration of PA will provide more definitive answers to the dose-response question, providing information relevant to achieving maximal anxiety reduction and maintenance of PA. As discussed by Ekkekakis (in press), further elucidation of factors affecting the enjoyment of exercise, and applying this information to exercise prescriptions, represents a major growth area for exercise science.

References

Abrantes, A. M., Strong, D. R., Cohn, A., Cameron, A. Y., Greenberg, B. D., Mancebo, M. C., & Brown, R. A. (2009). Acute changes in obsessions and compulsions following moderate-intensity aerobic exercise among patients with obsessive-compulsive disorder. *Journal of Anxiety Disorders, 23*(7), 923–927. doi:10.1016/j.janxdis.2009.06.008

Arnold, P. D., Zai, G., & Richter, M. A. (2004). Genetics of anxiety disorders. *Current Psychiatry Reports, 6*, 243–254.

Atalay, A., & Gençöz, T. (2008). Critical factors of social physique anxiety: Exercising and body image satisfaction. *Behaviour Change, 25*(3), 178–188. doi:10.1375/bech.25.3.178

Bahrke, M. S., & Morgan, W. P. (1978). Anxiety reduction following exercise and meditation. *Cognitive Therapy and Research, 2*, 323–333.

Bibeau, W. S., Moore, J. B., Mitchell, N. G., Vargas-Tonsing, T., & Bartholomew, J. B. (2010). Effects of acute resistance training of different intensities and rest periods on anxiety and affect. *Journal of Strength & Conditioning Research, 24*(8), 2184–2191.

Blumenthal, J. A., Williams, R. S., Needels, T. L., & Wallace, A. G. (1982). Psychological changes accompany aerobic exercise in healthy middle-aged adults. *Psychosomatic Medicine, 44*, 529–536.

Broman-Fulks, J. J., Berman, M. E., Rabian, B. A., & Webster, M. J. (2004). Effects of aerobic exercise on anxiety sensitivity. *Behaviour Research and Therapy, 42*(2), 125–136.

Broman-Fulks, J. J., & Storey, K. M. (2008). Evaluation of a brief aerobic exercise intervention for high anxiety sensitivity. *Anxiety, Stress & Coping: An International Journal, 21*(2), 117–128. doi:10.1080/10615800701762675

Broocks, A., Bandelow, B., Pekrun, G., George, A., Meyer, T., Bartmann, U., Hillmer-Vogel, U., & Ruther, E. (1998). Comparison of aerobic exercise, clomipramine, and placebo in the treatment of panic disorder. *American Journal of Psychiatry, 155*(5), 603–609.

Brown, R. A., Abrantes, A. M., Strong, D. R., Mancebo, M. C., Menard, J., Rasmussen, S. A., & Greenberg, B. D. (2007). A pilot study of moderate-intensity aerobic exercise for obsessive compulsive disorder. *Journal of Nervous and Mental Disease, 195*(6), 514–520. doi:10.1097/01.nmd.0000253730.31610.6c

Brownley, K. A., Hinderliter, A. L., West, S. G., Girdler, S. S., Sherwood, A., & Light, K. C. (2003). Sympathoadrenergic mechanisms in reduced hemodynamic stress responses after exercise. *Medical Science Sports and Exercise, 35*, 978–986.

Cassilhas, R. C., Antunes, H. K., Tufik, S., & de Mello, M. T. (2010). Mood, anxiety and serum IGF-1 in elderly men given 24 weeks of high resistance exercise. *Perceptual and Motor Skills, 110*, 265–276.

Conn, V. S. (2010). Depressive symptom outcomes of physical activity interventions: Meta-analysis finding. *Annals of Behavioral Medicine, 39*, 128–138.

De Moor, M. H., Boosma, D. I., Stubbe, J. H., Willemsen, G., & Geus, E. J. (2008). Testing causality in the association between regular exercise and symptoms of anxiety and depression. *Archives of General Psychiatry, 65*, 897–905.

Diaz, A. B., & Motta, R. (2008). The effects of an aerobic exercise program on posttraumatic stress disorder symptom severity in adolescents. *International Journal of Emergency Mental Health, 10*(1), 49–60.

DiLorenzo, T. M., Bargman, E. P., Stucky-Ropp, R., Brassington, G. S., Frensch, P. A., & LaFontaine, T. (1999). Long-term effects of aerobic exercise on psychological outcomes. *Preventive Medicine: An International Journal Devoted to Practice and Theory, 28*(1), 75–85. doi:10.1006/pmed.1998.0385

Dunn, A. L., Trivedi, M. H., & O'Neal, H. A. (2001). Physical activity dose-response effects on outcomes of depression and anxiety. *Medicine & Science in Sports & Exercise, 33*(6, Suppl), S587–S597. doi:10.1097/00005768-200106001-00027

Egan, M. F., Kojima, M., Callicott, J. H., Goldberg, T. E., Kolachana, B. S., Bertolino, A., . . . Weinberger, D. R. (2003) The BDNF Val66met polymorphism affects activity-dependent secretion of BDNF and human memory and hippocampal function. *Cell*, *112*, 257–269.

Ekkekakis, P. (in press). Redrawing the model of the exercising human in exercise prescriptions: From headless manikin to a creature with feelings! In J. M. Rippe (Ed.), *Lifestyle medicine* (2nd ed.). Hoboken, NJ: Wiley-Blackwell.

Ekkekakis, P. (2003). Pleasure and displeasure from the body: Perspectives from exercise. *Cognition and Emotion*, *17*, 213–239.

Ekkekakis, P. P., & Lind, E. E. (2006). Exercise does not feel the same when you are overweight: The impact of self-selected and imposed intensity on affect and exertion. *International Journal of Obesity*, *30*, 652–660. doi:10.1038/sj.ijo.0803052

Ekkekakis, P., Lind, E., & Vazou, S. (2010). Affective responses to increasing levels of exercise intensity in normal-weight, overweight, and obese middle-aged women. *Obesity*, *18*(1), 79–85. doi:10.1038/oby.2009.204

Ekkekakis, P., Parfitt, G., & Petruzzello, S. J. (2011). The pleasure and displeasure people feel when they exercise at different intensities: Decennial update and progress towards a tripartite rationale for exercise intensity prescription. *Sports Medicine*, *41*, 641–671.

Ekkekakis, P., & Petruzzello, S. J. (1999). Acute aerobic exercise and affect: Current status, problems and prospects regarding dose-response. *Sports Medicine*, *28*(5), 337–374.

Esquivel, G., Diaz-Galvis, J., Schruers, K., Berlanga, C., Lara-Munoz, C., & Griez, E. (2008). Acute exercise reduces the effects of a 35% CO2 challenge in patients with panic disorder. *Journal of Affective Disorders*, *107*, 217–220.

Esquivel, G., Schruers, K., Kuipers, H., & Griez, E. (2002). The effects of acute exercise and high lactate levels on 35% CO2 challenge in healthy volunteers. *Acta Psychiatrica Scandinavica*, *106*(5), 394–397.

Focht, B. C. (2002). Pre-exercise anxiety and the anxiolytic responses to acute bouts of self-selected and prescribed intensity resistance exercise. *Journal of Sports Medicine and Physical Fitness*, *42*, 217–223.

Goodwin, R. D. (2003). Association between physical activity and mental disorders among adults in the United States. *Preventive Medicine*, *36*(6), 698–703.

Hale, B. S., & Raglin, J. S. (2002). State anxiety responses to acute resistance training and step aerobic exercise across eight weeks of training. *Journal of Sports Medicine and Physical Fitness*, *42*, 108–112.

Hart, E. A., Leary, M. R., & Rejeski, W. (1989). The measurement of social physique anxiety. *Journal of Sport and Exercise Psychology*, *11*(1), 94–104.

Hassmen, P., Koivula, N., & Uutela, A. (2000). Physical exercise and psychological well-being: A population study in Finland. *Preventive Medicine*, *30*(1), 17–25.

Hayes, S. D., Crocker, P. E., & Kowalski, K. C. (1999). Gender differences in physical self-perceptions, global self-esteem and physical activity: Evaluation of the physical self-perception profile model. *Journal of Sport Behavior*, *22*(1), 1–14. Retrieved from EBSCOhost.

Herring M. P., Jacob, M. L., Suveg, C., Dishman, R. K., O'Connor, P. J. (2012). Feasibility of exercise training for the short-term treatment of generalized anxiety disorder: A randomized controlled trial. *Psychotherapy and Psychosomatics*, *81*(1), 21–28.

Kessler, R. C., Davis, C. G., & Kendler, K. S. (1997). Childhood adversity and adult psychiatric disorder in the US National Comorbidity Survey. *Psychological Medicine*, *27*(5), 1101–1119.

Knapen, J., Sommerijns, E., Vancampfort, D., Sienaert, P., Pietersm G., Haake, P. et al. (2009). State anxiety and subjective well-being responses to acute bouts of aerobic exercise in patients with depressive and anxiety disorders. *British Journal of Sports Medicine*, *43*, 756–759.

Lantz, C. D., Hardy, C. J., & Ainsworth, B. E. (1997). Social physique anxiety and perceived exercise behavior. *Journal of Sport Behavior*, *20*(1), 83–93.

Last, C. G., Barlow, D. H., & O'Brien, G. T. (1984). Cognitive changes during in vivo exposure in an agoraphobic. *Behavior Modification*, *8*, 93–113. doi:10.1177/01454455840081006

Lind, E., Joens-Matre, R. R., & Ekkekakis, P. (2005). What intensity of physical activity do previously sedentary middle-aged women select? Evidence of a coherent pattern from physiological, perceptual, and affective markers. *Preventive Medicine*, *40*, 407–419.

Lindwall, M., & Lindgren, E. (2005). The effects of a 6-month exercise intervention programme on physical self-perceptions and social physique anxiety in non-physically active adolescent Swedish girls. *Psychology of Sport and Exercise*, *6*(6), 643–658. doi:10.1016/j.psychsport.2005.03.003

Long, B. C., & van Stavel, R. (1995). Effects of exercise training on anxiety: A meta-analysis. *Journal of Applied Sport Psychology*, *7*(2), 167–189.

Lu, B. (2003). BDNF and activity-dependent synaptic modulation. *Learning and Memory, 10*, 86–98.

Manger, T. A., & Motta, R. W. (2005). The impact of an exercise program on posttraumatic stress disorder, anxiety, and depression. *International Journal of Emergency Mental Health, 7*(1), 49–57.

Martinsen, E. W., Raglin, J. S., Hoffart, A., & Friis, S. (1998). Tolerance to intensive exercise and high levels of lactate in panic disorder. *Journal of Anxiety Disorders, 12*(4), 333–342.

Mata, J., Thompson, R. J., & Gotlib, I. H. (2010). BDNF genotype moderates the relation between physical activity and depressive symptoms. *Health Psychology, 29*, 130–133.

McNally, R. J. (2002). Anxiety sensitivity and panic disorder. *Biological Psychiatry, 52*(10), 938–946.

Merom, D., Phongsavan, P., Wagner, R., Chey, T., Marnane, C., Steel, Z., . . . Bauman, A. (2008). Promoting walking as an adjunct intervention to group cognitive behavioral therapy for anxiety disorders—A pilot group randomized trial. *Journal of Anxiety Disorders, 22*(6), 959–968. doi:10.1016/j.janxdis.2007.09.010

Newman, C. L., & Motta, R. W. (2007). The effects of aerobic exercise on childhood PTSD, anxiety, and depression. *International Journal of Emergency Mental Health, 9*(2), 133–158.

Ofir, D., Laveneziana, P., Webb, K. A., & O' Donnell, D. E. (2007) Ventilatory and perceptual responses to cycle exercise in obese women. *Journal of Applied Physiology, 102*(6), 2217–2226.

Parfitt, G., Rose, E. A., & Burgess, W. M. (2006). The psychological and physiological responses of sedentary individuals to prescribed and preferred intensity exercise. *British Journal of Health Psychology, 11*: 39–53. PMID: 19186932.

Petruzzello, S. J., Landers, D. M., Hatfield, B. D., Kubitz, K. A., & Salazar, W. (1991). A meta-analysis on the anxiety-reducing effects of acute and chronic exercise. Outcomes and mechanisms. *Sports Medicine, 11*(3), 143–182.

Raglin, J. S., Turner, P. E., & Eksten, F. (1993). State anxiety and blood pressure following 30 min of leg ergometry or weight training. *Medicine and Science in Sports and Exercise, 25*(9), 1044–1048. doi:10.1249/00005768-199309000-00012

Raglin, J. S., & Wilson, M. (1996). State anxiety following 20 minutes of bicycle ergometer exercise at selected intensities. *International Journal of Sports Medicine, 17*, 467–471.

Reiss, S., Peterson, R. A., Gursky, D. M., & McNally, R. J. (1986). Anxiety sensitivity, anxiety frequency and the prediction of fearfulness. *Behaviour Research and Therapy, 24*, 1–8.

Rejeski, W., Thompson, A., Brubaker, P. H., & Miller, H. S. (1992). Acute exercise: Buffering psychosocial stress responses in women. *Health Psychology, 11*(6), 355–362. doi:10.1037/0278-6133.11.6.355

Rose, E. A., & Parfitt, G. (2007). A quantitative analysis and qualitative explanation of the individual differences in affective responses to prescribed and self-selected exercise intensities. *Journal of Sport and Exercise Psychology, 29*, 281–309.

Rose, E. A., & Parfitt, G. (2008). Can the feeling scale be used to regulate exercise intensity? *Medicine and Science in Sports and Exercise, 40*, 1852–1860.

Smits, J. A. J., Berry, A. C., Rosenfield, D., Powers, M. B., Behar, E., & Otto, M. W. (2008a). Reducing anxiety sensitivity with exercise. *Depression and Anxiety, 25*, 689–699.

Smits, J. A. J., Berry, A. C., Tart, C. D., & Powers, M. B. (2008b). The efficacy of cognitive-behavioral interventions for reducing anxiety sensitivity: A meta-analytic review. *Behaviour Research and Therapy, 46*, 1047–1054.

Smits, J. A., Meuret, A. E., Zvolensky, M. J., Rosenfield, D., & Seidel, A. (2009). The effects of acute exercise on CO2 challenge reactivity. *Journal of Psychiatric Research, 43*, 446–454.

Smits, J. A., Tart, C. D., Presnell, K., Rosenfield, D., & Otto, M. W. (2010). Identifying potential barriers to physical activity adherence: Anxiety sensitivity and body mass as predictors of fear during exercise. *Cognitive Behaviour Therapy, 39*(1), 28–36.

Smits, J. J., Tart, C. D., Rosenfield, D., & Zvolensky, M. J. (2011). The interplay between physical activity and anxiety sensitivity in fearful responding to carbon dioxide challenge. *Psychosomatic Medicine, 73*, 498–503.

Sothmann, M. S., Buckworth, J., Claytor, R. P., Cox, R. H., White-Welkley, J. E., & Dishman, R. K. (1996). Exercise training and the cross-stressor adaptation hypothesis. *Exercise and Sport Sciences Reviews, 24*, 267–287.

Spink, K. S. (1992). Relation of anxiety about social physique to location of participation in physical activity. *Perceptual and Motor Skills, 74*(3, Pt 2), 1075–1078. doi:10.2466/PMS.74.4

Stathopoulou, G., Powers, M. B., Berry, A. C., Smits, J. J., & Otto, M. W. (2006). Exercise interventions for mental health: A quantitative and qualitative review. *Clinical Psychology: Science and Practice, 13*, 179–193. doi:10.1111/j.1468-2850.2006.00021

Stephens, T. (1988). Physical activity and mental health in the United States and Canada: Evidence from four population surveys. *Preventive Medicine, 17*(1), 35–47.

Steptoe, A., Kimbell, J., & Basford, P. (1998). Exercise and the experience and appraisal of daily stressors: A naturalistic study. *Journal of Behavioral Medicine, 21*, 363–374.

Streeter, C. C., Whitfield, T. H., Owen, L., Rein, T., Karri, S. K., Yakhkind, A., . . . Jensen, J. (2010). Effects of yoga versus walking on mood, anxiety, and brain GABA levels: A randomized controlled MRS study. *The Journal of Alternative and Complementary Medicine, 16*(11), 1145–1152. doi:10.1089/acm. 2010.0007

Strohle, A., Feller, C., Onken, M., Godemann, F., Heinz, A., & Dimeo, F. (2005). The acute antipanic activity of aerobic exercise. *American Journal of Psychiatry, 162*(12), 2376–2378.

Ströhle, A., Graetz, B., Scheel, M., Wittmann, A., Feller, C., Heinz, A., & Dimeo, F. (2009). The acute antipanic and anxiolytic activity of aerobic exercise in patients with panic disorder and healthy control subjects. *Journal of Psychiatric Research, 43*(12), 1013–1017. doi:10.1016/j.jpsychires.2009.02.004

Ströhle, A., Höfler, M., Pfister, H., Müller, A., Hoyer, J., Wittchen, H., & Lieb, R. (2007). Physical activity and prevalence and incidence of mental disorders in adolescents and young adults. *Psychological Medicine: A Journal of Research in Psychiatry and the Allied Sciences, 37*(11), 1657–1666. doi:10.1017/S003329170 700089X

Tsutsumi, T., Don, B. M., Zaichowsky, L. D., & Delizonna, L. L. (1997). Physical fitness and psychological benefits of strength training in community dwelling older adults. *Applied Human Science, 16*, 257–266.

U.S. Department of Health and Human Services (2008). *2008 Physical Activity Guidelines for Americans.* Retrieved January 22, 2012 from http://www.health.gov/PAGuidelines/pdf/paguide.pdf

Wipfli, B. M., Rethorst, C. D., & Landers, D. M. (2008). The anxiolytic effects of exercise: A meta-analysis of randomized trials and dose-response analysis. *Journal of Sport & Exercise Psychology, 30*(4), 392–410.

6

MECHANISMS UNDERLYING THE RELATIONSHIP BETWEEN PHYSICAL ACTIVITY AND ANXIETY

Human data

Katharina Gaudlitz, Brigitt-Leila von Lindenberger, Elisabeth Zschucke, and Andreas Ströhle

Anxiety disorders are among the most common mental disorders. Overall prevalence of anxiety disorders is high, with a lifetime prevalence of 28.8% and a 12-month prevalence of 18.1% in the United States (Kessler et al., 2005; Kessler, Chiu, Demler, Merikangas, & Walters, 2005) and comparable 12-month prevalences (14%) in European countries (Wittchen et al., 2011).

Among psychiatric disorders, anxiety disorders constitute a particularly high burden for the health care system, since patients suffering from anxiety disorders tend to be high care utilizers (Lépine, 2002). The economic burden includes psychiatric and nonpsychiatric care, emergency care, hospitalization, drug prescription, reduced productivity, absenteeism from work, and suicide (Lépine, 2002).

Population-based studies (Goodwin, 2003; Stephens, 1988) showed that, even after controlling for confounding variables, self-reported levels of physical activity (both recreational and at work) are associated with better mental health, lower prevalences of anxiety and mood disorders, and fewer symptoms of anxiety. Also, longitudinal studies provide evidence for protective effects of physical activity with regard to the development of anxiety disorders (Pasco et al., 2011; Ströhle et al., 2007).

Numerous meta-analyses have been published on the effect of exercise on anxiety, although only a few examined the effects on individuals with increased anxiety levels (Petruzzello, Landers, Hatfield, Kubitz, & Salazar, 1991; Stich, 1999), revealing moderate to high effect sizes. Similarly, studies investigating the effect of exercise on anxiety in people with high trait anxiety (McEntee & Halgin, 1999; Steptoe, Edwards, Moses, & Mathews, 1989) or anxiety disorders (Broocks et al., 1998; Merom et al., 2008; Sexton, Maere, & Dahl, 1989; Wedekind et al., 2010) are rare. Acute and chronic exercise have been effective in reducing anxiety in healthy individuals as well as in people with anxiety disorders (Broocks et al., 1998; Esquivel, Schruers, Kuipers, & Griez, 2002; Ströhle et al., 2005; Wedekind et al., 2010). However, only a few studies have attempted to investigate the underlying mechanisms, which might partly be due to a failure to measure plausible mediators (Cerin, 2010).

Underlying mechanisms

Generally, psychological and biological mechanisms can be differentiated. Especially when it comes to underlying psychological mechanisms, results are sparse. We will cover this topic first, describing results from studies investigating exposure, changes in anxiety sensitivity, self-efficacy and self-esteem, and distraction from negative thoughts as being potential mediators. Then we will turn to the possible underlying biological mechanisms like changes in metabolism and the availability of central neurotransmitters, hormones, and neurotrophins, focusing exclusively on human data. Finally, we will briefly outline future directions and needs.

Psychological mechanisms

Exposure

Exercise provides repeated confrontation with internal bodily sensations such as sweating, racing heart, rapid breathing, etc. without the anticipated negative consequences the patients fear. This is important especially for patients with panic disorder (PD), whose anxiety mainly focuses on bodily symptoms being interpreted as dangerous.

Early uncontrolled case reports on phobic patients being successfully treated by exposure to the phobic stimulus after exhaustive exercise (Mueller & Armstrong, 1975; Orwin, 1973) were explained as systematic desensitization. Other early accounts suggested that exercise may facilitate a benign attribution of the arousal induced by the phobic stimulus and thereby prevent fear or panic (Clark, 1986).

Particularly, moderate to vigorous exercise has been shown to be a powerful interoceptive exposure strategy (Broman-Fulks, Berman, Rabian, & Webster, 2004; Martinsen, Raglin, Hoffart, & Friis, 1998) that results in a reattribution of somatic cues to nonpathological vegetative functions and allows the patient to relearn safety (Otto, Smits, & Reese, 2004). Additionally, experiencing exercise has been found to influence dysfunctional cognitions, especially those related to somatic concerns (Broocks & Bandelow, 1999; Broocks et al., 1998).

Anxiety sensitivity

Anxiety sensitivity (AS) is conceptualized as a permanent fear of anxiety and anxiety-related sensations, resulting from the belief that certain bodily sensations may have harmful physical, psychological, or social consequences (Reiss, Peterson, Gursky, & McNally, 1986). Evidence shows that AS is a risk factor (McNally, 2002) and a maintaining factor (McNally, 2002; Smits, Powers, Cho, & Telch, 2004) for anxiety-related psychopathology. Schmidt, Zvolensky, and Maner (2006) found that AS predicts the incidence of any anxiety disorder and overall Axis I disorders. Therefore, reducing AS potentially reduces the experience of panic attacks and the risk of developing anxiety disorders.

The association between AS and exercise frequency has cross-sectionally been studied in a sample of undergraduate students, revealing an inverse relationship (McWilliams & Asmundson, 2001). Furthermore, physically inactive patients with PD displayed both greater AS and greater symptom severity (Smits & Zvolensky, 2006). A causal link between exercise and reduced anxiety sensitivity was suggested by Broman-Fulks and coworkers (2004), who assigned individuals with elevated AS to six aerobic exercise sessions at either high or low intensity. In both groups, AS decreased, but high-intensity exercise caused more rapid reductions in a global measure of AS and additionally reduced fear of anxiety-related bodily sensations (Broman-Fulks et al., 2004). These results were replicated in a different study comparing six 20-minute high-intensity treadmill sessions with a no-exercise control condition. No significant change of AS scores was found in the control condition, whereas exercise again was associated with a reduction of AS scores (Broman-Fulks & Storey, 2008).

Similarly, Smits et al. (2008) reported larger anxiety-reducing effects of exercise compared to a waitlist control condition in subjects with elevated AS. Additionally, the study revealed that the positive effect of exercise on anxious and depressed mood was mediated by changes in AS (Smits et al., 2008). However, this finding has not yet been replicated in individuals meeting the criteria for anxiety disorders.

Two pathways are conceivable explanations of the role of exercise in decreasing fear of anxiety sensations: decreases in cognitive catastrophizing may subsequently decrease anxious affect, or the decline in anxious affect resulting from habituation may diminish catastrophizing on the potential consequences of physiological arousal (Sabourin et al., 2008). Furthermore, it is possible that the two explanations apply differentially across individuals (Sabourin et al., 2008).

Self-efficacy

Within the field of psychological-cognitive anxiety-reducing mechanisms of exercise, Bandura's (1997) self-efficacy theory has received some empirical support as a mediator of affective and behavioral change. Perceived self-efficacy is defined as "beliefs in one's capabilities to organize and execute the courses of action required to produce a given attainment" (Bandura, 1997, p. 3). Self-efficacy is a key concept of the social cognitive theory (Bandura, 1986, 1997) assuming that perceived control over potentially threatening events plays a crucial role in the experience of anxiety.

In a study in anxious individuals, Steptoe et al. (1989) found a significant increase in perceived coping self-efficacy and significant reductions of anxiety in subjects who engaged in moderate-intensity aerobic exercise compared to the placebo control condition.

Similarly, Bodin and Martinsen (2004) showed that exercise targeting self-efficacy (e.g., martial arts) corresponded with significantly greater improvements in positive affect and state anxiety compared to exercise not targeting self-efficacy. Using a false-feedback procedure to increase exercise-efficacy in one condition and to decrease it in the other, Marquez, Jerome, McAuley, Snook, and Canaklisova (2002) found reduced state anxiety after exercise in the high efficacy group.

Katula, Blissmer, and McAuley (1999) found that changes in self-efficacy in healthy older adults were related to anxiety responses only in a moderate-intensity exercise condition, which the authors see, in line with other studies, as suggesting that self-efficacy exerts its greatest influence in optimally challenging situations.

Self-esteem

The relationship between changes in physical self-concept/global self-esteem and negative affect in a population of psychiatric inpatients was investigated by Knapen et al. (2005). Self-concept is a multidimensional system of constructs, which contains more specific perceptions in different areas, e.g., perceptions about the body and physical abilities, the physical self-concept. In this context, self-esteem is defined as the "way in which an individual is able to express a positive idea about him/herself" (Knapen et al., 2005, p. 354), including a personal evaluation, based on cognitive comparison, and it is considered to be the evaluative component of self-concept.

Knapen et al. (2005) showed that an improvement in physical self-concept correlated with increased global self-esteem and decreased anxiety levels. The authors concluded that this supports a causal relationship between changes in physical self-concept and improved mental health. Further evidence is provided by a quantitative review revealing that participation in exercise leads to a change in global self-esteem, even though only small effects were observed (Spence, McGannon, & Poon, 2005).

Knapen et al. (2005) found no significant correlations between changes in physical fitness and changes in physical self-concept, indicating that the patient's perception of fitness changes rather than the objective fitness gains are responsible for enhancing the individual's physical self-concept. This is in line with earlier findings that emotional correlates of regular exercise cannot simply be attributed to fitness (Plante, 1999; Salmon, 2001) and that training which is sufficiently intensive to increase fitness is less effective in relieving anxiety, while anxious mood is reduced by exercise insufficient to increase fitness (Moses, Steptoe, Mathews, & Edwards, 1989).

Changes in accessibility or intensity of ruminations, worries, and anxiety

The idea that anxiety reduction is simply due to distraction from negative thoughts was suggested and tested by Bahrke and Morgan (1978). They compared the effects of acute physical activity, meditation, and a quiet rest control session on anxiety and showed that the conditions were equally effective in reducing state anxiety. This was found for participants within the normal range of anxiety as well as for participants with elevated state and/or trait anxiety (Bahrke & Morgan, 1978). However, since state anxiety was only measured immediately following the session and ten minutes later, these results did not rule out the possibility that anxiety decrease or tension reductions may have lasted for a longer period following exercise (Morgan, 1985). Szabo, Ainsworth, and Danks (2005) showed that statistically significant decreases in state anxiety were equally observed in four conditions: stationary cycling, watching a humorous video, listening to music, and sitting quietly. Again, though, state anxiety was only assessed five minutes after the treatment.

Goode and Roth (1993) found that it was not distraction per se, but the content of the distraction techniques that is associated with changes in emotional well-being: runners who focused on nonassociative thoughts (thoughts not relating to exercise) showed less fatigue and, in some cases, decreases in anxiety, compared to those who focused on associative thoughts (monitoring the body and the exercise itself).

Inconsistent with the distraction hypothesis are studies revealing a higher anxiolytic effect of physical activity when compared to other active treatments (e.g., relaxation/meditation or stress management education) (see Wipfli, Rethorst, & Landers, 2008), suggesting that distraction per se is not sufficient to explain the anxiolytic effect of exercise.

Furthermore, even though the distraction hypothesis can offer a reasonable account for the robust finding of reduced state anxiety and negative affect after exercise, it fails to offer a rationale why exercise induces positive affect and it remains largely inadequate in explaining the mechanisms driving affective changes (Barnes, Coombes, Armstrong, Higgins, & Janelle, 2010). Barnes and coworkers (2010) therefore focused on attentional adaptations that may be elicited by acute bouts of exercise and suggested that exercise facilitates a broadening of attentional scope in high trait anxious participants. So, one underlying mechanism of the exercise-induced increases in positive affect and decreases in negative affect and state anxiety might be the amelioration of maladaptive attention allocation.

Modification of action tendencies

Exercise may also serve to modify emotional action tendencies. More specifically, physical activity involves an action (activation, approach) that is inconsistent with the action tendency associated with anxiety and sustaining the disorder, namely avoidance. Therapeutic approaches that emphasize the replacement of action tendencies with actions consistent with alternative emotions have been shown to be effective for a variety of disorders, including anxiety disorders (Barlow, Allen, & Choate, 2004). Similarly, Otto et al. (2007) state that it is a common psychotherapeutic approach for anxiety disorders to make patients desist from avoiding behaviors and take actions that are inconsistent with their anxious feelings.

Social contact/social engagement

Higher levels of habitual physical activity have been shown to be protective against the development of anxiety disorders and leisure-time physical activity contributed substantially to the overall physical activity score (Pasco et al., 2011). The authors suggested that components of leisure-time physical activity such as social engagement may have contributed to the beneficial effects of exercise, but found that neither marital status nor employment status confounded the relationship (Pasco et al., 2011). Therefore, social engagement might explain why exercise can help to reduce the risk for the development of anxiety (disorders), but there are no studies directly investigating the role of social engagement in the acute anxiolytic effect of exercise.

Recently, support was found for the assumption that social support and social engagement are important in explaining the inverse relationship between leisure activity and symptoms of depression (Harvey, Hotopf, Øverland, & Mykletun, 2010), whereas for anxiety, evidence was less clear. However, improved interpersonal skills, positive social norms, and membership of prosocial peer groups that are promoted by organized sports are suggested to positively influence mental health, at least if sport is carried out during adolescence (Fletcher, Nickerson, & Wright, 2003).

Biological mechanisms

Serotonin (central serotonergic receptor sensitivity)

Several indices of abnormal serotonergic function have been reported in patients suffering from anxiety disorders. In PD and/or agoraphobic patients, there is evidence for an increased sensitivity of the 5-HT_{2C} subsystem (e.g., Benjamin, Geraci, McCann, Greenberg, & Murphy, 1999). On the other hand, stimulation of 5-HT_{1A} receptors has been shown to be associated with attenuated hypothermic and neuroendocrine responses in these patients (e.g., Broocks et al., 2000). Furthermore, the observation that serotonin reuptake inhibitors (SSRIs) are of particular benefit in the treatment of anxiety disorders (e.g., Otto, Tuby, Gould, McLean, & Pollack, 2001; Roy et al., 2001) provides additional evidence for the role of serotonergic pathways in their pathophysiology.

Broocks et al. (1999, 2001, 2003) suggested that exercise may lead to an adaptive downregulation of postsynaptic serotonin receptors, in particular 5-HT_{2C} receptors. Support for this hypothesis comes from a neuroendocrine challenge study, where marathon runners were compared to sedentary controls (Broocks et al., 1999). In both groups, responses to meta-chlorophenylpiperazine (m-CPP), a serotonin agonist producing anxiogenic symptoms by means of its action on 5-HT_{2C} receptors, were assessed, revealing a reduced cortisol response to m-CPP in marathon runners (Broocks et al., 1999). This reduced hormonal reaction suggests that anxiolytic effects of exercise may be mediated by the downregulation of 5-HT_{2C} receptors.

Furthermore, acute physical exercise has been shown to increase the availability of the enzyme tryptophan in the brain, which stimulates serotonin synthesis (Chaouloff, 1997).

Opioids

Based on the observation that physical activity causes a release of endogenous opioids (Morgan, 1985; Ransford, 1982), it has been hypothesized that the inhibitory effects of beta-endorphins on the central nervous system are partly responsible for the anxiolytic effects of exercise (Thorén, Floras, Hoffman, & Seals, 1990). Several studies demonstrated that participants engaging in exercise were calmer after administration of an opiate antagonist relative to sedentary participants (e.g., Allen & Coen, 1987). Other authors, however, did not find this effect (Markoff, Ryan, & Young, 1982).

It has been speculated that methodological problems may have accounted for these conflicting results: all assumptions about the involvement of brain-derived endorphinergic mechanisms were based on endorphin measurements from peripheral blood (Boecker et al., 2008), but plasma concentrations may not accurately reflect endorphin levels in the central nervous system (North, McCullagh, & Tran, 1990; Thorén et al., 1990).

However, recently, the central opioidergic mechanisms of the "runner's high" (a state of euphoria during running; Wagemaker & Goldstein, 1980) have been investigated and related to perceived euphoria (Boecker et al., 2008). The authors compared runners' brains at rest and after two hours of running, finding reductions in opioid receptor availability especially in prefrontal and limbic/paralimbic structures (Boecker et al., 2008). The perceived levels of euphoria were significantly increased after running and inversely correlated with opioid binding in frontolimbic brain areas (Boecker et al., 2008).

Stress hormone system

The hypothalamic–pituitary–adrenal (HPA) system (see Figure 6.1) is the body's major physiological stress response system and consists of a complex set of direct influences and feedback interactions among the hypothalamus, the pituitary gland, and the adrenal glands, mediated by the hormones CRH (corticotrophin-releasing hormone), ACTH (adrenocorticotropic hormone), and cortisol (e.g., Ströhle & Holsboer, 2003). Cortisol levels have been variously studied as an indicator of the stress response.

During panic attacks, patients experience a range of bodily symptoms perceived as dangerous, excessive fear, and massive stress, often combined with fear of losing control or even fear of death. Therefore, a strong activation of the HPA stress system in these patients could be expected, but findings are heterogeneous (see Abelson, Khan, Liberzon, & Young (2007) for a survey of conflicting results concerning HPA dysregulations).

Studies reported different hormonal responses to psychosocial stress depending on levels of regular physical activity in healthy participants (Rimmele et al., 2007, 2009). Rimmele et al. (2009) found significantly lower cortisol levels after a standardized psychosocial laboratory stressor in elite sportsmen compared to untrained men. However, amateur sportsmen did not differ significantly from untrained men with regard to their cortisol responses (Rimmele et al., 2009). In an earlier study, Kraemer et al. (1999) provided results for a significant decline in resting cortisol levels after 10 weeks of a strength-power training program in older, but not in younger, men.

Taken together, the involvement of the HPA system in pathophysiology of anxiety disorders needs to be further clarified before suggestions about the HPA system's role as a mediator between exercise and anxiety reduction can be made.

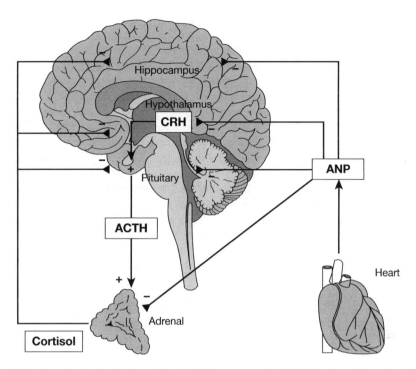

Figure 6.1 The hypothalamic–pituitary–adrenal (HPA) system and its inhibition by atrial natriuretic peptide (ANP).

Atrial natriuretic peptide

Atrial natriuretic peptide (ANP) is a cardiac hormone that was first discovered in mammalian atria (de Bold, 1985). ANP inhibits the HPA system (Kellner, Herzog, Holsboer, & Wiedemann, 1995; Kellner, Wiedemann, & Holsboer, 1992; Ströhle, Kellner, Holsboer, & Wiedemann, 1998; see Figure 6.1) and exhibits anxiolytic activity (Wiedemann, Jahn, Yassouridis, & Kellner, 2001). Ströhle and coworkers studied cholecystokinin-tetrapeptide (CCK-4)-induced panic attacks in patients with PD, demonstrating that pretreatment with ANP resulted in significantly lower anxiety symptoms than pretreatment with placebo (Ströhle, Kellner, Holsboer, & Wiedemann, 2001). This finding argues for the antipanic activity of ANP and is in line with results of an earlier preclinical study (Ströhle et al., 1997).

Since ANP concentrations were shown to increase with physical activity (Mandroukas et al., 1995, 2011), Ströhle, Feller, Strasburger, Heinz, and Dimeo (2006) suggested a potential role of ANP in modulating the exercise-induced anxiolytic activity. To test this hypothesis, panic attacks were induced by CCK-4 in healthy participants after either quiet rest or aerobic exercise. Results showed that after previous exercise, less anxiety was induced by CCK-4, and plasma ANP concentrations were increased, compared to the rest condition (Ströhle et al., 2006). Furthermore, the anxiolytic activity of exercise was positively correlated with increases in plasma ANP concentration (Ströhle et al., 2006).

As the exercise-induced increase in ANP concentration is more pronounced in untrained than in trained individuals (Rogers, Tyce, Bailey, & Bove, 1991), further studies will have to determine if different mechanisms are involved in the anxiolytic effects of acute versus chronic exercise.

Brain-derived neurotrophic factor

Brain-derived neurotrophic factor (BDNF), a secretory protein of the neurotrophin family, is believed to at least partly mediate the regulation of cell proliferation, migration, differentiation, and death, and therefore to be critically involved in regulating the plasticy of adult brain structures (Groves, 2007).

BDNF has been linked to depression and anxiety, mainly based on associations between decreased hippocampal BDNF levels and stress-induced depressive behaviors (Duman & Monteggia, 2006) and an enhancement of BDNF expression following antidepressant drug treatment (Sen, Duman, & Sanacora, 2008). It has also been shown that BDNF expression can be augmented by exercise (e.g., Gómez-Pinilla, Vaynman, & Ying, 2008), although studies in healthy participants provided heterogeneous results (see Ströhle et al., 2010). Furthermore, low BDNF serum concentrations have been linked to poor treatment responses to cognitive behavioral therapy in patients with PD (Kobayashi et al., 2005).

Ströhle et al. (2010) studied serum BDNF levels in PD patients and healthy controls before and after 30 minutes of moderate exercise. They demonstrated that patients had significantly reduced BDNF concentrations at baseline, which increased after acute exercise, whereas they remained unchanged by exercise in controls (Ströhle et al., 2010). These findings suggest that stimulation of BDNF concentrations might be associated with the beneficial effect of exercise on anxiety.

It remains unclear if this effect also holds true for long-term exercise training in patients. At least in healthy young men, 5 weeks of endurance training were shown to increase BDNF concentrations (Zoladz et al., 2008). However, these findings need to be replicated in larger samples, and it remains an open question whether increases in BDNF levels relate to therapeutic outcomes. Additionally, it is not proven yet that serum BDNF levels reflect BDNF concentrations in the brain, although preliminary results in rats as well as in humans favor this assumption (Karege, Schwald, & Cisse, 2002; Lang, Hellweg, Seifert, Schubert, & Gallinat, 2007; Pan, Banks, Fasold, Bluth, & Kastin, 1998).

Genetics

In order to investigate causal effects of exercise on anxious symptoms, De Moor and coworkers (De Moor, Boomsma, Stubbe, Willemsen, & de Geus, 2008) used a genetically informative design with both cross-sectional and longitudinal data from monozygotic and dizygotic twin pairs. Their results corroborated earlier findings linking lower levels of regular exercise to higher levels of anxiety, but a causal link could not be confirmed (De Moor et al., 2008). Instead, the authors suggested that negative associations between exercise and anxious and depressive symptoms (both cross-sectional and prospective) were best explained by common genetic factors (De Moor et al., 2008). Until now it has been unknown which genes play a role, but genes involved in the dopaminergic, norepinephrenergic, opioidergic, or serotonergic pathways are likely candidates (De Moor et al., 2008), which is in line with previous sections of this chapter. Furthermore, there were some limitations to the study, including the fact that only leisure-time exercise was affected by genetic factors, which does not necessarily preclude the potential preventive or therapeutic use of everyday physical activity and exercise interventions (Wolff & Ströhle, 2012).

Conclusion

Although physical activity and exercise training have been linked to reduced anxiety, and although there are clear recommendations to integrate physical activity into our everyday lives and into therapies of anxiety, many questions remain unsolved concerning why and how physical activity causes these benefits.

Currently discussed mechanisms can broadly be divided into psychological and biological factors. The most relevant psychological factors cover exposure, changes in anxiety sensitivity, self-efficacy and self-esteem, and distraction from negative thoughts. The most intensively studied biological factors include changes in metabolism and availability of central neurotransmitters, hormones, and neurotrophins.

To date, the most likely explanation for the anxiolytic effect of physical activity is a multi-factoral model combining several mechanisms and taking into account psychological as well as biological factors and their interactions.

Future directions and needs

In order to elucidate the mechanisms of the beneficial effects of physical activity on mental health, there is need for further well-designed studies. Concerning the identification of underlying mechanisms via statistical mediation analyses, an overview of appropriate methods is given by Cerin (2010). Beyond recommendations for cross-sectional studies and longitudinal mediation models, the author suggests study designs for the identification of mediators. The strongest empirical support for causal mediation processes is provided by experimental studies using double randomization, but also blockage, enhancement, purification, and pattern matching designs can help to clarify mediating effects of variables (Cerin, 2010). Blockage designs are defined as designs blocking the effects of a mediator, so that possibly mediating processes can be detected only in the unblocked experimental condition. Enhancement designs aim at enhancing rather than blocking the effects of a mediator in certain experimental groups. Purification studies can be used when multiple mechanisms of influence are present, as they focus on the identification and selection of components activating the most potent mechanisms of influence. The main aim of the pattern matching approach, finally, is to establish the convergent and divergent validity of a mediational hypothesis by studying specific mediation effects in different samples and contexts, at different times, and by using different outcome measures.

References

Abelson, J. L., Khan, S., Liberzon, I., & Young, E. A. (2007). HPA axis activity in patients with panic disorder: Review and synthesis of four studies. *Depression and Anxiety, 24*(1), 66–76.

Allen, M. E., & Coen, D. (1987). Naloxone blocking of running-induced mood changes. *Annals of Sports Medicine, 3*, 190–195.

Bahrke, M. S., & Morgan, W. P. (1978). Anxiety reduction following exercise and meditation. *Cognitive Therapy and Research, 2*(4), 323–333.

Bandura, A. (1986). *Social foundations of thought and action.* Englewood Cliffs, NJ: Prentice-Hall.

Bandura, A. (1997). *Self-efficacy: The exercise of control.* New York: Freeman.

Barlow, D. H., Allen, L. B., & Choate, M. L. (2004). Toward a unified treatment for emotional disorders. *Behavior Therapy, 35*, 205–230.

Barnes, R. T., Coombes, S. A., Armstrong, N. B., Higgins, T. J., & Janelle, C. M. (2010). Evaluating attentional and affective changes following an acute exercise bout using a modified dot-probe protocol. *Journal of Sports Sciences, 28*(10), 1065–1076.

Benjamin, J., Geraci, M., McCann, U., Greenberg, B. D., & Murphy, D. L. (1999). Attenuated response to m-CPP and to pentagastrin after repeated m-CPP in panic disorder. *Psychopharmacology, 143*(2), 215–216.

Bodin, T., & Martinsen, E. W. (2004). Mood and self-efficacy during acute exercise in clinical depression: A randomized, controlled study. *Journal of Sport & Exercise Psychology, 26*, 623–633.

Boecker, H., Sprenger, T., Spilker, M. E., Henriksen, G., Koppenhoefer, M., Wagner, K. J., . . . Tolle, T. R. (2008). The runner's high: opioidergic mechanisms in the human brain. *Cerebral Cortex, 18*(11), 2523–2531.

Bold, A. J. de (1985). Atrial natriuretic factor: a hormone produced by the heart. *Science, 230*(4727), 767–770.

Broman-Fulks, J. J., Berman, M. E., Rabian, B. A., & Webster, M. J. (2004). Effects of aerobic exercise on anxiety sensitivity. *Behaviour Research and Therapy, 42*(2), 125–136.

Broman-Fulks, J. J., & Storey, K. M. (2008). Evaluation of a brief aerobic exercise intervention for high anxiety sensitivity. *Anxiety, Stress, and Coping, 21*(2), 117–128.

Broocks, A., & Bandelow, B. (1999). Treatment of panic disorder: Reply. *American Journal of Psychiatry, 156*(7), 1129–1130.

Broocks, A., Bandelow, B., George, A., Jestrabeck, C., Opitz, M., Bartmann, U., . . . Hajak, G. (2000). Increased psychological responses and divergent neuroendocrine responses to m-CPP and ipsapirone in patients with panic disorder. *International Clinical Psychopharmacology, 15*(3), 153–161.

Broocks, A., Bandelow, B., Pekrun, G., George, A., Meyer, T., & Bartmann, U. (1998). Comparison of aerobic exercise, clomipramine, and placebo in the treatment of panic disorder. *American Journal of Psychiatry, 155*(5), 603–609.

Broocks, A., Meyer, T., George, A., Hillmer-Vogel, U., Meyer, D., Bandelow, B., . . . Ruether, E. (1999). Decreased neuroendocrine responses to meta-chlorophenylpiperazine (m-CPP) but normal responses to ipsapirone in marathon runners. *Neuropsychopharmacology, 20*(2), 150–161.

Broocks, A., Meyer, T., Gleiter, C. H., Hillmer-Vogel, U., George, A., Bartmann, U., & Bandelow, B. (2001). Effect of aerobic exercise on behavioral and neuroendocrine responses to meta-chlorophenylpiperazine and to ipsapirone in untrained healthy subjects. *Psychopharmacology, 155*(3), 234–241.

Broocks, A., Meyer, T., Opitz, M., Bartmann, U., Hillmer-Vogel, U., George, A., . . . Bandelow, B. (2003). 5-HT1A responsivity in patients with panic disorder before and after treatment with aerobic exercise, clomipramine or placebo. *European Neuropsychopharmacology, 13*(3), 153–164.

Cerin, L. (2010). Ways of unraveling how and why physical activity influences mental health through statistical mediation analyses. *Mental Health and Physical Activity, 3*, 51–60.

Chaouloff, F. (1997). Effects of acute physical exercise on central serotonergic systems. *Medicine & Science in Sports & Exercise, 29*(1), 58–62.

Clark, D. M. (1986). A cognitive approach to panic. *Behaviour Research and Therapy, 24*(4), 461–470.

De Moor, M. H. M., Boomsma, D. I., Stubbe, J. H., Willemsen, G., & Geus, E. J. C. de (2008). Testing causality in the association between regular exercise and symptoms of anxiety and depression. *Archives of General Psychiatry, 65*(8), 897–905.

Duman, R. S., & Monteggia, L. M. (2006). A neurotrophic model for stress-related mood disorders. *Biological Psychiatry, 59*(12), 1116–1127.

Esquivel, G., Schruers, K., Kuipers, H., & Griez, E. (2002). The effects of acute exercise and high lactate levels on 35% CO2 challenge in healthy volunteers. *Acta Psychiatrica Scandinavica, 106*(5), 394–397.

Fletcher, A. C., Nickerson, P. F., & Wright, K. L. (2003). Structured leisure activities in middle childhood: Links to well-being. *Journal of Community Psychology, 31*, 641–659.

Gomez-Pinilla, F., Vaynman, S., & Ying, Z. (2008). Brain-derived neurotrophic factor functions as a metabotrophin to mediate the effects of exercise on cognition. *European Journal of Neuroscience, 28*(11), 2278–2287.

Goode, K. T., & Roth, D. L. (1993). Factor analysis of cognitions during running: Association with mood change. *Journal of Sport & Exercise Psychology, 15*, 375–389.

Goodwin, R. (2003). Association between physical activity and mental disorders among adults in the United States. *Preventive Medicine, 36*, 698–703.

Groves, J. O. (2007). Is it time to reassess the BDNF hypothesis of depression? *Molecular Psychiatry, 12*(12), 1079–1088.

Harvey, S. B., Hotopf, M., Øverland, S., & Mykletun, A. (2010). Physical activity and common mental disorders. *British Journal of Psychiatry, 197*, 357–364.

Karege, F., Schwald, M., & Cisse, M. (2002). Postnatal developmental profile of brain-derived neurotrophic factor in rat brain and platelets. *Neuroscience Letters, 328*(3), 261–264.

Katula, J. A., Blissmer, B. J., & McAuley, E. (1999). Exercise intensity and self-efficacy effects on anxiety reduction in healthy, older adults. *Journal of Behavioral Medicine, 22*(3), 233–247.

Kellner, M., Herzog, L., Holsboer, F., & Wiedemann, K. (1995). Circadian changes in the sensitivity of the corticotropin-releasing hormone-stimulated HPA system after arginine vasopressin and atrial natriuretic hormone in human male controls. *Psychoneuroendocrinology, 20*(5), 515–524.

Kellner, M., Wiedemann, K., & Holsboer, F. (1992). Atrial natriuretic factor inhibits the CRH-stimulated secretion of ACTH and cortisol in man. *Life Sciences, 50*(24), 1835–1842.

Kessler, R. C., Berglund, P., Demler, O., Jin, R., Merikangas, K. R., & Walters, E. E. (2005). Lifetime prevalence and age-of-onset distributions of DSM-IV disorders in the National Comorbidity Survey Replication. *Archives of General Psychiatry, 62*(6), 593–602.

Kessler, R. C., Chiu, W. T., Demler, O., Merikangas, K. R., & Walters, E. E. (2005). Prevalence, severity, and comorbidity of 12-month DSM-IV disorders in the National Comorbidity Survey Replication. *Archives of General Psychiatry, 62*(6), 617–627.

Knapen, J., van de Vliet, P., van Coppenolle, H., David, A., Peuskens, J., Pieters, G., & Knapen, K. (2005). Comparison of changes in physical self-concept, global self-esteem, depression and anxiety following two different psychomotor therapy programs in nonpsychotic psychiatric inpatients. *Psychotherapy and Psychosomatics, 74*(6), 353–361.

Kobayashi, K., Shimizu, E., Hashimoto, K., Mitsumori, M., Koike, K., Okamura, N., . . . Iyo, M. (2005). Serum brain-derived neurotrophic factor (BDNF) levels in patients with panic disorder: As a biological predictor of response to group cognitive behavioral therapy. *Progress in Neuro-Psychopharmacology & Biological Psychiatry, 29*(5), 658–663.

Kraemer, W. J., Häkkinen, K., Newton, R. U., Nindl, B. C., Volek, J. S., McCormick, M., . . . Evans, W. J. (1999). Effects of heavy-resistance training on hormonal response patterns in younger vs. older men. *Journal of Applied Physiology, 87*(3), 982–992.

Lang, U. E., Hellweg, R., Seifert, F., Schubert, F., & Gallinat, J. (2007). Correlation between serum brain-derived neurotrophic factor level and an in vivo marker of cortical integrity. *Biological Psychiatry, 62*(5), 530–535.

Lépine, J.-P. (2002). The epidemiology of anxiety disorders: Prevalence and societal costs. *Journal of Clinical Psychiatry, 63 Suppl 14*, 4–8.

Mandroukas, A., Metaxas, T. I., Heller, J., Vamvakoudis, E., Christoulas, K., Riganas, C. S., . . . Mandroukas, K. (2011). The effect of different exercise-testing protocols on atrial natriuretic peptide. *Clinical Physiology and Functional Imaging, 31*(1), 5–10.

Mandroukas, K., Zakas, A., Aggelopoulou, N., Christoulas, K., Abatzides, G., & Karamouzis, M. (1995). Atrial natriuretic factor responses to submaximal and maximal exercise. *British Journal of Sports Medicine, 29*(4), 248–251.

Markoff, R. A., Ryan, P., & Young, T. (1982). Endorphins and mood changes in long-distance running. *Medicine & Science in Sports & Exercise, 14*(1), 11–15.

Marquez, D. X., Jerome, G. J., McAuley, E., Snook, E. M., & Canaklisova, S. (2002). Self-efficacy manipulation and state anxiety responses to exercise in low active women. *Psychology and Health, 17*(6), 783–791.

Martinsen, E. W., Raglin, J. S., Hoffart, A., & Friis, S. (1998). Tolerance to intensive exercise and high levels of lactate in panic disorder. *Journal of Anxiety Disorders, 12*(4), 333–342.

McEntee, D. J., & Halgin, R. P. (1999). Cognitive group therapy and aerobic exercise in the treatment of anxiety. *Journal of College Student Psychotherapy, 13*(3), 39–58.

McNally, R. J. (2002). Anxiety sensitivity and panic disorder. *Biological Psychiatry, 52*(10), 938–946.

McWilliams, L. A., & Asmundson, G. J. (2001). Is there a negative association between anxiety sensitivity and arousal-increasing substances and activities? *Journal of Anxiety Disorders, 15*(3), 161–170.

Merom, D., Phongsavan, P., Wagner, R., Chey, T., Marnane, C., Steel, Z., . . . Bauman, A. (2008). Promoting walking as an adjunct intervention to group cognitive behavioral therapy for anxiety disorders—a pilot group randomized trial. *Journal of Anxiety Disorders, 22*(6), 959–968.

Morgan, W. P. (1985). Affective beneficence of vigorous physical activity. *Medicine & Science in Sports & Exercise, 17*(1), 94–100.

Moses, J., Steptoe, A., Mathews, A., & Edwards, S. (1989). The effects of exercise training on mental well-being in the normal population: A controlled trial. *Journal of Psychosomatic Research, 33*(1), 47–61.

Mueller, B., & Armstrong, H. E. (1975). A further note on the running treatment for anxiety. *Psychotherapeutic Theory Research Practise, 12*, 385–387.

North, T. C., McCullagh, P., & Tran, Z. V. (1990). Effect of exercise on depression. *Exercise and Sport Science Reviews, 18*, 379–415.

Orwin, A. (1973). "The running treatment": A preliminary communication on a new use for an old therapy (physical activity) in the agoraphobic syndrome. *British Journal of Psychiatry, 122*(567), 175–179.

Otto, M. W., Church, T. S., Craft, L. L., Greer, T. L., Smits, J. A. J., & Trivedi, M. H. (2007). Exercise for mood and anxiety disorders. *Journal of Clinical Psychiatry, 68*(5), 669–676.

Otto, M. W., Smits, J. A. J., & Reese, H. E. (2004). Cognitive-behavioral therapy for the treatment of anxiety disorders. *Journal of Clinical Psychiatry, 65 Suppl 5*, 34–41.

Otto, M. W., Tuby, K. S., Gould, R. A., McLean, R. Y., & Pollack, M. H. (2001). An effect-size analysis of the relative efficacy and tolerability of serotonin selective reuptake inhibitors for panic disorder. *American Journal of Psychiatry*, *158*(12), 1989–1992.

Pan, W., Banks, W. A., Fasold, M. B., Bluth, J., & Kastin, A. J. (1998). Transport of brain-derived neurotrophic factor across the blood-brain barrier. *Neuropharmacology*, *37*(12), 1553–1561.

Pasco, J. A., Williams, L. J., Jacka, F. N., Henry, M. J., Coulson, C. E., Brennan, S. L., . . . Berk, M. (2011). Habitual physical activity and the risk for depressive and anxiety disorders among older men and women. *International Psychogeriatrics*, *23*(2), 292–298.

Petruzzello, S. J., Landers, D. M., Hatfield, B. D., Kubitz, K. A., & Salazar, W. (1991). A meta-analysis on the anxiety-reducing effects of acute and chronic exercise. Outcomes and mechanisms. *Sports Medicine*, *11*(3), 143–182.

Plante, T. G. (1999). Could the perception of fitness account for many of the mental and physical health benefits of exercise? *Advances in Mind-Body Medicine*, *15*(4), 291–301.

Ransford, C. P. (1982). A role for amines in the antidepressant effect of exercise: A review. *Medicine & Science in Sports & Exercise*, *14*(1), 1–10.

Reiss, S., Peterson, R. A., Gursky, D. M., & McNally, R. J. (1986). Anxiety sensitivity, anxiety frequency and the prediction of fearfulness. *Behaviour Research and Therapy*, *24*(1), 1–8.

Rimmele, U., Seiler, R., Marti, B., Wirtz, P. H., Ehlert, U., & Heinrichs, M. (2009). The level of physical activity affects adrenal and cardiovascular reactivity to psychosocial stress. *Psychoneuroendocrinology*, *34*(2), 190–198.

Rimmele, U., Zellweger, B. C., Marti, B., Seiler, R., Mohiyeddini, C., Ehlert, U., & Heinrichs, M. (2007). Trained men show lower cortisol, heart rate and psychological responses to psychosocial stress compared with untrained men. *Psychoneuroendocrinology*, *32*(6), 627–635.

Rogers, P. J., Tyce, G. M., Bailey, K. R., & Bove, A. A. (1991). Exercise-induced increases in atrial natriuretic factor are attenuated by endurance training. *Journal of the American College of Cardiology*, *18*(5), 1236–1241.

Roy, B. P., Clary, C. M., Miceli, R. J., Colucci, S. V., Xu, Y., & Grudzinski, A. N. (2001). The effect of selective serotonin reuptake inhibitor treatment of panic disorder on emergency room and laboratory resource utilization. *Journal of Clinical Psychiatry*, *62*(9), 678–682.

Sabourin, B., Stewart, S. H., Sherry, S. B., Watt, M. C., Wald, J., & Grant, V. V. (2008). Physical exercise as interoceptive exposure within a brief cognitive-behavioral treatment for anxiety-sensitive women. *Journal of Cognitive Psychotherapy*, *22*(4), 303–320.

Salmon, P. (2001). Effects of physical exercise on anxiety, depression, and sensitivity to stress: A unifying theory. *Clinical Psychology Review*, *21*(1), 33–61.

Schmidt, N. B., Zvolensky, M. J., & Maner, J. K. (2006). Anxiety sensitivity: Prospective prediction of panic attacks and Axis I pathology. *Journal of Psychiatric Research*, *40*(8), 691–699.

Sen, S., Duman, R., & Sanacora, G. (2008). Serum brain-derived neurotrophic factor, depression, and antidepressant medications: Meta-analyses and implications. *Biological Psychiatry*, *64*(6), 527–532.

Sexton, H., Maere, A., & Dahl, N. H. (1989). Exercise intensity and reduction in neurotic symptoms. A controlled follow-up study. *Acta Psychiatrica Scandinavica*, *80*(3), 231–235.

Smits, J. A. J., Berry, A. C., Rosenfield, D., Powers, M. B., Behar, E., & Otto, M. W. (2008). Reducing anxiety sensitivity with exercise. *Depression and Anxiety*, *25*(8), 689–699.

Smits, J. A. J., Powers, M. B., Cho, Y., & Telch, M. J. (2004). Mechanism of change in cognitive-behavioral treatment of panic disorder: Evidence for the fear of fear mediational hypothesis. *Journal of Consulting and Clinical Psychology*, *72*(4), 646–652.

Smits, J. A. J., & Zvolensky, M. J. (2006). Emotional vulnerability as a function of physical activity among individuals with panic disorder. *Depression and Anxiety*, *23*(2), 102–106.

Spence, J. C., McGannon, K. R., & Poon, P. (2005). The effect of exercise on global self-esteem: A quantitative review. *Journal of Sport & Exercise Psychology*, *27*(3), 311–334.

Stephens, T. (1988). Physical activity and mental health in the United States and Canada: Evidence from four popular surveys. *Preventive Medicine*, *17*, 35–47.

Steptoe, A., Edwards, S., Moses, J., & Mathews, A. (1989). The effects of exercise training on mood and perceived coping ability in anxious adults from the general population. *Journal of Psychosomatic Research*, *33*(5), 537–547.

Stich, F. A. (1999). A meta-analysis of physical exercise as a treatment for symptoms of anxiety and depression. *Dissertation Abstracts International: Section B: The Sciences and Engineering*, *59*(8-B), 4487.

Ströhle, A., Feller, C., Onken, M., Godemann, F., Heinz, A., & Dimeo, F. (2005). The acute antipanic activity of aerobic exercise. *American Journal of Psychiatry*, *162*(12), 2376–2378.

Ströhle, A., Feller, C., Strasburger, C. J., Heinz, A., & Dimeo, F. (2006). Anxiety modulation by the heart? Aerobic exercise and atrial natriuretic peptide. *Psychoneuroendocrinology*, *31*(9), 1127–1130.

Ströhle, A., Hoefler, M., Pfister, H., Mueller, A.-G., Hoyer, J., Wittchen, H.-U., & Lieb, R. (2007). Physical activity and prevalence and incidence of mental disorders in adolescents and young adults. *Psychological Medicine*, *37*(11), 1657–1666.

Ströhle, A., & Holsboer, F. (2003). Stress responsive neurohormone in depression and anxiety. *Pharmacopsychiatry*, *36*(3), S207–S214.

Ströhle, A., Jahn, H., Montkowski, A., Liebsch, G., Boll, E., Landgraf, R., & Wiedemann, K. (1997). Central and peripheral administration of atriopeptin is anxiolytic in rats. *Neuroendocrinology*, *65*(3), 210–215.

Ströhle, A., Kellner, M., Holsboer, F., & Wiedemann, K. (1998). Atrial natriuretic hormone decreases endocrine response to a combined dexamethasone-corticotropin-releasing hormone test. *Biological Psychiatry*, *43*(5), 371–375.

Ströhle, A., Kellner, M., Holsboer, F., & Wiedemann, K. (2001). Anxiolytic activity of atrial natriuretic peptide in patients with panic disorder. *American Journal of Psychiatry*, *158*(9), 1514–1516.

Ströhle, A., Stoy, M., Graetz, B., Scheel, M., Wittmann, A., Gallinat, J., . . . Hellweg, R. (2010). Acute exercise ameliorates reduced brain-derived neurotrophic factor in patients with panic disorder. *Psychoneuroendocrinology*, *35*(3), 364–368.

Szabo, A., Ainsworth, S. E., & Danks, P. K. (2005). Experimental comparison of the psychological benefits of aerobic exercise, humor, and music. *Humor: International Journal of Humor Research*, *18*(3), 235–246.

Thorén, P., Floras, J. S., Hoffmann, P., & Seals, D. R. (1990). Endorphins and exercise: Physiological mechanisms and clinical implications. *Medicine & Science in Sports & Exercise*, *22*(4), 417–428.

Wagemaker, H., & Goldstein, L. (1980). The runner's high. *Journal of Sports Medicine and Physical Fitness*, *20*(2), 227–229.

Wedekind, D., Broocks, A., Weiss, N., Engel, K., Neubert, K., & Bandelow, B. (2010). A randomized, controlled trial of aerobic exercise in combination with paroxetine in the treatment of panic disorder. *World Journal of Biological Psychiatry*, *11*(7), 904–913.

Wiedemann, K., Jahn, H., Yassouridis, A., & Kellner, M. (2001). Anxiolyticlike effects of atrial natriuretic peptide on cholecystokinin tetrapeptide-induced panic attacks: Preliminary findings. *Archives of General Psychiatry*, *58*(4), 371–377.

Wipfli, B. M., Rethorst, C. D., & Landers, D. M. (2008). The anxiolytic effects of exercise: A meta-analysis of randomized trials and dose-response analysis. *Journal of Sport & Exercise Psychology*, *30*, 392–411.

Wittchen, H. U., Jacobi, F., Rehm, J., Gustavsson, A., Svensson, M., Jönsson, B., . . . Steinhausen, H.-C. (2011). The size and burden of mental disorders and other disorders of the brain in Europe 2010. *European Neuropsychopharmacology*, *21*, 655–679.

Wolff, E., & Ströhle, A. (2010). Causal associations of physical activity/exercise and symptoms of depression and anxiety. *Archives of General Psychiatry*, *67*(5), 540–541.

Zoladz, J. A., Pilc, A., Majerczak, J., Grandys, M., Zapart-Bukowska, J., & Duda, K. (2008). Endurance training increases plasma brain-derived neurotrophic factor concentration in young healthy men. *Journal of Physiology and Pharmacology*, *59 Suppl 7*, 119–132.

7

MECHANISMS UNDERLYING THE RELATIONSHIP BETWEEN PHYSICAL ACTIVITY AND ANXIETY

Animal data

Benjamin N. Greenwood and Monika Fleshner

It is well established that physical activity can reduce the incidence and severity of anxiety disorders (see Chapter 5 by Utschig et al., this volume). Despite the anxiolytic effects of physical activity in humans, the underlying mechanisms remain unknown. Identification of these mechanisms could enhance our understanding of anxiety and lead to more effective therapeutic or preventative strategies.

The limited understanding of the mechanisms underlying the anxiolytic effects of exercise could be due, in part, to the mixed results of animal studies on the effects of exercise on anxiety. Indeed, the effects of exercise in rodent models of anxiety is far from clear, with both anxiolytic and anxiogenic effects being reported. Despite the confusion, progress has been made toward understanding the mechanisms by which physical activity prevents anxiety. In the current chapter, we attempt to interpret the data on the behavioral effects of exercise on animal models of anxiety. We will offer a perspective on the available data that suggest specific experimental conditions under which anxiolytic effects of exercise are maximally revealed. The hope is that understanding the sometimes subtle behavioral impact of exercise in animal models will help uncover the neurobiological mechanisms underlying the effects of exercise on anxiety states. To this end, potential mechanisms will be discussed in the context of the behavioral effects of exercise on various rodent models of anxiety, including tests of learned anxiety, unlearned anxiety, and stress-induced anxiety.

Learned anxiety

Models of learned anxiety are based on assessing conditioned responses to stimuli previously associated with aversive events. During a typical rodent fear conditioning paradigm, a neutral, conditioned stimulus (e.g., a context or a tone) is paired with an aversive stimulus (such as a shock), so that subsequent exposure to the context or tone elicits a fear response in the absence of the aversive stimulus. The fear response in these experiments is most readily assessed using freezing or potentiation of the acoustic startle reflex. Freezing, the absence of all movement except that required for respiration, is a species-typical defensive reaction that is elicited by exposure to a conditioned stimulus. An exaggerated conditioned fear response (be it freezing or startle) to the conditioned stimulus or a fear response elicited by a stimulus that only vaguely resembles the conditioned stimulus (i.e., fear generalization) are thought to be inappropriate fear responses and thus representative of anxiety (Maier & Watkins, 1998).

Behavioral effects of exercise on animal models of learned anxiety

The majority of the literature suggests that exercise facilitates contextual fear conditioning. When a rat with a history of prior wheel running is conditioned to fear a context, the exercised rat displays more freezing behavior than his sedentary counterpart when re-exposed to the conditioned context. This basic observation has been replicated by numerous investigators in both male and female rats and mice. The effects of exercise on fear conditioning are difficult to interpret in terms of anxiety. The increase in conditioned freezing elicited by exercise can be viewed as an inappropriate fear response (i.e., anxiety) or as a consequence of enhanced memory processes that cannot be distinguished from anxiety during a simple fear conditioning test.

Several experimental observations support the second interpretation. First, the effect of exercise on conditioned fear is relatively specific to freezing elicited during re-exposure to a conditioned context and is not generalized to all forms of conditioning. For example, exercise has no effect on freezing immediately following shock (Baruch, Swain, & Helmstetter, 2004; Burghardt, Pasumarthi, Wilson, & Fadel, 2006; Greenwood, Foley, Burhans, Maier, & Fleshner, 2005; Greenwood et al., 2003; J. D. Van Hoomissen, Holmes, Zellner, Poudevigne, & Dishman, 2004) or to a tone previously paired with shock (Baruch et al., 2004; Hopkins & Bucci, 2010); however, see Falls, Fox, & MacAulay, 2010. These data support the idea that exercise enhances function of a mechanism supporting contextual memory rather than one supporting fear, per se. The hippocampus normally supports context memory (Rudy, Barrientos, & O'Reilly, 2002), whereas other structures such as the amygdala can support freezing immediately following shock (Kim, Rison, & Fanselow, 1993) and CS-US associations (Huff & Rudy, 2004; Phillips & LeDoux, 1992). Consistent with exercise enhancement of contextually conditioned fear being a consequence of improved hippocampal-dependent learning and memory and not blatant anxiety, are the observations that both wheel running and treadmill training improve learning in other hippocampus-dependent tasks including the Morris water maze and object recognition (e.g., Clark et al., 2008; Garcia-Capdevila, Portell-Cortes, Torras-Garcia, Coll-Andreu, & Costa-Miserachs, 2009; Grace, Hescham, Kellaway, Bugarith, & Russell, 2009; Vaynman, Ying, & Gomez-Pinilla, 2004). Finally, if the increase in conditioned fear produced by exercise represents anxiety, we might expect to observe other signs of anxiety such as generalization of fear to environments different from the conditioned context. Indeed, over-consolidation of fear memories has been suggested to underlie symptoms of anxiety, such as phobias, intrusive thoughts, nightmares, and generalization of fear (Elzinga & Bremner, 2002). Instead, quite the opposite is observed in physically active rats. When a sedentary rat previously conditioned to fear one context is exposed to a different context sharing only limited features with the original context, it displays a small amount of freezing, which is representative of generalization of fear from the conditioned context to the new one. A rat previously allowed voluntary access to a running wheel, on the other hand, displays similar (J. Van Hoomissen et al., 2011) or less (Greenwood, Strong, Foley, & Fleshner, 2009) freezing in the new context compared to a sedentary rat, despite freezing more when placed back into the original conditioned context. These data suggest that exercise specifically improves the memory of the conditioned context, as well as the ability of the hippocampus to discriminate between contexts (Mizumori, Smith, & Puryear, 2007).

Based on these data, we offer the following interpretation of the effects of exercise on learned anxiety. Exercise does not enhance fear per se, but improves memory of the conditioned context. Improved memory of the conditioned context could be adaptive as the organism is more likely to avoid that environment in the future. Fear is particularly inappropriate when it is expressed in environments that were not previously paired with an aversive stimulus (i.e., generalization). Excessive generalization of fear could lead to avoidance of novel environments or experiences that might otherwise be safe. Here is where the anxiolytic effect of exercise can be observed. Enhanced ability to discriminate safe from dangerous contexts could aid physically active organisms from displaying excessive fear responses during relatively innocuous situations, such as exposure to environmental novelty. Consistent with this idea, exercise also attenuates the hypothalamic–pituitary–adrenal axis response to exposure to a novel environment (Campeau et al., 2010; Dishman et al., 1998). One implication of this interpretation is that the anxiolytic effects of exercise in models of learned anxiety are subtle and can only be revealed using experiments designed specifically to uncover them, such as tests of context discrimination.

Potential mechanisms

Although the mechanism by which exercise facilitates context discrimination is unknown, the facilitation of context discrimination could be a direct consequence of the enhanced memory of the conditioned context. Indeed, generalization can be inversely related to the strength of the original contextual memory, such as occurs as memories age (Wiltgen & Silva, 2007). Understanding how exercise enhances context memory could, therefore, provide insight into the mechanisms by which exercise improves context discrimination and reduces anxiety.

Potential mechanisms underlying the anxiolytic effect of exercise in models of learned anxiety are depicted in Figure 7.1. Because the effects of exercise on fear conditioning seem to be relatively selective to behaviors dependent upon hippocampus-dependent memory, and specifically the consolidation phase of memory (Falls et al., 2010; Greenwood et al., 2009), exercise-induced neuroplasticity in the hippocampus could contribute to the anxiolytic effect of exercise. Exercise increases the birth and survival of new neurons in the adult hippocampus (van Praag, Kempermann, & Gage, 1999), a process that could be important for some behavioral effects of antidepressant drugs (Santarelli et al., 2003). Clark et al. (2008), however, reported that the enhancement of contextual memory produced by wheel running in mice is independent of adult hippocampal neurogenesis (Clark et al., 2008). Although neurogenesis could remain important for the improvement in context discrimination provided by exercise, data are consistent with important roles for other factors relating to memory consolidation, such as neurotrophic factors and other regulators of synaptic plasticity.

Brain-derived neurotrophic factor (BDNF) is a neurotrophic factor implicated in hippocampus-dependent learning and memory and the consolidation phase of contextual fear conditioning (Poo, 2001; Tyler, Alonso, Bramham, & Pozzo-Miller, 2002). Genetic increases in BDNF can improve spatial learning and memory (Yukako et al., 2008), and neutralization of BDNF with intra-hippocampal injection of a BDNF antibody eliminates the beneficial effects of exercise on hippocampus-dependent memory tasks (Ding, Ying, & Gomez-Pinilla, 2011; Vaynman et al., 2004). BDNF, therefore, could be an important player in the mechanisms underlying exercise-facilitation of memory consolidation and context discrimination. Voluntary wheel running increases BDNF mRNA and protein in the hippocampus (Berchtold, Chinn, Chou, Kesslak, & Cotman, 2005; Greenwood, Strong, Foley, Thompson, & Fleshner, 2007; Neeper, Gomez-Pinilla,

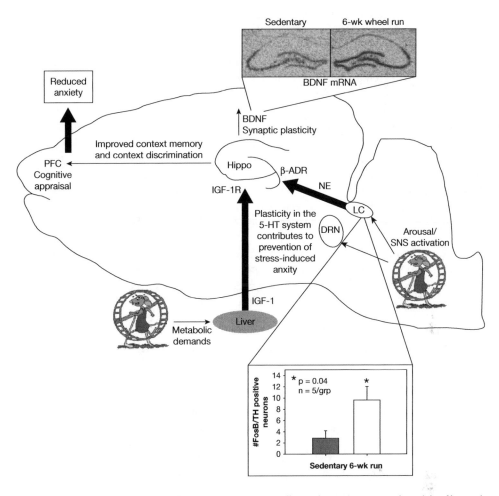

Figure 7.1 Potential mechanisms underlying the anxiolytic effects of exercise in animal models of learned anxiety. β-ADR, β-adrenergic receptor; BDNF, brain-derived neurotrophic factor; DRN, dorsal raphe nucleus; IGF-1, insulin-like growth factor-1; IGF-1R, insulin-like growth factor-1 receptor; LC, locus coeruleus; NE, norepinephrine; PFC, prefrontal cortex; TH, tyrosine hydroxylase.

Choi, & Cotman, 1995), including the ventral portion of the hippocampus (Greenwood et al., 2009), which has been particularly implicated in emotion regulation. For in-depth discussions on the potential role of BDNF in the beneficial effects of exercise, see Cotman, Berchtold, & Christie, 2007; Ding et al., 2011; Russo-Neustadt & Chen, 2005.

An interesting topic of inquiry is identification of the signal by which the experience of exercise is communicated to the brain resulting in alterations in anxiety or other behavioral effects of exercise. Such a signal could be peripherally or centrally derived. One potential peripherally derived signal is insulin-like growth factor-1 (IGF-1). Centrally derived signals could include the catecholamine neurotransmitter norepinephrine (NE). Both IGF-1 (Scofield et al., 2011), as a result of metabolic demands and growth hormone signaling to liver, and central NE (Kitaoka et al., 2010; Meeusen et al., 1997), as a result of increased arousal and sympathetic nervous system activation, can be elevated following exercise. Peripheral IGF-1 begets central IGF-1 (Ding, Vaynman, Akhavan, Ying, & Gomez-Pinilla, 2006; Yan et al., 2011), where IGF-1 acts as a neurotrophin similar to BDNF. Reducing central IGF-1 prevents the exercise-induced increase in BDNF while leaving BDNF levels in sedentary rats intact (Ding et al., 2006). Moreover, genetic deletion (Trejo, Llorens-Martin, & Torres-Aleman, 2008), as well as immuno-neutralization (Trejo, Carro, & Torres-Aleman, 2001) of peripheral IGF-1 prevents the beneficial effects of exercise on hippocampus-dependent learning and memory.

In addition to IGF-1, NE signaling in the hippocampus could also contribute to BDNF elevations through a β-ADR-mediated mechanism (R. S. Duman, Heninger, & Nestler, 1997; R. S. Duman & Monteggia, 2006). Consistent with a role for the β-ADR, blockade of β-ADRs prevents the exercise-induced increase in BDNF (Ivy, Rodriguez, Garcia, Chen, & Russo-Neustadt, 2003) and the improved contextual conditioning typically observed following six weeks of wheel running (J. D. Van Hoomissen et al., 2004). The majority of the NE innervation to the hippocampus comes from the brain stem locus coeruleus (LC). We have observed that six weeks of wheel running increases ΔFosB/FosB protein in catecholaminergic neurons of the rat LC (Figure 7.1). Because ΔFosB/FosB accumulates following repeated neural activation, these data suggest that long-term wheel running repeatedly activates noradrenergic neurons in the LC. Consistent with these data, Garcia, Chen, Garza, Cotman, & Russo-Neustadt (2003) reported that N-(2-chloroethyl)-N-ethyl-2-bromobenzylamine lesions of the LC reduce BDNF mRNA in the hippocampus of exercised rats to a level equivalent to sedentary rats, which are unaffected by DSP-4 lesions (Garcia et al., 2003).

Together, these data suggest that IGF-1 and NE could improve hippocampus function through increases in BDNF, synaptic plasticity, and neuroprotection, resulting in enhanced context discrimination and anxiety reduction. A role for IGF-1 or NE in the hippocampus does not preclude the involvement of other brain regions in the improved context memory and context discrimination produced by exercise. The prefrontal cortex (PFC) is another region implicated in the pathophysiology and treatment of anxiety. Although exercise could affect the PFC directly, exercise-induced plasticity in the hippocampus could indirectly improve PFC function (Peters, Dieppa-Perea, Melendez, & Quirk, 2010). The hippocampus provides contextual information to the PFC, which may facilitate PFC-mediated cognitive appraisal of anxiety-producing situations in order to constrain inappropriate or exaggerated fear responses.

Unlearned anxiety

Models of unlearned anxiety in rodents involve exposure to a stimulus that elicits innate fear or conflict. Innate fear is often generated in rodents by exposure to an open field, light/dark box, or elevated plus maze. In these examples, the rodent experiences conflict between the drive for exploration and the fear of open or brightly lit spaces. In all of these cases, the fear response is an unlearned response to a natural threat.

The effects of exercise on anxiety in tests of unlearned anxiety remain equivocal. Exercise has been reported to produce no effects (Chaouloff, 1994; Mello, Benetti, Cammarota, & Izquierdo, 2009; Pietropaolo, Feldon, Alleva, Cirulli, & Yee, 2006), anxiogenic effects (R. S. Duman, 2002; Fuss, Ben Abdallah, Hensley, et al., 2010; Fuss, Ben Abdallah, Vogt, et al., 2010; Garcia-Capdevila et al., 2009; Grace et al., 2009), and anxiolytic effects (Binder, Droste, Ohl, & Reul, 2004; C. H. Duman, Schlesinger, Russell, & Duman, 2008; Salam et al., 2009; Trejo et al., 2008) in animal models of unlearned anxiety. The discrepancy is present in both sexes of rats and mice. Neither alterations in general activity (C. H. Duman et al., 2008), fatigue (C. H. Duman et al.,

2008; Salam et al., 2009), nor pain sensitivity (C. H. Duman et al., 2008; Falls et al., 2010; Fuss et al., 2009) seem to influence the effects of exercise in tests of unlearned anxiety. Other factors including type of exercise (i.e., forced vs. voluntary; Burghardt, Fulk, Hand, & Wilson, 2004; Dishman et al., 1996; Leasure & Jones, 2008), housing conditions (Dubreucq, Marsicano, & Chaouloff, 2011), duration of prior exercise (Burghardt et al., 2004), time of day of testing (Hopkins & Bucci, 2010), and duration of behavioral test (Binder et al., 2004), however, may partially explain the discrepancy in the literature. Several studies reporting anxiogenic effects of exercise in the open field and elevated plus maze tests, for example, perform relatively short, five-minute tests (Burghardt et al., 2004; R. S. Duman, 2002; Fuss, Ben Abdallah, Vogt, et al., 2010; Garcia-Capdevila et al., 2009). Binder et al. (2004), however, observed that the anxiogenic effect (reduced center exploration) of wheel running present during the first 10 minutes of an open field test was made up for during the final 20 minutes of the test. The cautious behavior displayed by exercised animals during the beginning of the anxiety test could reflect greater cognitive appraisal of the environment. Consistent with this interpretation are the observations that exercised, compared to sedentary, animals spend more time in the center (the border between the closed and open arms) of the plus maze (Garcia-Capdevila et al., 2009), a behavior that has been related to decision-making (Wall & Messier, 2001). Later in the test, when exercised animals seem to display anxiolytic profiles, prior exercise could facilitate a shift from risk assessment to exploration. This strategy of caution followed by enhanced exploration, although only revealed under appropriate testing conditions, could be an adaptive response to conflict that could enhance survival.

Another factor that influences the effect of exercise on unconditioned anxiety is the stress status of the animals. Indeed, Figure 7.2 suggests that the effect of exercise on unconditioned anxiety depends upon history of prior stressor exposure. In this experiment, male F344 rats remained sedentary or were allowed access to wheels for six weeks prior to exposure to uncontrollable tail shock stress (see Greenwood et al., 2003), which produces robust learned and unlearned anxiety (Baratta et al., 2007; Maier & Watkins, 1998). Twenty-four hours later, rats were exposed to a novel open field (Figure 7.2A) for five minutes. Results indicate that although wheel running does not alter the total movement in the open field (Figure 7.2B), wheel running does reduce the time spent in the center of the field during the five-minute test (Figure 7.2C). Uncontrollable stress also reduces the time spent in the center of the open field. Interestingly, the anxiogenic effect of stress is specific to sedentary rats. In physically active rats, exposure to stress actually increases the time spent in the center of the open field (Figure 7.2C). Van Hoomissen et al. (2011) reported a similar effect of exercise. This group reported that rats allowed to run in running wheels for three weeks following olfactory bulbectomy displayed a robust anxiolytic profile as measured by entries into the center of a novel environment (J. Van Hoomissen et al., 2011). Interestingly, it was only the exercised rats lacking an olfactory bulb who displayed the anxiolytic profile. Exercised sham rats behaved similarly to sedentary rats. Although the mechanisms underlying the interaction between exercise and stress in tests of unlearned anxiety are not yet clear, these data suggest that researchers should be especially sensitive to the stress status of their animals, as even subtle, unintentional differences in stress status may influence the effects of exercise on these tests. Until the behavioral effects of exercise in these tests are better characterized, it will be difficult to use these tests to investigate mechanisms underlying the effects of exercise on anxiety.

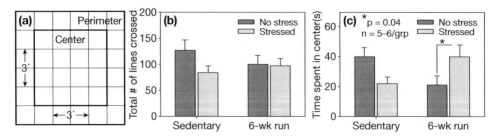

Figure 7.2 Effects of exercise on open field behavior.

Stress-induced anxiety

In addition to demonstrating that the behavioral effects of exercise in animal models of unlearned anxiety depend on the history of stressor exposure, the data in Figure 7.2 also provide an example of the powerful protective effect of exercise against stress-induced anxiety. Moreover, Figure 7.2 and prior data (Greenwood, Foley, Burhans, et al., 2005; Greenwood et al., 2003) suggest that the anxiolytic effects of exercise may be even more likely revealed following exposure to an event that can facilitate the development of anxiety, such as stressor exposure. Indeed, human data suggest the anxiolytic effects of exercise are more robust in individuals who are most susceptible to anxiety (Smits, Tart, Rosenfield, & Zvolensky, 2011). It may therefore be most appropriate to investigate the anxiolytic effects of exercise in animal models of anxiety following exposure to a manipulation (be it genetic, pharmacological, or environmental) that is known to lead to anxiety-like behaviors in sedentary organisms. One such manipulation is exposure to stress. Indeed, stressor exposure is an important causal factor in the development of human anxiety disorders. Animal models utilizing exposure to stressors may have the greatest potential for identification of the neurobiological mechanisms underlying the anxiolytic effects of exercise.

Behavioral effects of exercise on animal models of stress-induced anxiety

It is now well established that the behavioral consequences of stress that resemble anxiety are sensitive to physical activity status. Sedentary rats exposed to an uncontrollable stressor display behaviors that resemble symptoms of human anxiety, including social avoidance, exaggerated conditioned fear, and interference with instrumental learning (Christianson et al., 2008; Greenwood et al., 2003; Maier, 1990). Rats and mice allowed access to running wheels prior to uncontrollable stressor exposure are protected against later deficits in instrumental learning measured in the shuttle box escape task (Dishman et al., 1997; C. H. Duman et al., 2008; Greenwood, Foley, Burhans, et al., 2005; Greenwood et al., 2003; Greenwood et al., 2007), as well as the anxiety measured by social exploration (Greenwood et al., 2012) and conditioned fear (Greenwood, Foley, Burhans, et al., 2005; Greenwood et al., 2003; Greenwood et al., 2007).

Exercise protection against stress–induced anxiety extends beyond uncontrollable stressors and psychological stressors in general. Using a variety of anxiety tests including open field, light/dark box, the hole-board test, shock-probe defensive burying, and acoustic startle, exercise has been observed to prevent anxiety elicited by 24 hours of sleep deprivation (Vollert et al., 2011), oxidative stress (Salim et al., 2010), experimentally induced colitis (Kasimay et al., 2006), acute administration of a β-carboline (Sciolino, Dishman, & Holmes, 2012), a selective serotonin (5-HT) reuptake inhibitor (Greenwood, Strong, Brooks, & Fleshner, 2008), a non-selective 5-HT$_2$ receptor agonist (Fox, Hammack, & Falls, 2008), and a selective 5-HT$_{2C}$ receptor agonist (Greenwood, Strong, et al., 2012). The protective effect of exercise against stress-induced anxiety thus appears to be a relatively consistent observation that extends across many stressors and anxiety tests.

Potential mechanisms

Mechanisms that could contribute to the protective effect of exercise against stress-induced anxiety include changes in brain monoamines (Dishman et al., 1997; Greenwood & Fleshner, 2011; Greenwood et al., 2005b) and circuits involved in reward (Greenwood et al., 2011) or entrainment of circadian rhythms (Edgar & Dement, 1991; Solberg, Hortaon, & Turek, 1999), and enhanced neurotrophic (Russo-Neustadt & Chen, 2005), anti-inflammatory (Cotman et al., 2007; Gleeson et al., 2011), or antioxidant (Salim et al., 2010; Vollert et al., 2011) support. The literature on the effects of exercise on these systems is rather difficult to interpret due to the use of various exercise paradigms (i.e., forced swimming, treadmill training, and wheel running), which vary in their degree of stress, in addition to exercise duration, intensity, pattern, and controllability. Because many of these systems are also sensitive to stress, it has been difficult to separate the effects of stress from those of exercise, per se. This is especially true of forced exercise paradigms such as swimming or treadmill training, which are inherently stress-evoking (Brown et al., 2007; Moraska, Deak, Spencer, Roth, & Fleshner, 2000). Moreover, a recent study indicates that 6 weeks of treadmill training was unable to prevent stress-induced anxiety measured with conditioned fear (Greenwood, Spence, et al., 2012). For these reasons, future studies would be well served to focus on the effects of voluntary exercise, or at least a forced exercise paradigm demonstrated to prevent stress-induced anxiety (Greenwood, Spence, et al., 2012), on central changes associated with anxiety reduction.

We have been interested in the effects of voluntary exercise on the central 5-HT system. The focus on 5-HT is appropriate, given the involvement of 5-HT in reward (Hayes & Greenshaw, 2011), circadian entrainment (Meyer-Bernstein & Morin, 1996), and anxiety (Graeff, Guimaraes, De Andrade, & Deakin, 1996; Lowry, Johnson, Hay-Schmidt, Mikkelsen, & Shekhar, 2005). Moreover, accumulating data indicate that an increase in 5-HT is causal in anxiety and is critical for the social avoidance, exaggerated fear conditioning, and interference with instrumental learning produced by uncontrollable stress (Maier & Watkins, 2005). Exercise produces neuroplasticity in the central 5-HT system at multiple levels including (1) brain regions that modulate 5-HT activity during stressor exposure, (2) 5-HT cell body regions, such as the dorsal raphe nucleus, and (3) 5-HT projection sites, such as reduced expression or sensitivity of postsynaptic 5-HT receptors in brain regions critical for the expression of stress-induced anxiety. We have presented evidence supporting a role for each of these possibilities in the protective effect of exercise against stress-induced anxiety (Greenwood & Fleshner, 2011; Greenwood, Foley, Burhans, et al., 2005; Greenwood, Foley, Day, et al., 2005; Greenwood et al., 2003, 2012). Together, available data support the idea that limiting the behavioral impact of acute increases in 5-HT during stressor exposure contributes to the protection against stress-induced anxiety produced by exercise.

Exercise-induced plasticity in the central 5-HT system could contribute to anxiolytic effects of exercise in several types of anxiety. For example, 5-HT can modulate BDNF in the hippocampus, where 5-HT2 receptor activation contributes to stress-induced reductions in BDNF (Vaidya, Terwilliger, & Duman, 1999). Voluntary exercise prevents the reduction in

BDNF mRNA and protein in the hippocampus produced by stressor exposure (Adlard & Cotman, 2004; Greenwood et al., 2007), an observation that would be expected if exercise constrained stress-induced activation of 5-HT neurons or reduced sensitivity or expression of 5-HT2 receptors in the hippocampus. The effects of exercise on 5-HT and neurotrophic systems might, therefore, interact to produce anxiolytic effects under a variety of conditions (Figure 7.1).

Conclusions and future directions

Exercise is anxiolytic in tests of context discrimination and stress-induced anxiety. Mechanisms underlying the anxiolytic effects of exercise could include plasticity in neurotrophic and/or 5-HT systems that modulate learning and memory processes and behavioral responses to stress. The behavioral effects of exercise on animal models of unlearned anxiety are not yet clear, but seem to depend upon the history of stressor exposure. Investigators, therefore, should be especially attentive to the stress status of their animals when investigating mechanisms underlying the anxiolytic effects of exercise. This applies especially to the use of forced exercise paradigms such as swimming or treadmill training, which inherently introduce aspects of repeated stress. The mechanisms by which the experience of exercise is communicated to the brain to reduce anxiety could include peripheral IGF-1 or central NE, and is an important area of future inquiry. To identify these mechanisms, future studies should utilize exercise paradigms demonstrated to produce significant behavioral effects in animal models of anxiety.

References

Adlard, P. A., & Cotman, C. W. (2004). Voluntary exercise protects against stress-induced decreases in brain-derived neurotrophic factor protein expression. *Neuroscience, 124*(4), 985–992.

Baratta, M. V., Christianson, J. P., Gomez, D. M., Zarza, C. M., Amat, J., Masini, C. V., . . . Maier, S. F. (2007). Controllable versus uncontrollable stressors bi-directionally modulate conditioned but not innate fear. *Neuroscience, 146*(4), 1495–1503.

Baruch, D. E., Swain, R. A., & Helmstetter, F. J. (2004). Effects of exercise on Pavlovian fear conditioning. *Behavioral Neuroscience, 118*(5), 1123–1127.

Berchtold, N. C., Chinn, G., Chou, M., Kesslak, J. P., & Cotman, C. W. (2005). Exercise primes a molecular memory for brain-derived neurotrophic factor protein induction in the rat hippocampus. *Neuroscience, 133*(3), 853–861.

Binder, E., Droste, S. K., Ohl, F., & Reul, J. M. (2004). Regular voluntary exercise reduces anxiety-related behaviour and impulsiveness in mice. *Behavioural Brain Research, 155*(2), 197–206.

Brown, D. A., Johnson, M. S., Armstrong, C. J., Lynch, J. M., Caruso, N. M., Ehlers, L. B., . . . Moore, R. L. (2007). Short-term treadmill running in the rat: what kind of stressor is it? *Journal of Applied Physiology, 103*(6), 1979–1985.

Burghardt, P. R., Fulk, L. J., Hand, G. A., & Wilson, M. A. (2004). The effects of chronic treadmill and wheel running on behavior in rats. *Brain Research, 1019*(1–2), 84–96.

Burghardt, P. R., Pasumarthi, R. K., Wilson, M. A., & Fadel, J. (2006). Alterations in fear conditioning and amygdalar activation following chronic wheel running in rats. *Pharmacology Biochemistry and Behavior, 84*(2), 306–312.

Campeau, S., Nyhuis, T. J., Sasse, S. K., Kryskow, E. M., Herlihy, L., Masini, C. V., . . . Day, H. E. (2010). Hypothalamic pituitary adrenal axis responses to low-intensity stressors are reduced after voluntary wheel running in rats. *Journal of Neuroendocrinology, 22*(8), 872–888.

Chaouloff, F. (1994). Influence of physical exercise on 5-HT1A receptor- and anxiety-related behaviours. *Neuroscience Letters, 176*(2), 226–230.

Christianson, J. P., Paul, E. D., Irani, M., Thompson, B. M., Kubala, K. H., Yirmiya, R., . . . Maier, S. F. (2008). The role of prior stressor controllability and the dorsal raphe nucleus in sucrose preference and social exploration. *Behavioural Brain Research, 193*(1), 87–93.

Clark, P. J., Brzezinska, W. J., Thomas, M. W., Ryzhenko, N. A., Toshkov, S. A., & Rhodes, J. S. (2008).

Intact neurogenesis is required for benefits of exercise on spatial memory but not motor performance or contextual fear conditioning in C57BL/6J mice. *Neuroscience, 155*(4), 1048–1058.

Cotman, C. W., Berchtold, N. C., & Christie, L. A. (2007). Exercise builds brain health: key roles of growth factor cascades and inflammation. *Trends in Neuroscience, 30*(9), 464–472.

Ding, Q., Vaynman, S., Akhavan, M., Ying, Z., & Gomez-Pinilla, F. (2006). Insulin-like growth factor I interfaces with brain-derived neurotrophic factor-mediated synaptic plasticity to modulate aspects of exercise-induced cognitive function. *Neuroscience, 140*(3), 823–833.

Ding, Q., Ying, Z., & Gomez-Pinilla, F. (2011). Exercise influences hippocampal plasticity by modulating brain-derived neurotrophic factor processing. *Neuroscience, 192*, 773–780.

Dishman, R. K., Bunnell, B. N., Youngstedt, S. D., Yoo, H. S., Mougey, E. H., & Meyerhoff, J. L. (1998). Activity wheel running blunts increased plasma adrenocorticotrophin (ACTH) after footshock and cage-switch stress. *Physiology and Behavior, 63*(5), 911–917.

Dishman, R. K., Dunn, A. L., Youngstedt, S. D., Davis, J. M., Burgess, M. L., Wilson, S. P., & Wilson, M. A. (1996). Increased open field locomotion and decreased striatal GABAA binding after activity wheel running. *Physiology and Behavior, 60*(3), 699–705.

Dishman, R. K., Renner, K. J., Youngstedt, S. D., Reigle, T. G., Bunnell, B. N., Burke, K. A., ... Meyerhoff, J. L. (1997). Activity wheel running reduces escape latency and alters brain monoamine levels after footshock. *Brain Research Bulletin, 42*(5), 399–406.

Dubreucq, S., Marsicano, G., & Chaouloff, F. (2011). Emotional consequences of wheel running in mice: which is the appropriate control? *Hippocampus, 21*(3), 239–242.

Duman, C. H., Schlesinger, L., Russell, D. S., & Duman, R. S. (2008). Voluntary exercise produces antidepressant and anxiolytic behavioral effects in mice. *Brain Research*, 1199, 148–158.

Duman, R. S. (2002). Synaptic plasticity and mood disorders. *Molecular Psychiatry, 7(Suppl 1)*, S29–S34.

Duman, R. S., Heninger, G. R., & Nestler, E. J. (1997). A molecular and cellular theory of depression. *Archives of General Psychiatry, 54*(7), 597–606.

Duman, R. S., & Monteggia, L. M. (2006). A neurotrophic model for stress-related mood disorders. *Biological Psychiatry*, 59(12), 1116–1127.

Edgar, D. M., & Dement, W. C. (1991). Regularly scheduled voluntary exercise synchronizes the mouse circadian clock. *American Journal of Physiology, 261*(4 Pt 2), R928–933.

Elzinga, B. M., & Bremner, J. D. (2002). Are the neural substrates of memory the final common pathway in posttraumatic stress disorder (PTSD)? *Journal of Affective Disorders, 70*(1), 1–17.

Falls, W. A., Fox, J. H., & MacAulay, C. M. (2010). Voluntary exercise improves both learning and consolidation of cued conditioned fear in C57 mice. *Behavioural Brain Research, 207*(2), 321–331.

Fox, J. H., Hammack, S. E., & Falls, W. A. (2008). Exercise is associated with reduction in the anxiogenic effect of mCPP on acoustic startle. *Behavioral Neuroscience, 122*(4), 943–948.

Fuss, J., Ben Abdallah, N. M., Hensley, F. W., Weber, K. J., Hellweg, R., & Gass, P. (2010). Deletion of running-induced hippocampal neurogenesis by irradiation prevents development of an anxious phenotype in mice. *PloS ONE, 5*(9): e12769.

Fuss, J., Ben Abdallah, N. M., Vogt, M. A., Touma, C., Pacifici, P. G., Palme, R., ... Gass, P. (2010). Voluntary exercise induces anxiety-like behavior in adult C57BL/6J mice correlating with hippocampal neurogenesis. *Hippocampus, 20*(3), 364–376.

Garcia, C., Chen, M. J., Garza, A. A., Cotman, C. W., & Russo-Neustadt, A. (2003). The influence of specific noradrenergic and serotonergic lesions on the expression of hippocampal brain-derived neurotrophic factor transcripts following voluntary physical activity. *Neuroscience, 119*(3), 721–732.

Garcia-Capdevila, S., Portell-Cortes, I., Torras-Garcia, M., Coll-Andreu, M., & Costa-Miserachs, D. (2009). Effects of long-term voluntary exercise on learning and memory processes: dependency of the task and level of exercise. *Behavioural Brain Research, 202*(2), 162–170.

Gleeson, M., Bishop, N. C., Stensel, D. J., Lindley, M. R., Mastana, S. S., & Nimmo, M. A. (2011). The anti-inflammatory effects of exercise: mechanisms and implications for the prevention and treatment of disease. *Nature Reviews. Immunology, 11*(9), 607–615.

Grace, L., Hescham, S., Kellaway, L. A., Bugarith, K., & Russell, V. A. (2009). Effect of exercise on learning and memory in a rat model of developmental stress. *Metabolic Brain Disease, 24*(4), 643–657.

Graeff, F. G., Guimaraes, F. S., De Andrade, T. G., & Deakin, J. F. (1996). Role of 5-HT in stress, anxiety, and depression. *Pharmacology Biochemistry and Behavior, 54*(1), 129–141.

Greenwood, B. N., & Fleshner, M. (2011). Exercise, stress resistance, and central serotonergic systems. *Exercise and Sport Sciences Reviews, 39*(3), 140–149.

Greenwood, B. N., Foley, T. E., Burhans, D., Maier, S. F., & Fleshner, M. (2005a). The consequences of uncontrollable stress are sensitive to duration of prior wheel running. *Brain Research*, *1033*(2), 164–178.

Greenwood, B. N., Foley, T. E., Day, H. E., Burhans, D., Brooks, L., Campeau, S., & Fleshner, M. (2005b). Wheel running alters serotonin (5-HT) transporter, 5-HT(1A), 5-HT(1B), and alpha(1b)-adrenergic receptor mRNA in the rat raphe nuclei. *Biological Psychiatry*, *57*(5), 559–568.

Greenwood, B. N., Foley, T. E., Day, H. E., Campisi, J., Hammack, S. H., Campeau, S., . . . Fleshner, M. (2003). Freewheel running prevents learned helplessness/behavioral depression: role of dorsal raphe serotonergic neurons. *Journal of Neuroscience*, *23*(7), 2889–2898.

Greenwood, B. N., Foley, T. E., Le, T. V., Strong, P. V., Loughridge, A. B., Day, H. E., & Fleshner, M. (2011). Long-term voluntary wheel running is rewarding and produces plasticity in the mesolimbic reward pathway. *Behavioural Brain Research*, *217*(2), 354–362.

Greenwood, B. N., Spence, K. G., Crevling, D. M., Clark, P. J., Craig, W. C., & Fleshner, M. (2012). Exercise-induced stress resistance is independent of exercise controllability and the medial prefrontal cortex. *European Journal of Neuroscience*. In press.

Greenwood, B. N., Strong, P. V., Brooks, L., & Fleshner, M. (2008). Anxiety-like behaviors produced by acute fluoxetine administration in male Fischer 344 rats are prevented by prior exercise. *Psychopharmacology*, *199*(2), 209–222.

Greenwood, B. N., Strong, P. V., Foley, T. E., & Fleshner, M. (2009). A behavioral analysis of the impact of voluntary physical activity on hippocampus–dependent contextual conditioning. *Hippocampus*, *19*(10), 988–1001.

Greenwood, B. N., Strong, P. V., Foley, T. E., Thompson, R. S., & Fleshner, M. (2007). Learned helplessness is independent of levels of brain–derived neurotrophic factor in the hippocampus. *Neuroscience*, *144*(4), 1193–1208.

Greenwood, B. N., Strong, P. V., Loughridge, A. B., Day, H. E., Clark, P. J., Mika, A., . . . Fleshner, M. (2012). 5-HT(2C) Receptors in the basolateral amygdala and dorsal striatum are a novel target for the anxiolytic and antidepressant effects of exercise. *PloS One*, *7*(9), e46118.

Hayes, D. J., & Greenshaw, A. J. (2011). 5-HT receptors and reward-related behaviour: a review. *Neuroscience and Biobehavioral Reviews*, *35*(6), 1419–1449.

Hopkins, M. E., & Bucci, D. J. (2010). Interpreting the effects of exercise on fear conditioning: the influence of time of day. *Behavioral Neuroscience*, *124*(6), 868–872.

Huff, N. C., & Rudy, J. W. (2004). The amygdala modulates hippocampus–dependent context memory formation and stores cue-shock associations. *Behavioral Neuroscience*, *118*(1), 53–62.

Ivy, A. S., Rodriguez, F. G., Garcia, C., Chen, M. J., & Russo-Neustadt, A. A. (2003). Noradrenergic and serotonergic blockade inhibits BDNF mRNA activation following exercise and antidepressant. *Pharmacology Biochemistry and Behavior*, *75*(1), 81–88.

Kasimay, O., Guzel, E., Gemici, A., Abdyli, A., Sulovari, A., Ercan, F., & Yegen, B. C. (2006). Colitis-induced oxidative damage of the colon and skeletal muscle is ameliorated by regular exercise in rats: the anxiolytic role of exercise. *Experimental Physiology*, *91*(5), 897–906.

Kim, J. J., Rison, R. A., & Fanselow, M. S. (1993). Effects of amygdala, hippocampus, and periaqueductal gray lesions on short- and long-term contextual fear. *Behavioral Neuroscience*, *107*(6), 1093–1098.

Kitaoka, R., Fujikawa, T., Miyaki, T., Matsumura, S., Fushiki, T., & Inoue, K. (2010). Increased noradrenergic activity in the ventromedial hypothalamus during treadmill running in rats. *Journal of Nutritional Science and Vitaminology*, *56*(3), 185–190.

Leasure, J. L., & Jones, M. (2008). Forced and voluntary exercise differentially affect brain and behavior. *Neuroscience*, *156*(3), 456–465.

Lowry, C. A., Johnson, P. L., Hay-Schmidt, A., Mikkelsen, J., & Shekhar, A. (2005). Modulation of anxiety circuits by serotonergic systems. *Stress*, *8*(4), 233–246.

Maier, S. F. (1990). Role of fear in mediating shuttle escape learning deficit produced by inescapable shock. *Journal of Experimental Psychology: Animal and Behavior Processes*, *16*(2), 137–149.

Maier, S. F., & Watkins, L. R. (1998). Stressor controllability, anxiety, and serotonin. *Cognitive Therapy and Research*, *22*(6), 595–613.

Maier, S. F., & Watkins, L. R. (2005). Stressor controllability and learned helplessness: the roles of the dorsal raphe nucleus, serotonin, and corticotropin-releasing factor. *Neuroscience and Biobehavioral Reviews*, *29*(4–5), 829–841.

Meeusen, R., Smolders, I., Sarre, S., de Meirleir, K., Keizer, H., Serneels, M., . . . Michotte, Y. (1997). Endurance training effects on neurotransmitter release in rat striatum: an in vivo microdialysis study. *Acta Physiologica Scandinavica*, *159*(4), 335–341.

Mello, P. B., Benetti, F., Cammarota, M., & Izquierdo, I. (2009). Physical exercise can reverse the deficit in fear memory induced by maternal deprivation. *Neurobiology of Learning and Memory, 92*(3), 364–369.

Meyer-Bernstein, E. L., & Morin, L. P. (1996). Differential serotonergic innervation of the suprachiasmatic nucleus and the intergeniculate leaflet and its role in circadian rhythm modulation. *Journal of Neuroscience, 16*(6), 2097–2111.

Mizumori, S. J., Smith, D. M., & Puryear, C. B. (2007). Hippocampal and neocortical interactions during context discrimination: electrophysiological evidence from the rat. *Hippocampus, 17*(9), 851–862.

Moraska, A., Deak, T., Spencer, R. L., Roth, D., & Fleshner, M. (2000). Treadmill running produces both positive and negative physiological adaptations in Sprague-Dawley rats. *American Journal of Physiology: Regulatory, Integrative and Comparative Physiology, 279*(4), R1321–R1329.

Neeper, S. A., Gomez-Pinilla, F., Choi, J., & Cotman, C. (1995). Exercise and brain neurotrophins. *Nature, 373*(6510), 109.

Peters, J., Dieppa-Perea, L. M., Melendez, L. M., & Quirk, G. J. (2010). Induction of fear extinction with hippocampal-infralimbic BDNF. *Science, 328*(5983), 1288–1290.

Phillips, R. G., & LeDoux, J. E. (1992). Differential contribution of amygdala and hippocampus to cued and contextual fear conditioning. *Behavioral Neuroscience, 106*(2), 274–285.

Pietropaolo, S., Feldon, J., Alleva, E., Cirulli, F., & Yee, B. K. (2006). The role of voluntary exercise in enriched rearing: a behavioral analysis. *Behavioral Neuroscience, 120*(4), 787–803.

Poo, M. M. (2001). Neurotrophins as synaptic modulators. *Nature Reviews Neuroscience, 2*(1), 24–32.

Rudy, J. W., Barrientos, R. M., & O'Reilly, R. C. (2002). Hippocampal formation supports conditioning to memory of a context. *Behavioral Neuroscience, 116*(4), 530–538.

Russo-Neustadt, A. A., & Chen, M. J. (2005). Brain-derived neurotrophic factor and antidepressant activity. *Current Pharmaceutical Design, 11*(12), 1495–1510.

Salam, J. N., Fox, J. H., Detroy, E. M., Guignon, M. H., Wohl, D. F., & Falls, W. A. (2009). Voluntary exercise in C57 mice is anxiolytic across several measures of anxiety. *Behavioural Brain Research, 197*(1), 31–40.

Salim, S., Sarraj, N., Taneja, M., Saha, K., Tejada-Simon, M. V., & Chugh, G. (2010). Moderate treadmill exercise prevents oxidative stress-induced anxiety-like behavior in rats. *Behavioural Brain Research, 208*(2), 545–552.

Santarelli, L., Saxe, M., Gross, C., Surget, A., Battaglia, F., Dulawa, S., . . . Hen, R. (2003). Requirement of hippocampal neurogenesis for the behavioral effects of antidepressants. *Science, 301*(5634), 805–809.

Sciolino, N. R., Dishman, R. K., & Holmes, P. V. (2012). Voluntary exercise offers anxiolytic potential and amplifies galanin gene expression in the locus coeruleus of the rat. *Behavioural Brain Research, 233*(1), 191–200.

Scofield, D. E., McClung, H. L., McClung, J. P., Kraemer, W. J., Rarick, K. R., Pierce, J. R., . . . Nindl, B. C. (2011). A novel, noninvasive transdermal fluid sampling methodology: IGF-I measurement following exercise. *American Journal of Physiology. Regulatory, Integrative and Comparative Physiology, 300*(6), R1326–R1332.

Smits, J. A., Tart, C. D., Rosenfield, D., & Zvolensky, M. J. (2011). The interplay between physical activity and anxiety sensitivity in fearful responding to carbon dioxide challenge. *Psychosomatic Medicine, 73*(6), 498–503.

Solberg, L. C., Hortaon, T. H., & Turek, F. W. (1999). Circadian rhythms and depression: effects of exercise in an animal model. *American Journal of Physiology, 276*, R152–R161.

Trejo, J. L., Carro, E., & Torres-Aleman, I. (2001). Circulating insulin-like growth factor I mediates exercise-induced increases in the number of new neurons in the adult hippocampus. *Journal of Neuroscience, 21*(5), 1628–1634.

Trejo, J. L., Llorens-Martin, M. V., & Torres-Aleman, I. (2008). The effects of exercise on spatial learning and anxiety-like behavior are mediated by an IGF-I-dependent mechanism related to hippocampal neurogenesis. *Molecular and Cellular Neurosciences, 37*(2), 402–411.

Tyler, W. J., Alonso, M., Bramham, C. R., & Pozzo-Miller, L. D. (2002). From acquisition to consolidation: on the role of brain-derived neurotrophic factor signaling in hippocampal-dependent learning. *Learning and Memory, 9*(5), 224–237.

Vaidya, V. A., Terwilliger, R. M., & Duman, R. S. (1999). Role of 5-HT2A receptors in the stress-induced down-regulation of brain-derived neurotrophic factor expression in rat hippocampus. *Neuroscience Letters, 262*(1), 1–4.

Van Hoomissen, J. D., Holmes, P. V., Zellner, A. S., Poudevigne, A., & Dishman, R. K. (2004). Effects of beta-adrenoreceptor blockade during chronic exercise on contextual fear conditioning and mRNA for galanin and brain-derived neurotrophic factor. *Behavioral Neuroscience, 118*(6), 1378–1390.

141

Van Hoomissen, J., Kunrath, J., Dentlinger, R., Lafrenz, A., Krause, M., & Azar, A. (2011). Cognitive and locomotor/exploratory behavior after chronic exercise in the olfactory bulbectomy animal model of depression. *Behavioural Brain Research*, *222*(1), 106–116.

van Praag, H., Kempermann, G., & Gage, F. H. (1999). Running increases cell proliferation and neurogenesis in the adult mouse dentate gyrus. *Nature Neuroscience*, *2*(3), 266–270.

Vaynman, S., Ying, Z., & Gomez-Pinilla, F. (2004). Hippocampal BDNF mediates the efficacy of exercise on synaptic plasticity and cognition. *European Journal of Neuroscience*, *20*(10), 2580–2590.

Vollert, C., Zagaar, M., Hovatta, I., Taneja, M., Vu, A., Dao, A., . . . Salim, S. (2011). Exercise prevents sleep deprivation-associated anxiety-like behavior in rats: potential role of oxidative stress mechanisms. *Behavioural Brain Research*, *224*(2), 233–240.

Wall, P. M., & Messier, C. (2001). Methodological and conceptual issues in the use of the elevated plus-maze as a psychological measurement instrument of animal anxiety-like behavior. *Neuroscience and Biobehavioral Reviews*, *25*(3), 275–286.

Wiltgen, B. J., & Silva, A. J. (2007). Memory for context becomes less specific with time. *Learning and Memory*, *14*(4), 313–317.

Yan, H., Mitschelen, M., Bixler, G. V., Brucklacher, R. M., Farley, J. A., Han, S., . . . Sonntag, W. E. (2011). Circulating insulin-like growth factor (IGF)-1 regulates hippocampal IGF-1 levels and brain gene expression during adolescence. *Journal of Endocrinology*, *211*(1), 27–37.

Yukako, N., Susumu, M., Yoshikazu, N., Jing-Hui, X., Takuya, H., & Hiroji, Y. (2008). Genetic increase in brain-derived neurotrophic factor levels enhances spatial learning. *Brain Research*, *1241*, 103–109.

PART 3

Depression and mood disorders

Edited by
Lynette L. Craft

8

EXERCISE AND PHYSICAL ACTIVITY IN THE PREVENTION AND TREATMENT OF DEPRESSION

Patrick J. Smith and James A. Blumenthal

Depression is a term that refers both to a transient mood state and a clinical syndrome or disorder. As a mood state, depression is characterized by feeling despondent or unhappy, while depression as a mood disorder is a persistent set of symptoms as described in the fourth edition of the Diagnostic and Statistical Manual of Mental Disorders (DSM IV). Specifically, major depressive disorder (MDD) is a psychiatric condition in which diagnostic criteria require five or more depressive symptoms, one of which must include either depressed mood or loss of interest or pleasure. Other depressive symptoms include significant weight loss, sleep changes (i.e., insomnia or hypersomnia), psychomotor agitation or retardation, fatigue or loss of energy, feelings of worthlessness or excessive guilt, diminished ability to think or concentrate, and recurrent thoughts of death. MDD is also distinguished from normal symptoms of sadness by criteria for symptom severity and duration: symptoms of depression must have been present during the same two-week period, be present all or most of the time, and represent a *change* from a previous level of functioning.

Epidemiology of major depressive disorder

Although the estimates of depression prevalence vary between samples, community surveys generally find that up to 20% of adults and 50% of children and adolescents report depressive symptoms during the past 6 months (Kessler, Avenevoli, & Ries Merikangas, 2001; Kessler, Merikangas, & Wang, 2008) and 6.6% of U.S. adults experienced MDD during the last year (Kessler et al., 2003). Estimates vary depending primarily on whether the presence of depressive symptoms or clinical depression is assessed. Of the depressive episodes experienced by adults during the last year, nearly one-third were severe (Kessler, Chiu, Demler, Merikangas, & Walters, 2005). Depression is somewhat more common among whites compared to African Americans, and is twice as common among women in comparison to men (Kessler, Berglund, et al., 2005).

In the United States there has been recent concern that the prevalence of depression is increasing, particularly among teenagers and young adults. For example, compared with adults over the age of 60, 18–29-year-olds are 70% more likely to have experienced a major depressive episode in their lifetimes (Kessler, Berglund, et al., 2005). Depression is also commonly observed to co-occur in many medical conditions (Katon, 2003), including highly prevalent and costly diseases such as obesity (Roberts, Deleger, Strawbridge, & Kaplan, 2003), diabetes (Katon et al.,

2008), cardiovascular disease (Lichtman et al., 2008), and Alzheimer's disease (Ownby, Crocco, Acevedo, John, & Loewenstein, 2006), and has been associated with negative health behaviors such as physical inactivity (Roshanaei-Moghaddam, Katon, & Russo, 2009), poor dietary patterns (Katon et al., 2008), medical nonadherence (DiMatteo, Lepper, & Croghan, 2000), and substance use (Davis, Uezato, Newell, & Frazier, 2008).

Health consequences of depression

MDD is associated with poorer quality of life and is a significant burden on the healthcare system, increasing medical expenditures and healthcare utilization. In addition, depression is one of the leading sources of disability in the United States and is associated with significantly increased missed time at work. Although depression is a treatable condition, as many as 1 in 10 individuals with chronic depression may ultimately commit suicide (Wulsin, Vaillant, & Wells, 1999). MDD is a significant source of emotional suffering and a healthcare burden and is one of the leading causes of disability in the United States and internationally (Simon, 2003). According to the World Health Organization, depression is the leading cause of years lived with disability, the fourth leading cause of disability adjusted life years (DALYs), and is associated with greater health decrements in comparison with angina, arthritis, asthma, and diabetes (Moussavi et al., 2007). Depression is also associated with an increased risk for a variety of medical conditions, including diabetes and cardiovascular disease.

Conventional treatments for depression

Pharmacotherapy

Depression is most commonly treated with antidepressant medication (Olfson et al., 2002). Many randomized clinical trials (RCTs) have examined the effectiveness of various pharmacological compounds on depression outcomes (Lieberman et al., 2005). Antidepressants generally have been shown to have efficacy in improving depression and reducing relapse rates. The current recommendations for depression treatment typically involve treatment using a selective serotonin reuptake inhibitor (SSRI) (Trivedi, Fava, et al., 2006), although treatments with tricyclic antidepressants, benzodiazepines, and combined therapies are also common (Gelenberg et al., 2010). Approximately 50% of patients will have a clinical "response" to treatment (i.e., a 50% reduction in symptoms), whereas many individuals will require augmented treatment with more than one antidepressant agent (Hollon, Thase, & Markowitz, 2002).

Recent evidence suggests that the effects of antidepressant therapy may vary by severity of depression, with patients with more severe depressive symptomatology achieving the greatest benefit. This evidence is consistent with some treatment guidelines suggesting that patients with more severe depression are the most likely to benefit from pharmacotherapy treatment. In a meta-regression of randomized, placebo-controlled trials, Fournier and colleagues (Fournier et al., 2010) found differential effects of antidepressant therapy depending on the severity of depression at study entry among depressed adults. Patients with Hamilton Depression Rating Scale (HDRS) scores above 22 (suggesting moderate to severe levels of depression) at study entry were more likely to benefit from treatment compared to placebo, whereas participants with less severe levels of depression did not differ significantly from placebo controls.

Psychotherapy for depression

Depression is one of the most common presenting problems among outpatient psychiatric clinics and is highly prevalent in inpatient psychiatric settings. Accordingly, numerous studies have examined the effects of various forms of psychotherapy as a treatment for depression, which are reviewed in detail elsewhere in a number of publications (Cuijpers, van Straten, Andersson, & van Oppen, 2008). Multiple meta-analytic studies have attempted to combine the results of these RCTs to quantify the efficacy of various forms of psychotherapy (Cuijpers et al., 2008). Therapies typically involve individual treatment over the course of several months, although several studies of longer duration have been reported. The primary types of treatment examined are cognitive behavioral therapy (CBT), psychodynamic therapy, (nondirective) supportive treatment, behavioral activation treatment, problem-solving therapy, interpersonal psychotherapy, and social skills training. Among these, the most commonly used treatments for depression include CBT, which focuses on identifying and modifying maladaptive thought patterns, and interpersonal therapy (IPT), which is a structured, time-limited psychotherapy that emphasizes the social context in which depression occurs.

Previous reviews have documented the effectiveness of psychotherapy among individuals with depression, which appears to improve depression to a similar extent as pharmacotherapy (Robinson, Berman, & Neimeyer, 1990). In an early review, Robinson and colleagues (Robinson et al., 1990) combined results from 58 studies of psychotherapy for depression among adults in trials comparing psychotherapy versus a no-treatment control. In this case, the no-treatment control condition consisted of either waitlist controls or placebo treatments, including attention conditions or placebo drugs. Comparing participants at post-treatment, the authors found that psychotherapy was associated with substantial reductions in depressive symptoms (mean effect size improvement = 0.73) and that this improvement tended to be retained during follow-ups (mean effect size improvement = 0.68). In addition, there were no significant differences in depression outcomes between types of psychotherapeutic treatment in this study.

A recent meta-analytic study by Cuijpers and colleagues (Cuijpers et al., 2008) reported similar results in a comparison of various psychotherapeutic treatments of depression. Studies were included if they used a randomized allocation strategy, included only adults, compared two psychological treatments, and were conducted among individuals with MDD or elevated depressive symptoms. In order to examine the effects of various treatments separately, the authors conducted 7 separate meta-analytic analyses, including data from 53 primary trials among 2,757 participants with mild to moderate levels of depression. The authors found that all the major types of psychotherapy treatment were associated with improvements in depressive symptoms compared to control conditions. Although there was some indication that IPT was superior to other forms of therapy, all forms of therapy appeared to be equally efficacious. In addition to the above findings among patients with MDD, similar findings have been reported for patients with subclinical depression, e.g., depressive symptoms that do not meet criteria for MDD. In a meta-analytic study of 7 "high-quality trials," participants who received psychotherapy treatment showed greater improvements in depressive symptoms compared with control conditions and these results tended to persist in 4 studies that examined depressive symptoms among 533 participants at a 1-year follow-up time point, although the findings narrowly missed statistical significance (Cuijpers, Smit, & van Straten, 2007) (d = 0.16 [95% CI: -0.02 to 0.35]).

Summary of conventional treatments

Antidepressants and psychotherapy are effective for many patients, but not everyone benefits from treatment. Moreover, results of RCTs suggest that these conventional therapies do not always perform better than placebo controls, particularly in patients with less severe MDD. Also, these treatments are costly, time consuming, and, in the case of pharmacotherapy, are often associated with side effects. Novel approaches to treating depression are therefore needed. As described below, exercise may be one such approach.

Physical activity and exercise for depression

Epidemiological studies

Observational studies have found that higher levels of physical activity are associated with reduced incidence of depression and that more physically active individuals report lower levels of depressive symptoms compared to their sedentary counterparts (Brosse, Sheets, Lett, & Blumenthal, 2002; Camacho, Roberts, Lazarus, Kaplan, & Cohen, 1991). In one of the earliest observational studies, the first National Health and Nutritional Examination Survey (NHANES I) reported that participants who were not depressed at baseline but reported little or no physical activity were nearly twice as likely to report depressive symptoms during an 8-year follow-up examination compared to participants reporting more regular physical activity (Farmer et al., 1988). A dose-response relationship between physical activity and depression was also found in a 20-year follow-up study of 21,596 men in the Harvard alumni study (Paffenbarger, Lee, & Leung, 1994). In the Alameda County Study, Camacho and colleagues (Camacho et al., 1991) prospectively found that participants who were physically active were at lower risk for depression over an 18-year follow-up compared to less active participants. In addition, those participants who initially had higher levels of depression were at lower risk for later depression if they initiated exercise over the course of the study. Longitudinal studies suggest that exercise is associated with reduced rates of depression in non-depressed adults and also those who were initially depressed. For example, Harris and colleagues (Harris, Cronkite, & Moos, 2006) followed a cohort of 424 depressed adults for 10 years, conducting examinations of depression and physical activity at baseline, 1 year, 4 years, and 10 years. They found that greater levels of physical activity were associated with less concurrent depression. In addition, exercise appeared to be a buffer against negative life events, with physically active participants experiencing one negative life event reporting the same level of depression as sedentary participants without any negative life events.

There is preliminary evidence that the intensity of exercise may predict subsequent depressive symptoms. Lampinen and colleagues (Lampinen, Heikkinen, & Ruoppila, 2000) studied 663 Finnish older adults who were assessed in a baseline examination in 1988 and were reassessed in 1996. Results showed that approximately 50% of participants reported regular walking and approximately 20% reported participating in strenuous exercise. Participants who had decreased their intensity of exercise from baseline to follow-up examinations had significantly higher levels of depressive symptoms, whereas no increase was observed among individuals whose intensity remained unchanged. In a separate study, the authors found a similar relationship when they compared mobility-disabled and non-disabled individuals, with mobility-disabled participants having a greater likelihood of reporting depressive symptoms (Lampinen & Heikkinen, 2003). In contrast, Brown and colleagues (Brown, Ford, Burton, Marshall, & Dobson, 2005) found beneficial effects across a range of intensities in an analysis of 9,207 women participating in the Australian Longitudinal Study on Women's Health. Depressive symptoms were lower among participants who reported regular physical activity and this association remained significant even among individuals who reported "low" levels of physical activity, suggesting that any exercise is better than no exercise and that higher levels of exercise are not necessarily more beneficial compared to lower-intensity exercise.

Despite these positive findings, not all prospective studies have reported a protective effect of exercise on depressive symptoms. For example, Cooper-Patrick and colleagues (Cooper-Patrick, Ford, Mead, Chang, & Klag, 1997) did not observe a relationship between physical activity level and the development of subsequent depression in a sample of more than 700 former medical students. Participants' physical activity levels and depression status were assessed by self-report and review of medical records. Examination of follow-up data showed that the risk of depression was similar for exercisers and non-exercisers. Kritz-Silverstein and colleagues (Kritz-Silverstein, Barrett-Connor, & Corbeau, 2001) found a relationship between self-reported exercise and lower depressive symptoms among participants in the Rancho Bernardo Study in cross-sectional but not longitudinal studies. Participants were older men and women (aged 50–89 years) who were assessed at a baseline visit from 1984 to1987 and a follow-up visit from 1992 to 1995. Cross-sectionally, participants who were exercising had significantly lower depressed mood in comparison with their sedentary counterparts. However, longitudinal analyses found that participants who reported exercising during their baseline assessment did not show lower depression levels during their follow-up assessments. It is possible that these findings were influenced by sample selection causing a "floor effect," as participants who were clinically depressed at baseline were excluded and depression scores were higher among participants who failed to complete the follow-up assessment.

In sum, most, but not all, studies report an inverse association between physical activity and depressive symptoms, although it is noteworthy that observational studies cannot establish a causal relationship between higher levels of physical activity and fewer depressive symptoms. Intervention studies provide the highest level of evidence that exercise is causally related to reduced depression.

Interventional studies

The effects of exercise among individuals with clinical depression have been examined in over two dozen RCTs (Mead et al., 2009) and has been the topic of several systematic reviews (Stathopoulou, Power, Berry, & Smits, 2006), meta-analyses (Lawlor & Hopker, 2001), and one Cochrane review (Mead et al., 2009). Existing studies have varied substantially in size, type of control group, methodological rigor, length of follow-up, and even the type of exercise modality. Randomized trials have generally varied in length from 6 weeks to 4 months. At the time of this review, nearly 30 trials have examined the effects of exercise on depressive symptoms among adults with major depression. As reviewed elsewhere, there is also emerging evidence that exercise improves depression among adolescents (Larun, Nordheim, Ekeland, Hagen, & Heian, 2006), although little high-quality evidence is currently available that examines the effects of exercise in this age group. Although multiple trials have been conducted among adults with depression, few studies have utilized high-quality methodologies in which treatment allocation is concealed, intention-to-treat analyses are used, and assessment of depression is conducted by a trained psychologist instead of being based on self-report.

Several systematic reviews and meta-analytic studies have examined the effects of exercise on depression. In a quantitative and qualitative review, Stathopoulou and colleagues (Stathopoulou et al., 2006) examined the effects of randomized trials of exercise for depression in which only studies with non-active comparison conditions, such as waitlist controls, low-level exercise, and health education, were compared. In addition, only studies among individuals with elevated depressive symptoms were included in this analysis. This meta-analysis also examined the effects of exercise on other psychological disorders, including alcohol abuse, eating disorders, and anxiety disorders. Examining depression outcomes, 14 studies met their inclusion criteria and provided sufficient data to be included in analyses. Results showed large improvements in depression with exercise in comparison with nonactive controls (mean overall effect size of g = 1.39 [95% CI: .89 to 1.88] or d = 1.42 [95% CI: .92 to 1.93]).

Rethorst and colleagues (Rethorst, Wipfli, & Landers, 2009) also conducted a meta-analysis of the antidepressant effects of exercise. The authors combined data from 58 randomized trials, incorporating data from 2,982 individuals. In contrast to the Stathopoulou (Stathopoulou et al., 2006) study, the authors included all studies examining exercise as an intervention and did not limit their sample to depressed subjects. The authors found that exercise was associated with a −0.80 effect size (95% CI: −0.67 to −0.92) improvement in depressive symptoms, leading the authors to classify these findings as a level 1, Grade A quality for the effects of exercise on depression. In sensitivity analyses, the authors found that higher-quality studies, such as those using blinding, reported greater effects than lower-quality studies. Importantly, comparison of studies among depressed versus non-depressed samples showed a much stronger effect of treatment among depressed participants, with smaller benefits among non-depressed samples. Similar to other meta-analytic studies, the authors did not find a dose-response relationship between exercise volume and improvements in depression.

Lawlor and Hopker (2001) performed a meta-regression of aerobic exercise and depression among published randomized trials conducted among adults. Their literature search yielded 14 studies for inclusion, incorporating data from approximately 850 individuals. All studies had important methodological weaknesses, including inadequate concealment of randomization, failure to use intention-to-treat analyses, and lack of blinded assessment techniques. Using the Beck Depression Inventory as their outcome measure, the authors reported that exercise reduced depressive symptoms by −7.3 points (95% confidence interval −10.0 to −4.6), and that this effect was greater in trials with shorter follow-up periods. Despite the findings of improved depressive symptoms, the authors concluded that the effectiveness of exercise in treating depression could not be determined due to a lack of good research in clinical populations and a lack of appropriate follow-up assessments.

In a subsequent review, Mead and colleagues (Mead et al., 2009) conducted a comprehensive literature search of randomized controlled trials in adults in which exercise was compared to a standard treatment, no treatment, or a placebo control. Their search yielded 28 studies that met their inclusion criteria. Methodological quality varied substantially across studies, with a minority of studies adequately concealing treatment, using intention-to-treat analyses, and using objective (i.e., not self-reported) measures of depressive symptoms. Approximately half of the studies (n = 13) included used a two-arm design, comparing exercise with controls only. Many other studies utilized a three-arm design (n = 11), comparing exercise with one other treatment modality (e.g., pharmacotherapy, cognitive therapy, or a different intensity exercise group) and a control group. Most studies used jogging/running as their treatment modality, but some used walking, aerobic training with an instructor, stationary cycling, or mixed exercise (e.g., resistance training and stretching).

This Cochrane review limited the primary analyses to those trials comparing exercise treatment with no treatment or a control intervention (n = 25) and found a large, clinically meaningful improvement associated with exercise in comparison with controls (standardized mean difference [SMD] = −0.82 (95% CI −1.12 to −0.51). However, when the analyses were further limited to those trials using intention-to-treat analyses and blinded outcome assessment, the effect was modestly attenuated, and showed only a moderate benefit associated with exercise. In addition, when analyses were conducted among the five trials that collected long-term follow-up data, the effects of treatment were again slightly attenuated for a moderate clinical improvement (SMD −0.44 [95% CI −0.71 to −0.18]). The authors concluded that "exercise did seem to improve the symptoms of depression," which was somewhat surprising, given that only two new studies were included that were not part of their previous 2001 review (Blumenthal & Ong, 2009).

The beneficial effects of exercise have also been examined among individuals with heart failure. In the HF–ACTION (Heart Failure–A Controlled Trial Investigating Outcomes of Exercise Training) multicenter randomized trial, participants were randomized to either supervised aerobic exercise training for 1 to 3 months followed by home exercise, or to a guideline-based usual care group (O'Connor et al., 2009) and were followed for approximately 30 months. Depressive symptoms were assessed using the BDI-II every 3 months for a year (Blumenthal et al., 2012a). Depression scores were consistently lower in the aerobic exercise group compared to usual care controls at 3 months and 12 months. These improvements tended to be even greater among participants with clinically elevated depressive symptoms at baseline (BDI-II scores > 14). Volume of exercise was inversely related to depressive symptoms, such that participants reporting 90 minutes of exercise per week showed the greatest improvements in depression; there did not appear to be added benefit for exercise >90 minutes, however.

Comparative effectiveness

Several studies have compared exercise with other accepted forms of depression treatment, including psychotherapy and pharmacotherapy. The Mead meta-analysis (Mead et al., 2009) examined several of these comparative effectiveness analyses, conducting sensitivity analyses of those trials comparing these interventions directly. For example, the authors also reported the results when exercise was compared directly with CBT. Six trials examined this relationship, with data from 152 participants. Results showed no difference between exercise and cognitive therapy (SMD = −0.17 [95% CI −0.51, 0.18]).

An additional sensitivity analysis was conducted comparing the results of exercise compared with antidepressant medication. Only two studies, both from researchers at Duke University, compared the effectiveness of exercise with pharmacotherapy. No differences between exercise and antidepressant medication were noted (SMD = −0.04 [95% CI −0.31, 0.24]).

In the first Duke study, known as the SMILE study (Standard Medical Interventions and Longterm Exercise), we compared the effects of aerobic exercise to sertraline treatment among 156 older adults with MDD (Blumenthal et al., 1999). Participants were randomized to either aerobic exercise, sertraline, or a combined exercise and sertraline group. The treatment period of the trial lasted 16 weeks and participants' depression severity was assessed before and after treatment by a psychologist blinded to treatment condition. Participants in the exercise conditions exercised three times per week at 70–85% of their heart rate reserve. Importantly, participants exercised in groups, which were supervised by a study exercise physiologist. Participants in the sertraline condition were titrated for therapeutic response on sertraline by a study psychiatrist (50–200mg). Following 16 weeks of treatment, groups did not differ in their level of depressive symptoms. However, analysis of trajectory of change of depressive symptoms showed that patients receiving sertraline alone showed a faster initial response in the first 2 weeks compared with either the combination group or the exercise alone group. Interestingly, a follow-up examination of these participants conducted 10 months after the completion of the treatment period showed that participants in the exercise group showed lower rates of depression relapse in comparison with both the sertraline and combined groups (Babyak et al., 2000). The results were difficult to interpret, however, since many participants initiated exercise on their own following the completion of the 4-month trial. At the time of follow-up assessments, 48% of participants in the sertraline group began exercising, and 64% of participants in the exercise group and 66% of participants in the combination group continued to exercise following the trial intervention.

Regardless of group assignment during the active portion of the trial, participants who reported engaging in regular exercise during the follow-up period were more than 50% less likely to be depressed at their 10-month assessment.

In a second SMILE study, we extended these findings by including a placebo control group and by including a home-based exercise condition in which participants exercised at home on their own without supervision (Blumenthal et al., 2007). Participants were randomized to either home-based or supervised aerobic exercise, sertraline, or placebo pill for a 4-month period. Home-based exercisers were provided with the same exercise prescription as supervised participants and received an initial home visit to establish their exercise training routine, as well as instructions on how to monitor their heart rates accurately. Again, treatment allocation was concealed and participants' depressive symptoms were assessed by a psychologist blinded to treatment condition before and after the trial. Results revealed that participants in either exercise or sertraline groups tended to show greater improvement in comparison with placebo participants and these results became statistically significant when "early responders" (i.e., participants who experienced a self-reported improvement in depressive symptoms of >50% within the first week of treatment) were eliminated from analyses. In a recent follow-up analysis (Hoffman et al., 2011), participants' depression was reassessed one year following their completion of the active treatment phase of the intervention. Interestingly, neither group assignment nor antidepressant medication usage during the follow-up period was a significant predictor of depression at this follow-up time-point. Instead, the only significant predictor was self-reported exercise during the follow-up period. Regardless of group assignment or background characteristics, those individuals who engaged in regular exercise were less likely to be depressed at follow-up.

We also recently examined the impact of exercise or pharmacotherapy on depressive symptoms among individuals with coronary artery disease participating in the UPBEAT trial (Understanding the Prognostic Benefits of Exercise and Antidepressant Therapy) (Blumenthal et al., 2012b). One hundred and one participants were randomized to receive either supervised aerobic exercise, sertraline, or placebo treatment for 4 months. Participants in the exercise and sertraline groups showed improvements in depressive symptoms compared with the placebo group. Participants in the exercise and sertraline groups also showed improvements in heart rate variability compared with placebo participants.

Adjunctive therapy

Several studies have examined the effects of exercise as an adjunctive therapy among patients already being treated with antidepressants or psychotherapy. Mather and colleagues (Mather et al., 2002) examined this question in a randomized trial of 86 outpatients with depression and free from cognitive impairment. Importantly, in order to be considered eligible for the trial, all participants had to have been in receipt of a therapeutic dose of antidepressant therapy for at least 6 weeks without evidence of sustained response. Participants were then randomized to either exercise classes or health education for 10 weeks. Participants in the exercise group exercised for 45 minutes twice per week, performing strength training exercises. Clinical improvement in depressive symptoms (i.e., "response" to treatment) was defined as a >30% reduction in clinician-rated depressive symptoms. At the end of the 10-week intervention, 55% of participants in the exercise group showed improvements, compared to 33% in the control group. However, the groups did not show significant differences in mean levels of depressive symptoms. Several other trials have examined the effects of exercise alone versus exercise combined with antidepressant therapy, with results generally showing that exercise is equally effective when compared with a combined intervention. Martinsen and colleagues (Martinsen, Medhus, & Sandvik, 1985) examined the effects of exercise alone and combined with tricyclic antidepressants (TCAs). Specifically, 14 patients in the control group and 9 in the exercise group were given TCAs to augment treatment. Results showed that both groups exhibited similar improvements in depressive symptoms. In a second study, Martinsen and colleagues (Martinsen, Hoffart, & Solberg, 1989) compared aerobic and nonaerobic exercise in treating 99 inpatients with depression. Fourteen participants in each group were administered TCAs and results showed that exercise with TCA augmentation tended to show larger improvements in depression compared with exercise alone. As reviewed previously, Blumenthal and colleagues (Blumenthal et al., 1999) also examined the combined effects of aerobic exercise and sertraline versus either aerobic exercise or sertraline separately and found that all groups were equally effective in improving depression. Interestingly, a follow-up study 10 months after the completion of this intervention suggested that participants in the exercise alone group were the least likely to be depressed (Babyak et al., 2000).

One of the largest trials to examine exercise as an adjunctive treatment was the recently completed Treatment with Exercise Augmentation for Depression (TREAD) study (Trivedi, Greer, et al., 2006). In this randomized trial, 126 adults with unremitted depression following SSRI treatment were randomized to augmentation treatment with either 16 kcal/kg/week or 4 kcal/kg/week for 12 weeks. Although both groups showed lower remission rates with treatment, the higher-intensity exercise group showed greater rates of remission (28.3%) compared to the lower-intensity group (15.5%) (Trivedi et al., 2011).

Exercise prescriptions typically consider four critical elements: mode, frequency, duration, and intensity. Most studies have focused on aerobic exercise, but several studies have also considered resistance (strength) training alone or combined with an aerobic program. In the Mead meta-analysis both strength training and aerobic exercise interventions were effective in improving depression, but the aggregated effects of these different exercise modalities had a wide confidence interval, suggesting a large, heterogeneous effect of both types of training (Mead et al., 2009). Similarly, the Rethorst meta-analysis failed to find a relationship between exercise volume and improvement in depressive symptoms (Rethorst et al., 2009). In one of the more widely cited studies, Singh and colleagues (Singh et al., 2005) randomized 60 community-dwelling older adults with depression to either a high- or low-intensity progressive muscle training intervention, or a general practitioner control group. Following 8 weeks of intervention, depressive symptoms were most improved in the high-intensity group followed by the low-intensity group and then controls, demonstrating the value of strength training and suggesting a dose–response relationship between the intensity of strength training and the degree of improvement in depressive symptoms.

The issue of the intensity of aerobic exercise and whether greater intensity or duration of exercise is associated with dose–response improvements in depressive symptoms has also been the subject of both observational studies and RCTs. Observational studies have suggested a possible dose–response relationship between amount of physical activity and depressive symptoms (Hamer, Stamatakis, & Steptoe, 2009). Several RCTs have also examined this issue. In an early trial, DiLorenzo and colleagues (DiLorenzo et al., 1999) examined the effects of a variable intensity exercise intervention compared with a control condition on depressive symptoms among healthy adults. Exercise participants were randomized to either a 24-minute variable intensity exercise program four times per week or a 48-minute fixed intensity exercise program four times per week for a period of 12 weeks. Participants were assessed before and after the 12-week intervention and again at a 1-year follow-up. Exercise was found to have a beneficial effect on depressive symptoms in both exercise groups with no clear benefit of one exercise modality over another, and these findings persisted at one year.

In one of the more elegant RCTs that examined the optimal "dose" of exercise, Dunn and colleagues (Dunn, Trivedi, Kampert, Clark, & Chambliss, 2005) conducted a randomized, controlled trial of 80 young and middle-aged adults with mild to moderate MDD in which participants were randomized to treatment groups at varying levels of energy expenditure and frequency of exercise. Four aerobic exercise treatment groups were used, with two levels of energy expenditure (7 kcal/kg/week or 17.5 kcal/kg/week) and two levels of frequency (3 days per week or 5 days per week) for 12 weeks. 17.5 kcal/kg/week was selected because this level of energy expenditure corresponds to current public health recommendations. The authors found that participation in the 17.5 kcal/kg/week group was associated with the greatest improvements in depressive symptoms and remission rates, whereas the lower dose group was not significantly improved compared with control participants.

There is also some evidence to suggest that improvements in fitness may be associated with improvements in depressive symptoms among patients with cardiovascular disease, again suggesting a possible dose-response relationship. Among cardiac patients, for example, Milani and Lavie (Milani & Lavie, 2007) found that improvements in peak $\dot{V}O_2$ were associated with improvements in depression. In their retrospective analysis of cardiac rehabilitation participants, the authors found that those participants achieving modest (1–10%) or robust (>10%) increases in peak $\dot{V}O_2$ were likely to show reductions in depressive symptoms. Similarly, we have previously found that reductions in depression among individuals with hypertension were mediated by improvements in peak $\dot{V}O_2$ (Smith et al., 2007). However, in the Mead meta-analysis (Mead et al., 2009) only half of the trials showing improvements in fitness reported concurrent improvements in depressive symptoms.

Impact on depressive symptoms

Several studies have attempted to examine the effects of exercise on various clusters of depressive symptoms. Although depression is typified by depressed mood and anhedonia, many of the other symptoms are heterogeneous and may not present in any given depressed individual. Many previous factor analytic studies of depression inventories, for example, have identified different clusters of depressive symptoms. Although these vary somewhat between studies, they have generally clustered into three factors: affective factors (depressed mood, irritability, crying, etc.), somatic factors (sleep difficulties, fatigue, etc.), and cognitive factors (concentration difficulties, indecisiveness, etc.) (Vanheule, Desmet, Groenvynck, Rosseel, & Fontaine, 2008).

The impact of exercise on sleep has been examined in several studies, although none, to our knowledge, have examined aerobic exercise as a treatment for disturbed sleep among depressed adults. Observational studies have shown that regular physical activity is associated with better sleep (Penedo & Dahn, 2005). In addition, several intervention studies have shown that aerobic and strength training exercises improve sleep compared with a waitlist condition. King and colleagues (King, Oman, Brassington, Bliwise, & Haskell, 1997), for example, found that 16 weeks of four 30–40-minute aerobic exercise sessions improved sleep duration by 42 minutes among 48 community-dwelling adults. These findings were recently replicated using polysomnography to objectively measure sleep (King et al., 2008). Similar findings for aerobic exercise were reported among individuals with insomnia, as Reid and colleagues (Reid et al., 2010) have shown that a 16-week aerobic exercise intervention with sleep hygiene improved sleep duration by 75 minutes in the intervention group, while participants in the control condition improved by only 13 minutes. Although no studies of aerobic exercise on sleep have been conducted among depressed adults, Singh and colleagues (Singh et al., 2005) demonstrated that high-intensity weight training was associated with improved sleep duration, efficiency, and latency, although low-intensity training and a control group also showed similar, albeit weaker improvements.

There is some evidence that exercise may also improve cognitive functioning, including memory, concentration, and executive functions, although few studies have examined this relationship. In a substudy from the SMILE study described earlier (Blumenthal et al., 1999), Khatri and colleagues (Khatri et al., 2001) found that several measures of memory and executive function were modestly improved following a 16-week exercise intervention as compared to antidepressant medication, although no improvements were observed in attention/concentration or psychomotor speed. In contrast, a more recent substudy (Blumenthal et al., 2007) by Hoffman and colleagues (Hoffman et al., 2008) failed to find cognitive benefits associated with exercise compared with placebo participants following a 16-week intervention. Although exercise may not impact cognitive function among individuals with depression directly, there is evidence that cognitive coping thoughts may be improved with exercise (Stathopoulou et al., 2006). Quasi-experimental studies have shown that women participating in exercise reported higher coping self-efficacy, greater use of distraction, and lower depression compared with control participants (Craft, 2005), and similar findings have been suggested for anxiety (Steptoe, Edwards, Moses, & Mathews, 1989). Interventions targeting self-efficacy appear to have particularly strong effects in improving positive affect (Bodin & Martinsen, 2004), which is associated with lower levels of depression.

Other populations

Although the majority of existing evidence has examined the effects of exercise among adults with depression, several trials have been conducted among other populations, including adolescents, women with post-partum depression, and older adults (Greer & Trivedi, 2009). Few studies have been conducted among adolescents and the only available quantitative review of these studies found no high-quality trials examining this question (Larun et al., 2006). Preliminary evidence, however, suggests benefits associated with exercise among depressed youth. For example, Brown and colleagues (Brown, Welsh, Labbe, Vitulli, & Kulkarni, 1992) found that supplemental aerobic exercise training improved depressive symptoms among hospitalized psychiatric patients over the course of a 9-week intervention. Most recently, Nabkasorn and colleagues (Nabkasorn et al., 2006) found that group jogging improved depressive symptoms among 49 females aged 18–20 with mild-to-moderate depressive symptoms. Participants were randomized to either five 50-minute jogging sessions or to usual daily activities for 8 weeks. Following the intervention, participants in the exercise group showed reduced depressive symptoms in comparison with control participants, as well as reduced cortisol and epinephrine levels assessed from 24-hour urinary excretions.

Another area of interest has been the effects of exercise in women following childbirth. Postpartum depression is common and associated with poorer quality of life. Although few studies have examined the effects of exercise in postpartum depression, preliminary evidence suggests improvements in depressive symptoms. Participation in physical activity following childbirth has been associated with improved mood and reduced anxiety (Koltyn & Schultes, 1997) and two randomized trials have suggested positive benefits of increased physical activity during the postnatal period (Armstrong & Edwards, 2004; Heh, Huang, Ho, Fu, & Wang, 2008). Heh and colleagues (Heh et al., 2008) alternately assigned 80 first-time mothers with depressive symptoms to an exercise support group or control group beginning 6 weeks after childbirth. Participants in the exercise group participated in 1 hour of exercise per week at the hospital and two exercise sessions at home per week using an audio-guided regimen for 3 months. Following the 3-month intervention, participants in the exercise group were less likely to have elevated depression scores in comparison with control participants. Armstrong and colleagues (Armstrong & Edwards, 2004) conducted a similar randomized intervention of pram-walking among mothers who had given birth within the last 12 months. Participants assigned to pram-walking, who exercised twice per week for 40 minutes at 60–75% of age-predicted heart rate, showed improvements in both fitness and depressive symptoms compared to a social support control group.

Several randomized trials have been conducted among depressed older adults. In the UPLIFT trial, Sims and colleagues (Sims, Hill, Davidson, Gunn, & Huang, 2006) randomized adults aged 65 and older with depressive symptoms to progressive resistance training three times per week for 10 weeks, or to a brief advice control group. Participants in the exercise group tended to have lower Geriatric Depression Scale scores (P = .08) and a strong correlation was found between improvement in depressive status and number of exercise sessions completed in post hoc analyses (r = -0.8). In the Depression in Late Life Intervention Trial of Exercise (DeLLITE) (Kerse et al., 2008), participants aged 75 years and older with depressive symptoms were randomized to either an individualized physical activity program or to a social visit control condition. The exercise condition used moderate-intensity balance training, progressive resistance exercises, and walking, which were conducted three times a week for 30 minutes. Both groups showed improvements in psychosocial outcomes, without significant between-group differences, suggesting that both interventions were beneficial on psychosocial outcomes. As reviewed earlier, Blumenthal and colleagues (Blumenthal et al., 1999) also conducted an aerobic exercise, sertraline, or combined intervention among depressed adults. Results of this trial showed that all groups had improvement in depression severity, without significant between-group differences. In addition, a follow-up study from this trial suggested that regular physical activity was associated with significantly improved rates of remission (Babyak et al., 2000).

Proposed mechanisms

A number of potential biologic, social, and psychological mechanisms for the antidepressant effect of exercise have been proposed and are beyond the scope of this chapter. They are described in detail in the next two chapters.

Summary and future directions

In summary, available evidence suggests that exercise is an effective treatment for depression, improving depressive symptoms to a comparable degree as pharmacotherapy and psychotherapy. Observational studies generally have shown that individuals who are more physically active have lower rates of depression, although it is less clear whether greater physical activity levels protect against the subsequent development of depression. The majority of evidence supports aerobic exercise as a treatment for depression among adults, although a growing body of evidence supports its use as a treatment among adolescents as well, and also that other forms of exercise, including resistance training, may be effective. It appears that any level of exercise is better than no exercise. There have been relatively few studies that have examined the optimal dose of exercise, although available evidence suggests that 12–16 weeks of treatment may be necessary for therapeutic benefit and that the total volume of exercise may be more important than either frequency or intensity. A number of possible mechanisms have been suggested to explain how exercise may reduce depression, and examination of putative mechanisms is an important area for future research. In addition, more rigorous RCTs are needed in order to assess the beneficial effects of exercise for depression in adolescents and young adults. Other patient populations, including patients with coronary disease, should also be the focus of further research, especially in light of the accumulating evidence that depression in cardiac patients is a risk factor for increased morbidity and mortality, as well as for reduced quality of life.

References

Armstrong, K., & Edwards, H. (2004). The effectiveness of a pram-walking exercise programme in reducing depressive symptomatology for postnatal women. *International Journal of Nursing Practice, 10*(4), 177–194.

Babyak, M., Blumenthal, J. A., Herman, S., Khatri, P., Doraiswamy, M., Moore, K., et al. (2000). Exercise treatment for major depression: Maintenance of therapeutic benefit at 10 months. *Psychosomatic Medicine, 62*(5), 633–638.

Blumenthal, J. A., Babyak, M. A., Doraiswamy, P. M., Watkins, L., Hoffman, B. M., Barbour, K. A., et al. (2007). Exercise and pharmacotherapy in the treatment of major depressive disorder. *Psychosomatic Medicine, 69*(7), 587–596.

Blumenthal, J. A., Babyak, M. A., Moore, K. A., Craighead, W. E., Herman, S., Khatri, P., et al. (1999). Effects of exercise training on older patients with major depression. *Archives of Internal Medicine, 159*(19), 2349–2356.

Blumenthal, J. A., & Ong, L. (2009). A commentary on 'Exercise and Depression' (Mead et al., 2008): And the verdict is. *Mental Health and Physical Activity, 2*(2), 97–99.

Blumenthal, J. A., Babyak, M. A., O'Connor, C., Keteyian, S., Landzberg, J., Howlett, J., . . . Whellan, D. J. (2012a). Effects of exercise training on depressive symptoms in patients with chronic heart failure: The HF-ACTION randomized trial. *Journal of the American Medical Association, 308*(5), 465–474.

Blumenthal, J. A., Sherwood, A., Babyak, M. A., Watkins, L. L., Smith, P. J., Hoffman, B. M., . . . Hinderliter, A. L. (2012b). Exercise and pharmacological treatment of depressive symptoms in patients with coronary heart disease: Results from the UPBEAT (Understanding the Prognostic Benefits of Exercise and Antidepressant Therapy) study. *Journal of the American College of Cardiology, 60*(12):1053–1063.

Bodin, T., & Martinsen, E.W. (2004). Mood and self-efficacy during acute exercise in clinical depression: A randomized, controlled study. *Journal of Sport and Exercise Psychology, 26*, 623–633.

Brosse, A. L., Sheets, E. S., Lett, H. S., & Blumenthal, J. A. (2002). Exercise and the treatment of clinical depression in adults: Recent findings and future directions. *Sports Medicine (Auckland, NZ), 32*(12), 741–760.

Brown, S. W., Welsh, M. C., Labbe, E. E., Vitulli, W. F., & Kulkarni, P. (1992). Aerobic exercise in the psychological treatment of adolescents. *Perceptual and Motor Skills, 74*(2), 555–560.

Brown, W. J., Ford, J. H., Burton, N. W., Marshall, A. L., & Dobson, A. J. (2005). Prospective study of physical activity and depressive symptoms in middle-aged women. *American Journal of Preventive Medicine, 29*(4), 265–272.

Camacho, T. C., Roberts, R. E., Lazarus, N. B., Kaplan, G. A., & Cohen, R. D. (1991). Physical activity and depression: Evidence from the Alameda County Study. *American Journal of Epidemiology, 134*(2), 220–231.

Cooper-Patrick, L., Ford, D. E., Mead, L. A., Chang, P. P., & Klag, M. J. (1997). Exercise and depression in midlife: A prospective study. *American Journal of Public Health, 87*(4), 670–673.

Craft, L. L. (2005). Exercise and clinical depression: Examining two psychological mechanisms. *Psychology of Sport and Exercise, 6*, 151–171.

Cuijpers, P., Smit, F., & van Straten, A. (2007). Psychological treatments of subthreshold depression: A meta-analytic review. *Acta Psychiatrica Scandinavica, 115*(6), 434–441.

Cuijpers, P., van Straten, A., Andersson, G., & van Oppen, P. (2008). Psychotherapy for depression in adults: A meta-analysis of comparative outcome studies. *Journal of Consulting and Clinical Psychology, 76*(6), 909–922.

Davis, L., Uezato, A., Newell, J. M., & Frazier, E. (2008). Major depression and comorbid substance use disorders. *Current Opinion in Psychiatry, 21*(1), 14–18.

DiLorenzo, T. M., Bargman, E. P., Stucky-Ropp, R., Brassington, G. S., Frensch, P. A., & LaFontaine, T. (1999). Long-term effects of aerobic exercise on psychological outcomes. *Preventive Medicine, 28*(1), 75–85.

DiMatteo, M. R., Lepper, H. S., & Croghan, T. W. (2000). Depression is a risk factor for noncompliance with medical treatment: Meta-analysis of the effects of anxiety and depression on patient adherence. *Archives of Internal Medicine, 160*(14), 2101–2107.

Dunn, A. L., Trivedi, M. H., Kampert, J. B., Clark, C. G., & Chambliss, H. O. (2005). Exercise treatment for depression: Efficacy and dose response. *American Journal of Preventive Medicine, 28*(1), 1–8.

Farmer, M. E., Locke, B. Z., Moscicki, E. K., Dannenberg, A. L., Larson, D. B., & Radloff, L. S. (1988). Physical activity and depressive symptoms: The NHANES I epidemiologic follow-up study. *American Journal of Epidemiology, 128*(6), 1340–1351.

Fournier, J. C., DeRubeis, R. J., Hollon, S. D., Dimidjian, S., Amsterdam, J. D., Shelton, R. C., et al. (2010). Antidepressant drug effects and depression severity: A patient-level meta-analysis. *Journal of the American Medical Association, 303*(1), 47–53.

Gelenberg, A., Freeman, M. P., Markowitz, J. C., Rosenbaum, J. F. , Thase, M. E., Trivedi, M. H., & van Rhoads, R. S. of the Work Group on Major Depressive Disorder. (2010). *Practice Guidelines for the Treatment of Patients with Major Depressive Disorder* (3rd ed.). Arlington, VA: American Psychiatric Association.

Greer, T. L., & Trivedi, M. H. (2009). Exercise in the treatment of depression. *Current Psychiatry Reports, 11*(6), 466–472.

Hamer, M., Stamatakis, E., & Steptoe, A. (2009). Dose–response relationship between physical activity and mental health: The Scottish Health Survey. *British Journal of Sports Medicine, 43*(14), 1111–1114.

Harris, A. H., Cronkite, R., & Moos, R. (2006). Physical activity, exercise coping, and depression in a 10-year cohort study of depressed patients. *Journal of Affective Disorders, 93*(1–3), 79–85.

Heh, S. S., Huang, L. H., Ho, S. M., Fu, Y. Y., & Wang, L. L. (2008). Effectiveness of an exercise support program in reducing the severity of postnatal depression in Taiwanese women. *Birth, 35*(1), 60–65.

Hoffman, B. M., Babyak, M. A., Craighead, W. E., Sherwood, A., Doraiswamy, P. M., Coons, M. J., et al. (2011). Exercise and pharmacotherapy in patients with major depression: One-year follow-up of the SMILE study. *Psychosomatic Medicine, 73*(2), 127–133.

Hoffman, B. M., Blumenthal, J. A., Babyak, M. A., Smith, P. J., Rogers, S. D., Doraiswamy, P. M., et al. (2008). Exercise fails to improve neurocognition in depressed middle-aged and older adults. *Medicine and Science in Sports and Exercise, 40*(7), 1344–1352.

Hollon, S. D., Thase, M. E., & Markowitz, J. C. (2002). Treatment and prevention of depression. *Psychological Science in the Public Interest, 3*(2), 39–77.

Katon, W., Fan, M. Y., Unutzer, J., Taylor, J., Pincus, H., & Schoenbaum, M. (2008). Depression and diabetes: A potentially lethal combination. *Journal of General Internal Medicine, 23*(10), 1571–1575.

Katon, W. J. (2003). Clinical and health services relationships between major depression, depressive symptoms, and general medical illness. *Biological Psychiatry, 54*(3), 216–226.

Kerse, N., Falloon, K., Moyes, S. A., Hayman, K. J., Dowell, T., Kolt, G. S., et al. (2008). DeLLITE depression in late life: An intervention trial of exercise. Design and recruitment of a randomised controlled trial. *BMC Geriatrics, 8*, 12.

Kessler, R. C., Avenevoli, S., & Ries Merikangas, K. (2001). Mood disorders in children and adolescents: An epidemiologic perspective. *Biological Psychiatry, 49*(12), 1002–1014.

Kessler, R. C., Berglund, P., Demler, O., Jin, R., Koretz, D., Merikangas, K. R., et al. (2003). The epidemiology of major depressive disorder: Results from the National Comorbidity Survey Replication (NCS-R). *Journal of the American Medical Association, 289*(23), 3095–3105.

Kessler, R. C., Berglund, P., Demler, O., Jin, R., Merikangas, K. R., & Walters, E. E. (2005). Lifetime prevalence and age-of-onset distributions of DSM-IV disorders in the National Comorbidity Survey Replication. *Archives of General Psychiatry, 62*(6), 593–602.

Kessler, R. C., Chiu, W. T., Demler, O., Merikangas, K. R., & Walters, E. E. (2005). Prevalence, severity, and comorbidity of 12-month DSM-IV disorders in the National Comorbidity Survey Replication. *Archives of General Psychiatry, 62*(6), 617–627.

Kessler, R. C., Merikangas, K. R., & Wang, P. S. (2008). The prevalence and correlates of workplace depression in the national comorbidity survey replication. *Journal of Occupational and Environmental Medicine, 50*(4), 381–390.

Khatri, P., Blumenthal, J. A., Babyak, M. A., Craighead, W. E., Herman, S., Baldewicz, T., et al. (2001). Effects of exercise training on cognitive functioning among depressed older men and women. *Journal of Aging and Physical Activity, 9*, 43–57.

King, A. C., Oman, R. F., Brassington, G. S., Bliwise, D. L., & Haskell, W. L. (1997). Moderate-intensity exercise and self-rated quality of sleep in older adults. A randomized controlled trial. *Journal of the American Medical Association, 277*(1), 32–37.

King, A. C., Pruitt, L. A., Woo, S., Castro, C. M., Ahn, D. K., Vitiello, M. V., et al. (2008). Effects of moderate-intensity exercise on polysomnographic and subjective sleep quality in older adults with mild to moderate sleep complaints. *Journals of Gerontology. Series A, Biological Sciences and Medical Sciences, 63*(9), 997–1004.

Koltyn, K. F., & Schultes, S. S. (1997). Psychological effects of an aerobic exercise session and a rest session following pregnancy. *Journal of Sports Medicine and Physical Fitness, 37*(4), 287–291.

Kritz-Silverstein, D., Barrett-Connor, E., & Corbeau, C. (2001). Cross-sectional and prospective study of exercise and depressed mood in the elderly: The Rancho Bernardo study. *American Journal of Epidemiology, 153*(6), 596–603.

Lampinen, P., & Heikkinen, E. (2003). Reduced mobility and physical activity as predictors of depressive symptoms among community-dwelling older adults: An eight-year follow-up study. *Aging Clinical and Experimental Research, 15*(3), 205–211.

Lampinen, P., Heikkinen, R. L., & Ruoppila, I. (2000). Changes in intensity of physical exercise as predictors of depressive symptoms among older adults: An eight-year follow-up. *Preventive Medicine, 30*(5), 371–380.

Larun, L., Nordheim, L. V., Ekeland, E., Hagen, K. B., & Heian, F. (2006). Exercise in prevention and treatment of anxiety and depression among children and young people. *Cochrane Database of Systematic Reviews* (3), CD004691.

Lawlor, D. A., & Hopker, S. W. (2001). The effectiveness of exercise as an intervention in the management of depression: Systematic review and meta-regression analysis of randomised controlled trials. *British Medical Journal, 322*(7289), 763–767.

Lichtman, J. H., Bigger, J. T., Jr., Blumenthal, J. A., Frasure-Smith, N., Kaufmann, P. G., Lesperance, F., et al. (2008). Depression and coronary heart disease: Recommendations for screening, referral, and treatment: A science advisory from the American Heart Association Prevention Committee of the Council on Cardiovascular Nursing, Council on Clinical Cardiology, Council on Epidemiology and Prevention, and Interdisciplinary Council on Quality of Care and Outcomes Research: Endorsed by the American Psychiatric Association. *Circulation, 118*(17), 1768–1775.

Lieberman, J. A., Greenhouse, J., Hamer, R. M., Krishnan, K. R., Nemeroff, C. B., Sheehan, D. V., et al. (2005). Comparing the effects of antidepressants: Consensus guidelines for evaluating quantitative reviews of antidepressant efficacy. *Neuropsychopharmacology, 30*(3), 445–460.

Martinsen, E. W., Hoffart, A., & Solberg, O. (1989). Comparing aerobic with nonaerobic forms of exercise in the treatment of clinical depression: A randomized trial. *Comprehensive Psychiatry, 30*(4), 324–331.

Martinsen, E. W., Medhus, A., & Sandvik, L. (1985). Effects of aerobic exercise on depression: A controlled study. *British Medical Journal, 291*(6488), 109.

Mather, A. S., Rodriguez, C., Guthrie, M. F., McHarg, A. M., Reid, I. C., & McMurdo, M. E. (2002). Effects of exercise on depressive symptoms in older adults with poorly responsive depressive disorder: Randomised controlled trial. *British Journal of Psychiatry, 180*, 411–415.

Mead, G. E., Morley, W., Campbell, P., Greig, C. A., McMurdo, M., & Lawlor, D. A. (2009). Exercise for depression. *Cochrane Database of Systematic Reviews, 2009* (3), CD004366.

Milani, R. V., & Lavie, C. J. (2007). Impact of cardiac rehabilitation on depression and its associated mortality. *American Journal of Medicine, 120*(9), 799–806.

Moussavi, S., Chatterji, S., Verdes, E., Tandon, A., Patel, V., & Ustun, B. (2007). Depression, chronic diseases, and decrements in health: Results from the World Health Surveys. *Lancet, 370*(9590), 851–858.

Nabkasorn, C., Miyai, N., Sootmongkol, A., Junprasert, S., Yamamoto, H., Arita, M., et al. (2006). Effects of physical exercise on depression, neuroendocrine stress hormones and physiological fitness in adolescent females with depressive symptoms. *European Journal of Public Health, 16*(2), 179–184.

O'Connor, C. M., Whellan, D. J., Lee, K. L., Keteyian, S. J., Cooper, L. S., Ellis, S. J., . . . HF-ACTION Investigators (2009). Efficacy and safety of exercise training in patients with chronic heart failure: HF-ACTION randomized controlled trial. *Journal of the American Medical Association, 301*(14), 1439–1450.

Olfson, M., Marcus, S. C., Druss, B., Elinson, L., Tanielian, T., & Pincus, H. A. (2002). National trends in the outpatient treatment of depression. *Journal of the American Medical Association, 287*(2), 203–209.

Ownby, R. L., Crocco, E., Acevedo, A., John, V., & Loewenstein, D. (2006). Depression and risk for Alzheimer disease: Systematic review, meta-analysis, and metaregression analysis. *Archives of General Psychiatry, 63*(5), 530–538.

Paffenbarger, R. S., Jr., Lee, I. M., & Leung, R. (1994). Physical activity and personal characteristics associated with depression and suicide in American college men. *Acta Psychiatrica Scandinavica. Supplementum, 377*, 16–22.

Penedo, F. J., & Dahn, J. R. (2005). Exercise and well-being: A review of mental and physical health benefits associated with physical activity. *Current Opinion in Psychiatry, 18*(2), 189–193.

Reid, K. J., Baron, K. G., Lu, B., Naylor, E., Wolfe, L., & Zee, P. C. (2010). Aerobic exercise improves self-reported sleep and quality of life in older adults with insomnia. *Sleep Medicine, 11*(9), 934–940.

Rethorst, C. D., Wipfli, B. M., & Landers, D. M. (2009). The antidepressive effects of exercise: A meta-analysis of randomized trials. *Sports Medicine, 39*(6), 491–511.

Roberts, R. E., Deleger, S., Strawbridge, W. J., & Kaplan, G. A. (2003). Prospective association between obesity and depression: Evidence from the Alameda County Study. *International Journal of Obesity and Related Metabolic Disorders, 27*(4), 514–521.

Robinson, L. A., Berman, J. S., & Neimeyer, R. A. (1990). Psychotherapy for the treatment of depression: A comprehensive review of controlled outcome research. *Psychological Bulletin, 108*(1), 30–49.

Roshanaei-Moghaddam, B., Katon, W. J., & Russo, J. (2009). The longitudinal effects of depression on physical activity. *General Hospital Psychiatry, 31*(4), 306–315.

Simon, G. E. (2003). Social and economic burden of mood disorders. *Biological Psychiatry, 54*(3), 208–215.

Sims, J., Hill, K., Davidson, S., Gunn, J., & Huang, N. (2006). Exploring the feasibility of a community-based strength training program for older people with depressive symptoms and its impact on depressive symptoms. *BMC Geriatrics, 6*, 18.

Singh, N. A., Stavrinos, T. M., Scarbek, Y., Galambos, G., Liber, C., & Fiatarone Singh, M. A. (2005). A randomized controlled trial of high versus low intensity weight training versus general practitioner care for clinical depression in older adults. *The Journals of Gerontology. Series A, Biological Sciences and Medical Sciences, 60*(6), 768–776.

Smith, P. J., Blumenthal, J. A., Babyak, M. A., Georgiades, A., Hinderliter, A., & Sherwood, A. (2007). Effects of exercise and weight loss on depressive symptoms among men and women with hypertension. *Journal of Psychosomatic Research, 63*(5), 463–469.

Stathopoulou, G., Power, M. B., Berry, A. C., Smits, J. A. J. (2006). Exercise interventions for mental health: A quantitative and qualitative review. *Clinical Psychology: Science and Practice, 13*, 179–193.

Steptoe, A., Edwards, S., Moses, J., & Mathews, A. (1989). The effects of exercise training on mood and perceived coping ability in anxious adults from the general population. *Journal of Psychosomatic Research, 33*(5), 537–547.

Trivedi, M. H., Fava, M., Wisniewski, S. R., Thase, M. E., Quitkin, F., Warden, D., et al. (2006). Medication augmentation after the failure of SSRIs for depression. *New England Journal of Medicine, 354*(12), 1243–1252.

Trivedi, M. H., Greer, T. L., Church, T. S., Carmody, T. J., Grannemann, B. D., Galper, D. I., et al. (2011). Exercise as an augmentation treatment for nonremitted major depressive disorder: A randomized, parallel dose comparison. *Journal of Clinical Psychiatry, 72*(5), 677–684.

Trivedi, M. H., Greer, T. L., Grannemann, B. D., Church, T. S., Galper, D. I., Sunderajan, P., et al. (2006). TREAD: TReatment with Exercise Augmentation for Depression: Study rationale and design. *Clinical Trials, 3*(3), 291–305.

Vanheule, S., Desmet, M., Groenvynck, H., Rosseel, Y., & Fontaine, J. (2008). The factor structure of the Beck Depression Inventory-II: An evaluation. *Assessment, 15*(2), 177–187.

Wulsin, L. R., Vaillant, G. E., & Wells, V. E. (1999). A systematic review of the mortality of depression. *Psychosomatic Medicine, 61*(1), 6–17.

9

POTENTIAL PSYCHOLOGICAL MECHANISMS UNDERLYING THE EXERCISE AND DEPRESSION RELATIONSHIP

Lynette L. Craft

Understanding the ways in which exercise reduces the symptoms of clinical depression is an important step in determining the role for exercise in the standard of care for depression treatment. It can be argued that medicine is filled with examples of treatments coming well before the understanding of how the treatments worked. Antidepressant medications, for example, were being used with patients long before scientists and clinicians had a clear understanding of precisely how they exerted their antidepressant effects (Mayze, 2012). However, there will remain scientists, clinicians, and patients themselves who question the utility of incorporating exercise into the treatment of depression until the mechanisms underlying this relationship have been elucidated. Further, in order to develop the most effective exercise interventions, it is important to understand how exercise elicits its effect.

Several hypotheses have been proposed to explain the mechanisms by which exercise reduces depressive symptoms. These hypotheses are both psychological and neurobiological in nature. This chapter will focus on the potential psychological mechanisms, while the following chapter will cover proposed neurobiological mechanisms. Unfortunately, there is insufficient evidence at this time to support or refute most of the psychological mechanisms that have been proposed. Thus, this chapter will highlight the research in this area and suggest additional mechanisms for future researchers to consider.

The self-efficacy hypothesis

One of the most well-known psychological mechanisms proposed to explain the exercise–depression relationship is the enhancement of self-efficacy. Self-efficacy refers to the belief that one possesses the necessary skills to complete a task, as well as the confidence that the task can actually be completed with the desired outcome obtained. Depressed individuals often feel inefficacious to bring about positive desired outcomes in their lives and have low efficacy to cope with the symptoms of their depression (Bandura, 1997). This can lead to negative self-evaluation, negative ruminations, and faulty styles of thinking. Conversely, enhanced feelings of self-efficacy are associated with reduced catecholamine response to stress, lower perceived vulnerability to threat, reduced anxiety, and increased cognitive control (Bandura, 1997).

It is generally thought that there are four primary sources of information that influence an individual's perceptions of self-efficacy. These include mastery experiences, vicarious experience, verbal persuasion, and physiological and affective states. As an example, it has been suggested that exercise may enhance self-efficacy based on its ability to provide the individual with a meaningful mastery experience. Specifically, exercise programs teach an important health-related skill, utilization of the skill to achieve personal goals, and to attribute improved mental health to the mastery and use of the skills. A second example is that observing someone similar to oneself learn to exercise, and to utilize exercise as a means to manage symptoms, may increase one's own self-efficacy to use exercise for symptom management (i.e., via vicarious experience).

Research examining the association between exercise and self-efficacy in the general population has focused predominantly on the enhancement of overall self-efficacy following exercise participation. That is, studies have examined whether involvement in a program of regular exercise leads to either enhanced feelings of overall confidence or increased feelings of self-efficacy to engage in exercise behaviors. This has been examined in a variety of clinical samples (e.g., cancer survivors, persons with HIV, persons with multiple sclerosis) and healthy volunteers (Elavsky et al., 2005; Fillipas, Oldmeadow, Bailey, & Cherry, 2006; Hughes et al., 2010; Motl & Snook, 2008). In general, these studies find that exercise is associated with improved feelings of self-efficacy pre- to post-intervention and this, in turn, is associated with better quality of life (QOL). In addition, many of these exercise intervention studies have found that enhanced feelings of exercise self-efficacy, following an exercise intervention, are predictive of increased time spent in physical activity.

While it is highly relevant that exercise promotes enhanced feelings of efficacy, the afore-mentioned studies did not address the relationships of exercise and self-efficacy with depression. Clinical depression has received far less attention in the exercise and self-efficacy literature. Few studies have actually examined the effects of exercise interventions on self-efficacy among those with depression and the findings of these studies have been equivocal as to whether exercise leads to an enhancement of generalized feelings of efficacy (Brown, Welsh, & Labbe, 1992; Martinsen, Hoffart, & Solberg, 1989; Shin, Kang, Park, & Heitkemper, 2009; Singh et al., 2005).

While generalized feelings of self-efficacy are important, it is also essential that we understand whether exercise leads to an enhanced feeling of ability to cope with or manage one's symptoms of depression (i.e., coping self-efficacy). One longitudinal cross-sectional study was conducted to examine the relationships among physical activity, exercise coping, and depression (Harris, Cronkite, & Moos, 2006). Depressed patients (N = 452) were followed for 10 years and completed assessments at study entry, and 1, 4, and 10 years post-entry. A limited assessment of physical activity was utilized, with participants indicating whether or not they engaged in swimming, tennis, or long hikes or walks with family or friends during the past month. Exercise coping, or how often the person exercised more to cope with an important problem or stressful event (i.e., a form of coping self-efficacy), as well as the presence of stressful life events and medical conditions were assessed. Results indicated that every one increment increase in physical activity was associated with a 2.24-point reduction in depression. Further, exercise coping was associated with a 1.23-point reduction in depression. Each medical condition was associated with a 3.00-point increase in depression, but every increment increase in physical activity decreased depression by .90 points and exercise coping decreased depression by .67 points. Finally, each negative life event increased depression by ~3.50 points, but every increment in physical activity decreased this by .89 points and exercise coping decreased depression by .66 points. Therefore, physical activity and exercise coping both appear to be helpful in managing life stressors and medical conditions, providing some support for the role of self-efficacy as a mechanism to explain the exercise–depression relationship.

There is a paucity of exercise intervention studies that have examined the potential role of coping self-efficacy in both depressed and non-depressed samples. For example, we conducted a study to examine the relationship between involvement in an exercise program and enhanced feelings of coping self-efficacy (i.e., confidence to cope with one's symptoms of depression) in depressed women (Craft, 2005). Women (N = 19) with moderate depression, taking anti-depressant medications, were assigned to either a 9-week moderate-intensity aerobic exercise intervention or a control group. Those in the intervention arm exercised three times/week, at 50–75% heart rate reserve, for 30 minutes. We found that coping self-efficacy was significantly higher in the exercise group (as compared to controls) at 3 weeks and this significant difference between groups was maintained at 9 weeks. Further, coping self-efficacy was inversely related to and the best predictor of depressive symptoms at both 3 and 9 weeks, after controlling for baseline values of depression and coping self-efficacy (Craft, 2005).

Surkan and colleagues (Surkan, Gottlieb, McCormick, Hunt, & Peterson, 2012) conducted a randomized controlled trial to examine the effect of a healthy lifestyle intervention (aimed at improving dietary and physical activity behaviors) on depressive symptoms in 679 low-income postpartum women. While not all women were experiencing depressive symptoms at baseline, the authors report that improvement in self-efficacy score for at least one health behavior (e.g., physical activity, eat more fruits and vegetables) appeared to mediate the overall effect of the intervention on depressive symptoms. Conversely, a study implementing an exercise and educational program among non-depressed persons with rheumatoid arthritis (N = 34) found no benefit with respect to coping self-efficacy. Specifically, the exercise intervention increased aerobic capacity and muscle strength but there were no improvements in self-efficacy for arthritis disease management (Breedland, van Scheppingen, Leijsma, Verheij-Jansen, & van Weert, 2011).

While self-efficacy is by far the most widely studied of the proposed psychological mechanisms, the majority of studies in this area have examined relationships between exercise and overall feelings of efficacy, rather than examining the mediating role of self-efficacy in the exercise–depression relationship. Consequently, although the enhancement of self-efficacy to lower depressive symptoms fits within current models of depression treatment, we have insufficient evidence at this time to be convinced that the self-efficacy hypothesis is valid.

The affect regulation hypothesis

The use of exercise to regulate affect may play a key role in how exercise alleviates depressive symptoms. Acute or individual bouts of exercise can reduce negative mood states and enhance positive mood states (Miller, Bartholomew, & Springer, 2005). Thus, exercise may act to provide temporary depressive symptom relief. Bartholomew and colleagues (Bartholomew, Morrison, & Ciccolo, 2005) found that a single bout of moderate-intensity exercise significantly improved negative aspects of mood and elevated feelings of general well-being and vigor in adults diagnosed with major depressive disorder (MDD). Participants (N = 40) were randomly assigned to either aerobic exercise for 30 minutes or to a 30-minute period of quiet rest. Mood and well-being were assessed 5 minutes before exercise or control and 5, 30, and 60 minutes following. Both conditions were associated with sustained improvements in mood in those with MDD. However, the exercise condition was also associated with significant and sustained improvements in feelings of well-being and vigor. Thus, acute exercise bouts may lessen depressive symptoms by allowing patients a means to more immediately regulate their mood and to experience brief periods of relief from their depression.

A second study has examined the effects of an acute bout of exercise on mood in individuals diagnosed with MDD or minor depressive disorder (Weinstein, Deuster, Francis, Beadling, & Kop, 2010). In this study, 14 individuals with depression and 16 controls (without a diagnosis of depression) engaged in an acute bout of exercise following a 30-minute rest period. The exercise bout was conducted at 70–85% of $\dot{V}O_2$max. Mood assessments were conducted prior to the exercise, immediately post-exercise, and 30 minutes after completion of exercise. Mood was assessed with the Profile of Mood States–Short Form inventory. Results indicated a significant reduction in depressed mood immediately post-exercise in participants with depression as compared to the control group, who had no change in depressed mood. Further, no group differences were found for fatigue or vigor immediately post-exercise. However, at 30 minutes following exercise, participants with depression experienced an increase in depressed mood, decreased vigor, and increased fatigue compared to baseline levels. Interestingly, severity of depression (as assessed by the Beck Depression Inventory-II at baseline) was significantly related to increases in depressed mood and fatigue at the 30 minutes post-exercise assessment. Thus, while an acute bout of exercise provided a mood benefit immediately post-exercise for those with depression, this mood benefit appears to be short-lived for some participants.

More work is needed with respect to this hypothesis. If affect regulation plays a role in the exercise–depression relationship, this has important implications for the timing and length of exercise interventions. Further, utilizing short, acute bouts of activity at multiple times during the day may be particularly important as those with depression often choose less healthy mood management strategies such as alcohol, tobacco, and drugs (Bartholomew, Morrison, & Ciccolo, 2005). It will be important for researchers to further examine the role that symptom severity plays in the effectiveness of acute exercise to manage mood and to investigate other person characteristics, such as age or race, that may influence the psychological response to an exercise bout (Hasson et al., 2011).

The distraction hypothesis

The distraction hypothesis has been commonly described in the exercise and depression literature since the 1970s (Barhrke & Morgan, 1978). This hypothesis proposes that exercise serves as a distraction from worries, stress, and depressive thoughts. Thus, distraction is a response style (Nolen-Hoeksema, 1991) or way of coping with depression in which the individual engages in distracting activities as a means to focus on something other than their depressed mood. Exercise has been compared to other distracting activities such as social contact, health education, relaxation, and assertiveness training, with mixed results (Doyne, Chambless, & Beutler, 1983; Klein et al., 1985; McNeil, LeBlanc, & Joyner, 1991; Singh, Clements, & Fiatarone, 1997). That is, exercise is superior to some of these activities and similar to others in its ability to alleviate depressive symptoms.

In our study of coping self-efficacy described previously (Craft, 2005), we also examined distraction as a potential mechanism underlying the exercise–depression relationship. In that study, we administered the Response Styles Questionnaire (RSQ) in order to assess an individual's tendency to use distraction as a coping mechanism, as opposed to using rumination (passively and repeatedly focusing on one's depressive feelings). Following the 9-week exercise intervention, both exercisers and control group members reported a reduction in their use of rumination but neither group reported an increase in their use of distraction. Thus, the data did not support our prediction that exercise would increase the use of distraction as a response style and that a distraction response style would be associated with lower depression scores among those in the exercise group.

The utility of this hypothesis remains unclear. Exercise may be a particularly distracting task when first being learned. Initially, individuals may be focused on somatic responses such as heart rate, breathing, fatigue, or sore muscles, as well as achieving exercise goals (Leith, 1994). However, once an activity is well learned, some might argue that one's mind is at liberty to problem solve or to further analyze one's troubles. Consequently, this hypothesis, in particular, may apply for some individuals at certain stages of an exercise program but have less relevance at other stages of exercise involvement.

Behavioral activation hypothesis

Behavioral activation is a psychotherapeutic process that encourages structured attempts at increases in behaviors that are likely to provide the patient with the opportunity for positive reinforcement and corresponding improvements in thoughts, mood, and quality of life (Hopko, Lejuez, Ruggiero, & Eifert, 2003). Depressed individuals often engage in maladaptive coping strategies such as inactivity and withdrawal. Within the process of behavioral activation, individuals are asked to begin replacing their inactive and passive activities with more active, enjoyable, and pleasurable activities. This theory would suggest that exercise is an action that is inconsistent with the natural tendencies associated with depression. Thus, it is thought that exercise represents an activity that has the potential to be rewarding and enjoyable, providing a sense of accomplishment. Consequently, depressive symptoms may be alleviated as the individual begins to replace passive activities with exercise and other more enjoyable activities.

This therapeutic approach involves teaching patients to formulate and accomplish behavioral goals. Further, in some types of behavioral activation therapy, the patient is asked to systematically increase the frequency of healthy behaviors (Hopko et al., 2003). Therapists may use a variety of behavioral strategies such as self-monitoring of activities and mood, activity scheduling, problem solving, social skill training, reward, and persuasion (Dimidjian, Barrera, Martell, Munoz, & Lewinsohn, 2011). For example, the patient may be asked to self-monitor his daily activities and then to identify relevant behavioral goals in major life areas in a hierarchical fashion (Hopko et al., 2003). This work often includes homework assignments, the use of self-identified rewards when goals are met, and opportunities for positive reinforcement. Over time, replacing depressive behaviors with activities and behaviors that are incompatible with depression should also result in a change in thoughts and mood (Dimidjian et al., 2011; Hopko et al., 2003).

There is no research to date that has explicitly tested this hypothesis within the context of exercise as a treatment for depression. However, these therapeutic processes are, in many ways, quite similar to what occurs within the context of an exercise training program. For example, exercise programs for depression often start with a self-monitoring exercise so that the study participant can understand the extent to which they currently engage in movement throughout the day. This is often accomplished with an activity log or a pedometer. Long-term goals for the exercise program are often established (e.g., working up to 30–45 min/week of moderate-intensity exercise on 5 or more days/week), while working collaboratively with the participant to set shorter-term weekly goals. In addition, participants are often asked to rate their mood during and after their exercise bouts so that they become more cognitively aware of how exercise affects mood. Participants are also generally encouraged to self-identify some personally meaningful reward that they will provide themselves should they meet their exercise goals. Finally, within the context of working with the exercise leader, there are also ample opportunities for positive feedback and positive social interactions.

Thus, an exercise program contains many of the same components of behavioral activation. Consequently, some may argue that exercise is simply a form of behavioral activation and, as a result, causes antidepressant benefits in a manner similar to that of behavioral activation. Studies are needed that directly compare exercise to behavioral activation and to other pleasant, reinforcing activities in individuals with depression, as well as studies that examine the importance of the "process" of learning to exercise (i.e., self-monitoring, goal setting, achieving exercise goals). It may be that the process of engaging in an exercise program and the cognitive behavioral characteristics of the program are as important in alleviating depressive symptoms as is the physical exercise that is completed.

As described, there is limited research examining the psychological mechanisms that have frequently been proposed during the past three decades. Many psychological mechanisms that have been proposed or mentioned in the literature have only one study, or in many cases, no studies empirically examining their worth. Consequently, it is an understatement to say that more work is needed.

To elucidate new, potentially relevant mechanisms, future researchers may find it helpful to more closely examine current evidence-based psychological therapies for depression. There are likely many commonalities between psychotherapy components and exercise programs. Understanding these commonalities may provide insight into mechanisms of treatment action. There has also been much written about the importance of the therapeutic relationship with respect to successful psychotherapy treatment outcomes. Primary aspects of the therapeutic relationship that have been identified as contributing to treatment success are goal consensus and collaboration. Goal consensus involves the patient and therapist coming to agreement about treatment goals and the processes by which the two will work together to achieve these goals. Collaboration refers to the process of the therapist and client working together to achieve the treatment goals (Swift & Callahan, 2009; Tryon & Winograd, 2011). Notably, the relationship between the exercise leader and depressed participant may also involve these specific therapeutic features as exercise goals are set and the dyad work collaboratively to achieve goals. As a result, these aspects of the therapeutic alliance may be important, independent of the actual exercise activity. Therefore, examining the ways in which psychotherapy "works" to alleviate depression may, in turn, allow us to postulate new mechanisms for how exercise effectively alleviates depressive symptoms.

Summary

In summary, more research is needed to determine which, if any, of the mechanisms described in this chapter underlie the effect of exercise on depression. It is highly likely that a combination of biological, psychological, and sociological factors influence the relationship between exercise and depression. This is consistent with current treatments for depression in which the effects of pharmacotherapy and psychotherapy on depression are often additive and address biological, psychological, and sociological aspects of the patient. Orlinsky and colleagues (Orlinsky, Ronnestad, & Willutzki, 2004), in their discussion of successful psychotherapy processes, state that "Both relationship variables and intervention procedures, patient participation and therapist influences, contribute jointly and variously to shaping the outcome of therapy" (p. 363). This is likely to also be true with respect to the effect of an exercise program on depressive symptoms. Future researchers must continue to identify and understand the various contributing mechanisms. Until we gain a better understanding of how exercise alleviates the symptoms of depression, we will likely continue to encounter difficulty in achieving a permanent place for exercise in mainstream depression treatment.

References

Bandura, A. (Ed.). (1997). *Self-efficacy: The exercise of control*. New York: W.H. Freeman and Company.
Barhrke, M. S., & Morgan, W. P. (1978). Anxiety reduction following exercise and meditation. *Cognitive Therapy and Research, 2*, 323–333.

Bartholomew, J. B., Morrison, D., & Ciccolo, J. T. (2005). Effects of acute exercise on mood and well-being in patients with major depressive disorder. *Medicine and Science in Sports and Exercise*, *37*(12), 2032–2037. doi:10.1249/01.mss.0000178101.78322.dd

Breedland, I., van Scheppingen, C., Leijsma, M., Verheij-Jansen, N. P., & van Weert, E. (2011). Effects of a group-based exercise and educational program on physical performance and disease self-management in rheumatoid arthritis: a randomized controlled study. *Physical Therapy*, *91*(6), 879–893. doi:10.2522/ptj.20090010

Brown, S. W., Welsh, M. C., & Labbe, E. E. (1992). Aerobic exercise in the psychological treatment of adolescents. *Perceptual and Motor Skills*, *74*(2), 555–560.

Craft, L. L. (2005). Exercise and clinical depression: examining two psychological mechanisms. *Psychology of Sport and Exercise*, *6*(2), 151–171. doi:10.1016/j.psychsport.2003.11.003

Dimidjian, S., Barrera, M., Jr., Martell, C., Munoz, R. F., & Lewinsohn, P. M. (2011). The origins and current status of behavioral activation treatments for depression. *Annual Review of Clinical Psychology*, 7, 1–38. doi:10.1146/annurev-clinpsy-032210-104535

Doyne, E. J., Chambless, D. L., & Beutler, L. E. (1983). Aerobic exercise as a treatment for depression in women. *Behavior Therapy*, *14*, 434–440.

Elavsky, S., McAuley, E., Motl, R. W., Konopack, J. F., Marquez, D. X., Hu, L., . . . Diener, E. (2005). Physical activity enhances long-term quality of life in older adults: efficacy, esteem, and affective influences. *Annals of Behavioral Medicine*, *30*(2), 138–145. doi:10.1207/s15324796abm3002_6

Fillipas, S., Oldmeadow, L. B., Bailey, M. J., & Cherry, C. L. (2006). A six-month, supervised, aerobic and resistance exercise program improves self-efficacy in people with human immunodeficiency virus: a randomised controlled trial. *Australian Journal of Physiotherapy*, *52*(3), 185–190.

Harris, A. H., Cronkite, R., & Moos, R. (2006). Physical activity, exercise coping, and depression in a 10-year cohort study of depressed patients. *Journal of Affective Disorders*, *93*(1–3), 79–85. doi:10.1016/j.jad.2006.02.013

Hasson, R. E., Granados, K. E., Marquez, D. X., Bennett, G., Freedson, P., & Braun, B. (2011). Psychological responses to acute exercise in sedentary black and white individuals. *Journal of Physical Activity and Health*, *8*(7), 978–987.

Hopko, D. R., Lejuez, C. W., Ruggiero, K. J., & Eifert, G. H. (2003). Contemporary behavioral activation treatments for depression: procedures, principles, and progress. *Clinical Psychology Review*, *23*(5), 699–717. doi:S0272735803000709

Hughes, D., Baum, G., Jovanovic, J., Carmack, C., Greisinger, A., & Basen-Engquist, K. (2010). An acute exercise session increases self-efficacy in sedentary endometrial cancer survivors and controls. *Journal of Physical Activity and Health*, *7*(6), 784–793.

Klein, M. H., Greist, J. H., Gurman, A. S., Neimeyer, R. A., Lesser, D. P., Bushnell, N. J., & Smith, R. E. (1985). A comparative outcome study of group psychotherapy vs. exercise treatments for depression. *International Journal of Mental Health*, *13*, 148–177.

Leith, L. M. (Ed.). (1994). *Foundations of exercise and mental health*. Morgantown, WV: Fitness Information Technology.

Martinsen, E. W., Hoffart, A., & Solberg, O. (1989). Comparing aerobic with nonaerobic forms of exercise in the treatment of clinical depression – a randomized trial. *Comprehensive Psychiatry*, *30*(4), 324–331.

Mayze, T. (2012). How antidepressants work. *CNS Forum*, *6*. Retrieved from http://www.cnsforum.com/clinicalresources/articles/annualreviews/antidepressants/

McNeil, J. K., LeBlanc, E. M., & Joyner, M. (1991). The effect of exercise on depressive symptoms in the moderately depressed elderly. *Psychology and Aging*, *6*(3), 487–488.

Miller, B. M., Bartholomew, J. B., & Springer, B. A. (2005). Post-exercise affect: the effect of mode preference. *Journal of Applied Sport Psychology*, *17*, 263–272.

Motl, R. W., & Snook, E. M. (2008). Physical activity, self-efficacy, and quality of life in multiple sclerosis. *Annals of Behavioral Medicine*, *35*(1), 111–115. doi:10.1007/s12160-007-9006-7

Nolen-Hoeksema, S. (1991). Responses to depression and their effects on the duration of depressive episodes. *Journal of Abnormal Psychology*, *100*(4), 569–582.

Orlinsky, D. E., Ronnestad, M. H., & Willutzki, U. (2004). Fifty years of psychotherapy process-outcome research: continuity and change. In M. Lambert (Ed.) *Handbook of psychotherapy and behavior change* (5th ed.). New York: John Wiley & Sons.

Shin, K. R., Kang, Y., Park, H. J., & Heitkemper, M. (2009). Effects of exercise program on physical fitness, depression, and self-efficacy of low-income elderly women in South Korea. *Public Health Nursing*, *26*(6), 523–531. doi:10.1111/j.1525-1446.2009.00812.x

Singh, N. A., Clements, K. M., & Fiatarone, M. A. (1997). A randomized controlled trial of the effect of exercise on sleep. *Sleep, 20*(2), 95–101.

Singh, N. A., Stavrinos, T. A., Scarbek, Y., Galambos, G., Liber, C., & Singh, M. A. F. (2005). A randomized controlled trial of high versus low intensity weight training versus general practitioner care for clinical depression in older adults. *Journals of Gerontology Series A: Biological Sciences and Medical Sciences, 60*(6), 768–776.

Surkan, P. J., Gottlieb, B. R., McCormick, M. C., Hunt, A., & Peterson, K. E. (2012). Impact of a health promotion intervention on maternal depressive symptoms at 15 months postpartum. *Maternal and Child Health Journal, 16*(1), 139–148. doi:10.1007/s10995-010-0729-x

Swift, J., & Callahan, J. (2009). Early psychotherapy processes: an examination of client and trainee clinician perspective convergence. *Clinical Psychology and Psychotherapy, 16*(3), 228–236. doi:10.1002/cpp.617

Tryon, G. S., & Winograd, G. (2011). Goal consensus and collaboration. *Psychotherapy (Chic), 48*(1), 50–57. doi:10.1037/a0022061

Weinstein, A. A., Deuster, P. A., Francis, J. L., Beadling, C., & Kop, W. J. (2010). The role of depression in short-term mood and fatigue responses to acute exercise. *International Journal of Behavioral Medicine, 17*(1), 51–57. doi:10.1007/s12529-009-9046-4

10

THE NEUROBIOLOGY OF DEPRESSION AND PHYSICAL EXERCISE

Michael J. Chen

Chronic severe stress often culminates in major depression. Whereas stress/depression atrophies neurons and dendrites, enjoyable physical exercise restores them. Exercise, therefore, is conducive to neuronal survival and is considered antidepressant. Herein, I start with discussing neurotransmitters and gradually progress to how depression and exercise are involved in systemic diseases, such as metabolic disorders.

The monoamine hypothesis of depression and the neurotrophin hypothesis of depression

The earliest putative biological underpinnings regarding the etiology of depression were in a deficiency of monoaminergic neural transmission, historically giving rise to the monoamine hypothesis of depression (Chopra, Kumar, & Kuhad, 2011; Duman, Heninger, & Nestler, 1997; Krishnan & Nestler, 2008; Russo-Neustadt & Chen, 2005). With less norepinephrine and/or serotonin (5HT) to bind their respective postsynaptic receptors, the postsynaptic neuron is, in turn, stimulated less than normal. The overall result is a higher excitation threshold and, therefore, depressive symptoms. To reverse this trend, therefore, antidepressant drugs increase or restore the levels of synaptic monoamines either by preventing their metabolism or re-uptake into the presynaptic neuron. In depression, neurons will homeostatically respond to low synaptic levels of monoaminergic neurotransmitters by up-regulating postsynaptic receptors in an effort to compensate. This is in part supplemented by an antidepressant drug, which, likewise, prevents any further metabolism or re-uptake of any more neurotransmitter. In the event of chronic administration of antidepressant, and consequent higher levels of synaptic neurotransmitter, monoaminergic receptors begin to down-regulate or desensitize.

It soon became apparent, however, that major depression cannot be solely explained by a mere shortage of neurotransmitters in the synapse; other influences must be at work, such as increased hypothalamic-pituitary-adrenal (HPA) activity, and differential genetic (Chopra et al., 2011; Thakker-Varia & Alder, 2009) and epigenetic (Elsner et al., 2011; Gomez-Pinilla, Zhuang, Feng, Ying, & Fan, 2011) expression of receptors, transporters, and metabolic enzymes. Evidence implicating the role of these other variables contributing to the complex etiology of depression was accumulating, thereby underscoring the time-consuming plastic changes that might account for the long therapeutic lag consumed by antidepressant drugs.

Borne out of antidepressant-induced plasticity, was mounting evidence that neurotrophins, specifically brain-derived neurotrophic factor (BDNF) plays a central role in psychiatric disorders, learning, and development (Dwivedi, 2009; Greenwood & Fleshner, 2008; Russo-Neustadt & Chen, 2005; Zoladz & Pilc, 2010). According to the neurotrophin hypothesis (Chopra et al., 2011; Krishnan & Nestler, 2008; Russo-Neustadt & Chen, 2005), BDNF is a putative signaling molecule transcribed from its immediate early gene as a downstream result of monoaminergic receptor binding and which subsequently activates a wide variety of intracellular survival signaling pathways (Chen, Nguyen, Pike, & Russo-Neustadt, 2007; Stone, Quartermain, Yin, & Lehmann, 2007), resulting in gene expression-mediated synaptic plasticity.

Despite the oversimplification regarding the complex etiology of depression via the two aforementioned hypotheses (Russo-Neustadt & Chen, 2005; Krishnan & Nestler, 2008), there is much evidence that physical exercise is significantly linked to a reduction of depression and anxiety disorders (Greenwood & Fleshner, 2008; Ströhle, 2009; Young, 2007). Via increased HPA and sympathetic nervous system activity, exercise releases neurotransmitter into the blood (Eisenhofer, Kopin, & Goldstein, 2004) and increases the levels of circulating synaptic norepinephrine (Russo-Neusstadt & Chen, 2005) and 5HT (Chaouloff, 1997; Dishman, Renner, White-Welkley, Burke, & Bunnel, 2000; Meeusen & De Meirleer, 1995). Therefore, vesicle proteins, such as synapsin I (Ding, Vaynman, Akhavan, Ying, & Gomez-Pinilla, 2006), synaptophysin (Vaynman, Ying, Yin, & Gomez-Pinilla, 2006), and SNAP-25 (Hu, Ying, Gomez-Pinilla, & Frautschy, 2009) involved in presynaptic neurotransmitter release, would be induced by exercise and therefore, BDNF; conversely, TrkB with IgG prevents their increase (Vaynman et al., 2006).

Monoaminergic receptors and projections in depression and exercise

Besides monoamines themselves, receptors may also play pivotal roles in mediating the effects of exercise on depression. The effects of depression and exercise on beta-adrenergic receptors (βAR), alpha-adrenergic receptors (αAR), and 5HT receptors across studies are not consistent. Generally, however, depression increases, while antidepressant drugs decrease βAR binding and/or number; like antidepressant drugs, exercise also decreases βAR number (reviewed by Russo-Neustadt & Chen, 2005; Stanford, 2001). Antidepressant drugs increase α_1ARs (Stone et al., 2007) and decrease α_2ARs (Lucki & O'Leary, 2004; Russo-Neustadt & Chen, 2005; Stanford, 2001). Stress increases corticosterone levels, which decreases norepinephrine release from the locus coeruleus and leads to α_1AR desensitization and/or decreased activation, which, in turn, lead to depression (Ressler & Nemeroff, 1999; Stone & Quartermain, 1999). While Morishima et al. (2006) found that high-intensity running down-regulated α_2AR, Greenwood and Fleshner (2008) reviewed no significant differences in α_2AR mRNA between sedentary and exercising rats. And finally, depression increases $5HT_{1A}$ and $5HT_{2A}$ receptor numbers, whereas anti-depressants decrease them (Carr & Lucki, 2011). In exercise-primed experienced rats, however, compared to those in sedentary controls, $5HT_{1A}$ mRNA increased (Greenwood & Fleshner, 2008) in the dorsal raphé, while also decreasing stress-induced activation of norepinephrine from the locus coeruleus. Exercise also decreases $5HT_{2C}$ receptor subtype (Broocks, Ahrendt, & Sommer, 2007), thereby augmenting norepinephrine and dopamine release from limbic areas (Pytliak, Vargová, Mechírová, & Felsöci, 2011) and increasing monoaminergic synaptic activity and counteracting the stress-to-depression response.

Gross morphological changes associated with depression and exercise

Numerous studies have indicated that in depressed humans, overall decreased brain volumes reflect severe neuronal and glial cell loss (Manji et al., 2003). Specifically, the hippocampal formation is one of several brain structures directly impacted by stress and depression. In patients suffering from major depression or post-traumatic stress disorder, a significant decrease in hippocampal volume (Bremner et al., 2000; Gerritsen et al., 2011; MacQueen et al., 2003; Stockmeier et al., 2004) or change in shape (Tae et al., 2011) has been reported, although it may not be necessarily due to neuronal loss per se, as interventions that ameliorate stress, allowing animals to recover, have been shown to restore such volume changes (Lucassen et al., 2010). Such volume changes may result from factors other than that of cell death, such as mere somatodendritic atrophy (which can be reversed) (Xiao, Feng, & Chen, 2010) or changes in glia or extracellular fluid volume (Lucassen et al., 2010). Thus, the decreased hippocampal volume was asymmetric and only transient (Ahdidan et al., 2011). However, whether volumetric reductions in motor and limbic structures in humans are strictly due to depression is unknown (Canbeyli, 2010).

Exercise increases neurogenesis and dendritic complexity

The gross morphological changes resulting from stress/depression or age on one hand and the ameliorative reversal, or at least, maintenance effects, of exercise on the other, can be partly attributed to altered levels and/or patterns of neurogenesis. Physical exercise has been shown to increase neurogenesis in the hippocampus (Bjφnebekk, Mathé, & Brené, 2005; Ernst, Olson, Pinel, Lam, & Christie, 2006; Kitamura, Mishina, & Sugiyama, 2003) and dentate gyrus (Åberg, Perlman, Olson, & Brené, 2008; Fuss et al., 2010; Kitamura & Sugiyama, 2006; Pereira et al., 2007; Redila & Christie, 2006; Snyder, Glover, Sanzone, Kamhi, & Cameron, 2009). In addition, exercise increases mossy fiber density (da Silva et al., 2012), both hippocampal and entorhinal cortical dendritic spines (Stranahan, Khalil, & Gould, 2007) and synaptic transmission (Kobayashi, Ikeda, & Suzuki, 2006). Consequently, exercise can increase, or at least maintain, hippocampal volume in older adults (Erickson et al., 2009, 2011). Highly correlated with neurogenesis is BDNF, which is up-regulated in the well-known environmental enrichment protocols (Russo–Neustadt & Chen, 2005) in which running, dietary restriction (Kitamura, Mishina, & Sugiyama, 2006), and possibly the other varied stimuli increase hippocampal angiogenesis (Ekstrand, Hellsten, & Tingström, 2008) and neurogenesis (Kitamura et al., 2006), dendritic length and arborization complexity of parietal cortical pyramidal neurons (Leggio et al., 2005), and hippocampal mossy fibers (Toscano–Silva et al., 2010), compared to those in rats housed in standard conditions. Conversely, in trkB knock-out mice, exercise resulted in no neurogenesis of hippocampal neuroprogenitor cells (Li, Jarvis, Alvarez-Borda, Lim, & Nottebohm 2000; Li et al., 2008).

Antidepressant medications and physical exercise engage the same neuroprotective, prosurvival pathways

According to the neurotrophin hypothesis, plastic changes, resulting from antidepressant drug treatment and/or exercise, begin with enhanced synaptic monoamine concentrations allowing for increased norepinephrine and/or 5HT binding (above) to their respective G-protein coupled receptors, which activate adenylate cyclase to produce cAMP, which activates protein kinase A. A major target of the cAMP cascade is the cAMP response element binding (CREB) protein, a transcription factor that regulates gene expression by binding to cAMP response element (CRE)—a cis-acting enhancer element in the regulatory region of various genes (Meyer and Habener, 1993; Montminy, Gonzalez, & Yamamoto, 1990). The increase in phosphorylated CREB up-regulates BDNF, which activates neuronal survival signaling pathways (Chen et al., 2007; Chen & Russo-Neustadt, 2005; Russo-Neustadt & Chen, 2005) against various forms of stress, such as trauma, ischemia, and diabetes mellitus (Dishman et al., 2006; Greenwood & Fleshner, 2008; Kazanis, Giannakopoulou, Philippidis, & Stylianopoulou, 2004; Matsuzaki, Namikawa, Kiyama, Mori, & Sato, 2004; Schabitz, Schwab, Spranger, & Hacke, 1997; Schabitz et al., 2000; Yamashita, Wiessner, Lindholm, Thoenen, & Hossmann, 1997; Zhang & Pardridge, 2001).

Stress, physical exercise, and BDNF

The hippocampus is particularly vulnerable to cortisol (Lee, Ogle, & Sapolsky, 2002), which is increased during times of prolonged unremitting stress (Lee et al., 2002; Uno, Ross, Else, Suleman, & Sapolsky, 1989). Conversely, an antidepressant regimen, which includes exercise, ameliorates stress and/or depression via BDNF (da Silva et al., 2012; Duman & Monteggia, 2006; Dwivedi, 2009; Marais, Stein, & Daniels, 2009; Mata, Thompson, & Gotlib, 2010; Sartori et al., 2011; Siefert et al., 2010; Zheng et al., 2006) and TrkB (da Silva et al., 2012; Widenfalk, Olson, & Thorén, 1999) expression and subsequent intracellular signaling-mediated plasticity (Vaynman et al., 2006) and therefore, cell survival (Chen & Russo-Neustadt, 2007; Li, Jarvis, Alvarez-Borda, Lim, & Nottebolm, 2000). And when running stops, both BDNF and TrkB mRNAs down-regulate (Widenfalk et al., 1999).

Depression, metabolism, and exercise

There is ample evidence that major depressive disorder and obesity are linked (Anderson, Cohen, Naumova, Jacques, & Must, 2007; Dong, Sanchez, & Price, 2004; Herva et al., 2006; Roberts, Deleger, Strawbridge, & Kaplan, 2003). In fact, many diseases for which overeating is a risk factor (e.g., cardiovascular disease, diabetes mellitus, cancer) tend to cluster with neurodegenerative and psychiatric diseases (Mattson, 2005; Pedersen et al., 2009). Conversely, regular exercise and/or dietary restriction can regulate neuronal plasticity through the expression and activation of BDNF and release of 5HT (Mattson, Maudsley, & Martin, 2004). Indeed, BDNF levels are relatively low in those with metabolic diseases (Pederson et al., 2009). Further, the link between depression and obesity may reside with the hormone leptin, to which many obese people may be resistant (Klok, Jakobsdottir, & Drent, 2007). Thus, leptin may be antidepressant, as leptin increases hippocampal BDNF in diet-control mice, but not in diet-induced obese mice (Yamada et al., 2011) in which obesity could be directly attributed to decreased leptin (Mainardi et al., 2010). Similarly, the antidepressant effects of leptin were abolished by the presence of a TrkB inhibitor; therefore, leptin activity in the hippocampus may at least partly explain the depression–obesity connection (Yamada et al., 2011).

The benefits derived from physical exercise (Dishman et al., 2006) and dietary restriction (Mattson, 2000) have revealed that both increase resistance to oxidative stress involving ROS-mediated damage to proteins, lipids, and nucleic acids. With dietary restriction, nutrient metabolism is more efficiently utilized, thereby promoting neuronal mitochondrial function (Mattson, Gleichmann, & Cheng, 2008), activating and deactivating cell survival and apoptotic cascades, respectively (Mattson, 2000; Mattson, Duan, & Gao, 2003). Chronic mild stress, however, has been shown to inhibit respiration rates and dissipate the membrane potential of hippocampal mitochondria in mice (Gong, Chai, Ding, Sun, & Hu, 2011).

The opposite of dietary restriction is overeating, which, as mentioned above, clusters with depression (Pederson et al., 2009). Following a carbohydrate-rich meal and release of insulin, there is a decrease in both glucose and amino acids in the blood. However, blood tryptophan levels remain steady, because branched-chain amino acids (BCAAs) prevent tryptophan from being taken up into the brain, which drastically decreases the ability of this organ to synthesize 5HT. The resultant lower brain 5HT levels then can lead to or contribute to depression (Wurtman, 1993). Depressive symptoms can then, in turn, lead to over-eating, completing the vicious cycle. Such a cycle, over a span of decades, would eventually lead to insulin resistance. To break this cycle, therefore, (more) 5HT must be able to enter the brain and/or the brain must be able to synthesize it *de novo*. Thus, 5HT-selective re-uptake inhibitors (SSRI)s have been shown to increase insulin sensitivity; specifically, citalopram leads to increased glucose tolerance and a decrease in cardio-vascular response to stress and attendant decrease in hyperglycemia (Mattson, 2005). Therefore, medications often used to treat obesity target the same neurotransmitter system (5HT) as those used to treat depression (Bello & Liang, 2011). Thus, because there is initially a deficiency in 5HT (say, before SSRI administration and as a result of carbohydrate indulging), there is a defect in the ability of 5HT to regulate hypothalamic function, which may underlie the inability of patients with insulin resistance to effectively cope with stress/depression. On the other hand, dietary restriction increases 5HT hypothalamic signaling, which may decrease oxidative stress and enhance mood (Mattson, 2005). Moreover, exercise has been shown to reverse many of the afore-mentioned trends. During exercise, there is an increase in plasma BCAAs, which are taken up by muscle, thereby nullifying their inhibitory effect of tryptophan (which is also increased by exercise) uptake into various brain regions (Fernstrom & Fernstrom, 2006; Newsholme & Blomsbrand, 2006). As a result, central 5HT synthesis and release are increased (Fernstrom & Fernstrom, 2006).

Because exercise is antidepressant, it might confer the same antioxidant neuroprotective effects that treatment with SSRIs and antioxidants produced. Regular exercise in both young and middle-aged rats led to decreased accumulation of oxidatively damaged proteins (protein carbonyls) (Radak et al., 2001). And by increasing BDNF, exercise reverses the deleterious effects of a high-fat diet, such as increases in reactive oxygen species (ROSs). On its own, without exercise, BDNF injected chronically into the paraventricular nucleus of the hypothalamus reverses obesity brought about by a high-fat diet (Wang, Godar, Billington, & Kotz, 2010). Conversely, deletion of the *bdnf* gene in the ventral medial hypothalamus (VMH) results in hyperphagia and obesity (Unger, Calderon, Bradley, Sena-Esteves, & Rios, 2007), which, in turn, decreases hippocampal BDNF (Park et al., 2010; Wu, Molteni, Ying, & Gomez-Pinilla, 2003), and impairs neurogenesis. Both effects are associated with increased lipid peroxidation (Park et al., 2010), thereby compromising these plastic changes.

The antidepressant effects of exercise, namely increased BDNF release, combined with dietary restriction, can suppress feeding (Klok et al., 2007; Lebrun, Bariohay, Moyse, & Jean, 2006), thereby increasing glucose metabolism and energy expenditure (Pederson et al., 2009). Intracerebroventricular infusion of BDNF has led to increased peripheral insulin sensitivity in normal rodents, a reduction in diabetes in mice (Mattson, 2005), decreased leptin resistance, and decreased obesity (Kernie, Liebl, & Parada, 2000). Without BDNF (or exercise), there is increased sensitivity to stress, increased plasma glucose (Pederson et al., 2009) and insulin (Maniam & Morris, 2010) levels, and obesity (Kernie et al., 2000). Exercise plus dietary restriction, therefore, will lead to increased BDNF signaling, which, in turn, may stimulate signaling pathways that increase glucose metabolism and cellular resistance, leading to protection against stress–associated diseases such as cardiovascular disease, diabetes mellitus, and obesity.

Normally, glucose is a satiety signal, inducing BDNF and TrkB in the VMH (Unger et al., 2007). Below a certain brain glucose level, however, leptin is released from adipose stores and then acts on neuropeptide Y (NPY) receptors in the VMH, culminating in decreased leptin binding to leptin receptors. NPY receptor activation increases feeding and body weight and decreases resting metabolic rate, all of which then increase adipose tissue mass. Increased adipose then absorbs more glucose, again depriving the brain of glucose, and thereby completing the cycle (Noble, Billington, Kotz, & Wang, 2011; Peters et al., 2004). On the other hand, physical exercise increases adipose tissue metabolism, thereby releasing higher amounts of leptin into the circulation (higher than that released during severe depression, above). Leptin then binds its receptors residing on neurons in the arcuate nucleus and VMH. In the latter, α-melanocyte-stimulating hormone (α-MSH) increases leptin binding to leptin receptors. Alpha-MSH then binds to MC4 receptors, which increases BDNF binding to TrkB (Xu et al., 2003). Increased BDNF activity then suppresses feeding and decreases hyperglycemia, hyperinsulinemia, hyper-lipidemia, and GABA receptor binding; this last effect then increases excitation, which then increases physical exercise, thereby completing the cycle (Mainardi et al., 2010; Noble et al., 2011).

Oxidative damage and exercise

It has been suggested that exercise can ameliorate the effects of stress-induced ROS production (Mattson, 2000), perhaps by maintaining a redox homeostasis conducive to brain function. However, exercise itself is a stressor. The type of exercise (running vs swimming), protocol intensity, length of running (acute vs chronic), voluntary vs forced, species, brain region, and physiological status (age, gender, overweight, diabetic) of the animal all interact in determining whether exercise is beneficial (enjoyable) or stressful (aversive). Thus, one must consider the activity of various antioxidant enzymes, as well as the oxidative damage to lipids, proteins, and DNA, which occur as by-products of routine cellular metabolism. These free radicals are extremely reactive and have been implicated in various neurodegenerative disorders (Chrissobolis, Miller, Drummond, Kemp-Harper, & Sobey, 2011; Genovese et al., 2011; Hegde, Hegde, Rao, & Mitra, 2011). Generally, exercise was shown to decrease such damage (Radak, Kumagai, Taylor, Naito, & Goto, 2007). More recently, Radak, Chung, and Goto (2008) found that as a result of an acute, stressful bout of forced exercise, there is increased production of free radicals, oxidative damage, antioxidant enzyme activity, and decreased resistance to oxidative stress and declining physiological function. Chronic exercise, on the other hand, generally results in decreased levels of these measures, except for antioxidant enzyme activity and oxidative damage, which both acute and chronic exercise increase (Radak et al., 2008). The central player in exercise-mediated amelioration of brain health during depression is BDNF. Earlier studies from our lab have shown that nitric oxide production (Boveris & Navarro, 2008) is related to exercise-induced and norepinephrine-induced increases in BDNF expression *in vivo* (Chen, Ivy, & Russo-Neustadt., 2006) and *in vitro* (Chen & Russo-Neustadt, 2007).

Glutamate

One of the ways by which exercise can rapidly and robustly increase BDNF is via glutamatergic activation (Castrén, Berninger, Leingärtner, & Lindholm, 1998) and nitric oxide signaling (Chen et al., 2006; Chen & Russo-Neustadt, 2007). General physical activity not only increases release of norepinephrine (above), but also glutamate (Richter-Levine, Canevari, & Bliss, 1998). While antidepressant drugs and exercise activate intrasynaptic norepinephrine and/or 5HT-induced increased CREB-mediated BDNF transcription (Russo-Neustadt & Chen, 2005), increased glutamate release (Lonart & Johnson, 1995) activates nitric oxide synthesis (Fedele, Marchi, &

Raiteri, 2001), which, in turn, may lead to more norepinephrine release (Lonart, Wang, & Johnson, 1992; Stout & Woodward, 1994) and up-regulated NMDAR1 mRNA (Dietrich et al., 2005; Lou, Liu, Chang, & Chen, 2008), NMDAR2B (Dietrich et al., 2005; Farmer et al., 2004; Hu et al., 2009), glutamate receptors GluR1, GluR2/3 (Dietrich et al., 2005), and GluR5 (Farmer et al., 2004), and AMPA receptors (Real, Ferreira, Hernandez, Britto, & Pires, 2010). This would result in a rapid positive feedback and potentiation of the norepinephrine-to-BDNF signal (Chen et al., 2007; Mattson, 2008), perhaps by induction of PSD-95 (Hu et al., 2009). In addition, nitric oxide activates the PI-3K pathway directly via ras (Deora, Win, Vanhaesebroeck, & Lander, 1998) and the subsequent transcription of many pro-survival genes involved in neurite outgrowth and synaptogenesis (Mattson, 2008).

Research concerns in depression/exercise experimentation

Methodological issues of research of the neurobiological mechanisms of exercise and depression were addressed earlier by Dishman et al. (2006). One of the most disconcerting issues facing the practice of using animal models of human depression is its content validity. Because we are assuming that the various behavioral tests and therefore biochemical measures we use (e.g., forced swim, tail suspension) are indeed valid models of depression, it is difficult to imagine that a full understanding of the complex mechanisms involved in the etiology of this disorder will ever be achieved. Such behavioral tests fail to take into account the emotional contribution of the animal to the observed results. Additionally, there may be simpler interpretations, such as lack of motivation or simple fatigue resulting from so much struggling (tail suspension test). Assuming that a lack of struggling is not due to fatigue or lack of motivation, how long must a rat *not* struggle before it is considered a valid model of human depression, which can last for years, long-term? Because it is neither practical nor ethical to effect a proportional length of time a rat must struggle to mirror a human depressive episode, there is a paucity of human studies demonstrating whether such long-term changes in synaptic efficacy induced by stress/depression can be partially reversed by antidepressant treatment/exercise (Popoli, Gennarelli, & Racagni, 2002). Further, there are often distinct differences between voluntary exercise (enjoyable) vs that which is forced (aversive and stressful). Just as it does in humans, exercise in other animals, therefore, may carry an emotional component with it.

Is depression anatomically localized?

Most of the neurobiological research of depression and exercise has examined the hippocampus and cortex, where most of the brain BDNF is expressed. Much of the pathophysiology of depression, however, also occurs in the ventral tegmental area-nucleus accumbens (Nestler & Carlezon, 2006); anhedonia indicates problems with this mesolimbic reward pathway, where disturbances may also cause decreased BDNF (Angelucci, Brenè, & Matheé, 2005).

Genetic models of depression

Other animal models of depression may provide new information and warrant further consideration. For example, the Flinders sensitive/resistant line has exhibited increased BDNF. This could mean that there is a compensatory increased BDNF expression in response to down-regulated TrkB signaling (Angelucci et al., 2005); it could also mean a decreased BDNF turnover with a higher pool of BDNF in the tissue that is not released (Angelucci et al., 2005). Such a pool of BDNF could be released as a result of exercise-induced increases in monoaminergic activation (Chen et al., 2007) and could shorten the length of time required for plastic changes to occur and therefore, therapeutic efficacy would be reached sooner.

Sedentary lifestyle is not normal

Standard laboratory conditions of sedentary lifestyles are those of deprivation and lack of stimulation (Gould, Tanapat, Rydel, & Hastings, 2000; Würbel, 2001). Sedentary rodents may not be the most valid models of human disease. It has been noted, therefore, that rodents should perhaps have access to a running wheel in their cages (Van Praag, Barlow, & Gage, 2001), thereby simulating as closely as possible what their lives would be outside captivity. Because runners are often compared to their sedentary controls, the baseline of various molecules, such as that of BDNF, is already rather low. Therefore, it often does not take much running stimulation to increase this already very low amount of BDNF. The vast majority of studies use young adult rodents starting at 2–3 months of age. Voluntary running usually entails a running wheel accessible 24 hr/day for the pre-specified length of the study, the objectives of which will determine the exercise protocol. Exercise durations, therefore, vary widely and can range from only an acute bout of running for, say, 6 hours (Chen & Russo-Neustadt, 2009) to as long as 28 or even 90 days (Berchtold et al., 2005). Between these extremes, access to running wheels, depending on the objectives of the study, typically lasts 1, 2, 3, or 4 weeks (Russo-Neustadt & Chen, 2005). In addition, it is common practice to initially allow the rodents a brief period of 3–5 days of voluntary running, followed by a period of 7–10 days of wheel removal from their cages, followed by the beginning of the running protocol itself. This brief priming or training period allows the rodents to gain dexterity while also decreasing the effects of novelty and learning during the actual treatment period (Russo-Neustadt, Ha, Ramirez, & Kesslak, 2001; Berchtold, Kesslak, & Cotman, 2002; Vaynman et al., 2006). Running distances and speeds are computer-monitored and calculated as meters run per night, typically 2–6 km/night, although these distances also vary widely across labs, strains, and species (mice vs rats). Other investigators have used forced running, in which rodents are placed on a treadmill for, say, 7 sessions/10 days at 30 min/session/day and in which the speed of the treadmill gradually increased (Soya et al., 2007).

Interpretive hurdles

Applying the observation that exercise increases neurogenesis in rodents to human major depressive disorder is, at best, suggestive. Whether exercise-induced increases in neurogenesis in humans are actually therapeutic for major depression remains to be seen. Establishing a direct connection between exercise and neurogenesis in humans would be difficult, unless BDNF activity could somehow be tracked in a way similar to that of glucose in fMRI.

Future research directions

Because of the potential validity issues facing the use of animal models for studying mood disorders (above), a major challenge for future research would be to conduct more human studies, addressing the genetics of major depressive disorder, such as polymorphisms of the genes of the 5HT receptor subtypes, BDNF, and other monoaminergic receptors and transporters.

In addition, exercise should be prescribed in doses, gradually increasing over time. Such a practice might serve to overcome the inertia that depressed individuals often find daunting in starting an exercise regimen; treating exercise and diet the same as one would any other drug provides a systematic and predictable outcome measure – whether or not mood improves.

Moreover, researchers and clinicians should both recognize that emotions play a significant role. The critical difference seems to lie in whether the activity is enjoyable. Physical activity can be aversive and exercise can be enjoyable. Often, it is the "intent" of the activity that distinguishes these two. Physical activity relates more strongly to daily movements, and exercise more to structured, purposeful, or planned activity with the aim of increasing strength, cardiovascular fitness, etc. Just as it has been observed that an increase in BDNF and neurogenesis is associated with voluntary running (enjoyable, exercise), these biological measures are not increased with treadmill (stressful, forced) running. Although these interventions increase central expression of BDNF, it is possible that intense exercise raises body temperature enough to allow BDNF to exchange between the CNS and the periphery (Goekint, Roelands, Heyman, Njemini, & Meeusen, 2011).

Finally, specific human characteristics, such as age, gender, health/disease state, etc. should be considered when evaluating the effects of leisure-time physical exercise on depression.

References

Åberg, E., Perlman, T., Olson, L., & Brené, S. (2008). Running increases neurogenesis without retinoic acid receptor activation in the adult mouse dentate gyrus. *Hippocampus, 18*(8), 785–792.

Ahdidan, J., Hviid, L. B., Chakravarty, M. M., Ravnkilde, B., Rosenberg, R., Rodell, A., . . . Videbech, P. (2011). Longitudinal MR study of brain structure and hippocampus volume in major depressive disorder. *Acta Psychiatrica Scandinavica, 123*(3), 211–219.

Anderson, S. E., Cohen, P., Naumova, E. N., Jacques, P. F., & Must, A. (2007). Adolescent obesity and risk for subsequent major depressive disorder and anxiety disorder: Prospective evidence. *Psychosomatic Medicine, 69*(8), 740–747.

Angelucci, F., Brenè, S., & Matheé, A. A. (2005). BDNF in schizophrenia, depression and corresponding animal models. *Molecular Psychiatry, 10*(4), 345–352.

Bello, N. T., & Liang, N-C. (2011). The use of serotonergic drugs to treat obesity – Is there any hope? *Drug Design, Development and Therapy, 5*, 95–109.

Berchtold, N. C., Chinn, G., Chou, M., Kesslak, J. P., & Cotman, C. W. (2005). Exercise primes a molecular memory for brain-derived neurotrophic factor protein induction in the rat hippocampus. *Neuroscience, 133*(3), 853–861.

Berchtold, N. C., Kesslak, J. P., & Cotman, C. W. (2002). Hippocampal brain-derived neurotrophic factor gene regulation by exercise and the medial septum. *Journal of Neuroscience Research, 68*(5), 511–521.

Bjφnebekk, A., Mathé, A. A., & Brené, S. (2005). The antidepressant effect of running is associated with increased hippocampal cell proliferation. *International Journal of Neuropsychopharmacology, 8*, 1–12.

Boveris, A., & Navarro, A. (2008). Systemic and mitochondrial adaptive responses to moderate exercise in rodents. *Free Radical Biology and Medicine, 44*(2), 224–229.

Bremner, J., Narayan, M., Anderson, E. R., Staib, L. H., Miller, H., &Charney, D. S. (2000). Hippocampal volume reduction in major depression. *American Journal of Psychiatry, 157*(1), 115–118.

Broocks, A., Ahrendt, U., & Sommer, M. (2007). Physical training in the treatment of depressive disorders. *Psychiatry Prax, 34*, S300–S304.

Canbeyli, R. (2010). Sensorimotor modulation of mood and depression: An integrative review. *Behavioural Brain Research, 207*(2), 249–264.

Carr, G. V., & Lucki, I. (2011). The role of serotonin receptor subtypes in treating depression: A review of animal studies. *Psychopharmacology, 213*(2–3), 265–287.

Castrén, E., Berninger, B., Leingärtner, A., & Lindholm, D. (1998). Regulation of brain-derived neurotrophic factor mRNA levels in hippocampus by neuronal activity. *Progress in Brain Research, 117*, 57–64.

Chaouloff, F. (1997). Effects of acute physical exercise on central serotonergic systems. *Medicine and Science in Sports and Exercise, 29*(1), 58–62.

Chen, M. J., Ivy, A. S., & Russo-Neustadt, A. A. (2006). Nitric oxide synthesis is required for exercise-induced increases in hippocampal BDNF and phosphatidylinositol 3′ kinase. *Brain Research Bulletin, 68*(4), 257–268.

Chen, M. J., Nguyen, T. V., Pike, C. J., & Russo-Neustadt, A. A. (2007). Norepinephrine induces BDNF and activates the PI-3K and MAPK cascades in embryonic hippocampal neurons. *Cellular Signalling, 19*(1), 114–128.

Chen, M. J., & Russo-Neustadt, A. A. (2005). Exercise activates the phosphatidylinositol 3-kinase pathway. *Molecular Brain Research, 135*(1–2), 181–193.

Chen, M. J., & Russo-Neustadt, A. A. (2007). Nitric oxide signaling participates in norepinephrine-induced activity of neuronal intracellular survival pathways. *Life Sciences, 81*(16), 1280–1290.

Chen, M. J., & Russo-Neustadt, A. A. (2009). Running exercise-induced up-regulation of hippocampal brain-derived neurotrophic factor is CREB-dependent, *Hippocampus, 19*(10), 962–972.

Chopra, K., Kumar, B., & Kuhad, A. (2011). Pathobiological targets of depression. *Expert Opinion in Therapeutic Targets, 15*(4), 379–400.

Chrissobolis, S., Miller, A. A., Drummond, G. R., Kemp-Harper, B. K., & Sobey, C.G. (2011). Oxidative stress and endothelial dysfunction in cerebrovascular disease. *Frontiers in Bioscience, 16,* 1733–1745.

da Silva, S. G., Unsain, N., Mascó, D. H., Toscano-Silva, M., de Amorim, H. A., Araújo, B. H. S., . . . Arida, R. M. (2012). Early exercise promotes positive hippocampal plasticity and improves spatial memory in the adult life of rats. *Hippocampus, 22*(2), 347–358.

Deora, A. A., Win, T., Vanhaesebroeck, B., & Lander, H. M. (1998). A redox-triggered ras-effector interaction. Recruitment of phosphatidylinositol 3′-kinase to Ras by redox stress. *Journal of Biological Chemistry, 273*(45), 29923–29928.

Dietrich, M. O., Mantese, C. E., Porciuncula, L. O., Ghisleni, G., Vinade, L., Souza, D. O., & Portela, L. V. (2005). Exercise affects glutamate receptors in postsynaptic densities from cortical mice brain. *Brain Research, 1065*(1–2), 20–25.

Ding, Q., Vaynman, S., Akhavan, M., Ying, Z., & Gomez-Pinilla, F. (2006). Insulin-like growth factor I interfaces with brain-derived neurotrophic factor-mediated synaptic plasticity to modulate aspects of exercise-induced cognitive function. *Neuroscience, 140*(3), 823–833.

Dishman, R. K., Berthoud, H-R., Booth, F. W., Cotman, C. W., Edgerton, V. R., Fleshner, M. R., . . . & Zigmond, M. J. (2006). Neurobiology of exercise. *Obesity, 14*(3), 345–356.

Dishman, R. K., Renner, K. J., White-Welkley, J. E., Burke, K. A., & Bunnell, B. N. (2000). Treadmill exercises training augments brain norepinephrine response to familiar and novel stress. *Brain Research Bulletin, 52*(5), 337–342.

Dong, C., Sanchez, L. E., & Price, R. A. (2004). Relationship of obesity to depression: A family-based study. *International Journal of Obesity and Related Metabolic Disorders, 28*(6), 790–795.

Duman, R. S., Heninger, G. R., & Nestler, E. J. (1997). A molecular and cellular theory of depression. *Archives of General Psychiatry, 54*(7), 597–606.

Duman, R. S., & Monteggia, L. M. (2006). A neurotrophic model for stress-related mood disorders. *Biological Psychiatry, 59*(12), 1116–1127.

Dwivedi, Y. (2009). Brain-derived neurotrophic factor: A role in depression and suicide. *Neuropsychiatric Disease and Treatment, 5,* 433–449.

Eisenhofer, G., Kopin, I. J., & Goldstein, D. S. (2004). Leaky catecholamine stores: Undue waste or a stress response coping mechanism? *Annals of the New York Academy of Sciences, 1018,* 224–230.

Ekstrand, J., Hellsten, J., & Tingström, A. (2008). Environmental enrichment, exercise and corticosterone affect endothelial cell proliferation in adult rat hippocampus and prefrontal cortex. *Neuroscience Letters, 442*(3), 203–207.

Elsner, V. R., Lovatel, G. A., Bertoldi, K., Vanzella, C., Santos, F. M., Spindler, C., . . . Siqueira, I. R. (2011). Effect of different exercise protocols on histone acetyltransferases and histone deacetylases activities in rat hippocampus. *Neuroscience, 192,* 580–587.

Erickson, K. I., Prakash, R. S., Voss, M. W., Chaddock, L., Hu, L., Morris, K. S., . . . Kramer, A. F. (2009). Aerobic fitness is associated with hippocampal volume in elderly humans. *Hippocampus, 19*(10), 1030–1039.

Erickson, K. I., Voss, M. W., Prakash, R. S., Basak, C., Szabo, A., Chaddock, L., . . . Kramer, A. F. (2011). Exercise training increases size of hippocampus and improves memory. *Proceedings of the National Academy of Sciences USA, 108*(7), 3017–3022.

Ernst, C., Olson, A. K., Pinel, J. P. J., Lam, R. W., & Christie, B. R. (2006). Antidepressant effects of exercise: Evidence for an adult-neurogenesis hypothesis? *Reviews in Psychiatric Neuroscience, 31,* 84–91.

Farmer, J., Zhao, X., van Praag, H., Woodke, K., Gage, F. H., & Christie, B. R. (2004). Effects of voluntary exercise on synaptic plasticity and gene expression in the dentate gyrus of adult male Sprague-Dawley rats in vivo. *Neuroscience, 124*(1), 71–79.

Fedele, E., Marchi, M., & Raiteri, M. (2001). In vivo NO/cGMP signaling in the hippocampus. *Neurochemical Research, 26*(8–9), 1069–1078.

Fernstrom, J. D., & Fernstrom, M. H. (2006). Exercise, serum free tryptophan, and central fatigue. *Journal of Nutrition, 136*(2), 553S–559S.

Fuss, J., Abdallah, N. M.-B. B., Vogt, M. A., Touma, C., Pacifici, G., Palme, R., . . . Gass, P. (2010). Voluntary exercise induces anxiety-like behavior in adult C57BL/6J mice correlating with hippocampal neurogenesis. *Hippocampus, 20*(3), 364–376.

Genovese, T., Mazzon, E., Paterniti, I., Esposito, E., Bramanti, P., & Cuzzocrea, S. (2011). Modulation of NADPH oxidase activation in cerebral ischemia/reperfusion injury in rats. *Brain Research, 1372,* 92–102.

Gerritsen, L., Comijs, H. C., van der Graaf, Y., Knoops, J. G., Penninx, B. W. J. H., & Geerlings, M. I. (2011). Depression, hypothalamic pituitary adrenal axis, and hippocampal and entorhinal cortex volumes – The SMART Medea Study. *Biological Psychiatry, 70*(4), 373–380.

Goekint, M., Roelands, B., Heyman, E., Njemini, R., & Meeusen, R. (2011). Influence of citalopram and environmental temperature on exercise-induced changes in BDNF. *Neuroscience Letters, 494*(2), 150–154.

Gomez-Pinilla, F., Zhuang, Y., Feng, J., Ying, Z., & Fan, G. (2011). Exercise impacts brain-derived neurotrophic factor plasticity by engaging mechanisms of epigenetic regulation. *European Journal of Neuroscience, 33*(3), 383–390.

Gong, Y., Chai, Y., Ding, J-H., Sun, X-L., & Hu, G. (2011). Chronic mild stress damages mitochondrial ultrastructure and function in mouse brain. *Neuroscience Letters, 488*(1), 76–80.

Gould, E., Tanapat, P., Rydel, T., & Hastings, N. (2000). Regulation of hippocampal neurogenesis in adulthood. *Biological Psychiatry, 48*(8), 715–720.

Greenwood, B. N., & Fleshner, M. K. (2008). Exercise, learned helplessness, and the stress-resistant brain. *Neuromolecular Medicine, 10*(2), 81–98.

Hegde, M. L., Hegde, P. M., Rao, K. S., & Mitra, S. (2011). Oxidative genome damage and its repair in neurodegenerative diseases: Function of transition metals as a double-edged sword. *Journal of Alzheimers Disease, 24*(Supplement 2), 183–198.

Herva, A., Laitinen, J., Miettunen, J., Veijola, J., Karvonen, J. T., Läksy, K., & Joukamaa, M. (2006). Obesity and depression: Results from the longitudinal Northern Finland 1966 Birth Cohort Study. *International Journal of Obesity London, 30*(3), 520–527.

Hu, S., Ying, Z., Gomez-Pinilla, F., & Frautschy, S. A. (2009). Exercise can increase small heat shock proteins (sHSP) and pre- and postsynaptic proteins in the hippocampus. *Brain Research, 1249,* 191–201.

Kazanis, I., Giannakopoulou, M., Philippidis, H., & Stylianopoulou, F. (2004). Alterations in IGF-I, BDNF and NT-3 levels following experimental brain trauma and the effect of IGF-I administration. *Experimental Neurology, 186*(2), 221–234.

Kernie, S. G., Liebl, D. J., & Parada, L. F. (2000). BDNF regulates eating behavior and locomotor activity in mice. *EMBO Journal, 19*(6), 1290–1300.

Kitamura, T., Mishina, M., & Sugiyama, H. (2003). Enhancement of neurogenesis by running wheel exercise is suppressed in mice lacking NMDA receptor (1 subunit). *Neuroscience Research, 47*(1), 55–63.

Kitamura, T., Mishina, M., & Sugiyama, H. (2006). Dietary restriction increases hippocampal eurogenesis by molecular mechanisms independent of NMDA receptors. *Neuroscience Letters, 393*(2–3), 94–96.

Kitamura, T., & Sugiyama, H. (2006). Running wheel exercises accelerate neuronal turnover in mouse dentate gyrus. *Neuroscience Research, 56*(1), 45–52.

Klok, M. D., Jakobsdottir, S., & Drent, M. L. (2007). The role of leptin and ghrelin in the regulation of food intake and body weight in humans: A review. *Obesity Reviews, 8*(1), 21–34.

Kobayashi, K., Ikeda, Y., & Suzuki, H. (2006). Locomotor activity correlates with modifications of hippocampal mossy fibre synaptic transmission. *European Journal of Neuroscience, 24*(7), 1867–1873.

Krishnan, V., & Nestler, E. J. (2008). The molecular neurobiology of depression. *Nature, 455*(7215), 894–902.

Lebrun, B., Bariohay, B., Moyse, E., & Jean, A. (2006). Brain-derived neurotrophic factor (BDNF) and food intake regulation: A minireview. *Autonomic Neuroscience: Basic and Clinical, 126*(127), 30–38.

Lee, A. L., Ogle, W. O., & Sapolsky, R. M. (2002). Stress and depression: Possible links to neuronal death in the hippocampus. *Bipolar Disorders, 4*(2), 117–128.

Leggio, M. G., Mandolesi, L., Federico, F., Spirito, F., Ricci, B., Gelfo, F., & Petrosini L. (2005). Environmental enrichment promotes improved spatial abilities and enhanced dendritic growth in the rat. *Behavioural Brain Research, 163*(1), 78–90.

Li, X. C., Jarvis, E. D., Alvarez-Borda, B., Lim, D. A., & Nottebohm F. (2000). A relationship between behavior, neurotrophin expression, and new neuron survival. *Proceedings of the National Academy of Sciences, USA, 97*(15), 8584–8589.

Li, Y., Luikart, B. W., Birnbaum, S., Chen, J., Kwon, C-H., Kernie, S. G., . . . Parada, L. F. (2008). TrkB regulates hippocampal neurogenesis and governs sensitivity to antidepressive treatment. *Neuron, 59*(3), 399–412.

Lonart, G., & Johnson, K. M. (1995). Characterization of nitric oxide generator-induced hippocampal [3H]norepinephrine release. I. The role of glutamate. *Journal of Pharmacology and Experimental Therapeutics, 275*(1), 7–13.

Lonart, G., Wang, J., & Johnson, K. M. (1992). Nitric oxide induces neurotransmitter release from hippocampal slices. *European Journal of Pharmacology, 220*(2–3), 271–272.

Lou, S. J., Liu, J. Y., Chang, H., & Chen, P. J. (2008). Hippocampal neurogenesis and gene expression depend on exercise intensity in juvenile rats. *Brain Research, 1210*, 48–55.

Lucassen, P. J., Meerlo, P., Naylor, A. S., van Dam, A. M., Dayer, A. G., Fuchs, E., . . . Czéh, B. (2010). Regulation of adult neurogenesis by stress, sleep disruption, exercise and inflammation: Implications for depression and antidepressant action. *European Neuropsychopharmacology, 20*(1), 1–17.

Lucki, I., & O'Leary, O. F. (2004). Distinguishing roles for norepinephrine and serotonin in the behavioral effects of antidepressant drugs. *Journal of Clinical Psychiatry, 65*(Suppl 4), 11–24.

MacQueen, G. M., Campbell, S., McEwens, B. S., Macdonald, K., Amano, S., Joffe, J. T., . . . Young, L. T. (2003). Course of illness, hippocampal function, and hippocampal volume in major depression. *Proceedings of the National Academy of Sciences, USA, 100*(3), 1387–1392.

Mainardi, M., Scabia, G., Vottari, T., Santini, F., Pinchera, A., Maffei, L., . . . Maffei, M. (2010). A sensitive period for environmental regulation of eating behavior and leptin sensitivity. *Proceedings of the National Academy of Sciences, USA, 107*(38), 16673–16678.

Manium, J., & Morris, M. J. (2010). Voluntary exercise and palatable high-fat diet both improve behavioral profile and stress responses in male rats exposed to early life stress: Role of hippocampus. *Psychoneuroendocrinology, 35*(10), 1553–1564.

Manji, H. K., Quiroz, J. A., Sporn, J., Payne, J. L., Denicoff, K., Gray, N. A., . . . Charney, D. S. (2003). Enhancing neuronal plasticity and cellular resistance to develop novel, improved therapeutics for difficult-to-treat depression. *Biological Psychiatry, 53*(8), 707–742.

Marais, L., Stein, D. J., & Daniels, M. M. U. (2009). Exercise increases BDNF levels in the striatum and decreases depressive-like behavior in chronically stressed rats. *Metabolic Brain Disease, 24*(4), 587–597.

Mata, J., Thompson, R. J., & Gotlib, I. H. (2010). BDNF genotype moderates the relation between physical activity and depressive symptoms. *Health Psychology, 29*(2), 130–133.

Matsuzaki, H., Namikawa, K., Kiyama, H., Mori, N., & Sato, K. (2004). Brain-derived neurotrophic factor rescues neuronal death induced by methamphetamine. *Biological Psychiatry, 55*(1), 52–60.

Mattson, M. P. (2000). Neuroprotective signaling and the aging brain: Take away my food and let me run. *Brain Research, 886*(1–2), 47–53.

Mattson, M. P. (2005). Energy intake, meal frequency, and health: A neurobiological perspective. *Annual Review of Nutrition, 25*, 237–260.

Mattson, M. (2008). Glutamate and neurotrophic factors in neuronal plasticity and disease. *Annals of the New York of Academy of Sciences, 1144*, 97–112.

Mattson, M. P., Duan, W., & Gao, Z. (2003). Meal size and frequency affect neuronal plasticity and vulnerability to disease: Cellular and molecular mechanisms. *Journal of Neurochemistry, 84*(3), 417–431.

Mattson, M. P., Gleichmann, M., & Cheng A. (2008). Mitochondria in neuroplasticity and neurological disorders. *Neuron, 60*(5), 748–766.

Mattson, M. P., Maudsley, S., & Martin, B. (2004). BDNF and 5-HT: A dynamic duo in age-related neuronal plasticity and neurodegenerative disorders. *Trends in Neurosciences, 27*(10), 589–594.

Meeusen, R., & De Meirleir, K. (1995). Exercise and brain neurotransmission. *Sports Medicine, 20*(3), 160–188.

Meyer, T. E., & Habener, J. F. (1993). Cyclic adenosine 3′,5′-monophosphate response element-binding protein (CREB) and related transcription-activating deoxyribonucleic acid-binding proteins. *Endocrine Reviews, 14*, 269–290.

Montminy, M. R., Gonzalez, G. A., & Yamamoto, K. K. (1990). Regulation of cAMP-inducible genes by CREB. *Trends in Neurosciences, 13*(5), 184–188.

Morishima, M., Harada, N., Hara, S., Sano, A., Seno, H., Takahashi, A., . . . Nakaya, Y. (2006). Monoamine oxidase A activity and norepinephrine level in hippocampus determine hyperwheel running in SPORTS rats. *Neuropsychopharmacology, 31*(12), 2627–2638.

Nestler, E. J., & Carlezon, W. A. Jr. (2006). The mesolimbic dopamine reward circuit in depression. *Biological Psychiatry, 59*(12), 1151–1159.

Newsholme, E. A., & Blomstrand, E. (2006). Branched-chain amino acids and central fatigue. *Journal of Nutrition, 136*(1 Supplement), 274S–276S.

Noble, E. E., Billington, C. J., Kotz, C. M., & Wang, C. F. (2011). The lighter side of BDNF. *American Journal of Physiology – Regulatory, Integrative and Comparative Physiology, 300*(5), R1053–R1069.

Park, H. R., Park, M., Choi, J., Park, K. Y., Chung, H. Y., & Lee, J. (2010). A high-fat diet impairs neurogenesis: Involvement of lipid peroxidation and brain-derived neurotrophic factor. *Neuroscience Letters, 482*(3), 235–239.

Pedersen, B. K., Pedersen, M., Krabbe, K. S., Bruunsgaard, H., Matthews, V. B., & Febbraio, M. A. (2009). Role of exercise-induced brain-derived neurotrophic factor production in the regulation of energy homeostasis in mammals. *Experimental Physiology, 94*(12), 1153–1160.

Pereira, A. C., Huddleston, D. E., Brickman, A. M., Sosunov, A. A., Hen, R., McKhann, G. M., . . . Small, S. A. (2007). An in vivo correlate of exercise-induced neurogenesis in the adult dentate gyrus. *Proceedings of the National Academy of Sciences, USA, 104*(13), 5638–5643.

Peters, A., Schweiger, U., Pellerin, L., Hubold, C., Oltmanns, K. M., Conrad, M., . . . Fehm, H, L. (2004). The selfish brain: Competition for energy resources. *Neuroscience and Biobehavior Reviews, 28*(2), 143–180.

Popoli, M., Gennarelli, M., & Racagni, G. (2002). Modulation of synaptic plasticity by stress and antidepressants. *Bipolar Disorders, 4*(3), 166–182.

Pytliak, M., Vargová, V., Mechírová, V., & Felsöci, M. (2011). Serotonin receptors: From molecular biology to clinical applications. *Physiological Research, 60*(1), 15–25.

Radák, Z., Chung, H. Y., & Goto, S. (2008). Systemic adaptation to oxidative challenge induced by regular exercise. *Free Radical Biology & Medicine, 44*(2), 153–159.

Radák, Z., Kaneko, T., Tahara, S., Nakamoto, H., Puscok, J., Sasvári, M., . . . Goto, S. (2001). Regular exercise improves cognitive function and decreases oxidative damage in rat brain. *Neurochemistry International, 38*(1), 17–23.

Radák, Z., Kumagai, S., Taylor, A. W., Naito, H., & Goto, S. (2007). Effects of exercise on brain function: Role of free radicals. *Applied Physiology, Nutrition, and Metabolism, 32*(5), 942–947.

Real, C., Ferreira, A. F. B., Hernandes, M. S., Britto, L. R. G., & Pires, R. S. (2010). Exercise-induced plasticity of AMPA-type glutamate receptor subunits in the rat brain. *Brain Research, 1363*, 63–71.

Redila, V. A., & Christie, B. R. (2006). Exercise-induced changes in dendritic structure and complexity in the adult hippocampal dentate gyrus. *Neuroscience, 137*(4), 1299–1307.

Ressler, K. J., & Nemeroff, C. B. (1999). Role of norepinephrine in the pathophysiology and treatment of mood disorders. *Biological Psychiatry, 46*(9), 1219–1233.

Richter-Levine, G., Canevari, L., & Bliss, T. V. (1998). Spatial training and high-frequency stimulation engage a common pathway to enhance glutamate release in the hippocampus. *Learning and Memory, 4*(6), 445–450.

Roberts, R. E., Deleger, S., Strawbridge, W. J., & Kaplan, G. A. (2003). Prospective association between obesity and depression: Evidence from the Alameda County Study. *International Journal of Obesity, 27*(4), 514–521.

Russo-Neustadt, A. A., & Chen, M. J. (2005). Brain-derived neurotrophic factor and antidepressant activity. *Current Pharmaceutical Design, 11*(12), 1495–1510.

Russo-Neustadt, A. A., Ha, T., Ramirez, R., & Kesslak, J. P. (2001). Physical activity-antidepressant treatment combination: Impact on brain-derived neurotrophic factor and behavior in an animal model. *Behavioural Brain Research, 120*(1), 87–95.

Sartori, C. R., Vieira, A. S., Ferrari, E. M., Langone, F., Tongiorgi, E., & Parada, C. A. (2011). The antidepressive effect of the physical exercise correlates with increased levels of mature BDNF, and proBDNF proteolytic cleavage-related genes, p11 and tPA. *Neuroscience, 180*, 9–18.

Schabitz, W. R., Schwab, S., Spranger, M., & Hacke, W. (1997). Intraventricular brain-derived neurotrophic factor reduces infarct size after focal cerebral ischemia in rats. *Journal of Cerebral Blood Flow and Metabolism, 17*(5), 500–506.

Schabitz, W. R., Sommer, C., Zoder, W., Kiessling, M., Schwaninger, M., & Schwab, S. (2000). Intravenous brain-derived neurotrophic factor reduces infarct size and counterregulates Bax and Bcl-2 expression after temporary focal cerebral ischemia. *Stroke, 31*(9), 2212–2217.

Siefert, T., Brassard, P., Wissenberg, M., Rasmussen, P., Nordby, P., Stallknecht, B., . . . Secher, N. H. (2010). Endurance training enhances BDNF release from the human brain. *Journal of Physiology – Regulatory, Integrative and Comparative Physiology, 298*(2), R372–R377.

Snyder, J. S., Glover, L. R., Sanzone, K. M., Kamhi, J. F., & Cameron, H. A. (2009). The effects of exercise and stress on the survival and maturation of adult-generated granule cells. *Hippocampus, 19*(10), 898–906.

Soya, H., Nakamura, T., Deocaris, C. C., Kimpara, A., Iimura, M., Fujikawa, T., . . . Nishijima, T. (2007). BDNF induction with mild exercise in the rat hippocampus. *Biochemical Biophysical Research Communications, 358*(4), 961–967.

Stanford, C. (2001) Depression. In R. A. Webster (Ed.), *Neurotransmitters, Drugs and Brain Function* (pp. 425–452). Chichester: Wiley.

Stockmeier, C. A., Mahajan, G. J., Konick, L. C., Overholser, J. C., Jurjus, G. J., Meltzer, H. Y., . . . Rajkowska, G. (2004). Cellular changes in the postmortem hippocampus in major depression. *Biological Psychiatry, 56*(9), 640–650.

Stone, E. A., & Quartermain, D. (1999). Alpha-1-noradrenergic neurotransmission, corticosterone, and behavioral depression. *Biological Psychiatry, 46*(9), 1287–1300.

Stone, E. A., Quartermain, D., Lin, Y., & Lehmann, M. L. (2007). Central α1-adrenergic system in behavioral activity and depression. *Biochemical Pharmacology, 73*(8), 1063–1075.

Stout, A. K., & Woodward, J. J. (1994). Differential effects of nitric oxide gas and nitric oxide donors on depolarization-induced release of [3H]norepinephrine from rat hippocampal slices. *Neuropharmacology, 33*(11), 1367–1374.

Stranahan, A. M., Khalil, D., & Gould, E. (2007). Running induces widespread structural alterations in the hippocampus and entorhinal cortex. *Hippocampus, 17*(11), 1017–1022.

Ströhle, A. (2009). Physical activity, exercise, depression and anxiety disorders. *Journal of Neural Transmission, 116*(6), 777–784.

Tae, W. S., Kim, S. S., Lee, K. U., Nam, E. C., Choi, J. W., & Park, J. I. (2011). Hippocampal shape deformation in female patients with unremitting major depressive disorder. *American Journal of Neuroradiology, 32*(4), 671–676.

Thakker-Varia, S., & Adler, J. (2009). Neuropeptides in depression: Role of VGF. *Behavioural Brain Research, 197*(2), 262–278.

Toscano-Silva, M., da Silva, S. G., Scorza, F. A., Bonvent, J. J., Cavalheiro, E. A., & Arida, R. M. (2010). Hippocampal mossy fiber sprouting induced by forced and voluntary physical exercise. *Physiology and Behavior, 101*(2), 302–308.

Unger, T. J., Calderon, G. A., Bradley, L. C., Sena-Esteves, M., & Rios, M. (2007). Selective deletion of BDNF in the ventromedial and dorsomedial hypothalamus of adult mice results in hyperphagic behavior and obesity. *Journal of Neuroscience, 27*(52), 14265–14274.

Uno, H., Ross, T., Else, J., Suleman, M., & Sapolsky, R. (1989). Hippocampal damage associated with prolonged and fatal stress in primates. *Journal of Neuroscience, 9*(5), 1705–1711.

Van Praag, H., Barlow, C., & Gage, F. H. (2001). Are drug targets missed owing to lack of physical activity? *Drug Discovery Today, 6*(12), 615–617.

Vaynman, S., Ying, Z., Yin, D., & Gomez-Pinilla, F. (2006). Exercise differentially regulates synaptic proteins associated to the function of BDNF. *Brain Research, 1070*(1), 124–130.

Wang, C. F., Godar, R. J., Billington, C. J., & Kotz, C. M. (2010). Chronic administration of brain-derived neurotrophic factor in the hypothalamic paraventricular nucleus reverses obesity induced by high-fat diet. *Journal of Physiology – Regulatory, Integrative, and Comparative Physiology, 298*(5), R1320–R1332.

Widenfalk, J., Olson, L., & Thorén, P. (1999). Deprived of habitual running, rats downregulate BDNF and TrkB messages in the brain. *Neuroscience Research, 34*(3), 125–132.

Wu, A., Molteni, R., Ying, Z., & Gomez-Pinilla, F. (2003). A saturated-fat diet aggravates the outcome of traumatic brain injury on hippocampal plasticity and cognitive function by reducing brain-derived neurotrophic factor. *Neuroscience, 119*(2), 365–375.

Würbel, H. (2001). Ideal homes? Housing effects on rodent brain and behaviour. *Trends in Neurosciences, 24*(4), 207–211.

Wurtman, J. J. (1993). Depression and weight gain: The serotonin connection. *Journal of Affective Disorders, 29*(2–3), 183–192.

Xiao, L., Feng, C., & Chen, Y. (2010). Glucocorticoid rapidly enhances NMDA-evoked neurotoxicity by attenuating the NR2A-containing NMDA receptor-mediated ERK1/2 activation. *Molecular Endocrinology, 24*(3), 497–510.

Xu, B., Goulding, E. H., Zang, K., Cepoi, D., Cone, R. D., Jones, K. R., . . . Reichardt, L. F. (2003). Brain-derived neurotrophic factor regulates energy balance downstream of melanocortin-4 receptor. *Nature Neuroscience, 6*(7), 736–742.

Yamada, N., Katsuura, G., Ochi, Y., Ehihara, K., Kusakabe, T., Hosoda, K., & Nakao, K. (2011). Impaired CNS leptin action is implicated in depression associated with obesity. *Endocrinology, 152*(7), 2634–2643.

Yamashita, K., Wiessner, C., Lindholm, D., Thoenen, H., & Hossmann, K. A. (1997). Post-occlusion treatment with BDNF reduces infarct size in a model of permanent occlusion of the middle cerebral artery in rat. *Metabolic Brain Disease, 12*(4), 271–280.

Young, S. N. (2007). How to increase serotonin in the brain without drugs. *Journal of Psychiatry & Neuroscience, 32*(6), 394–399.

Zhang, Y., & Pardridge, W. M. (2001). Neuroprotection in transient focal brain ischemia after delayed intravenous administration of brain-derived neurotrophic factor conjugated to a blood–brain barrier drug targeting system. *Stroke, 32*(6), 1378–1384.

Zheng, H., Liu, Y., Li, W., Yang, B., Chen, D., Wang, X., . . . Halberg, F. (2006). Beneficial effects of exercise and its molecular mechanisms on depression in rats. *Behavioral Brain Research, 168*(1), 47–55.

Zoladz, J. A., & Pilc, A. (2010). The effect of physical activity on brain-derived neurotrophic factor: From animal to human studies. *Journal of Physiology and Pharmacology*, 61(5), 533–541.

PART 4

Self-perceptions and self-evaluations

Edited by
Kathleen A. Martin Ginis

11

PHYSICAL ACTIVITY AND SELF-PERCEPTIONS AMONG CHILDREN AND ADOLESCENTS

Lindsay E. Kipp and Maureen R. Weiss

Physical activity has the potential to enhance children's and adolescents' mental health and overall well-being (Smith & Biddle, 2008; Weiss, 2004). One important aspect of well-being is positive self-perceptions, or favorable beliefs about oneself and one's abilities (Horn, 2004). Positive self-perceptions are associated with adaptive cognitive, affective, and behavioral outcomes, such as enjoyment, self-determined motivation, and physical activity (Crocker, Kowalski, & Hadd, 2008). It is important to understand the underlying mechanisms for improving self-perceptions and physical activity levels because this knowledge can help researchers and practitioners envision interventions to simultaneously promote both outcomes among youth.

We conceptualize physical activity within structured settings, such as organized programs, school physical education, and out–of–school–time sports, which have been primary contexts in which self-perceptions have been studied. We highlight structured physical activities because they maximize opportunities for skill mastery and positive interactions with significant others, which can foster enhanced self-perceptions. Physical activity is thus inclusive of variations in frequency, intensity, duration, and type found in structured school and out–of–school–time programs.

We discuss knowledge about and implications for promoting self-perceptions and physical activity for youth. First, we review theoretical approaches for understanding the significance of self-perceptions. Second, we synthesize robust research findings on the linkage between physical activity and self-perceptions, including correlational, longitudinal, and intervention studies. Finally, we conclude with limitations of current research and recommendations for future studies on the self-perception/physical activity link.

Definitions and terminology

Numerous terms and types of self-perceptions have been specified in the physical activity literature (Horn, 2004). Self-perceptions and self-concept will be used interchangeably and refer to one's judgments, evaluations, and beliefs about oneself. Self-perceptions can take on global, domain-specific, and situation-specific forms. At the broadest level, self-esteem or self-worth refers to evaluations of one's significance or value as a person. Self-esteem is multidimensional in that perceptions of ability in different domains (e.g., academic, physical, social) contribute to overall self-esteem (Fox, 1997; Harter, 1999). However, self-esteem is not simply an aggregate of one's perceived abilities; starting around age 8 children begin to form global self-evaluations independent of domain-specific judgments (Harter, 1999).

At a domain-specific level, perceived competence is one's evaluation of his or her *ability* in a particular domain (e.g., physical, academic) or subdomain (e.g., soccer, math) (Harter, 1999; Horn, 2004). Perceptions of competence in domains that are developmentally relevant and personally important contribute to one's global self-esteem. For example, perceived physical competence and physical appearance are consistently related to cognitive, affective, and behavioral outcomes among youth (Weiss, Amorose, & Kipp, 2012).

Extending Harter's (1985, 1988) construct of perceived *physical* competence, Fox (1997) customized the construct *physical self-worth*, defined as evaluation of one's physical self. Physical self-worth is the overarching construct and is made up of perceived athletic competence, physical appearance, physical strength, and physical conditioning. The significance of this approach is in deconstructing global self-worth (physical self-worth) and perceived physical competence (athletic, appearance, strength, conditioning) to refined ways of investigating physical activity as a context for promoting self-perceptions.

At the most specific level, self-efficacy is a situational form of confidence or belief that one can successfully complete a task (Bandura, 1986). For example, *self-efficacy to be active* and *self-efficacy to overcome barriers to being active* have been typical ways of assessing youths' self-perceptions (e.g., Motl, Dishman, Saunders, Dowda, & Pate, 2007; Motl et al., 2005).

Theoretical perspectives for understanding self-perceptions among children and adolescents in the physical domain

We briefly review social–cognitive theories and other conceptual approaches that are useful for describing and explaining the relationship between youth physical activity and self-perceptions.

Model of global self-worth

Harter's (1987, 1999) model of global self-worth provides a developmental framework for understanding antecedents and consequences of self-esteem. Antecedents include perceived competence and perceived social regard (e.g., reflected appraisals by significant others), whereas consequences include affect and motivation. In the physical domain, significant others such as parents, coaches, and teammates can impact youths' self-perceptions that, in turn, influence emotional responses and motivation for physical activity.

Harter's (1987, 1999) model considers changes in the structure, content, and processes of self-judgments from early childhood through adolescence (Harter, 1999; Horn, 2004). First, the number and type of competence subdomains vary over the childhood years. During early childhood (ages 4–7), children evaluate themselves in five subdomains (cognitive, physical, social, appearance, behavior), but these are not clearly differentiated. Young children have not yet constructed a sense of global self-worth because they do not have the cognitive capacity to integrate domain-specific abilities into a broad perception. As youth move into middle to late childhood (ages 8–11), they differentiate the five competence subdomains as well as a sense of global self-worth. Adolescence (ages 12–18) is a time of increasing cognitive maturity and further differentiation of three new competence subdomains: job, close friendships, and romantic relationships.

Second, developmental differences in cognitive processes involve changes in sources of competence information (Horn, 2004; Horn & Amorose, 1998). Younger children rely on simple task accomplishment, effort, and feedback from significant adults to judge their physical abilities, whereas youth in middle to late childhood use additional sources like performance outcome, peer comparison, and skill improvement. Adolescents experience greater differentiation of information sources (e.g., delineation of feedback from others) and use self-referenced sources more frequently (e.g., improvement, enjoyment) than those who are younger.

Third, the social environment also contributes strongly to judgments about the self (Horn, 2004; Weiss, Bhalla, & Price, 2008). During early and middle childhood, parents are a predominant source of competence information. In late childhood and adolescence, teachers, coaches, and peers are used more frequently as credible sources, and youth may place more emphasis on outperforming others and social comparison. This shift in emphasis helps explain youths' increasing use of norm-referenced criteria to judge their ability as they get older. However, older adolescents are able to integrate multiple sources, which should facilitate positive self-perceptions (e.g., Horn, Glenn, & Wentzell, 1993; Weiss & Amorose, 2005). Thus, significant others who emphasize multiple sources for judging physical ability (e.g., effort and improvement in addition to social comparison) should contribute to adaptive competence beliefs.

Social cognitive theory

Bandura's (1986) social cognitive theory has been useful for understanding self-perceptions and physical activity behavior among youth (Ward, Saunders, & Pate, 2007). According to this theory, characteristics of the person (notably self-efficacy), their environment, and their behavior influence one another reciprocally. Physical activity can be explained by personal characteristics like self-efficacy to be active, environmental characteristics like social support from teachers and peers, and behavioral characteristics like goal-setting and self-regulation skills. In turn, being active can affect personal, environmental, and behavioral characteristics (e.g., regular physical activity can improve self-efficacy for future activity).

Positive youth development

The positive youth development framework (PYD) focuses on promoting potential in children and adolescents, with a focus on external assets (social-environmental enablers) and internal assets (social, psychological, and physical competencies) (Eccles & Gootman, 2002; Lerner, Almerigi, Theokas, & Lerner, 2005). Internal assets include self-perceptions (global self-esteem, perceived competence, self-efficacy) and physical abilities and health (activity level, fitness, motor skills). Although conceived within mainstream psychology that emphasizes school and family contexts, researchers have customized the PYD framework in *physical activity contexts* (Weiss, 2008; Weiss & Wiese-Bjornstal, 2009). School physical education and after-school sport programs connote settings in which caring and knowledgeable adults can nurture physical and psychosocial assets.

Prevention science

Prevention science is an interdisciplinary approach focused on preventing unhealthy, maladaptive behaviors and promoting healthy, adaptive outcomes, including self-perceptions and physical activity (Coie et al., 1993; O'Connell, Boat, & Warner, 2009). Scholars have shifted away from the traditional disease model to one that includes prevention *and* promotion. Prevention science emphasizes holistic health, or the idea that mental and physical health are inseparable. Youth who are regularly active should experience greater perceived competence and self-esteem, and youth who display positive self-perceptions should be more active (e.g., Fredricks & Eccles, 2005). Prevention science and PYD are useful approaches to the problem of declining physical activity levels because interventions can help prevent sedentary behavior while at the same time promoting physical activity and positive self-perceptions. Conceptual approaches described have served as the basis for research on self-perceptions and physical activity among youth.

Research on physical activity and self-perceptions among children and adolescents

To make sense of research findings, this section is divided into correlational, longitudinal, and intervention studies. Correlational studies reinforce positive associations between physical activity and self-perceptions but do not specify directional influence. Longitudinal studies provide insight into the temporal ordering of self-perceptions and physical activity, and intervention studies have been conducted to determine whether structured physical activity can promote self-perceptions and other outcomes.

Correlational research

Studies support meaningful relationships between global and physical self-evaluations and physical activity for youth ages 10–17 (Fridlund Dunton, Atienza, Tscherme, & Rodriguez, 2006; Smith, 1999; Tremblay, Inman, & Willms, 2000). For example, Fridlund Dunton et al. assessed relationships among moderate and vigorous physical activity (measured by self-report), physical fitness (measured by oxygen consumption), and specific and global self-perceptions among female adolescents. Physical fitness was more strongly related to physical self-worth and self-esteem than was physical activity level. They concluded that physical activity might impact global self-perceptions through improvements in fitness, so interventions should include activities that improve fitness levels.

A number of studies support perceived competence as a correlate of physical activity for youth ages 10–18 (Crocker, Eklund, & Kowalski, 2000; Eriksson, Nordqvist, & Rasmussen, 2008; Sabiston & Crocker, 2008; Shen, McCaughtry, & Martin, 2007). For instance, Eriksson et al. found that 12-year-old children's perceived athletic competence was strongly related to their sport participation and vigorous physical activity, and partially mediated the relationship between parent and child physical activity levels. When parents were more active, children reported greater perceived competence and physical activity.

Several studies have examined the relationship between self-efficacy and physical activity. For youth ages 10–18, self-efficacy to be active and self-efficacy to overcome activity barriers are significant correlates of activity level (Martin, McCaughtry, Flory, Murphy, & Wisdom, 2011; Motl et al., 2007; Spence et al., 2010). For example, Spence and colleagues found that self-efficacy to be active was significantly related to physical activity for grade 7–10 boys and girls. When youth felt confident about their ability to be active, they engaged in physical activity more frequently.

Cross-sectional studies show consistent relationships between self-perceptions and physical activity, but the mechanisms of influence are not transparent. As we saw from theories discussed earlier, significant others strongly influence youths' self-perceptions and physical activity motivation and behavior. Several studies examined parental beliefs and behaviors (e.g., Davison, Symons Downs, & Birch, 2006), peer influence (e.g., Smith, 1999), and coach/teacher behaviors (e.g., Weiss, Amorose, & Wilko, 2009) in relation to self-perceptions and physical activity. Youths' perceptions of parent, peer, coach, and teacher behaviors are related to perceptions of competence, self-worth, and physical activity behavior. For example, Smith found that, among 12- to 15-year-old students, perceptions of peer acceptance were associated with greater physical self-worth, positive affect, intrinsic motivation, and physical activity. Sabiston and Crocker (2008) found that perceived physical competence mediated the relationship between parent and peer influence with self-reported physical activity level among 15- to 18-year-olds.

Longitudinal research

It is important to determine direction of causality to identify interventions for improving self-perceptions and physical activity levels. Among girls, perceived physical competence and self-esteem tend to decline starting in early adolescence (Horn, 2004). Both girls and boys show a decrease in physical activity throughout adolescence, with girls consistently at lower levels than boys (Findlay, Garner, & Kohen, 2009; Pate et al., 2009). Thus, understanding factors that promote self-perceptions and physical activity is key for maximizing mental and physical well-being.

Some studies have not supported *global self-perceptions* as a predictor of physical activity (e.g., Crocker, Sabiston, Kowalski, McDonough, & Kowalski, 2006; Crocker et al., 2003; Inchley, Kirby, & Currie, 2011), but *domain-specific self-perceptions* are consistent predictors of activity level. Inchley and colleagues conducted a 5-year longitudinal study with youth ages 11–15. For boys, baseline activity and perceived competence increased the odds of being active at 2 and 4 years later. For girls, baseline activity, perceived competence, exercise self-efficacy, and physical self-worth increased the odds of being active 2 years later, and exercise self-efficacy and physical self-worth increased the odds of being active 4 years later. Youth who reported greater physical self-perceptions were more likely to engage in physical activity over time.

Some researchers have explored direction of causality between self-perceptions and physical activity by testing multiple models (Schmalz, Deane, Birch, & Davison, 2007; Trautwein, Gerlach, & Lüdtke, 2008). Schmalz and colleagues studied physical activity and self-esteem with girls at age 9, 11, and 13. Higher physical activity at ages 9 and 11 predicted higher self-esteem at ages 11 and 13. Trautwein et al. showed support for bidirectional relationships with 8- to 10-year-olds: perceived competence predicted physical activity, *and* physical activity predicted perceived competence 15 months later. Discrepant findings of these studies may be due to differing measurement periods, age groups, self-construct, and mode of assessing physical activity. It could be that domain-specific self-perceptions predict physical activity, and physical activity has long-term effects on youths' global self-esteem.

Longitudinal studies have shown that perceived competence is a predictor of physical activity (Baker & Davison, 2011; Crocker et al., 2003, 2006; Fridlund Dunton et al., 2011). Fridlund Dunton et al. assessed physical activity and global and domain-specific self-perceptions of 10th-grade girls two times, one year apart. Physical activity in 11th grade was highest for participants who were active and had higher perceived sport competence in 10th grade. Crocker et al. (2006) assessed physical activity, physical self-perceptions, and global self-esteem over a 24-month period with adolescent girls, and found that perceived physical conditioning was the only self-perception predicting change in physical activity.

Other longitudinal studies show support for self-efficacy as a predictor of physical activity level (Dishman, Saunders, Motl, Dowda, & Pate, 2009; Motl et al., 2005). Dishman et al. found that self-efficacy moderated the relationship between social support and physical activity for girls in 8th, 9th, and 12th grades. Girls who reported higher self-efficacy and social support showed less of a decline in physical activity compared to girls with higher self-efficacy and lower social support.

Intervention research

Theories discussed earlier inform age-appropriate interventions to promote self-perceptions and physical activity. Experimental designs in which an intervention is introduced and outcomes are evaluated reveal mechanisms involved in promoting health and well-being.

School-based physical activity

Interventions have been implemented in school physical education using several mechanisms to effect change in youths' self-perceptions. Researchers have been successful at promoting social support, self-efficacy, enjoyment, and physical activity (Dishman et al., 2005; Neumark-Sztainer, Story, Hannan, & Rex, 2003; Pate et al., 2005; Taymoori & Lubans, 2008). Based on social cognitive theory, the Lifestyle Education for Activity Project (LEAP) was an intervention to enhance self-efficacy and enjoyment, teach physical and behavioral skills to adopt a healthy lifestyle, and promote adolescent girls' moderate-to-vigorous physical activity (Dishman et al., 2005; Pate et al., 2005; Ward et al., 2006). These goals were accomplished through changes in the school environment, such as providing girls-only classes, providing choice in activities, encouraging social interactions, promoting lifelong activities, and providing activity opportunities in the community. Intervention schools also provided health education, staff health promotion, and family involvement. LEAP was effective in increasing participants' moderate-to-vigorous activity both in and out of physical education class (Pate et al., 2005) and revealed that self-efficacy, enjoyment, and social support are important mechanisms for increasing activity levels (Dishman et al., 2005). LEAP studies provide evidence that a theory-driven intervention, including a deliberate curriculum and trained teachers, can increase youths' self-efficacy to be active and their physical activity behavior.

Another approach to promoting self-perceptions in schools has been cooperative and team-building interventions in physical education classes (Ebbeck & Gibbons, 1998; Gibbons, Ebbeck, Concepcion, & Li, 2010; Marsh & Peart, 1988). Ebbeck and Gibbons trained middle school teachers to implement physical challenges using a cooperative-style approach with their students over 8 months. Teachers implemented activities that challenged youth to devise strategies to complete each task (e.g., helping all group members climb through an obstacle course) and reflect on group involvement. At postintervention, boys and girls in the experimental group were significantly higher on global self-worth and perceptions of athletic competence, physical appearance, and social acceptance than the control group (who participated in regular physical education activities). Gibbons et al. conducted a follow-up study with the same team-building curriculum with middle school boys and girls. The experimental group was higher in global self-worth and perceived academic competence, social acceptance, athletic competence, and behavioral conduct compared to the control group. Thus, a team-building intervention that featured positive peer interactions and group interdependence to achieve collaborative goals was successful in enhancing global and domain-specific self-evaluations.

Interventions for preschool and kindergarten children have been effective at promoting physical self-perceptions (Robinson, 2011; Robinson, Rudisill, & Goodway, 2009; Valentini & Rudisill, 2004). Robinson et al. examined the effect of instructional style during a 9-week motor skill program on preschoolers' perceived physical competence. At-risk participants (e.g, single-parent household, poverty, parental unemployment) were randomly assigned to a mastery climate, low-autonomy, or comparison group. Children in the mastery climate group were afforded experiences to explore multiple tasks, choose activities and group members, assume leadership roles, and be evaluated on effort and improvement rather than norm-referenced criteria. The low-autonomy group experienced less variety in tasks, no choice in selecting tasks or group members, no leadership opportunities, and evaluation based on performance outcome. The comparison group engaged in unstructured free play. The mastery climate group significantly improved in perceived competence from pre- to posttest, had higher perceived competence than the low-autonomy and control group at posttest, and retained their improvement 9 weeks later. The low-autonomy and comparison groups showed no significant improvements.

School-based interventions have also focused on optimally challenging and enjoyable physical activities to promote global self-evaluations (Petty, Davis, Tkacz, Young-Hyman, & Waller, 2009; Schneider, Fridlund Dunton, & Cooper, 2008). In a randomized controlled trial, Petty and colleagues tested dose-response effects of a 3-month physical activity program with overweight, sedentary Black and White children ages 7–11 years. During the school day, youth participated in either no activity (control), 20 minutes (low-dose), or 40 minutes (high-dose) of physical activity. Activities were chosen based on their ability to elicit a heart rate of at least 150 beats per minute (e.g., running games, jump rope, basketball). Results revealed a race-by-group interaction where only White children's global self-worth improved with increased activity dosage. The authors suggested that, for Black children, the relation between self-worth and obesity may not be as strong—race may be a protective factor over weight-related self-worth. In sum, physical activity interventions in schools have successfully promoted global and domain-specific self-perceptions through mechanisms such as teacher support, a mastery motivational climate, opportunities for skill building, cooperation and team building, and engaging in enjoyable, physically intense activities.

Out-of-school-time physical activity

Programs outside school provide unique settings in which to promote self-evaluations and physical activity behavior. One approach to promoting self-esteem and perceived competence has been training coaches to provide appropriate reinforcement and feedback and then assessing change in participants' psychosocial outcomes over the course of a season (e.g., Barnett, Smoll, & Smith, 1992; Smoll, Smith, Barnett, & Everett, 1993). Smoll and colleagues employed a coach-training intervention with boys' baseball coaches designed to emphasize (a) reinforcement for good performances and effort, (b) mistake-contingent encouragement, and (c) corrective and technical instruction given in a non-judgmental way. Coaches were also encouraged to avoid or minimize using punitive instruction. At the end of the season, boys who played for the trained coaches and started the season with low self-esteem showed significant increases in self-esteem, while those in the control group did not. Thus, children who have the most to gain from a positive sport experience benefit greatly from having a coach who uses positive forms of instruction. In addition, players of trained coaches reported greater baseball competence, enjoyment, and liking of teammates compared to controls. These variables should relate to continued physical activity participation. Indeed, in a follow-up study 1 year later (Barnett et al.), players for the trained coaches exhibited a lower attrition rate than players in the control group (5% versus 26%).

Positive self-perceptions also result when coaches and instructors emphasize a mastery motivational climate and demonstrate autonomy-supportive behaviors (Coatsworth & Conroy, 2006, 2009; Theeboom, De Knop, & Weiss, 1995). Theeboom et al. randomly assigned 8–12-year-old youth to an experimental (mastery climate) or control group (traditional approach) for learning martial arts skills during 3 weeks of a summer program. The experimental group instructor highlighted effort and improvement rather than social comparison, used a variety of tasks with skill progressions rather than traditional drills, and provided participants with activity choices rather than teacher-determined drills. At postintervention, youth in the mastery climate group reported greater enjoyment and demonstrated better skills than the traditional group, and interviews indicated increased perceived competence and intrinsic motivation in connection with the intervention. The mastery motivational climate was successful in enhancing perceptions of competence, intrinsic motivation, and motor skills, which should relate to continued physical activity.

Some out-of-school-time programs have focused on promoting girls' self-perceptions and physical activity attitudes and behaviors. Girls on the Run (www.girlsontherun.org) is a 12-week physical activity-based youth development program for 8–13-year-old girls, aimed at teaching skills to lead a physically active lifestyle and achieve favorable self-perceptions. Coaches attend a two-day training to learn how to deliver the deliberate curriculum in a developmentally appropriate way. Sessions include lessons on running, other physical activities, and life skills, including psychological, social, and physical assets (e.g., positive relationships, healthy eating). Evaluation studies show significant increases from pre- to postintervention for self-esteem, physical self-perceptions, body size satisfaction, and physical activity attitudes and level (DeBate, Gabriel, Zwald, Huberty, & Zhang, 2009; DeBate & Thompson, 2005; DeBate, Zhang, & Thompson, 2007; Martin, Waldron, McCabe, & Choi, 2009).

Other out-of-school-time skill-building programs have been effective at improving self-perceptions for boys and girls (Annesi, Westcott, Faigenbaum, & Unruh, 2005; Bruening, Dover, & Clark, 2009). Taking a PYD approach, Bruening and colleagues conducted a 12-week physical activity program for pre-adolescent girls of color, incorporating a curriculum that included physical activities, life skills (e.g., resisting peer pressure), and healthy choices, and utilized social assets in the form of female college-athlete role models. At postintervention, interviews revealed that girls improved in self-esteem and knowledge and application of life skills to healthy living. This intervention improved self-perceptions and physical activity behavior among at-risk pre-adolescent girls.

Another physical activity-based youth development program, The First Tee (www.thefirsttee. org), uses golf as a vehicle to promote life skills and developmental outcomes, including positive self-perceptions and healthy behaviors. The program involves a motivating context (golf), external assets (trained coaches who teach golf and life skills using positive instructional behaviors) and internal assets (interpersonal, self-management, goal-setting skills). Weiss and colleagues evaluated the impact of The First Tee on positive youth development through a 4-year longitudinal study (Weiss, 2008; Weiss, Bhalla, Bolter, & Price, 2008; Weiss, Bolter, Bhalla, & Price, 2007; Weiss, Stuntz, Bhalla, Bolter, & Price, 2012). Survey and interview data with 10–18-year-old participants showed improved confidence in academic, physical, social, and moral domains over time, such as meeting new people and being socially responsible. In addition, youth in The First Tee compared favorably to youth in other programs on self-efficacy to resist peer pressure for high-risk behaviors and self-efficacy to regulate learning. The intentional curriculum and trained coaches using a mastery-oriented approach were contributors to positive self-perceptions and associated life skills.

In sum, out-of-school-time programs are unique settings to incorporate physical activities, life skills, health education, and instructors who communicate lessons within a mastery climate. Successful interventions in and out of schools reveal common mechanisms to improve self-perceptions and physical activity levels, and provide support for theories and non-experimental studies that suggest the powerful influence of social-environmental factors.

Recommendations for future research

Our review suggests there is much to be encouraged by—robust findings show that self-evaluations and physical activity are strongly associated. Still, limitations exist that can be considered in future studies to elevate knowledge about physical activity as a context for promoting self-perceptions. First, given the diverse ways in which "the self" is conceived—global self-worth, perceived competence, self-efficacy—researchers should carefully consider which construct is most appropriate to measure in relation to their research questions. A good example is a fitness intervention study by Marsh and Peart (1988) with adolescent girls. They hypothesized that (a) girls in the cooperative group would be superior to competitive and control groups at postintervention on perceived physical ability and physical appearance and (b) there would be no between-group differences on nonphysical self-perceptions (e.g., academic, social). Given the short duration (6 weeks) and nature of the intervention (physical fitness), identifying physical self-perceptions as the target variables, and not global self-worth or nonphysical self-perceptions, made sound conceptual sense. Thus, level of self-perception construct is an important consideration in conjunction with the research question and study design.

Choice of self-perception instrument should be developmentally appropriate (Brustad, 1998). Harter (1985, 1988) validated global and domain-specific measures of self-perceptions for children and adolescents based on extensive psychometric testing. Yet some studies modified these measures by altering item content and response format without providing validity data for modifications. Without such information, we do not know whether results can be attributed to study variables or measurement error. In addition, studies used a wide range of age groups for examining self-perceptions and physical activity. Because children and adolescents vary in cognitive, social, and physical development, researchers should provide a rationale for the specific ages they include in their study (Brustad, 1998). It is advisable to limit the age bandwidth so that findings are not confounded by cognitive and physical developmental differences. Depending on the ages included, an assessment of physical maturity (i.e., pubertal status) would control for developmental differences within chronological age and be helpful for explaining study findings (e.g., Baker & Davison, 2011; Kipp & Weiss, 2012; Smith, 1999).

Another consideration is variation in modes of assessing physical activity. Conflicting findings may have emerged across studies because different methods were used to assess activity, including accelerometers, self-report, parent report, and pedometers. Accelerometers are relatively objective and capable of quantifying movements, but the downside is that they are expensive and multiple data points are necessary to obtain valid assessments of activity level. These limitations make it a challenge to use with large samples. Self-report surveys, while accessible and conducive to large samples, are more subjective and prone to social desirability. In some studies, self-perceptions are assessed relative to participating in a physical activity-based program that is not quantified per se (e.g., yes/no response for sport participation). In the future, associations between physical activity and self-perceptions should account for how variations in frequency, intensity, duration, and type of activity are assessed and quantified.

Different data analytic methods have been used, which may contribute to variations in interpreting findings. Studies used analysis of variance, several regression techniques, structural equation modeling, multilevel modeling, and group classification methods. The data analysis should be a good "fit" to the research questions and hypotheses. For example, multilevel modeling is designed to account for dependencies among individuals' data within a group (e.g., participants within classes). This is conceptually accurate, but if there is little dependency in the data (as assessed by intraclass correlation), inadequate power due to insufficient sample size at the group level (level-2 cluster), and multiple outcome variables that should be analyzed simultaneously, then this technique may not be appropriate to accurately assess the self-perception/physical activity relationship. Researchers should remain focused on the research goal by conducting appropriate analyses that do not obscure what the data mean.

Finally, more longitudinal, intervention, and evaluation studies are needed to determine effectiveness of protocols and programs on youth self-perceptions. Such designs are capable of quantifying evidence of change, whether effects are immediate or enduring, and which mechanisms are responsible for successful outcomes. To this point, future studies must include control or comparison groups and multiple data points to establish causal effects of programs on self-perceptions and activity levels. Such designs can also untangle the proverbial chicken-and-egg question: do variations in physical activity predict change in self-perceptions or do modifications to self-perceptions translate to greater physical activity levels? Answers are important for determining which intervention components are most likely to promote physical and psychosocial well-being among youth.

Conclusion

Physical activity is important for children's and adolescents' physical and psychosocial well-being, including an active lifestyle and favorable self-perceptions. Structured settings such as school physical education and out-of-school-time sports have the potential to provide youth with opportunities to enhance self-efficacy, perceived competence, physical self-worth, and self-esteem. Heightened self-perceptions, in turn, are associated with initiating, maintaining, and enhancing physical activity frequency, duration, and intensity, which is seen in youths' choice to return to activity programs and exert sufficient effort to attain health benefits. Correlational studies provide support for relationships between self-perceptions and physical activity, whereas longitudinal and intervention studies help uncover direction of causality and mechanisms of influence. More theory-driven physical activity interventions that incorporate positive social-environmental factors and a curriculum that entails teaching life skills and healthy behaviors should continue to be conducted. Ultimately, definitive data-based evidence can reveal the power of physical activity to successfully enhance youths' sense of self and interest in embracing physical activity as a lifestyle choice.

References

Annesi, J.J., Westcott, W.L., Faigenbaum, A.D., & Unruh, J.L. (2005). Effects of a 12-week physical activity protocol delivered by YMCA after-school counselors (Youth Fit For Life) on physical and self-efficacy changes in 5–12 year-old boys and girls. *Research Quarterly for Exercise and Sport, 76*, 468–476.

Baker, B.L., & Davison, K.K. (2011). I know I can: A longitudinal examination of precursors and outcomes of perceived athletic competence among adolescent girls. *Journal of Physical Activity and Health, 8*, 192–199.

Bandura, A. (1986). *Social foundations of thought and action: A social cognitive theory.* Englewood Cliffs, NJ: Prentice-Hall, Inc.

Barnett, N.P., Smoll, F.L., & Smith, R.E. (1992). Effects of enhancing coach–athlete relationships on youth sport attrition. *The Sport Psychologist, 6*, 111–127.

Bruening, J.E., Dover, K.M., & Clark, B.S. (2009). Preadolescent female development through sport and physical activity: A case study of an urban after-school program. *Research Quarterly for Exercise and Sport, 80*, 87–101.

Brustad, R.J. (1998). Developmental considerations in sport and exercise psychology measurement. In J.L. Duda (Ed.), *Advances in sport and exercise psychology measurement* (pp. 461–470). Morgantown, WV: Fitness Information Technology.

Coatsworth, J.D., & Conroy, D.E. (2006). Enhancing self-esteem of youth swimmers through coach training: Gender and age effects. *Psychology of Sport and Exercise, 7*, 173–192.

Coatsworth, J.D., & Conroy, D.E. (2009). The effect of autonomy-supportive coaching, need satisfaction, and self-perceptions on initiative and identity in youth swimmers. *Developmental Psychology, 45*, 320–328.

Coie, J.D., Watt, N.F., West, S.G., Hawkins, J.D., Asarnow, J.R., Markman, H.J., . . . Long, B. (1993). The science of prevention: A conceptual framework and some directions for a national research program. *American Psychologist, 48*, 1013–1022.

Crocker, P.R.E., Eklund, R.C., & Kowalski, K.C. (2000). Children's physical activity and physical self-perceptions. *Journal of Sports Sciences, 18*, 383–394.

Crocker, P.R.E., Kowalski, K.C., & Hadd, V. (2008). The role of the self. In A.L. Smith & S.J.H. Biddle (Eds.), *Youth physical activity and sedentary behavior* (pp. 215–237). Champaign, IL: Human Kinetics.

Crocker, P., Sabiston, C., Forrestor, S., Kowalski, N., Kowalski, K., & McDonough, M. (2003). Predicting change in physical activity, dietary restraint, and physique anxiety in adolescent girls. *Canadian Journal of Public Health, 94*, 332–337.

Crocker, P.R.E., Sabiston, C.M., Kowalski, K.C., McDonough, M.H., & Kowalski, N. (2006). Longitudinal assessment of the relationship between physical self-concept and health-related behavior and emotion in adolescent girls. *Journal of Applied Sport Psychology, 18*, 185–200.

Davison, K.K., Symons Downs, D., & Birch, L.L. (2006). Pathways linking perceived athletic competence and parental support at age 9 years to girls' physical activity at age 11 years. *Research Quarterly for Exercise and Sport, 77*, 23–31.

DeBate, R.D., Gabriel, K.P., Zwald, M., Huberty, J., & Zhang, Y. (2009). Changes in psychosocial factors and physical activity frequency among 3rd to 8th grade girls who participated in a developmentally focused youth sport program: A preliminary study. *Journal of School Health, 79*, 478–484.

DeBate, R.D., & Thompson, S.H. (2005). Girls on the Run: Improvements in self-esteem, body size satisfaction, and eating attitudes/behaviors. *Eating and Weight Disorders, 10*, 25–32.

DeBate, R.D., Zhang, Y., & Thompson, S.H. (2007). Changes in commitment to physical activity among 8- to 11-year-old girls participating in a curriculum-based running program. *American Journal of Health Education, 38*, 277–284.

Dishman, R.K., Motl, R.W., Saunders, R., Felton, G., Ward, D.S., Dowda, M., & Pate, R.R. (2005). Enjoyment mediates effects of a school-based physical-activity intervention. *Medicine & Science in Sports & Exercise, 37*, 478–487.

Dishman, R.K., Saunders, R.P., Motl, R.W., Dowda, M., & Pate, R.R. (2009). Self-efficacy moderates the relation between declines in physical activity and perceived social support in high school girls. *Journal of Pediatric Psychology, 34*, 441–451.

Ebbeck, V., & Gibbons, S.L. (1998). The effect of a team building program on the self-conceptions of grade 6 and 7 physical education students. *Journal of Sport & Exercise Psychology, 20*, 300–310.

Eccles, J.S., & Gootman, J.A. (2002). Features of positive developmental settings. In J.S. Eccles & J.A. Gootman (Eds.), *Community programs to promote youth development* (pp. 86–118). Washington, DC: National Academy Press.

Eriksson, M., Nordqvist, T., & Rasmussen, F. (2008). Associations between parents' and 12-year-old children's sport and vigorous activity: The role of self-esteem and athletic competence. *Journal of Physical Activity and Health, 5*, 359–373.

Findlay, L.C., Garner, R.E., & Kohen, D.E. (2009). Children's organized physical activity patterns from childhood to adolescence. *Journal of Physical Activity and Health, 6*, 708–715.

Fox, K.R. (1997). The physical self and processes in self-esteem development. In K.R. Fox (Ed.), *The physical self: From motivation to well-being* (pp. 111–139). Champaign, IL: Human Kinetics.

Fredricks, J.A., & Eccles, J.S. (2005). Family socialization, gender, and sport motivation and involvement. *Journal of Sport & Exercise Psychology, 27*, 3–31.

Fridlund Dunton, G., Atienza, A.A., Tscherne, J., & Rodriguez, D. (2011). Identifying combinations of risk and protective factors predicting physical activity change in high school students. *Pediatric Exercise Science, 23*, 106–121.

Fridlund Dunton, G.F., Schnieder, M., Graham D.J., & Cooper, D.M. (2006). Physical activity, fitness, and physical self-concept in adolescent females. *Pediatric Exercise Science, 18*, 240–251.

Gibbons, S.L., Ebbeck, V., Concepcion, R.Y., & Li, K. (2010). The impact of an experiential education program on the self-perceptions and perceived social regard of physical education students. *Journal of Sport & Exercise Psychology, 32*, 786–804.

Harter, S. (1985). *Manual for the self-perception profile for children.* Denver, CO: University of Denver.

Harter, S. (1987). The determinants and meditational role of global self-worth in children. In N. Eisenberg (Ed.), *Contemporary topics in developmental psychology* (pp. 219–242). New York: Wiley.

Harter, S. (1988). *Manual for the self-perception profile for adolescents.* Denver, CO: University of Denver.

Harter, S. (1999). *The construction of the self: A developmental perspective.* New York: The Guilford Press.

Horn, T.S. (2004). Developmental perspectives on self-perceptions in children and adolescents. In M.R. Weiss (Ed.), *Developmental sport and exercise psychology: A lifespan perspective* (pp. 101–143). Morgantown, WV: Fitness Information Technology.

Horn, T.S., & Amorose, A.J. (1998). Sources of competence information. In J.L. Duda (Ed.), *Advances in sport and exercise psychology measurement* (pp. 49–64). Morgantown, WV: Fitness Information Technology.

Horn, T.S., Glenn, S.D., & Wentzell, A.B. (1993). Sources of information underlying personal ability judgments in high school athletes. *Pediatric Exercise Science, 5*, 263–274.

Inchley, J., Kirby, J., & Currie, C. (2011). Longitudinal changes in physical self-perceptions and associations with physical activity during adolescence. *Pediatric Exercise Science, 23*, 237–249.

Kipp, L.E., & Weiss, M.R. (2012). Social influences, psychological need satisfaction, and well-being among female adolescent gymnasts. *Sport, Exercise, and Performance Psychology*. Advance online publication. doi:10.1037/a0030236

Lerner, R.M., Almerigi, J.B., Theokas, C., & Lerner, J.V. (2005). Positive youth development: A view of the issues. *Journal of Early Adolescence, 25*, 10–16.

Marsh, H.W., & Peart, N.D. (1988). Competitive and cooperative physical fitness training programs for girls: Effects on physical fitness and multidimensional self-concepts. *Journal of Sport & Exercise Psychology, 10*, 390–407.

Martin, J.J., McCaughtry, N., Flory, S., Murphy, A., & Wisdom, K. (2011). Using social cognitive theory to predict physical activity and fitness in underserved middle school children. *Research Quarterly for Exercise and Sport, 82*, 247–255.

Martin, J.J., Waldron, J.J., McCabe, A., & Choi, Y.S. (2009). The impact of "Girls on the Run" on self-concept and fat attitudes. *Journal of Clinical Sport Psychology, 3*, 127–138.

Motl, R.W., Dishman, R.K., Saunders, R.P., Dowda, M., & Pate, R.R. (2007). Perceptions of physical and social environment variables and self-efficacy as correlates of self-reported physical activity among adolescent girls. *Journal of Pediatric Psychology, 32*, 6–12.

Motl, R.W., Dishman, R.K., Ward, D.S., Saunders, R.P., Dowda, M., Felton, G., & Pate, R.R. (2005). Perceived physical environment and physical activity across one year among adolescent girls: Self-efficacy as a possible mediator? *Journal of Adolescent Health, 37*, 403–408.

Neumark-Sztainer, D., Story, M., Hannan, P., & Rex, J. (2003). New Moves: A school-based obesity prevention program for adolescent girls. *Preventive Medicine, 37*, 41–51.

O'Connell, M.E., Boat, T., & Warner, K.E. (Eds.). (2009). *Preventing mental, emotional, and behavioral disorders among young people: Progress and possibilities*. National Research Council. Washington, DC: National Academy Press.

Pate, R.R., Stevens, J., Webber, L.S., Dowda, M., Murray, D.M., Young, D.R., & Going, S. (2009). Age-related change in physical activity in adolescent girls. *Journal of Adolescent Health, 44*, 275–282.

Pate, R.R., Ward, D.S., Saunders, R.P., Felton, G., Dishman, R.K., & Dowda, M. (2005). Promotion of physical activity among high-school girls: A randomized controlled trial. *American Journal of Public Health, 95*, 1582–1587.

Petty, K.H., Davis, C.L., Tkacz, J., Young-Hyman, D., & Waller, J.L. (2009). Exercise effects on depressive symptoms and self-worth in overweight children: A randomized controlled trial. *Journal of Pediatric Psychology, 34*, 929–939.

Robinson, L.E. (2011). Effect of a mastery climate motor program on object control skills and perceived physical competence in preschoolers. *Research Quarterly for Exercise and Sport, 82*, 355–359.

Robinson, L.E., Rudisill, M.E., & Goodway, J.D. (2009). Instructional climates in preschool children who are at-risk. Part II: Perceived physical competence. *Research Quarterly for Exercise and Sport, 80*, 543–551.

Sabiston, C.M., & Crocker, P.R.E. (2008). Exploring self-perceptions and social influences as correlates of adolescent leisure-time physical activity. *Journal of Sport & Exercise Psychology, 30*, 3–22.

Schmalz, D.L., Deane, G.D., Birch, L.L., & Davison, K.K. (2007). A longitudinal assessment of the links between physical activity and self-esteem in early adolescent non-Hispanic females. *Journal of Adolescent Health, 41*, 559–565.

Schneider, M., Fridlund Dunton, G., & Cooper, D.M. (2008). Physical activity and physical self-concept among sedentary adolescent females: An intervention study. *Psychology of Sport and Exercise, 9*, 1–14.

Shen, B., McCaughtry, N., & Martin, J. (2007). The influence of self-determination in physical education on leisure-time physical activity behavior. *Research Quarterly for Exercise and Sport, 78*, 328–338.

Smith, A.L. (1999). Perceptions of peer relationships and physical activity participation in early adolescence. *Journal of Sport & Exercise Psychology, 21*, 329–350.

Smith, A.L., & Biddle, S.J.H. (Eds.). (2008). *Youth physical activity and sedentary behavior*. Champaign, IL: Human Kinetics.

Smoll, F.L., Smith, R.E., Barnett, N.P., & Everett, J.J. (1993). Enhancement of children's self-esteem through social support training for youth sport coaches. *Journal of Applied Psychology, 78*, 602–610.

Spence, J.C., Blanchard, C.M., Clark, M., Plotnikoff, R.C., Storey, K.E., & McCargar, L. (2010). The role of self-efficacy in explaining gender differences in physical activity among adolescents: A multilevel analysis. *Journal of Physical Activity and Health, 7*, 176–183.

Taymoori, P., & Lubans, D.R. (2008). Mediators of behavior change in two tailored physical activity interventions for adolescent girls. *Psychology of Sport and Exercise, 9*, 605–619.

Theeboom, M., De Knop, P., & Weiss, M.R. (1995). Motivational climate, psychosocial responses, and motor skill development in children's sport: A field-based intervention study. *Journal of Sport & Exercise Psychology, 17*, 294–311.

Trautwein, U., Gerlach, E., & Lüdtke, O. (2008). Athletic classmates, physical self-concept, and free-time physical activity: A longitudinal study of frame of reference effects. *Journal of Educational Psychology, 100*(4), 988–1001.

Tremblay, M.S., Inman, J.W., & Willms, J.D. (2000). The relationship between physical activity, self-esteem, and academic achievement in 12-year-old children. *Pediatric Exercise Science, 12*, 312–323.

Valentini, N., & Rudisill, M. (2004). Motivational climate, motor-skill development, and perceived competence: Two studies of developmentally delayed kindergarten children. *Journal of Teaching in Physical Education, 23*, 216–234.

Ward, D.S., Saunders, R., Felton, G.M., Williams, E., Epping, J.N., & Pate, R.R. (2006). Implementation of a school environment intervention to increase physical activity in high school girls. *Health Education Research, 21*, 896–910.

Ward, D.S., Saunders, R.P., & Pate, R.R. (2007). *Physical activity interventions in children and adolescents.* Champaign, IL: Human Kinetics.

Weiss, M.R. (Ed.). (2004). *Developmental sport and exercise psychology: A lifespan perspective.* Morgantown, WV: Fit Information Technology.

Weiss, M.R. (2008). "Field of dreams": Sport as a context for youth development. *Research Quarterly for Exercise and Sport, 79*, 434–449.

Weiss, M.R., & Amorose, A.J. (2005). Children's self-perceptions in the physical domain: Between- and within-age variability in level, accuracy, and sources of perceived competence. *Journal of Sport & Exercise Psychology, 27*, 226–244.

Weiss, M.R., Amorose, A.J., & Kipp, L.E. (2012). Youth motivation and participation in sport and physical activity. In R.M. Ryan (Ed.), *The Oxford handbook of human motivation* (pp. 520–553). New York: Oxford University Press.

Weiss, M.R., Amorose, A.J., & Wilko, A.M. (2009). Coaching behaviors, motivational climate, and psychosocial outcomes among female adolescent athletes. *Pediatric Exercise Science, 21*, 475–492.

Weiss, M.R., Bhalla, J.A., Bolter, N.D., & Price, M.S. (2008). Lessons learned and core values adopted in a sport-based youth development program: A longitudinal qualitative analysis [Abstract]. *Journal of Sport & Exercise Psychology, 30*, S208.

Weiss, M.R., Bhalla, J.A., & Price, M.S. (2008). Developing positive self-perceptions through youth sport participation. In H. Hebestreit & O. Bar-Or (Eds.), *The encyclopaedia of sports medicine, Vol. X: The young athlete* (pp. 302–318). Oxford: Blackwell Science.

Weiss, M.R., Bolter, N.D., Bhalla, J.A., & Price, M.S. (2007). Positive youth development through sport: Comparison of participants in The First Tee life skills programs with participants in other organized activities. *Journal of Sport & Exercise Psychology, 29*, S212.

Weiss, M.R., Stuntz, C.P., Bhalla, J.A., Bolter, N.D., & Price, M.S. (2012). "More than a game": Impact of The First Tee life skills programme on positive youth development: Project introduction and Year 1 findings. *Qualitative Research in Sport, Exercise, and Health.* doi:10.1080/2159676X.2012.712997

Weiss, M.R., & Wiese-Bjornstal, D.M. (2009). Promoting positive youth development through physical activity. *President's Council on Physical Fitness and Sports: Research Digest, 10*(3), 1–8.

12

PHYSICAL ACTIVITY
AND SELF-PERCEPTIONS
AMONG ADULTS

Peter R. E. Crocker, Carolyn E. McEwen, and Amber D. Mosewich

For over a century, theorists have recognized that self-processes are central in understanding human adaptation (Bandura, 1997; Baumeister, 1987; Harter, 1999; James, 1890). Self-processes are involved in guiding and motivating behavior, attention and self-regulation, influencing appraisals and emotion, as well as helping individuals buffer the effects of negative events (see Guindon, 2010; Leary & Tangney, 2003). The self develops through feedback, and person and social comparison processes, processes which are heavily influenced by the person's interactions with the world and by social relationships, shared cultural experiences, and self-reflexivity (our ability to think about and attend to our self; Harter, 1999; Stets & Burke, 2003). Aspects of self, such as self-esteem, are thought to be key markers of well-being. Therefore, it is hardly surprising that researchers are intrigued by the potential causal relationship between physical activity and self-processes (see Crocker, Kowalski, & Hadd, 2008; Fox, 2000).

This chapter will review the theoretical and empirical literature on self-representations and physical activity in adults. We begin with defining key self-constructs, as well as identifying the conceptual boundaries of the chapter. Since several other chapters in this book are related to self-processes, we will attempt to highlight unique topics while avoiding any unnecessary overlap. We then discuss how global self is multidimensional, the relevance of the physical self and associated subdomains, and the issue of domain identification. We briefly review measurement issues and how researchers have attempted to model physical activity and self-representations before reviewing the research literature linking physical activity and self. We pay special attention to gender and cultural differences. In the final section, we address the implications for practitioners as well as identify research challenges.

Conceptions of the self and definitions

A review of the sport and exercise psychology literature in the last 20 years would reveal the use of many self-related terms including self-identity, self-efficacy, self-esteem, self-worth, self-concept, self-compassion, self-perceptions, physical self, self-image, and self-representations. Leary and Tangney (2003) found over 60 self-related terms in the general psychology literature. Unfortunately these terms have not been used or measured consistently (Harter, 1999), making comparisons and developing theoretical and practical generalizations difficult.

This chapter will focus on self-representations and related constructs, such as self-esteem and self-concept. Self-representations are defined as "attributes or characteristics of the self that are consciously acknowledged by the individual through language – that is, how one describes oneself" (Harter, 1999, p. 3). Self-representations can vary in terms of globalism (i.e., self-evaluation of the person as a whole versus parts), domain specificity (i.e., social, physical, and intellectual self-representations), as well as stability across time and contexts. To clarify key terms used in this chapter, the following descriptions are provided:

- **Self-concept** refers to self-evaluations of personal attributes, such as abilities and characteristics, within discrete domains such as physical, social, and intellectual areas (Harter, 1999; Hattie, 1992). Some theorists believe self-concepts can vary in importance, valence (positive and negative), stability, and can change over the lifespan (see Kernis & Goldman, 2003).
- **Self-esteem** or **self-worth** is an emotionally laden self-evaluation reflecting how a person feels about him/herself: it captures a sense of worth (Leary & MacDonald, 2003). It can be conceptualized at both global and domain levels and can vary across the lifespan.
- **Self-efficacy** refers to beliefs in one's capabilities to organize and execute the courses of action required to produce given attainments (Bandura, 1997). Self-efficacy is influenced by self-concept but also other cognitive appraisals and situational demands. Self-efficacy is described in greater detail in Chapter 14 (McAuley, Mailey, Szabo, & Gothe, this volume).
- **Identity** is commonly used interchangeably with self-constructs. Identity often includes group affiliations, self-representations, and social roles (see Hogg, 2003) and frequently comprises goals, values, and beliefs a person is strongly committed to (Waterman, 1985). An individual may have multiple identities, which can include physical activity, sport, and exercise. Identity and physical activity are discussed in greater detail in Chapter 13 (Strachan & Whaley, this volume).

To a large extent, this chapter will focus on self-representations associated with the constructs of self-concept and self-esteem, and how they influence and are influenced by physical activity. We will also only briefly touch on the area of body image and body appearance because this area is covered in more detail in Chapter 15 (Martin Ginis, McEwan, & Bassett-Gunter, this volume). However, it is impossible to completely exclude this area since body appearance is an important aspect of self-concept and a strong correlate of self-worth (Fox, 2000; Harter, 1999). This becomes more apparent when we consider the multidimensional structure of self.

Multidimensional self

Both self-concept and self-esteem are implicated in the organization of motivated behaviors including physical activity, and are markers of mental health and well-being. There are literally thousands of studies on self-esteem and self-concept and their associations to psychological functioning, health, stress management, emotions, academic achievement, and sport and exercise involvement (see Fox, 1998; Kernis & Goldman, 2003; Kort-Butler & Hagewen, 2011; Leary & MacDonald, 2003). Clearly, these are important topics from both empirical and theoretical perspectives.

To appreciate the effects of physical activity and self-processes one must acknowledge that the structure of self is multidimensional. This view proposes that global self can consist of different levels or specific domains including such dimensions as physical, social, and academic (Harter, 1999; Shavelson, Hubner, & Stanton, 1976). Subdomains can be nested under the domains, with possible increasing differentiation. For example, the physical self can consist of subdomains like perceptions of physical conditioning, sport skills, flexibility, body fat, body appearance, and strength (see Fox & Corbin, 1989; Marsh, Richards, Johnson, Roche, & Tremaybe, 1994). A subdomain like strength might be further divided into facets like arm strength, leg strength, core strength, and the like. This multidimensional perspective of self becomes critical when considering whether (a) self-processes motivate physical activity behavior, (b) physical activity enhances self-processes, or (c) whether there is a reciprocal effect between physical activity and self-processes (Marsh & Craven, 2006).

When physical activity researchers are interested in the global level, they typically look at global self-esteem or global self-worth. At the domain or subdomain level there is greater attention on self-concept, although there are measures of domain self-worth like physical self-worth (Fox & Corbin, 1989). There is strong evidence that the physical self is strongly linked to an individual's perception of global self-esteem (e.g., Fox, 2000; Sonstroem & Morgan, 1989). As Fox (1997) stated, "For many theorists, the physical self has become the *major* component of our self-expression and interaction with the world, and it is seen to hold a key to our understanding of the total self" (p. v).

Domain identification and self-esteem enhancement

Given that so many dimensions can be nested under global self, what is the potential contribution of the physical self and the influence of physical activity interventions on enhancing self-esteem? Although it seems intuitive that lower levels of the multidimensional (sometimes referred to as hierarchical) structure should contribute to global self, the influence of various levels of the structure on other levels is much less clear (Hattie & Fletcher, 2005). A popular notion is that people may value or identify with particular domains and these valued domains should have a greater impact on higher self-structures like global self-esteem. Therefore, some researchers study domain identification, which is the extent that a person defines his or her higher level self through performance in a particular domain like school, sport, or exercise (see Marsh & Sonstroem, 1995; Osborne & Jones, 2011).

Based on the notion of domain identification, physical activity interventions could be directed towards increasing the value attached to physical activity (sport, exercise, dance, or lifestyle activity), as well as increasing competence in the particular physical self-subdomain. However, there is not strong evidence for domain identification process in enhancing self-esteem. Many researchers have found that the importance attached to a domain seems to have little influence on global self (Donnellan, Tzesniewski, Conger, & Conger, 2007; Hattie & Fletcher, 2005). However, others still hold that it is necessary to consider the perceived importance of specific domains in understanding global self-constructs (see Harter, 2003; Osborne & Jones, 2011). The contribution of domain identification to understanding global self is clearly a source of contention.

Measurement of global and physical self

Many instruments have been developed to measure self-concept and self-esteem, including the physical self (see Fox, 1997; Marsh, 1992). In the sport and exercise psychology literature, popular measures of global self-esteem include Rosenberg's global self-esteem measure (Rosenberg, 1965), Harter's General Self-worth subscale from the Adult Self-Perception Profile (Messer & Harter, 1986), as well as Marsh's self-worth subscale from the Self-Description Questionnaire (Marsh, 1992). All of these scales have strong psychometric properties, although Leary and MacDonald (2003) believe most measures of global self-esteem and self-worth are heavily weighted by self-concept items and do not primarily assess the affective reactions central to this construct.

Many different instruments have been used to assess the physical self, including measures of physical self-esteem and physical self-concept. Harter has developed measures for across the lifespan that compartmentalize physical self-perceptions into two primary domains: physical/athletic competence and physical appearance (Harter, 1988; Messer & Harter, 1986). Fox and Corbin (1989) developed the Physical Self-perception Profile (PSPP), which assesses four subdomains of physical self-concept (sport competence, attractive body, physical strength, and physical conditioning) and a global domain of physical self-worth. Marsh and colleagues' Physical Self-description Questionnaire (PSDQ; Marsh et al., 1994) assesses 10 physical self-concepts, in addition to including a global self-esteem dimension (strength, body fat, activity, endurance/fitness, sport competence, coordination, health, appearance, flexibility, and general physical self-concept). There are also physical self-concept measures for elite athletes (Elite Athlete Self-description Questionnaire; Marsh, Hey, Johnson, & Perry, 1997). All of these measures have demonstrated sound psychometric properties.

Modeling physical activity and the self

There has been a long debate about the nature of the relationship between self-representations and motivated behavior like physical activity (see Crocker et al., 2008; Fox, 2000). At a basic level, most researchers believe that physical self-representations are correlated more strongly, compared to global self-constructs, with physical activity (Fox, 1997). A more complex question, however, concerns the direction of causality. There are three potential directions of causality models to consider: bottom–up, top–down, and reciprocal. These causal models require the use of experimental and longitudinal designs, combined with more sophisticated data analysis strategies such as latent growth modeling and structural equation modeling (see Kort-Bulter & Hagewen, 2011; Marsh & Craven, 2006).

Many sport and exercise researchers have argued for a bottom–up causality model in that physical activity can enhance global self-esteem (Folkins & Sims, 1981; Opdendacker, Delecluse, & Boen, 2009). A bottom–up model holds that changes in a situation-specific experience (e.g., lifting weights) causes changes in a physical domain (e.g., strength), which produces modifications in physical self-worth, ultimately causing change in global self-esteem. An example of a specific bottom–up model is Sonstroem and Morgan's (1989) Exercise and Self-esteem Model (EXSEM). This model holds that interventions in physical activity cause changes in self-efficacy, which in turn influences change in physical self-perceptions and upwards to enhancing global self-esteem. Although the specific components in the EXSEM have been modified over the years, it has been a popular bottom–up model to examine exercise interventions, as well as the effects of sport participation on self-representations across the lifespan (see McAuley, Blissmer, Katula, Duncan, & Mihalko, 2000; Opdenacker et al., 2009; Sonstroem, 1997).

A top–down causal model holds that the flow of change is from global self-esteem to lower order domains like the physical self and then down to specific types of subdomains, which would then impact specific physical activity behavior (see Harter, 1999). Some sport and exercise researchers have examined how variables such as perceived physical competence or exercise identity influence engagement in physical activity (Whaley & Ebbeck, 2002). There are few systematic evaluations of the top–down model in the sport and exercise psychology literature (see Kowalski, Crocker, Kowalski, Chad, & Humbert, 2003).

Reciprocal effects causal models hold that prior self-concept influences subsequent motivated behavior and prior motivated behavior influences subsequent self-concept (Marsh & Craven, 2006). Evaluating this model requires the researcher to evaluate both self-concept and physical behavior across multiple time points. It is also critical to evaluate self-concept at the multidimensional level, since the evidence for reciprocal effects model is most prominent when the domain self-concept matches the achievement domain (Marsh & Craven, 2006). There are, however, only a limited number of studies that have examined this model in physical activity contexts, with none focusing on exercise behavior in adults (see Marsh, Gerlach, Trautwein, Lüdtke, & Brettschneider, 2007; Marsh & Perry, 2005).

Empirical evidence for physical activity and the self

There are numerous studies with emerging, young, middle-aged, and older adult populations that demonstrate a weak to moderate relationship between physical activity behavior and global and physical self-esteem/self-concept. But what is the evidence that physical activity interventions can enhance self-representations? Also, what is the evidence for various bottom-down, top-down, or reciprocal models? This section will review the empirical evidence about the relationship between physical activity involvement and aspects of global and physical self.

The literature indicates that global self-esteem and physical self-concepts like conditioning, sport skills, and strength are correlated with participation in physical activity contexts like exercise, sport, dance, and physical activity lifestyles (see Fox, 2000; Spence, McGannon, & Poon, 2005). However, many research studies have used cross-sectional correlational or simple non-experimental group comparison designs. These designs, although informative, make it difficult to determine the causal relationship between physical activity behaviors and self-representations. It is far more informative, however, to investigate the effectiveness of physical activity interventions. These studies are more common in exercise or lifestyle physical activity contexts.

Several authors have provided narrative or meta-analytic reviews of the effectiveness of physical activity interventions in adults (Fox, 2000; Leith, 2009; McDonald & Hodgdon, 1991; Spence et al., 2005; Sonstroem, 1984). These reviews reveal a number of challenges. First, the measurement of self-esteem or self-concept is problematic, with many studies using unidimensional measures of self, or using psychometrically weak measures. Thus, it is difficult for the reviews to clearly establish relationships between physical activity intervention and the effects on specific components of the self. Second, some reviews have included both children and adults and integrated both populations in their summary conclusions. Third, some reviews have focused on only global self-representations. Fourth, interventions vary widely in terms of the type of activity, program duration, intensity, and frequency (in many cases not reporting some of this key information). Given some of these challenges, we will highlight some key findings in regard to the effects of physical activity interventions on both global and multi-dimensional self-representations. This will be complemented with recent research on these relationships using various research designs.

Physical activity and global self-esteem

The majority of intervention studies have focused on global self-esteem or self-concept in all populations (see Crocker et al., 2008; Spence et al., 2005). Leith (2009) argued that exercise programs result in significant changes in global self-concept and self-esteem, with over 50% of intervention studies reporting significant intervention effects. Leith, Kerr, and Faulkner (2011) suggest that the greatest effects are found with running and weight-training activities. Fox (2000) also argued that about 50% of intervention studies reported between 1970 and 1995 found positive effects on some indicator of global self.

Meta-analytic procedures represent a more powerful means to evaluate the effects of interventions on global self-representations. An excellent example is the work of Spence et al.

(2005) who analyzed the effects of exercise interventions on global self and considered a number of potential moderating effects including age, sex, treatment (type of intervention and fitness measure, and mode of exercise), changes in fitness, initial level of global self, initial level of fitness, exercise mode, and exercise dose (frequency, duration, and intensity). They selected 113 studies, of which 42 were published, with adult populations. However, only 54 studies had random assignment. The dependent measure was an indicator of global self-concept ($n = 83$) or global self-esteem ($n = 44$). Their results indicated that the average weighted effect size was $d = 0.23$, suggesting a weak but significant effect of exercise on global self. The only significant moderators were fitness change and type of program (exercise and lifestyle versus skill development). The former effect suggests that changes in actual physical fitness are required for significant changes in either global self-esteem or global self-concept. There were, however, a number of limitations in the study. Many studies failed to report key information (e.g., intensity, fitness change), intervention duration widely varied, and only 21 studies were considered to be good quality. Nevertheless, the results suggested that exercise interventions have only a small impact on global self.

Sport involvement appears to be a strong medium to enhance self-esteem and self-concept because it not only involves physical activity but is also associated with social value and social support. However, intervention studies with sport are difficult, especially with adult populations. One interesting way to examine the effect of previous sport involvement on self is to use longitudinal designs. An interesting study by Kort-Butler and Hagewen (2011) examined changes in initial levels and growth of global self-esteem as a function of involvement in extracurricular school activities in sport and school clubs from youth to young adulthood. Their longitudinal findings with over 5300 participants were somewhat surprising. As expected, participants in sport-only, school club-only, and multiple involvement had higher initial global self-esteem compared to non-participants. However, although all participants increased in self-esteem over time, initial levels did not contribute to long-term differences. There were no sex or ethnicity effects for self-esteem trajectories. Thus, involvement in activities like sport in high school seems to have only a short-term effect during the school years. Although this study did have limitations (e.g., did not measure physical activity involvement on repeated waves), the growth curve methodology points to a promising way to examine self-processes over time in physical activity contexts where intervention designs are difficult.

Overall, research indicates that physical activity has relatively weak effects on improving global self-esteem. Conclusions about the strength of relationships must be tempered since there are several limitations in research, including a lack of systematic investigation of dose response and instrumentation problems. Nevertheless, the weak effect of physical activity interventions on improving global self-esteem is not surprising given the multidimensional nature of self. There are numerous self-representation domains that can contribute to global self. Models of multidimensional self strongly suggest that physical activity is more likely to have robust effects on the physical self-domain and its associated subdomains (see Fox, 2000).

Physical activity and the multidimensional self

The development of multidimensional models and associated measurement tools since the late 1980s allowed researchers to examine various causal models concerning self-representations and physical activity. A review of the literature indicates there are many studies that have now included multidimensional measures of the physical self in adult populations. Unfortunately, many of these investigations used research designs or explored specific research questions that do not allow us to determine causal relationships. Systematic reviews are also rare (see Fox, 2000).

Nevertheless, there are enough quality studies that suggest it is critical to consider domain-level effects in the link between physical activity and self-representations.

Fox (2000) noted that a majority of intervention studies (78%) indicated positive changes in some aspect of physical self-representations across various populations. On the surface, it appears that physical activity interventions have a more powerful effect on the physical self compared to the global self. However, Fox's conclusion needs to be tempered by the fact that few studies used psychometrically sound measures of the physical self; some measured only specific aspects of the physical self. In addition, many studies were underpowered, and treatment modality and dose varied widely. Since Fox's review, however, there have been several studies using relatively strong methodologies and statistical analysis procedures that do shed light on the effectiveness of interventions to change the physical, and sometimes global, self. Four of these studies are reviewed below.

Li and colleagues provided evidence that a low-intensity physical activity intervention like Tai Chi can produce changes in physical and global self (Li, Harmer, Chaumeton, Duncan, & Duncan, 2002). Using a randomized control trial design, they examined the effects of a 6-month Tai Chi intervention on physical self-dimensions and global self-esteem in older adults (> 64 yrs). The intervention consisted of 60-minute sessions (30 minutes of active Tai Chi) twice a week focusing on balance, postural alignment, and concentration. The authors used growth curve analysis to compare group differences, as well as within-person slope scores to calculate correlations among self-representation scores. The results indicated a significant increase in all physical self-concept scores (conditioning, body appearance, and strength), physical self-worth (PSW), and global self-esteem (GSE) scores in the intervention group compared to the control group. The strongest effect was for conditioning and the weakest effect was for physical appearance, with no difference between PSW and GSE. All physical self-domain slope scores were positively related to changes in PSW. Although the authors argued that PSW mediated the effects of subdomains on GSE (slope scores between PSW and GSE were statistically significant in the intervention group), there were no relationships between subdomains and GSE. Thus, although the Tai Chi intervention had similar effects on PSW and GSE, there did not seem to be a causal pathway between changes in subdomains and GSE. This indicated that the mechanisms of change may be dissimilar at the different levels of the self.

McAuley and colleagues (2000) demonstrated that various forms of physical activity can enhance aspects of the physical self in older adults (60–75 years). Comparing a walking group (*n* = 85) to a stretch and tone group (*n* = 89) in a randomized design, they examined aspects of Sonstroem's model (EXSEM) over 12 months (6-month intervention and 6-month follow-up). Unfortunately, they did not include a non-exercising control group. Nevertheless, their data did provide support for the EXSEM. Using growth modeling statistical techniques, the results indicated that both exercise groups improved at the end of the 6-month intervention in all aspects of physical self-concept (strength, body appearance, and conditioning), as well as physical self-worth. However, both exercise groups also showed significant decreases at follow-up in all self-representations. The modeling appeared to demonstrate that changes in physical fitness, body composition, and physical self-efficacy were related to changes in specific physical self-concepts and increased physical self-worth. Overall, the results indicated that various forms of activity can change physical self-representations.

Opdenacker and colleagues (2009) provided further evidence that various types of physical activity interventions can impact multidimensional self-representations in older adults. They examined the effects of a structured exercise program, a lifestyle exercise program, and a non-randomized control group. The structured intervention consisted of 60–90 minutes, three times per week of individualized programs including endurance, strength, flexibility, and balance training supervised by trainers in a fitness center. The lifestyle intervention had similar training components including home-based exercises adapted to the individual's lifestyle. Both programs lasted for 11 months, with a follow-up assessment at 22 months. In terms of multidimensional self-representations, both interventions improved conditioning and sport competence perceptions, with significant improvement also for physical appearance and physical self-worth in the lifestyle group. The use of the non-randomized design does create some challenges as group scores on some variables were not equivalent at baseline. Nevertheless, there were interesting data for examining the relationship between multidimensional self and activity. When examining the intervention groups and controlling for pre-test data using residualized change scores, the authors found that changes in physical self-subdomains were more strongly related to changes in PSW than GSE. At the end of the intervention, changes in physical activity were more strongly related to changes in PSW than GSE. This study does contribute to the literature by suggesting that physical activity has its greatest influence on the physical self-domain.

The three intervention studies reviewed thus far, although providing support for the effectiveness of physical activity on enhancing the physical self, assume a bottom-up causal model. Marsh and his colleagues, however, have provided evidence that self-concept and physical activity behavior might be best viewed as dynamic and reciprocal. Marsh and Perry (2005) examined the reciprocal effects of swimming performance and physical self-concept in 270 elite swimmers from 30 countries (mean age = 20.8 years; range = 14–35 years). The reciprocal model evaluated held that previous swimming achievement would influence swimming physical self-concept, which would in turn impact swimming achievement even after controlling for previous swimming achievement. Previous swimming achievement was determined by personal best performance. Swimming self-concept was assessed by adapting the Elite Athlete Self-description Questionnaire, which has five specific self-concepts (skill levels, body suitability, aerobic fitness, anaerobic fitness, and mental competence) and a global factor (overall performance). The results supported the reciprocal model in that the strongest predictor of performance was previous achievement, but self-concept did add about 10% to the overall prediction (which was a remarkable 83%).

The reciprocal effect model, which has been replicated in adolescent populations in physical activity and many academic achievement studies (see Marsh & Craven, 2006; Marsh, Chanal, & Sarrazin, 2006), has important practical and theoretical implications. First, the reciprocal model demonstrated that self-concept needs to be considered in motivated achievement behaviors. Second, it indicates that interventions need to target both self-concept and the specific achievement skills related to the domain of interest. Third, the research suggests that self-concept needs to be assessed at the logical level related to the motivated behavior. To a large extent, most of the reciprocal effects research has occurred in achievement settings, primarily in education. It will be important to replicate the reciprocal effects model in other physical activity contexts, such as exercise settings.

Culture and gender

Research has demonstrated that culture and gender influence physical activity behavior and self-representations (e.g., Cağlar & Aşçi, 2006; Hayes, Crocker, & Kowalski, 1999; Ramanathan & Crocker, 2009). This is hardly surprising since culture shapes individual and group attitudes, values, and behaviors and can impact development of both the global and physical self (Cross & Gore, 2003). Since gendered cognitions and roles are molded by social-cultural institutions, these forces will impact how males and females develop global and physical self-perceptions and engage in physical activity. The following section will discuss if there are meaningful cultural and gender differences in (a) self-representations and (b) the relationship between physical activity and self-representations.

There are a number of conceptual and measurement challenges to examining cultural differences in self-representations. First, current assumptions about global self-concept, self-esteem, and specific self-representations may not generalize across different cultural groups (Heine, Lehman, Markus, & Kitayama, 1990). Second, the same measurement tools may not generate valid scores, even if items are translated, because of differences in interpretation. Third, many researchers have used nationality as a proxy for culture. This is problematic since little knowledge is gained, because nationality differences may not reflect the influence of specific cultural values (Unger et al., 2002).

Few studies have specifically examined cultural differences in the multidimensional self. Most studies are descriptive, have little theoretical base, and almost all centered on nationality differences. For example, Hagger, Lindwall, and Aşçi (2004) found higher mean physical self-perceptions scores among British participants compared to Swedish or Turkish participants. In a subsequent study of Turkish university students, mean PSPP scores were lower than in previous studies with American, British, and Canadian samples, particularly on perceived body attractiveness and physical strength (Cağlar & Aşçi, 2006). Other studies have looked at differences in German and Turkish populations, with Germans scoring higher on some scales (i.e., health, coordination, physical activity, sport competence, flexibility, strength, and self-esteem), and Turkish participants scoring higher on other subscales of the PSDQ (i.e., appearance, body fat, and global physical self-worth; Aşçi, Alfermann, Gağar, & Stiller, 2008). There are also no studies that have specifically examined if there are cultural effects on the relation between physical self and physical activity. Overall, most studies provide little understanding of why there are cultural differences and whether the differences have implications for mental health and engagement in motivated behavior, specifically physical activity.

Unlike the mixed findings from cultural investigations, consistent gender differences in both global and physical self-representations (see Cağlar, 2009; Fox, 2000; Kling, Hyde, Showers, & Buswell, 1999) might have important ramifications for physical activity interventions. There are a number of studies that show gender differences in physical activity levels and the physical self, and that physical self-subdomains are correlated with physical activity (e.g., Cağlar and Aşçi, 2006; Hayes et al., 1999). Fox (2000) argued that exercise might have a greater benefit on self for females because they report both lower physical activity levels and lower physical self-representations. Intervention or longitudinal research, however, has failed to provide compelling evidence of gender differences in the link between physical activity and self-representations. In the meta-analysis on physical activity interventions and global self-esteem discussed earlier, Spence and colleagues (2005) found no evidence of gender differences. Similarly, in the study by Opdenacker and colleagues (2009) on lifestyle physical activity and exercise interventions with older adults, there were no gender effects for self-representations. Despite Fox's claim that exercise interventions may have greater impact for women's self-esteem, there is little evidence at either the global or physical self level. However, it is hard to draw strong conclusions in this area because there are few quality studies that have systematically examined gender differences.

Conclusions and implications

Physical activity interventions can increase self-concept and self-worth, with the strongest effect on the physical self. There is emerging evidence of a reciprocal effect between physical activity and self-concept (Marsh & Perry, 2005). Although the physical self is composed of multiple subdomains, research suggests that interventions have a generalized effect on these components. Since people use multiple sources of information to develop self-representations, such as evaluative feedback, and social and self-comparison, practitioners need to incorporate these factors into physical activity interventions. There is evidence of gender differences in the perceptions of physical self-subdomains, but no evidence that physical activity causes a differential gender effect on enhancing global or physical self. Nevertheless, practitioners need to be aware that women typically have lower perceptions of global and physical self and that these self-representations may influence their participation in physical activity. Although the cultural data is inconclusive, practitioners need to consider the complexity of a multicultural world and be sensitive to how cultural values might impact how a person sees themselves and the subsequent impact on physical activity and mental health.

There remain a number of research challenges in this area. First, the reciprocal effect model suggests that scholarly inquiry needs to scrutinize the effectiveness of simultaneous physical self-concept and physical activity interventions (Marsh & Craven, 2006). Second, investigators should consider if it is best to systematically examine dose responses in terms of frequency, intensity, and duration of physical activity. Research has found positive effects on the physical self across various levels of intensity and duration. This suggests that a dose response model might not be appropriate. Third, since self-concept and self-esteem are distinct constructs, researchers need to separate out their effects at multiple self levels (Marsh & Craven, 2006). Fourth, cultural investigations need to examine cultural values, not nationality. Finally, physical activity researchers need to be aware of ongoing work on theoretical and empirical developments on the self and related areas of motivation (see Guindon, 2010; Kernis, 2006; Leary & Tangney, 2003; Marsh & Craven, 2006). How people perceive and evaluate themselves is important for mental health and well-being. Understanding the reciprocal effects of self and physical activity and developing effective interventions should be a primary goal of researchers.

References

Aşçi, F. H., Alfermann, D., Gağar, E., & Stiller, J. (2008). Physical self-concept in adolescent and young adulthood: A comparison of Turkish and German students. *International Journal of Sport Psychology, 39*, 217–236.

Bandura, A. (1997). *Self-efficacy: The exercise of control*. New York: W. H. Freeman and Company.

Baumeister, R. F. (1987). How the self became a problem. A psychological review of historical research. *Journal of Personality and Social Psychology, 52*, 163–176.

Cağlar, E. (2009). Similarities and differences in physical self-concept of males and females during late adolescence and early adulthood. *Adolescence, 44*, 407–419.

Cağlar, E., & Aşçi, F. H. (2006). Gender and physical activity level differences in physical self-perception of university students: A case of Turkey. *International Journal of Sport Psychology, 37*, 58–74.

Crocker, P. R. E., Kowalski, K., & Hadd, V. (2008). The role of self and identity in physical (in)activity. In A. Smith & S. J. Biddle (Eds.), *Youth physical activity and inactivity: Challenges and solutions* (pp. 215–237). Champaign, IL: Human Kinetics.

Cross, S. E., & Gore, J. S. (2003). Cultural models of the self. In M. R. Leary & J. P. Tangney (Eds.), *Handbook of self and identity* (pp. 536–564). New York: Guilford Press.

Donnellan, M. B., Trzesniewski, K. H., Conger, K. J., & Conger, R. D. (2007). A three-wave longitudinal study of self-evaluations during young adulthood. *Journal of Research in Personality, 41*, 453–472.

Folkins, C. H., & Sime, W. E. (1981). Physical fitness training and mental health. *American Psychologist, 36*, 373–389.

Fox, K. R. (Ed.) (1997). *The physical self: From motivation to well-being*. Champaign, IL: Human Kinetics.

Fox, K. R. (1998). Advances in the measurement of the physical self. In J. L. Duda (Ed.), *Advances in sport and exercise psychology measurement* (pp. 295–310). Morgantown, WV: Fitness Information Technology.

Fox, K. R. (2000). The effects of exercise on self-perceptions and self-esteem. In S. J. H. Biddle, K. R. Fox, & S. H. Boutcher (Eds.), *Physical activity and psychological well-being* (pp. 88–117). London: Routledge.

Fox, K. R., & Corbin, C. B. (1989). The Physical Self-perception Profile: Development and preliminary validation. *Journal of Sport & Exercise Psychology, 11*, 408–430.

Guindon, M. H. (2010). *Self-esteem across the lifespan: Issues and interventions*. New York: Routledge.

Hagger, M. S., Lindwall, M., & Aşçi, F. H. (2004). A cross-cultural evaluation of a multidimensional and hierarchical model of physical self-perceptions in three national samples. *Journal of Applied Social Psychology*, *34*, 1075–1107.

Harter, S. (1988). *Manual of the Self-Perception Profile for Adolescents*. Denver, CO: University of Denver.

Harter, S. (1999). *The construction of the self: A developmental perspective*. New York: Guilford Press.

Harter, S. (2003). The development of self-representations during childhood and adolescence. In M. R. Leary & J. P. Tangney (Eds.), *Handbook of self and identity* (pp. 610–642). New York: Guilford Press.

Hattie, J. (1992). *Self-concept*. Hillsdale, NJ: Erlbaum.

Hattie, J., & Fletcher, R. (2005). Self-esteem = success/pretensions: Assessing pretensions/importance in self-esteem. In H. W. Marsh, R. G. Craven, & D. M. McInerney (Eds.), *International advances in self research: Vol. 2. New frontiers for self research* (pp. 123–152). Greenwich, CT: Information Age Publishers.

Hayes, S. D., Crocker, P. R. E., & Kowalski, K. C. (1999). Gender differences in physical self-perceptions, global self-esteem and physical activity: Evaluation of the physical self-perception profile model. *Journal of Sport Behavior*, *22*, 1–14.

Heine, S. H., Lehman, D. R., Markus, H. R., & Kitayama, S. (1990). Is there a universal need for positive self-regard? *Psychological Review*, *106*, 766–794.

Hogg, M. A. (2003). Social identity. In M. R. Leary & J. P. Tangney (Eds.), *Handbook of self and identity* (pp. 462–479). New York: Guilford Press.

James, W. (1890). *The principles of psychology*. Reprint (1963), New York: Holt, Rinehart, & Winston.

Kernis, M. H. (2006). *Self-esteem issues and answers: A sourcebook on current perspectives*. New York: Psychology Press.

Kernis, M. H., & Goldman, B. M. (2003). Stability and variability in self-concept and self-esteem. In M. R. Leary & J. P. Tangney (Eds.), *Handbook of self and identity* (pp. 106–127). New York: Guilford Press.

Kling, K. C., Hyde, J. S., Showers, C. J., & Buswell, B. N. (1999). Gender differences in self-esteem: A meta-analysis. *Psychological Bulletin*, *125*, 470–500.

Kort-Bulter, L. A., & Hagewen, K. J. (2011). School-based extracurricular activity involvement and adolescent self-esteem: A growth curve analysis. *Journal of Youth and Adolescence*, *40*, 568–581.

Kowalski, K. C., Crocker, P. R. E., Kowalski, N. P., Chad, K. E., & Humbert, M. L. (2003). Examining the physical self in adolescent girls over time: Further evidence against the hierarchical model. *Journal of Sport & Exercise Psychology*, *25*, 5–18.

Leary, M. R., & MacDonald, G. (2003). Individual differences in self-esteem: A review and theoretical integration. In M. R. Leary & J. P. Tangney (Eds.), *Handbook of self and identity* (pp. 401–418). New York: Guilford Press.

Leary, M. R., & Tangney, J. P. (2003). The self as an organizing construct in the behavioral and social sciences. In M. R. Leary & J. P. Tangney (Eds.), *Handbook of self and identity* (pp. 3–14). New York: Guilford Press.

Leith, L. M. (2009). *Foundations of exercise and mental health* (2nd ed.). Morgantown, WV: Fitness Information Technology.

Leith, L. M., Kerr, G. A., & Faulkner, G. E. (2011). Exercise and mental health. In P. R. E. Crocker (Ed.), *Sport and exercise psychology: A Canadian perspective* (pp. 306–336). Toronto: Pearson Canada.

Li, F. Z., Harmer, P., Chaumeton, N. R., Duncan. T. E., & Duncan, S. C. (2002). Tai chi as a means to enhance self-esteem: A randomized controlled trial. *Journal of Applied Gerontology*, *21*, 70–89.

Marsh, H. W. (1992). *Self-description Questionnaire II: Manual*. Publication Unit, Faculty of Education, University of Western Sydney.

Marsh, H. W., Chanal J. P., & Sarrazin P. G. (2006). Self-belief does make a difference: A reciprocal effects model of the causal ordering of physical self-concept and gymnastics performance. *Journal of Sport Sciences*, *24*, 101–111.

Marsh, H. W., & Craven, R. G. (2006). Reciprocal effects of self-concept and performance from a multidimensional perspective: Beyond seductive pleasure and unidimensional perspectives. *Perspectives on Psychological Science*, *1*, 133–162.

Marsh, H. W., Gerlach, E., Trautwein, U., Lüdtke, U., & Brettschneider, W. D. (2007). Longitudinal study of preadolescent sport self-concept and performance: Reciprocal effects and causal ordering. *Child Development*, *78*, 1640–1656.

Marsh, H. W., Hey, J., Johnson, S., & Perry, C. (1997). Elite Athlete Self Description Questionnaire: Hierarchical confirmatory factor analysis of responses by two distinct groups of elite athletes. *International Journal of Sport Psychology*, *28*, 237–258.

Marsh, H. W., & Perry, C. (2005). Self-concept contributes to winning gold medals: Causal ordering of self-concept and elite swimming performance. *Journal of Sport & Exercise Psychology*, *27*, 71–91.

Marsh, H. W., Richards, G. E., Johnson, S., Roche, L., & Tremayne, P. (1994). Physical Self-description Questionnaire: Psychometric properties and a multitrait-multimethod analysis of relations to existing instruments. *Journal of Sport & Exercise Psychology, 16,* 270–305.

Marsh, H. W., & Sonstroem, R. J. (1995). Importance ratings and specific components of physical self-concept: Relevance to predicting global components of self-concept and exercise. *Journal of Sport & Exercise Psychology, 17,* 84–104.

McAuley, E., Blissmer, B., Katula, J., Duncan, T. E., & Mihalko, S. L. (2000). Physical activity, self-esteem, and self-efficacy relationships in older adults: A randomized controlled trial. *Annals of Behavioral Medicine, 22,* 131–139.

McDonald, D. G., & Hodgdon, J. A. (1991). *Psychological effects of aerobic fitness training.* New York: Springer.

Messer, B., & Harter, S. (1986). *Manual for the Adult Self-perception Profile.* Denver, CO: University of Denver.

Opdenacker, J., Delecluse, C., & Boen, F. (2009). The longitudinal effects of lifestyle physical activity intervention and a structured exercise intervention on physical activity. *Journal of Sport & Exercise Psychology, 31,* 743–760.

Osborne, J. W., & Jones, B. D. (2011). Identification with academics and motivation to achieve in school: How the structure of the self influences academic outcomes. *Educational Psychology Review, 23,* 131–158.

Ramanathan, S., & Crocker, P. R. E. (2009). The influence of family and culture on physical activity among female adolescents from the Indian Diaspora. *Qualitative Health Research, 19,* 492–503.

Rosenberg, M. (1965). *Society and adolescent self-image.* Princeton, NJ: Princeton University Press.

Shavelson, R. J., Hubner, J. J., & Stanton, G. C. (1976). Self-concept: Validation of construct interpretations. *Review of Educational Research, 46,* 407–441.

Spence, J. C., McGannon, K. R., & Poon, P. (2005). The effects of exercise on global self-esteem: A quantitative review. *Journal of Sport & Exercise Psychology, 27,* 311–334.

Sonstroem, R. J. (1984). Exercise and self-esteem. *Exercise and Sport Sciences Reviews, 12,* 123–155.

Sonstroem, R. J. (1997). The physical self-system: A mediator of exercise and self-esteem. In K. R. Fox (Ed.), *The physical self: From motivation to well-being* (pp. 3–26). Champaign, IL: Human Kinetics.

Sonstroem, R. J., & Morgan, W. P. (1989). Exercise and self-esteem: Rationale and model. *Medicine and Science in Sports and Exercise, 21,* 329–337.

Stets, J. E., & Burke, P. J. (2003). A sociological approach to self and identity. In M. R. Leary & J. P. Tangney (Eds.), *Handbook of self and identity* (pp. 128–152). New York: Guilford Press.

Unger, J. B., Ritt-Olson, A., Teran, L., Huang, T., Hoffman, B. R., & Palmer, P. (2002). Cultural values and substance use in a multiethnic sample of California adolescents. *Addiction Research & Theory, 10,* 257–279.

Waterman, A. S. (1985). *Identity in adolescence; Process and contents.* San Francisco: Jossey-Bass.

Whaley, D. E., & Ebbeck, V. (2002). Self-schemata and exercise identity in older adults. *Journal of Aging & Physical Activity, 10,* 245.

13

IDENTITIES, SCHEMAS, AND DEFINITIONS

How aspects of the self influence exercise behavior

Shaelyn M. Strachan and Diane E. Whaley

A full understanding of human behavior requires consideration of how individuals view themselves. The proliferation of research addressing constructs such as self-esteem and self-efficacy exemplify this focus on self. Leary and Price Tangney (2003) posit self as an organizing construct that imposes order upon the numerous self-related constructs. According to these researchers, self is defined as the "psychological apparatus that allows organisms to think consciously about themselves" (Leary & Price Tangney, 2003, p. 8). How we view ourselves is recognized as more than a reservoir of self-knowledge and has implications for motivation and execution of goal-directed behavior (Stein & Markus, 1996). Through providing a reflexive core, the self is thought to enable individuals to experience, perceive, think, and feel in relation to themselves, as well as regulate themselves (Leary & Price Tangney, 2003).

Self-related variables have been applied in an attempt to understand exercise adherence (Fox & Wilson, 2008). The problem of exercise non-adherence has been consistently documented (e.g., Colley et al., 2011) leading to the proclamation that physical inactivity is a "major public health and human welfare problem" (Blair & Morris, 2009, p. 255). This problem is given further salience when one considers that through being sedentary, inactive individuals miss out on the extensive health benefits of physical activity (e.g., Haskell, Blair, & Hill, 2009; Kesäniemi, Riddoch, Reeder, Blair, & Sørensen, 2010). In an attempt to address the problem, the role of self in understanding exercise behavior has received increased research attention. In particular, identity has been implicated as an important self-related variable for understanding exercise behavior.

Conceptual views of identity

Identity has been viewed from cognitive (e.g., Markus, 1977) and sociological (e.g., Stets & Burke, 2003) perspectives. Fox (1997) defined identity as "the integration of beliefs, values, self-perceptions, and behaviors into a consistent, coherent, and recognizable self-package" (p. xii). With regard to adult development, Whitbourne and Collins (1998) add that identity is one's sense of self over time, incorporating content areas such as physical functioning, social relationships, and life experiences. Finally, Burke and Stets (2009) suggest that "an identity is the set of meanings that define who one is when one is an occupant of a particular role in society, a member of a particular group, or claims particular characteristics that identify him or her as a unique person" (p. 3). Thus, a composite of these definitions might be that identity is a complex yet organized integration of our beliefs, values, and behaviors into a self-package that develops and changes over time, guided by our social relationships and society at large.

The purpose of this chapter is to provide an overview of current knowledge pertaining to exercise identity. We focus on role identities related to exercise or physical activity, or related constructs that also capture self-definition around these behaviors. Identities include both implicit (outside conscious awareness) and explicit (known to the individual) components. Although both are important (e.g., Banting, Dimmock, & Lay, 2009), we focus on explicit identities. Our overview will include two theoretical perspectives that have been used to study exercise identities, followed by a review of the relevant literature associated with each perspective. We then describe Kendzierski and colleagues' physical activity self-definition model, which provides a potential mechanism for fostering and maintaining an exercise-related identity. We conclude with a discussion of future directions for research.

The use of theory in exercise identity research

The use of theory is important in advancing research (Biddle & Nigg, 2000; Brawley, 1993; Noar & Zimmerman, 2005). Exercise identity research has varied in the extent to which it has been theory-based. Some researchers acknowledge the theoretical backing of the exercise identity construct whereas others go further and test theoretical propositions offered by relevant theories. A number of theories have incorporated the identity construct including the theory of planned behavior (e.g., Sheeran & Orbell, 2000) and recently, self-determination theory (e.g., Strachan, Fortier, Perras, & Lugg, in press; Vlachopoulous, Kaperoni & Moustaka, 2010; Wilson & Muon, 2008). While the inclusion of exercise identity within these theories is well justified and useful, due to space restrictions, our review of relevant theories is limited to theoretical perspectives in which self-identification is the central construct. Namely, we provide overviews of self-schema theory and identity theory.

Self-schema theory

Markus (1977) described self-schemas as "cognitive generalizations about the self derived from past experience, that organize and guide the processing of self-related information contained in the individual's social experiences" (p. 64). Self-schemas are domain-specific; they represent the attributes, abilities, and experiences of an individual in a particular domain. The presence of a schema in a given domain facilitates encoding, evaluation, and retrieval of domain-relevant information (Cross & Markus, 1994). As a result, self-schemas are used as a basis for future decision-making, and theoretically, behavior (Whaley, 2004). Self-schema theory has its roots in the social cognitive perspective. Markus (1990) stated that, "while hypothesized to reside inside one individual's head or heart, self-schemas are in large measure interpersonal achievements" (p. 249). Thus, schemas are influenced by and in turn influence the context and our perceptions of others (Whaley, 2004). Research examining self-schema theory in exercise has focused on the presence of schemas, as well as links between schemas, intentions, and behavior.

Kendzierski (1988, 1990) first examined self-schemas related to exercise. She found that college-aged exerciser schematics (individuals who considered exercise extremely important and descriptive of their self-image) compared to nonexerciser schematics (important and nondescriptive) and aschematics (moderately important and moderately or nondescriptive) exercised more frequently, did more activities, were more likely to have exercised the previous semester, were more committed to exercising in the future, and had more strategies for remaining active (Kendzierski, 1988). These findings were substantiated in a concurrent multi-phase study (Kendzierski, 1990), where she found exerciser schematics could be distinguished from aschematics on a number of information processing tasks (endorsing more exercise-related descriptors, taking less time to make schema-consistent judgments, recalling more specific instances of past exercise, and predicting themselves more likely to exercise in the future). This attentional bias among exercise schematics has been more recently demonstrated (Berry & Spence, 2009. In a second study, Kendzierski used a prospective design to show that exerciser schematics were more likely to report adopting an exercise program than individuals without such a schema.

Since those influential studies, a number of researchers have examined the link between exercise schemas and behavior. Estabrooks and Courneya (1997) found partial evidence for the moderating effect of an exercise schema on the intention–behavior relationship, a finding confirmed in a longitudinal study (Sheeran & Orbell, 2000). Sheeran and Orbell suggested the importance dimension of self-schema was responsible for this moderator effect such that people who place greater value on exercise were most likely to follow through with their intention. Recently, Banting, Dimmock, and Lay (2009) found that implicit and explicit forms of self-schema were related to higher levels of exercise in adults. Although they did not find self-schema moderated the intention–behavior relationship, they did find that explicit exerciser self-schema was mediated by intention in its relationship with behavior. Kendzierski and her colleagues examined a potential explanation for the link between intention and behavior (Kendzierski & Sheffield, 2000; Kendzierski, Sheffield, & Morganstein, 2002). They found that exerciser schematics made less stable attributions for exercise lapses they imagined happened to them than aschematics, but both groups made similar attributions for lapses they imagined happened to others. A schema for exercise, then, seems to be related to more adaptive strategies that allow exerciser schematics to take the same situation and infer attributes that can be changed to allow for continued exercise participation.

Other researchers have examined correlates of exerciser schemas. For example, Boyd and Yin (1999) reported that exerciser schematics had more knowledge and enjoyment of sports than unschematics (i.e., aschematics and nonschematics), and Yin and Boyd (2000) found that exerciser schematics had higher levels of exercise self-efficacy and more positive perceptions of their physical fitness than non-exerciser schematics or aschematics. In an investigation of the relationship between exercise and depression in adult women (20–45 years), Clark (2002) found that exercise schemas mediated the relationship between physical self-efficacy and depression, and Harju and Reed (2003) discovered active college students who identified as an exerciser had higher levels of self-efficacy, longer workouts, and higher fitness levels. In contrast, those who identified as a nonexerciser were less fit and dwelled on negative thoughts related to their ability to exercise.

In the first qualitative examination of exercise self-schema, Whaley and Ebbeck (2002) interviewed 13 older adults who had been long-term exercisers. They hypothesized that older adults, and in particular older women, might be influenced in their perceptions of their exercise behavior because of ageist beliefs; descriptors embraced by younger populations (such as "exerciser") might not be accepted as relevant to their behavior. Consistent with this hypothesis, only six of the 13 individuals were schematic for exercise using Kendzierski's (1988) measure. Of the remaining seven, all but one rated their exercise behavior as very important to their sense of self, but not descriptive of the image they had of themselves. They preferred terms that hinted at age-related stereotypes such as "physically inclined." It seems that although self-schema is regarded as a cognitive construct, the social context plays a role in helping to shape perceptions of identities. Hardcastle and Taylor (2005) built on this work by conducting multiple interviews of middle-aged and older adult women over time in order to examine the potential for changes in perception of self and identity. Embracing an integrative view of identity (that is, across theories), they found that over time women developed new priorities and identities that included physical activity, and an identity of exerciser was associated with feelings of empowerment and well-being. Finally, Whaley and Schrider (2005) assessed current (self-schema) and future-oriented (possible selves) identities over a 10-week period in a group of older adult exercisers. Although future identities changed the most, changes also occurred in current selves. The idea that self-schemas can change is consistent with Markus' notion of the dynamic self (Markus & Wurf, 1987). This implies that interventions can be created to develop exercise-related identities, a point we will return to later in this chapter.

In the majority of studies described above, assessment of exercise schema uses the framework originally proposed by Markus (1977) and adapted to the exercise domain by Kendzierski (1988, 1990). Consistent with theory, three key questions focusing on importance and self-description related to physical activity are the basis of classification, with participants sorted into groups (schematic, aschematic, nonschematic, and unclassified) based on responses to those questions. The criticism of this approach is that a sizeable number of respondents typically remain unclassified (Sheeran & Orbell, 2000). Some researchers have opted to pool aschematics, nonschematics, and unclassified respondents into one category ("unschematics"), a technique that Kendzierski et al. (2002) demonstrated to be effective in distinguishing individuals possessing a specific schema from those who do not, and consistent with theory. Recently Mullen (2008), drawing from the work of Petersen, Stahlberg, and Dauenheimer (2000), added "self-certainty" as an additional schemata dimension in an investigation of adult fitness club members. Self-certainty is described as the certainty of people's self-views, with higher self-certainty related to positive outcomes. As part of a larger study of exercise identity, Mullen found through factor analysis that the revised measure had three distinct factors (self-description, importance, and certainty), and cluster analysis showed profiles consistent with Kendzierski's (1988) schema classifications. Although lower self-certainty was related to changes in exercise self-description and importance (suggesting a role in maintaining exercise identity), 25% of the sample still fell into the unclassified category. The issue of measurement is an important one, and additional research across groups is indicated. In the meantime, Kendzierski's measure remains the gold standard for evaluating exercise-related self-schemas.

In summary, the research to date utilizing self-schema theory in exercise contexts has produced significant and meaningful information on the importance of having an exerciser schema. Having a schema for exercise is related to a number of positive outcomes, including enjoyment, persistence, and higher rates of exercise behavior. Research indicates that individuals with an exercise schema make more facilitative attributions for their exercise behavior, and create more strategies to maintain their exercise program. Exercise schemas do appear to have the capacity for change, boding well for use in interventions. Finally, although there are some criticisms of the measurement of exercise schemas, the process has been shown to differentiate individuals who possess an exercise-related schema from those who do not.

Identity theory

Identity theory assumes that individuals acquire a shared knowledge about social categories, including roles, through socialization. This shared knowledge provides boundaries for individuals and results in relatively fixed and predictable behavior (Burke & Stets, 2009). Identity theory has branched out into various emphases (e.g., Burke, 1980; McCall & Simmons, 1978; Stryker, 1980; Thoits, 1983). The work of Burke and colleagues focuses on internal dynamics and outlines how identities function as self-regulating control systems (Burke, 2006) that link identities to behavior (e.g., Burke, 1980; Burke & Stets, 2009; Stets & Burke, 2003), which makes this stream of identity theory suited to understanding goal-directed exercise behavior.

According to identity theory (Burke, 1980), identities are associated with role meanings (e.g., what it means to be an exerciser) (Stets & Burke, 2003). Because of their link with meanings, identities serve as a personally relevant standard (Burke & Stets, 2009; Stryker & Burke, 2000) that encourages identity-consistent behavior (2006). As described elsewhere (e.g., Strachan & Brawley, 2008), individuals seek to behave consistently with their identity meanings. When individuals perceive they have behaved inconsistently with their exercise identity meaning (e.g., exercisers engage in regular exercise; I have not exercised in three days), the incongruence is thought to create negative affect and motivation to modify the situation so that behavior is brought in line with identity meanings (cf. Stets & Burke, 2003). If the comparison suggests no difference (I have engaged in regular exercise), identity verification has occurred, positive affect should result, and no change to the situation is necessary (Stryker & Burke, 2000). Finally, individuals can vary in the salience or strength of an identity (Ryan & Deci, 2003), which should influence the likelihood that individuals will engage in identity-relevant behavior (Anderson, Cychosz, & Franke, 2001).

Exercise researchers recognize the relevance of the identity construct for understanding exercise behavior. Anderson and Cychosz developed the exercise identity scale (Anderson & Cychosz, 1994), which measures the "salience of an individual's identification with exercise as an integral part of the concept of self" (p. 747). Norms for this scale have been established (Anderson, Cychosz, & Franke, 2001; Vlachopoulos, Kaperoni, Moustake, & Anderson, 2008) and this scale has been widely used to measure the exercise identity construct.

Initial exercise identity research, much of it using the exercise identity scale (Anderson & Cychosz, 1994), established a link between exercise identity and exercise behavior. In cross-sectional studies examining university and adult community samples, exercise identity was found to relate to minutes of weekly exercise (Anderson, Cychosz, & Franke, 1998; Storer, Cychosz, & Anderson, 1997), frequency of exercise (Miller, Ogletree, & Welshimer, 2002; Wilson & Muon, 2008), number of weeks of exercise, perceived exertion, and physiological outcomes (Anderson, Cychosz, & Franke, 1998). These findings with mostly young adults have been extended to older adults where a relationship between physical activity identity and weekly frequency of physical activity was supported (Strachan, Brawley, Spink, & Glazebrook, 2010).

While these studies support a concurrent association between exercise identity and exercise outcomes, stronger support is offered by prospective research. Cardinal and Cardinal (1997) followed female college students enrolled in either an exercise or non-exercise class for 14 weeks. Exercise identity increased over the course of the class exclusively among exercise class participants. These findings show that exercise identity can increase over a relatively short time period. A few studies have examined exercise identity along with social cognitive variables in the prediction of exercise outcomes. In a sample of college students, Petosa et al. (2003) found exercise identity contributed to a model that significantly predicted frequency of vigorous physical activity (Petosa, Suminski, & Hortz, 2003). Strachan and colleagues (2005) prospectively examined identification with running among a sample of maintenance runners and found this construct to predict weekly running frequency and duration when combined with self-efficacy variables (Strachan, Woodgate, Brawley, & Tse, 2005).

Exercise identity is also associated with variables known to be important in the self-regulation of exercise. In a sample of maintenance runners Strachan and colleagues (2005) found that, when compared with individuals with lower scores on runner identity, individuals with higher scores reported higher concurrent levels of task and self-regulatory efficacy for running. These researchers found exercise identity to be concurrently related to self-efficacy for future exercise

(Strachan & Brawley, 2008; Strachan, Brawley, Spink, & Jung, 2009) and suggest that self-regulatory efficacy may act as a mechanism that encourages identity-consistent exercise (Strachan et al., 2009). In a prospective study Strachan and colleagues found that self-regulatory efficacy mediated the relationship between exercise identity and both exercise behavior (Sweet et al., 2009) and perceptions of identity-behavior consistency (Strachan, Brawley, Spink, & Sweet, 2011). Carraro and Gaudreau (2010) found that physical activity identity predicted the extent to which people planned their exercise, which in turn predicted physical activity goal progress. In addition, planning and physical activity goal progress related to physical activity identification over time. Recently, researchers have found links between exercise identity and the satisfaction of psychological needs (Vlachopoulos, Kaperoni, & Moustaka, 2011; Wilson & Muon, 2008) and more autonomous forms of behavioral regulations (Strachan et al., in press; Vlachapoulos et al., 2011), which are both factors identified as important in the regulation of exercise (Ryan & Deci, 2003). Finally, a study with older adults suggests that physical activity identity is a significant predictor of strength of physical activity intentions and quality of life (Strachan et al., 2010). It appears that exercise identity may be a marker for psychological variables important in the self-regulation of exercise such as intentions, planning, and self-regulatory efficacy related to exercise. Further, some research suggests that exercise identity may exert its influence on exercise outcomes through some of these variables (e.g., planning, self-regulatory efficacy).

Research that supports a link between exercise identity and behavior is consistent with the identity theory notion that individuals seek to behave consistently with endorsed identities (Stets & Burke, 2003). However, identity theory makes additional propositions about how identities relate to behavior as outlined previously. Strachan and colleagues have tested some of these theoretical propositions. Drawing on Burke's identity theory (1980), these researchers examined how individuals react to hypothetical (Strachan & Brawley, 2008; Strachan, Flora, Brawley, & Spink, 2011) and real-life (Strachan, Brawley, Spink, & Jung, 2009) situations where individuals perceive that their recent exercise is inconsistent with their exercise identity. Individuals with strong exercise identities react to these situations in a manner consistent with identity theory predictions, which suggests they are seeking identity-behavior congruency. For example, strong exercise identity individuals report greater negative affect about the situation, and stronger intentions and self-regulatory efficacy for future exercise (Strachan & Brawley, 2008) regardless of the cause (personally controllable versus situationally caused) of the identity-inconsistent behavior (Strachan et al., 2011). In an experimental study, individuals receiving feedback from a confederate designed to challenge their exercise identity displayed greater negative affect and made more effort to present themselves differently from the identity-inconsistent feedback than did individuals who received feedback designed to confirm their identities (Stadig, Strachan, & Jung, 2010). Finally, affective reactions associated with perceptions of identity-consistent or inconsistent behavior appear to be moderated by strength of exercise identity (Strachan et al., 2009).

Taken together, research examining the exercise identity construct suggests that exercise identity is reliably related to exercise behavior. A criticism of the exercise identity research to date is that only a small body of research has examined whether identified correlates of identity that may be important in the self-regulation of exercise (e.g., affect, planning, self-regulatory exercise) serve as links between exercise identity and identity-consistent exercise behavior. This lack of research is surprising given that identity theory outlines specific internal dynamics thought to link identities to behavior (Burke & Stets, 2009; Stets & Burke, 2003). This type of research is necessary to advance our understanding of exercise identity's role in the self-regulation of exercise.

Both schema theory (Markus, 1977) and identity theory (Burke, 1980) serve as appropriate bases for research that seeks to understand identification with exercise and how this process may be linked to exercise outcomes. Research stemming from both of these theories provides converging support that self-identification as an exerciser is reliably related to exercise and exercise self-regulatory outcomes. A logical next step for researchers is to determine how exercise identities can be built, strengthened, and maintained so as to facilitate positive exercise outcomes.

Developing and maintaining an exercise identity

Although both Markus (1977) and Burke (1980) describe identities as robust and slow to change once formed, there is theoretical and empirical evidence that suggests identities can be created or strengthened. For example, Stets and Burke (2003) discuss how individuals can act as agents to create new roles and identities. Further, Stein and Markus (1996) describe how the self, as a dynamic, multifaceted structure, contains both stable, self-defining conceptions and less developed images of the self that can be shaped through ongoing social events. Researchers have found that exercise identity exhibits some change over time (Carraro & Gaudreau, 2010; Cardinal & Cardinal, 1997; Hardcastle & Taylor, 2005; Whaley & Schrider, 2005) supporting these theoretical notions. Until recently however, little work has examined *how* such identities might be formed. In particular, the process of forming an identity for an activity an individual freely chooses has received relatively little empirical attention (Kendzierski & Morganstein, 2009). The physical activity self-definition model (PASD; Kendzierski, Furr, & Schiavoni, 1998; Kendzierski & Morganstein, 2009) was created to explore identities for specific (e.g., tennis player, runner) and general (e.g., exerciser) physical activities. The development of the model focused on (a) what it might take for someone to "claim" an exercise-related identity (or self-definition) and (b) what the correlates of a physical activity self-definition are.

A number of applicable concepts and theories were examined in developing the preliminary model, including Bem's (1972) self-perception theory, the early work of Cooley (1902) and James (1890) related to the role of the social world in how we see ourselves, the more recent theorizing of identity (Stryker, 1987), and self-schema (Markus, 1977) theorists. According to these models, identity should include constructs that relate to perceptions about the behavior (effort, importance) and motivation to engage in the behavior (perceived competence, improvement, and enjoyment). A comment from someone in the individual's social world (e.g., "I'm impressed how consistent a runner you are") or a choice one is forced to make (e.g., complying with a doctor prescribing a cardiac rehabilitation program) are hypothesized to activate self-reflection about a PASD.

In a series of three studies, Kendzierski et al. (1998) examined these correlates in weightlifters, basketball players, and exercisers. Perceived effort, perceived competence, the extent that physical activity was made a priority, perceived competence relative to others, perceived improvement, perceived social acknowledgment of the self-definition, and the extent to which others mention one's activities were related to self-definition (enjoyment and self-definition was related to basketball and exercise but not weightlifting), and in open-ended responses far more behavioral than affective criteria were used to describe applicable identities. Kendzierski and Morganstein (2009) then tested and cross-validated the PASD model with runners and cyclists. Structural equation modeling supported a model whereby perceived commitment and perceived ability directly influenced self-definition, and perceived wanting, perceived trying, and enjoyment had indirect effects. The model suggests that although the context may necessitate changes in self-definitions (e.g., going from a walker to a runner self-definition over the course of a training program), the process by which individuals arrive at a self-definition should not. For example, runners might have different levels of enjoyment or commitment if they are working to increase their speed through interval training versus taking a cross-country run, but the process of developing their runner self-definition (e.g., developing perceived ability and commitment) will remain the same.

This model has great potential for interventions, but the authors acknowledge some limitations. More testing is needed to determine if the model generalizes across physical activities and across individual differences like age, ethnicity, or ability level. Longitudinal research is also needed in order to track the development and maintenance of PASD over time. Following up on what social factors specifically relate to PASD formation is also needed. Although social factors are hypothesized to prompt thoughts about one's PASD, research to date has focused primarily on the cognitive correlates. However, the model does provide a starting point for interventions designed to build applicable physical activity self-definitions. Whaley and Schroyer (2010) offered an action-plan that included ways practitioners could foster aspects of the PASD model such as perceived commitment, perceived ability, and identity acceptance. Consistent with those suggestions, we offer the following ideas. Exercise leaders could increase perceived commitment by instituting appropriate goal setting or setting up a social support network for participants. Much research has examined ways to increased perceived ability, such as using skill progression, allowing enough time for practice, and keeping an exercise log. Finally, to help participants accept and embrace their new self-definitions, exercise leaders should provide appropriate feedback and use applicable language (e.g., you are a runner!) so participants can more easily "see" themselves in these new identities.

Future directions for exercise identity research

We have reviewed the extant exercise-identity literature and in the process attempted to identify gaps in the literature. Next, we outline suggestions for future research in terms of theory, methodology, and new thematic research directions that are likely to contribute to the field's advancement.

Theory

There are numerous reasons why we encourage exercise-identity researchers to ground their research in theory (Biddle & Nigg, 2000; Brawley, 1993; Noar & Zimmerman, 2005). Researchers who choose self-schema theory or identity theory as a basis are positioned to posit theoretically based hypotheses and situate their findings in an established body of literature. We encourage researchers to continue to integrate the identity construct into established theories or use theories that pertain to identity in a complementary fashion (e.g., Sheeran & Orbell, 2000; Strachan & Brawley, 2008). For example, self-determination theory (Ryan & Deci, 2003) offers a complement to identity research owing to its articulation of how individuals vary in terms of the extent to which they internalize a behavior. Recent research supports the relevancy of this theory for identity researchers (Strachan et al., in press; Vlachapoulous et al., 2011; Wilson & Muon, 2008).

Methodology and research design

Much of the exercise-identity research is correlational and cross-sectional. This preliminary research provides a basis for research questions and designs (e.g., longitudinal, experimental) that will lead to a better understanding of how exercise identity leads to exercise behavior (e.g., Banting, Dimock & Lay, 2009; Carraro & Gaudreau, 2010; Sheeran & Orbell, 2000; Strachan et al., 2011). Additionally, although a few studies have used a qualitative approach (e.g., Hardcastle

& Taylor, 2005; Whaley & Ebbeck, 2002), more qualitative research is needed to further clarify the significance and meaning of identities to individuals engaged in exercise. Future research should continue to utilize research designs and analyses that help elucidate the relationships among exercise identity, self-regulatory processes, and exercise behavior.

New thematic research directions

The physical activity self-definition model (Kendzierski et al., 1998; Kendzierski & Morganstein, 2009) provides an opportunity to examine the creation of identities, as well as the evolution of identities over time. Researchers should take this opportunity to test the model in activity contexts in diverse populations. As described above, both quantitative and qualitative methodologies would be helpful in explicating the mechanisms that are critical for self-definition to occur, as well as the maintenance of these identities. This latter issue could be critical in furthering our understanding of exercise adherence.

Similarly, temporal aspects of identity deserve additional attention. We have focused on identities formed from past and present experiences (Markus, 1977); however, future-oriented selves, termed possible selves by Markus and Nurius (1986), have been shown to complement present selves and serve as motivational plans for future behavior (Stein & Markus, 1996; Whaley, 2004). Imagining oneself in the future (e.g., as a physically active person) allows people to explore different possible identities (Dunkel, 2000) and may serve as a tool for changing one's self-concept (Dunkel, Kelts, & Coon, 2006). Future research should explore the potential role of possible selves related to physical activity in relation to exercise identity.

Final thoughts

In this chapter we reviewed two theories that focus directly on identity. Schema and identity theories have more in common than differences, with schema theory focusing more on cognitions, where identity theory takes a decidedly social approach. In the exercise domain, schema and identity both capture the extent to which people view exercise as a part of who they are and focus on importance as a critical marker for the existence of a schema/identity. Empirical research based on the two theories has found schemas and identities related to exercise outcomes such as adherence, enjoyment, and self-regulatory mechanisms such as self-efficacy and stable attributions. We believe there is room for two theoretical approaches, as there is room for multiple overlapping theories of motivation, anxiety, or peer relationships. Rather than being considered as independent and unrelated, we suggest that researchers consider exercise schema and identity theory research together when seeking to understand exercise self-definition. In addition, Kendzierski and colleagues' physical activity self-definition model draws from both theoretical perspectives and describes how identities might be established and maintained. This model presents an opportunity to move beyond description and prediction to the creation of interventions to establish new identities for exercise. Finally, our suggestions for future research are intended to engage new investigators and pursue new directions in identity-related research. We fervently believe that understanding identity is key to understanding exercise behavior, and we invite others to investigate these issues for themselves.

References

Anderson, D.F., & Cychosz, C.M. (1994). Development of an exercise identity scale. *Perceptual and Motor Skills, 78,* 747–751.

Anderson, D.F., Cychosz, C.M., & Franke, W.D. (1998). Association of exercise identity with measures of exercise commitment and physiological indicators of fitness in a law enforcement cohort. *Journal of Sport Behavior, 21,* 233–241.

Anderson, D.F., Cychosz, C.M., & Franke, W.D. (2001). Preliminary exercise identity scale (EIS) norms for three adult samples. *Journal of Sport Behavior, 24,* 1–9.

Banting, L.K., Dimmock, J.A., & Lay, B.S. (2009). The role of implicit and explicit components of exerciser self-schema in the prediction of exercise behavior. *Psychology of Sport & Exercise, 10,* 80–86. doi:10.1016/j.psychsport.2008.07.007

Bem, D.J. (1972). Self-perception theory. In L. Berkowitz (Ed.), *Advances in experimental social psychology* (Vol. 6, pp. 1–62). New York: Academic Press.

Berry, T., & Spence, J.C. (2009). Automatic activation of exercise and sedentary stereotypes. *Research Quarterly for Sport and Exercise, 80,* 633–638.

Biddle, S.J., & Nigg, C.R. (2000). Theories of exercise behavior. *International Journal of Sport Psychology, 31,* 290–304.

Blair, S.N., & Morris, J.N. (2009). Healthy hearts – and the universal benefits of being physically active: Physical activity and health. *Annals of Epidemiology, 19,* 253–256. doi:10.1016/j.annepidem.2009.01.019

Boyd, M.P., & Yin, Z. (1999). Cognitive-affective and behavioral correlates of self-schemata in sport. *Journal of Sport Behavior, 22,* 288–302.

Brawley, L.R. (1993). The practicality of using social psychological theories for exercise and health research and intervention. *Journal of Applied Sport Psychology, 5,* 99–115. doi:10.1080/10413209308411309

Burke, P.J. (1980). The self: Measurement requirements from an interactionist perspective. *Social Psychology Quarterly, 43,* 18–29.

Burke, P.J. (2006). Identity change. *Social Psychology Quarterly, 69,* 81–96.

Burke, P.J., & Stets, J.E. (2009). *Identity theory.* New York: Oxford University Press.

Cardinal, B.J., & Cardinal, M.K. (1997). Changes in exercise behavior and exercise identity associated with a 14-week aerobic exercise class. *Journal of Sport Behavior, 20,* 377–386.

Carraro, N., & Gaudreau, P. (2010). The role of implementation planning in increasing physical activity identification. *American Journal of Health Behavior, 34,* 298–308.

Clark, C.G. (2002). Depression, exercise schemas, and physical self-efficacy. *Dissertation Abstracts International: Section B. Sciences and Engineering,* 5957.

Colley, R.C., Garriguet, D., Janssen, I., Craig, C.L., Clarke, J., & Tremblay, M.S. (2011). Physical activity of Canadian adults: Accelerometer results from the 2007 to 2009 Canadian Health Measures Survey. *(Statistics Canada) Health Reports, 22,* 7–14.

Cooley, C.H. (1902). *Human nature and social order.* New York: Scribner's.

Cross, S.E., & Markus, H.R. (1994). Self-schemas, possible selves, and competent performance. *Journal of Educational Psychology, 86,* 423–438.

Dunkel, C.S. (2000). Possible selves as a mechanism for identity exploration. *Journal of Adolescence, 23,* 519–529. doi:10.1006/jado.2000.0340

Dunkel, C.S., Kelts, D., & Coon, B. (2006). Possible selves as mechanisms of change in therapy. In C. Dunkel & J. Kerpelman (Eds.), *Possible selves: Theory, research and application* (pp. 187–204). New York: Nova Science Publishers.

Estabrooks, P., & Courneya, K.S. (1997). Relationships among self-schema, intention, and exercise behavior. *Journal of Sport & Exercise Psychology, 19,* 156–168.

Fox, K.R. (1997). Let's get physical. In K.R. Fox (Ed.), *The physical self: From motivation to well being* (pp. vii–xiii). Champaign, IL: Human Kinetics.

Fox, K.R., & Wilson, P.M. (2008). Self-perceptual systems and physical activity. In T.S. Horn (Ed.), *Advances in sport psychology* (3rd ed., pp. 46–64). Champaign, IL: Human Kinetics.

Hardcastle, S., & Taylor, A.H. (2005). Finding an exercise identity in an older body: "It's redefining yourself and working out who you are." *Psychology of Sport and Exercise, 6,* 173–188. doi:10.1016/j.psychsport.2003.12.002

Harju, B.L., & Reed, J.M. (2003). Potential clinical implications of implicit and explicit attitudes within possible exercise selves schemata: A pilot study. *Journal of Clinical Psychology in Medical Settings, 10,* 201–208. doi:10.1023/A:1025414913130

Haskell, W.L., Blair, S.N., & Hill, J.O. (2009). Physical activity: Health outcomes and importance for public health policy. *Preventive Medicine, 49,* 280–282. doi:10.1016j.ypmed.2009.05.002

James, W. (1890). *The principles of psychology* (Vols. 1 & 2). New York: Holt.

Kendzierski, D. (1988). Self-schemata and exercise. *Basic and Applied Social Psychology, 9,* 45–59.

Kendzierski, D. (1990). Exercise self-schemata: Cognitive and behavioral correlates. *Health Psychology, 9,* 69–82.

Kendzierski, D., Furr, M., & Schiavoni, J. (1998). Physical activity self-definitions: Correlates and perceived criteria. *Journal of Sport & Exercise Psychology, 20,* 176–193.

Kendzierski, D., & Morganstein, M.S. (2009). Test, revision, and cross-validation of the physical activity self-definition model. *Journal of Sport & Exercise Psychology, 31,* 484–504.

Kendzierski, D., & Sheffield, A. (2000). Self-schema and attributions for an exercise lapse. *Basic and Applied Social Psychology, 22,* 1–8. doi:10.1207/S15324834BASP2201_1

Kendzierski, D., Sheffield, A., & Morganstein, M.S. (2002). The role of self-schema in attributions for own versus other's exercise lapse. *Basic and Applied Social Psychology, 24,* 251–260. doi:10.1207/S15324834 BASP2404_1

Kesäniemi, A., Riddoch, C.J., Reeder, B., Blair, S.N., & Sørensen, T.I.A. (2010). Advancing the future of physical activity guidelines in Canada: An independent expert panel interpretation of the evidence. *International Journal of Behavioral Nutrition and Physical Activity, 7,* 1–14. doi:10.1186/1479-5868-7-41

Leary, M.R., & Price Tangney, J. (2003). The self as an organizing construct in the behavioral and social sciences. In M.R. Leary & J.P. Tangney (Eds.), *Handbook of self and identity* (pp. 3–14). New York: Guilford Press.

Markus, H. (1977). Self-schemata and processing information about the self. *Journal of Personality and Social Psychology, 35,* 63–78.

Markus, H. (1990). Unresolved issues of self-representation. *Cognitive Therapy and Research, 14,* 241–253.

Markus, H., & Nurius, P. (1986). Possible selves. *American Psychologist, 41,* 954–969. doi:10.1037/0003-066X.41.9.954

Markus, H. & Wurf, E. (1987). The dynamic self-concept: A social psychological perspective. *Annual Review of Psychology, 38,* 299–337. doi:10.1146/annurev.ps.38.020187.001503

McCall, G.J., & Simmons, J.L. (1978). *Identities and interactions: An examination of human associations in everyday life* (Rev. ed.). New York: Free Press.

Miller, K.H., Ogletree, R.J., & Welshimer, K. (2002). Impact of activity behaviors on physical activity identity and self-efficacy. *American Journal of Health Behavior, 26,* 323–330.

Mullen, S. (2008). *Factors involved in the development and maintenance of exercise identity across time* (Doctoral dissertation, University of Virginia). Retrieved from Dissertations & Theses at the University of Virginia (Publication No. AAT 3400964).

Noar, S.M., & Zimmerman, R.S. (2005). Health behavior theory and cumulative knowledge regarding health behaviors: Are we moving in the right direction? *Health Education Research, 20,* 275–290. doi:10.1093/her/cyg113

Perras, M.G.M., Strachan, S.M., Fortier, M.S., & Lugg, C. (2011, April). *Understanding variations in the strength of the exercise identity: An identity theory and self-determination theory perspective.* Poster presented at the 2011 Annual Meeting of the Society for Behavioral Medicine, Washington, DC.

Petersen, L.-E., Stahlberg, D., & Dauenheimer, D. (2000). Effects of self-schema elaboration on affective and cognitive reactions to self-relevant information. *Genetic, Social, and General Psychology Monographs, 126,* 25–42.

Petosa, R.L., Suminski, R., & Hortz, B. (2003). Predicting vigorous physical activity using social cognitive theory. *American Journal of Health Behaviour, 27,* 301–310.

Ryan, R.M., & Deci, E.L. (2003). On assimilating identities to the self: A self-determination theory perspective on internalization and integrity within cultures. In M.R. Leary & J. Price (Eds.), *Handbook of self and identity* (253–272). New York: The Guilford Press.

Sheeran, P., & Orbell, S. (2000). Self-schemas and the theory of planned behaviour. *European Journal of Social Psychology, 30,* 533–550. doi:10.1002/1099-0992(200007/08)30:4<533::AID-EJSP6>3.0.CO;2-F

Stadig, G., Strachan, S.M., & Jung, M.E. (2010). *Affective and self-presentational reactions to a public exercise identity challenge* (unpublished Master's thesis). University of Ottawa, Ottawa, ON.

Stein, K.F., & Markus, H.R. (1996). The role of the self in behavioral change. *Journal of Psychotherapy Integration, 6,* 349–384.

Stets, J.E., & Burke, P.J. (2003). A sociological approach to identity. In M.R. Leary & J.P. Tangney (Eds.), *Handbook of self and identity* (pp. 128–152). New York: Guilford Press.

Storer, J.H., Cychosz, C.M., & Anderson, D.F. (1997). Wellness behaviors, social identities, and health promotion. *American Journal of Health Behavior, 21*, 260–268.

Strachan, S.M., & Brawley, L.R. (2008). Reactions to a perceived challenge to identity: A focus on exercise and healthy eating. *Journal of Health Psychology, 13*, 575–588. doi:10.1177/1359105308090930

Strachan, S.M., Brawley, L.R., Spink, K.S., & Glazebrook, K. (2010). Older adults' physically-active identity: Relationships between social cognitions, physical activity and satisfaction with life. *Psychology of Sport and Exercise, 11*, 114–121. doi:10.1016/j.psychsport.2009.09.002

Strachan, S.M., Brawley, L.R., Spink, K.S., & Jung, M.E. (2009). Strength of exercise identity and identity-exercise consistency. *Journal of Health Psychology, 14*, 1196–1206. doi:10.1177/1359105309346340

Strachan, S.M., Brawley, L.R., Spink, K.S., & Sweet, S. (2013). Self-regulatory efficacy mediates the relationship between exercise identity and perceptions of identity behaviour consistency. Manuscript in preparation.

Strachan, S.M., Flora, P.K., Brawley, L.R., & Spink, K.S. (2011). Varying the cause of a challenge to exercise identity behaviour: Reactions of individuals of differing identity strength. *Journal of Health Psychology, 16*, 572–583. doi:10.1177/1359105310383602

Strachan, S.M., Fortier, S., Perras, G.M., & Lugg, C. (in press). Understanding variations in identity strength through identity theory and self-determination theory. *International Journal of Sport and Exercise Psychology*.

Strachan, S.M., Woodgate, J., Brawley, L.R., & Tse, A. (2005). The relationship of self-efficacy and self-identity to long-term maintenance of vigorous physical activity. *Journal of Applied Biobehavioral Research, 10*, 98–112. doi:10.1111/j.1751-9861.2005.tb00006.x

Stryker, S. (1980). *Symbolic interactionism: A social structural version*. Menlo Park, CA: Benamin/Cummings.

Stryker, S. (1987). Identity theory: Developments and extensions. In K. Yardley & T. Honess (Eds.), *Self and identity* (pp. 89–104). New York: Wiley.

Stryker, S., & Burke, P.J. (2000). The past, present, and future of an identity theory. *Social Psychology Quarterly, 63*, 284–297.

Sweet, S.N., Strachan, S.M., Brawley, L.R., Spink, K.S., Jung, M.E., & Wiseman, E. (2009). Does self-regulatory efficacy mediate the relationship between exercise identity and physical activity: A prospective investigation. Poster presented at the 2009 Annual Meeting of the Society for Behavioral Medicine, Montreal, QC. Abstract retrieved from http://www.springerlink.com/content/f5276143682q6421/fulltext.html

Thoits, P.A. (1983). Multiple identities and psychological well-being: A reformulation and test of the social isolation hypothesis. *American Sociological Review, 49*, 174–187.

Vlachopoulos, S.P., Kaperoni, M., & Moustaka, F.C. (2011). The relationship of self-determination theory variables to exercise identity. *Psychology of Sport and Exercise, 12*, 265–272. doi:10.1016/j.psychsport.2010.11.006

Vlachopoulos, S.P., Kaperoni, M., Moustaka, F.C., & Anderson, D.F. (2008). Psychometric evaluation of the exercise identity scale among Greek adults and cross-cultural validity. *Research Quarterly for Exercise and Sport, 79*, 283–299.

Whaley, D.E. (2004). Seeing isn't always believing: Self-perceptions and physical activity behaviors in adults. In M.R. Weiss (Ed.), *Developmental sport and exercise psychology: A lifespan perspective* (pp. 289–311). Morgantown, WV: Fitness Information Technology.

Whaley, D.E., & Ebbeck, V. (2002). Self-schemata and exercise identity in older adults. *Journal of Aging and Physical Activity, 10*, 245–259.

Whaley, D.E., & Schrider, A. (2005). The process of adult exercise adherence: Self-perceptions and competence. *The Sport Psychologist, 19*, 148–163.

Whaley, D.E., & Schroyer, R. (2010). I yam what I yam: The power of the self in exercise behavior. *Journal of Sport Psychology in Action, 1*, 25–32.

Whitbourne, S.K., & Collins, K.J. (1998). Identity processes and perceptions of physical functioning in adults: Theoretical and clinical implications. *Psychotherapy, 35*, 519–530.

Wilson, P.M., & Muon, S. (2008). Psychometric properties of the exercise identity scale in a university sample. *International Journal of Sport and Exercise Psychology, 6*, 115–131.

Yin, Z., & Boyd, M.P. (2000). Behavioral and cognitive correlates of exercise self-schemata. *Journal of Psychology, 134*, 269–282.

14

PHYSICAL ACTIVITY AND PERSONAL AGENCY

Self-efficacy as a determinant, consequence, and mediator

Edward McAuley, Emily L. Mailey, Amanda N. Szabo, and Neha Gothe

Social Cognitive Theory (SCT; Bandura, 1997, 2004) is a theoretical foundation that has served as the impetus for a considerable body of literature documenting the correlates and determinants of health behavior change. The core set of determinants underlying SCT (self-efficacy, outcome expectations, goals, and facilitators/impediments) and the manner in which they are theorized to influence behavior have been clearly articulated by Bandura (2004). The "active agent" in SCT is self-efficacy. Self-efficacy expectations are beliefs regarding one's capabilities to successfully carry out a course of action (Bandura, 1997) and in lay terms may be considered a situation-specific form of self-confidence. As self-efficacy expectations can be subject to external and internal influences, they are ideal targets for manipulation (McAuley, Talbot, & Martinez, 1999) and intervention (McAuley, Courneya, Rudolph, & Lox, 1994). The primary sources of efficacy information include past performance accomplishments (i.e., mastery experiences), social persuasion, social modeling, and the interpretation of physiological and emotional states (Bandura, 1997). Efficacy expectations are theorized to influence the activities individuals choose to pursue, the degree of effort they expend in pursuit of their goals, and the levels of persistence they demonstrate in the face of setbacks, failures, and difficulties. Clearly, choice, effort, and persistence are important elements of successful adoption and maintenance of physical activity behavior. Thus, self-efficacy would appear to be a very natural correlate of this complex health behavior and, indeed, it has been perhaps one of the most consistently reported correlates of exercise behavior and its outcomes (McAuley & Blissmer, 2000).

In the present chapter, we have elected to review the literature that has been published since the McAuley and Blissmer (2000) review. This review highlights not only the role that self-efficacy plays in physical activity but also in important health outcomes associated with physical activity. The first section begins with a review of the role self-efficacy plays in sustained physical activity. This literature ranges from correlational studies to more elaborate analyses of intervention effects on physical activity and new work combining social cognitive and cognitive neuroscience approaches to understanding adherence. This is followed by a section reviewing the effects that physical activity has on self-efficacy and details center-based intervention effects, print-media effects, and internet-delivered physical activity effects on efficacy expectations. Our final section briefly overviews the literature focusing on self-efficacy as a mediator of physical activity effects on health outcomes, in particular quality of life and functional limitations. This relatively contemporary literature has begun to identify physical activity models that view self-efficacy as a more proximal physical activity outcome that plays a mediating role between physical activity and outcomes that are more distal. The chapter concludes by addressing limitations in the literature and recommendations for future research.

Self-efficacy as a determinant of physical activity

Self-efficacy is one of the most consistently identified correlates and determinants of physical activity behavior. As noted by McAuley and Blissmer (2000), there exists a considerable corpus of cross-sectional, longitudinal, and intervention studies supporting the role of self-efficacy in understanding this complex behavior. In this section, we provide a brief overview of this literature.

Cross-sectional evidence of the self-efficacy and physical activity relationship has been replicated in samples ranging in age from college students to the elderly (Conn, Burks, Pomeroy, & Cochran, 2003; Sylvia-Bobiak & Caldwell, 2006). This relationship appears to be reliable regardless of how physical activity is measured. For example, Conn et al. (2003) found adherence self-efficacy to be the best predictor of not only exercise frequency, but also exercise intensity and duration. Similarly, in a sample of older adults, Harris, Owen, Victor, Adams, and Cook (2009) reported exercise self-efficacy to be positively associated with accelerometer-measured step count in a dose-dependent manner. This suggests that greater improvements in self-efficacy may translate to greater increases in objectively measured physical activity.

Longitudinal studies offer the opportunity to examine the temporal nature of the efficacy–physical activity relationship absent in cross-sectional studies. For example, Gyurcsik, Bray, and Brittain (2004) reported task self-efficacy during the first month of college to be a significant positive predictor of vigorous physical activity four weeks later in first-year students. Plotnikoff, Brez, and Hotz (2000) found self-efficacy assessed during the winter significantly predicted energy expenditure the following summer in adults with diabetes. However, it is self-efficacy's ability to predict long-term maintenance of physical activity that demonstrates it to be a rather powerful correlate. For example, McAuley, Morris, Motl, et al. (2007) assessed physical activity and self-efficacy 2 and 5 years after entry into a 6-month randomized exercise program for older adults. Results showed adherence self-efficacy assessed at year 2 was a significant predictor of physical activity 3 years later, even when controlling for past physical activity behavior. This latter finding is consistent with both McAuley's (1993) and Bandura's (1989) position that, under challenging circumstances (e.g., long-term maintenance of physical activity), higher cognitive control systems, such as self-efficacy, exert a significant influence on the execution of behavioral repertoires.

Data from physical activity interventions offer further support for self-efficacy as a consistent predictor of physical activity behavior. For example, pre-intervention self-efficacy has been identified as a significant predictor of adherence to goals for women participating in walking interventions (Wilbur, Miller, Chandler, & McDevitt, 2003; Williams, Bezner, Chesbro, & Leavitt, 2008). Linde, Rothman, Baldwin, and Jeffery (2006) assessed self-efficacy midway through an 8-week weight loss program for overweight adults reporting self-efficacy predicted blocks walked and stairs climbed at program end, as well as adherence to the exercise plan during weeks 5–8. Similar results have been observed in a 13-week physical activity intervention for primary care patients, with 6-week task and barrier self-efficacy significantly predicting post-intervention physical activity (Blanchard et al., 2007). In fact, one might argue that self-efficacy ratings during an intervention are more informative than baseline measures because participants have been exposed to the behavior and can draw on recent experiences to make more accurate judgments about the extent to which they will be successful in the future (McAuley et al., 2011).

It is equally important to consider how changes in self-efficacy predict changes in physical activity behavior. For example, Hankonen, Absetz, Ghisletta, Renner, and Uutela (2010) conducted a 3-month lifestyle intervention for overweight adults and found changes in self-efficacy across the intervention period positively predicted exercise behavior change. Hall et al. (2010) reported similar findings from a 12-month counseling intervention for older men. In addition to the direct relationship between self-efficacy changes and physical activity changes, they also found this relationship was partially mediated by changes in health-related goals. This is consistent with Bandura's assertions that targeting self-efficacy in interventions enhances behavior not only directly, but also indirectly through other social cognitive constructs.

Embedding strategies to enhance self-efficacy within exercise interventions also appears to be important for improving long-term maintenance of exercise regimens. The transition from a structured, supervised exercise program to independent exercise presents a significant challenge for most adults, and McAuley, Jerome, Elavsky, Marquez, and Ramsey (2003) have demonstrated self-efficacy beliefs at the end of a structured program reliably predict self-reported physical activity 6 and 18 months later. Importantly, these relationships hold when controlling for previous physical activity behavior. These findings have been replicated in a home-based physical activity intervention, in which adherence to a walking regimen during a 24-week maintenance phase was associated with self-efficacy ratings at the end of the initial 24-week intervention (Wilbur, Vassalo, Chandler, McDevitt, & Miller, 2005). Interestingly, results of this study also showed that levels of self-efficacy at baseline did not predict exercise adherence during the maintenance phase, but individuals who demonstrated improvements in self-efficacy across the initial intervention period did exhibit greater adherence during the maintenance phase. These findings underscore the influence that changes occurring during an intervention can have on future behavior. In particular, it may be useful to embed efficacy-building strategies into the final weeks of structured exercise programs in order to prepare participants for the challenges associated with the transition to maintaining regular exercise independently (McAuley et al., 2011).

It is important to acknowledge that although the relationship between self-efficacy and physical activity is relatively consistent, the strength of this relationship can vary based on the type of efficacy assessed, the behavior in question, the characteristics of the sample population, and the timing of self-efficacy and physical activity measurement. For example, Strachan, Woodgate, Brawley, and Tse (2005) found two measures of self-regulatory efficacy (i.e., barriers and scheduling) were significant predictors of running frequency, whereas task-specific efficacy was associated with running duration. In a large cross-sectional study of physical activity in Belgian adults, Van Dyck et al. (2010) reported a stronger association between self-efficacy and leisure-time physical activity than between self-efficacy and active transportation. They reasoned that performing leisure-time physical activity is a conscious individual choice and is more prone to mediation by psychosocial factors, whereas active transportation may largely be governed by environmental characteristics that are beyond the individual's control. Such results highlight the situation-specific nature of self-efficacy measures, and stress the importance of choosing measures that are closely aligned with the outcome(s) of interest.

Although self-efficacy is the more potent construct in Bandura's (2004) social cognitive model, it is important to consider that self-efficacy has direct, as well as indirect effects on behavior, outcome expectations, goals, and barriers/facilitators. Unfortunately, there have been few tests of the full social cognitive model. However, Ayotte, Margrett, and Hicks-Patrick (2010) demonstrated support for the hypothesized direct and indirect effects of self-efficacy in a community-dwelling sample of married adults aged 50–75. In a study of physical activity in college students (Rovniak, Anderson, Winett, & Stephens, 2002), self-efficacy had the greatest total effect on physical activity 8 weeks later, and this effect was largely mediated by self-regulation. In a recent prospective study of middle-aged and older adults, White, Wojcicki, and McAuley (2012) reported that changes in self-efficacy across an 18-month period were directly related to changes in outcome expectations, disability limitations, goals, and physical activity. In addition, changes in self-efficacy were indirectly related to changes in physical activity through changes in physical and social outcome expectations. Continued testing of Bandura's social cognitive model remains an important focus for our understanding of physical activity behavior and would help us determine which aspects of the model respond best to intervention targeting.

Evidence for the mediating role played by self-efficacy in interventions designed to increase physical activity behavior is present in media-based delivery systems such as print and the internet. For example, Dutton et al. (2009) reported that adult diabetics receiving a tailored, print media intervention were significantly more active than participants in a usual care control group 4 weeks later. This effect, however, was no longer significant when self-efficacy was included in the model, suggesting the intervention effect was mediated by changes in self-efficacy across the 4-week period. Luszczynska and Tryburcy (2008) conducted an internet-based intervention and found the effects of their 6-month intervention were mediated by changes in self-efficacy, but only in participants with cardiovascular disease or diabetes. The effect of the intervention on disease-free individuals was negligible. Such findings emphasize the importance of identifying subgroups of individuals who may respond differently to interventions. Finally, Roesch, Norman, Villodas, Sallis, and Patrick (2010) examined the effects of two year-long internet-based interventions to improve physical activity and diet in overweight adults. The interactive websites resulted in significantly higher physical activity levels among individuals in the intervention groups compared to those in the control groups at the end of the 12-month programs. Intervention participants also exhibited positive growth trajectories for self-efficacy, which were positively related to physical activity at 12 months. In their mediation model analyses, the direct effects of the intervention on physical activity were no longer significant when the self-efficacy growth trajectory was included in the model. These findings suggest that the intervention–physical activity effect was completely mediated by self-efficacy.

Physical activity effects on self-efficacy

Consistent with Bandura's perspective on reciprocal determinism, self-efficacy can also be a consequence of physical activity. That is, while self-efficacy acts as a determinant of physical activity behavior, participation in physical activity can change one's self-efficacy for exercise. Cross-sectional research has shown that the amount of physical activity in which one participates is significantly related to one's confidence in his or her ability to exercise on a regular basis (e.g., McAuley, Konopack, Motl, et al., 2006). However, in order to truly understand how participation in physical activity contributes to improvements in self-efficacy, one must examine how the physical activity–self-efficacy relationship changes over time, especially in the context of exercise interventions.

A number of physical activity interventions have shown that simply adhering to a regular exercise regimen as part of an intervention results in an increase in self-efficacy for exercise. This is likely due to the accumulation of mastery experiences, which acts as the primary source of efficacy information. Furthermore, theory-based interventions (e.g., those employing a social cognitive approach) have been shown to be more effective at increasing self-efficacy than non-theory-based interventions (Bock, Marcus, Pinto, & Forsyth, 2001; Hall et al., 2011; Hughes et al., 2004). Such theory-based interventions typically employ purposeful strategies to increase self-efficacy (i.e., provide mastery experiences, facilitate social modeling, utilize social persuasion) in accordance with the recommendations of Bandura (2004).

Although there is evidence of exercise programs increasing self-efficacy, this is not always the case. Indeed, McAuley and colleagues (McAuley et al. 2011) have argued that the timing of efficacy assessments in the early stages of interventions and the type of efficacy measured can have differential effects on efficacy trajectories. In this study, they assessed three types of self-efficacy – exercise self-efficacy, barriers self-efficacy, and self-efficacy – for walking, at four time points: baseline, 3 weeks into the trial, at 6 months, and then at the end of the 12-month program. Findings from this trial showed that exercise self-efficacy decreased from baseline to 3 weeks, followed by a significant upturn at 6 months, and then a second, steeper downturn at program end. Barriers self-efficacy showed a similar pattern, although the increase in self-efficacy between week 3 and month 6 was not significant. Finally, self-efficacy for walking showed a linear trend with a significant positive increase over time that was maintained at 12 months. This study was the first to take multiple measures of self-efficacy within an exercise intervention and demonstrate that a recalibration of self-efficacy occurs in the early weeks of an exercise program. It appears that when judging their capabilities to adhere to regular exercise, individuals may be overly optimistic at baseline, when they have not yet undertaken the behavior. Thus, the week 3 measure may be considered a "true baseline," and the increases in self-efficacy exhibited between week 3 and month 6 occur as a function of regular exercise participation (i.e., mastery experiences). The decrease in self-efficacy at 12 months is consistent with previous studies (Hughes et al., 2004; McAuley, Jerome, Marquez, Elavsky, & Blissmer, 2003; Moore et al., 2006) that have shown efficacy decreases at program end due to the impending challenge of maintaining an exercise regimen after the termination of the structured intervention.

To reinforce claims that exercise participation enhances self-efficacy, it is important to consider the role of adherence to exercise interventions. For example, D'Alonzo and colleagues (D'Alonzo, Stevenson, & Davis, 2004) compared low and high attendees of a 16-week site-based exercise intervention. They found that the high attendees had significantly higher exercise self-efficacy, as well as higher perceived benefits and reduced barriers to physical activity participation, compared to low attendees. Similarly, McAuley, Jerome, Marquez, et al. (2003) found that adherence or frequency of attendance to a 6-month exercise trial was significantly related to increased barriers self-efficacy and exercise self-efficacy. These results underscore the importance of regularly engaging in a specific behavior in order to enjoy mastery experiences from which efficacy improvements are derived. Interestingly, in both interventions, the authors found evidence to suggest that social support from exercising with a group may influence an individual's adherence to an exercise intervention. Thus, it may be valuable to provide participants with ways to stay in contact with other exercisers after an intervention in order to maintain physical activity and exercise self-efficacy.

Given that self-efficacy is a situation-specific evaluation of one's capabilities, one would expect increases in self-efficacy to be closely tied to the task, or type of physical activity being performed. Indeed, there is good evidence that this is the case. For example, Caldwell, Harrison, Adams, and Travis Triplett (2009) found college students who participated in a Pilates class showed significant increases in Pilates self-efficacy across the semester. Similarly, Katula and colleagues (Katula, Rejeski, & Marsh, 2008; Katula, Sipe, Rejeski, & Focht, 2006) found significant increases in self-efficacy for upper-body strength in older adults who participated in a power and strength training intervention. Li and colleagues (Li et al., 2002; Li, Fisher, Harmer, & McAuley, 2005) have conducted Tai Chi interventions in older adults and found increases in not only self-efficacy for Tai Chi, but also in falls self-efficacy. These increases in self-efficacy were also associated with increases in physical function. Importantly, these latter results suggest that by implementing physical activity interventions, which bolster older adults' confidence in their functional capabilities, one may also see improvements in functional performance.

In addition to site-based exercise interventions, a number of counseling interventions that teach behavioral strategies to promote physical activity and self-efficacy for physical activity have also been reported. In some cases, interventions with a counseling component have been shown to increase self-efficacy to a level above what is seen by physical activity participation alone (Hughes et al., 2004; Katula et al., 2006). Social cognitive theory (Bandura, 1997) would suggest that simply providing information about being physically active, however, may not be enough to significantly influence physical activity participation or self-efficacy (Bock, Marcus, Pinto, & Forsyth, 2001). That is, it may be necessary for participants to receive objective feedback about their progress. For example, Bennett, Young, Nail, Winters-Stone, and Hanson (2008) conducted a 6-month telephone-delivered intervention with one group receiving monthly phone calls only and the other receiving a pedometer in addition to the monthly calls. Results showed that the pedometer group maintained physical activity and increased self-efficacy, whereas the group receiving only telephone calls reported significant declines in both self-efficacy and activity levels.

With the advent of improved technology, web-based behavior change programs have shown promise for improving self-efficacy and physical activity levels. For example, Huang and colleagues (Huang, Hung, Chang, & Chang, 2009) reported improvements in self-efficacy for physical activity in college students who received a 2-month web-based physical activity intervention. The extent to which participants utilize the website, however, is an important consideration. Irvine and colleges (Irvine et al., 2011) examined repeat visits to a website providing information and support to develop a personalized physical activity plan. Participants randomized to receive the web intervention differed significantly from the control participants on multiple outcomes (e.g., physical activity minutes per day, perceived barriers, self-efficacy). Within the treatment group, however, those who visited the website multiple times demonstrated significant improvements in physical activity, motivation, self-efficacy, and intention compared to individuals who only visited one time. These results draw attention to one of the greatest challenges of web-based interventions: making the website interactive enough to promote sustained use. If participants are not engaged in the intervention, self-efficacy is likely to decline due to reduced physical activity involvement from which to evaluate their capabilities.

Self-efficacy as a mediator of physical activity and other health outcomes

Although established as a reliable determinant and outcome of physical activity behavior, self-efficacy is also theorized to be a mediator of physical and psychological outcomes associated with physical activity. An increasing body of research highlights the role of self-efficacy in the pathways between physical activity and quality of life (QOL) and functional limitations, and such findings suggest that researchers should integrate strategies for improving self-efficacy when delivering physical activity interventions in order to maximize improvements in disability outcomes and improve QOL among older adults. Given space constraints, we now provide a very brief overview of this literature.

Physical activity and quality of life

The relationship between physical activity and QOL tends to be weaker for global QOL (Netz, Wu, Becker, & Tenenbaum, 2005; Rejeski & Mihalko, 2001) than for intermediate outcomes such as functional status and well-being. This is not surprising given that global QOL is a relatively stable construct that would be likely to change only when intermediate variables that inform individuals' evaluations of their overall QOL also change. In order to design interventions to enhance QOL, it is critical to determine the factors that may moderate and/or mediate the relationship between physical activity and QOL. There is good evidence that physical activity can lead to improved QOL through meditational pathways, and self-efficacy appears to play a critical role.

Elvasky et al. (2005) tested whether physical activity effects on QOL were mediated by positive affect, self-esteem, and self-efficacy, both cross-sectionally and longitudinally over a 5-year period. They found that older adults who were more physically active had higher levels of self-efficacy and physical self-esteem and expressed more positive affect. In turn, self-efficacy and affect were associated with enhanced satisfaction with life. Over a 5-year period similar relationships emerged; that is, increased physical activity was associated with improved physical self-esteem and positive affect, and improvements in affect had a direct effect on satisfaction with life. These findings are consistent with the position that individuals do consider affective well-being when making judgments regarding satisfaction with life (Diener, Scollon, & Lucas, 2003). Recently, a social cognitive model of physical activity's relationship with QOL proposed by McAuley, Konopack, Motl, et al. (2006) has received support in the literature. In this model, physical activity is hypothesized to influence self-efficacy, which in turn indirectly influences global QOL through physical and mental health status. With self-efficacy occupying a central position in the model, the model fits well within a social cognitive framework, and also provides a logical pathway from more proximal and easily modifiable factors to more global and stable factors associated with QOL. The hypothesized model was supported in an initial sample of older women and has been replicated in a sample of community-dwelling older men and women (White, Wójcicki, & McAuley, 2009) and in the context of a longitudinal study (McAuley et al., 2008). These results, as well as other studies (e.g., Paxton, Motl, Aylward, & Nigg, 2010), have shown indicators of physical health status (e.g., functional limitations) and mental health status (e.g., affect, depression, perceived stress) mediate the relationship between physical activity and QOL. Importantly, self-efficacy is a key antecedent of changes in health status, which then influence global QOL perceptions.

Physical activity, function, and disability

Functional limitations in older adults are important risk factors for subsequent disability and institutionalization (Fried & Guralnik, 1997) and loss of independence is likely to diminish overall QOL. Fortunately, there is good evidence that functional declines are attenuated by engaging in protective behaviors such as physical activity (Keysor & Jette, 2001; Paterson & Warbuton, 2010). Thus, as the population becomes increasingly older, it will be important to discourage sedentary behavior and encourage physical activity to minimize functional limitations. Self-efficacy has been identified as an important factor mediating the relationship between physical activity and functional limitations (McAuley, Konopack, Morris, et al., 2006; McAuley, Morris, Doerksen, et al., 2007). As Bandura (1997) has consistently asserted, individuals who believe they are capable of accomplishing specific tasks are more likely to try harder to achieve their goals and persist longer when they encounter barriers. Thus, it makes good sense that functional self-efficacy judgments can be expected to exert important motivational influences on behavior and functional performance. McAuley and colleagues (2006) reported support for a model in which physical activity effects on functional performance and functional limitations were mediated by self-efficacy. McAuley et al. (2007) subsequently replicated this model and demonstrated that increases in physical activity over a 2-year period were associated with greater improvements in self-efficacy, which were associated with improved physical function performance and fewer functional limitations. As well as mediating the physical activity, functional performance, and functional limitations relationship, self-efficacy has also been demonstrated to mediate the relationship between physical activity behavior and the maintenance of mobility (Focht, Rejeski, Ambrosius, Katula, & Messier, 2005). Such findings underscore the importance of control beliefs in the disablement process and suggest any interventions designed to enhance physical functioning should incorporate efficacy-building strategies to enhance participants' confidence in their physical capabilities.

Physical activity and well-being

Several studies have specifically examined self-efficacy's role as a mediator of mental health outcomes. For instance, Anderson, King, Stewart, Camacho, and Rejeski (2005) conducted a randomized controlled trial to determine the effects of behavioral counseling on physical activity in inactive adults. Results showed participants who received the intervention reported significant decreases in perceived stress at the end of the 2-year study that were mediated by changes in self-efficacy. In a study of adults with diabetes, Sacco et al. (2007) found adherence to diabetes self-care behaviors (i.e., physical activity, diet, glucose testing, and medication) was inversely associated with depression. Once again, self-efficacy was a significant mediator of this relationship. Together, these studies suggest improvements in self-efficacy might help alleviate negative mental health outcomes such as stress and depression. Enhanced confidence in one's exercise capabilities might stimulate enhanced skills to cope with daily stressors and generate feelings of accomplishment, which counteract depressive thought patterns.

Limitations and future directions

Self-efficacy's role as a correlate of physical activity has been consistently demonstrated and there would seem to be little need for any more cross-sectional studies in this area. Rather, studies which further enhance our understanding of the physical activity–efficacy relationship by testing the full social cognitive model of physical activity behavior change, further exploring mediation, and examining how self-efficacy interacts with other variables to influence behavior are needed. Future studies should also attempt to replicate the findings of McAuley et al. (2011), as the recalibration of efficacy during the early weeks of an exercise intervention is a novel finding that highlights the complexity of the physical activity–self-efficacy relationship. It will also be important to explore how social cognitive theory might be combined with other disciplinary approaches to understand physical activity behavior change. For example, McAuley and colleagues (McAuley et al. 2011) recently combined social cognitive and neurocognitive approaches to better understand how self-regulatory processes influence physical activity over a 12-month period in older adults. Their findings indicate that executive function, specifically tasks that reflect one's ability to multi-task and inhibit habitual responses, as well as frequency of self-regulatory strategy use, influenced physical activity adherence across a 12-month trial via mediation by self-efficacy. Approaches such as this are likely to better inform us as to the complexity of the self-efficacy and physical activity relationship.

Additionally, future researchers should continue to develop interventions that use contemporary technologies to deliver physical activity programs, and examine how these programs uniquely contribute to an individual's self-efficacy to engage in physical activity and other health behaviors (Huang et al., 2009). The role of self-efficacy as a mediator of intervention effects has primarily been examined in the context of brief behavioral interventions designed within a social cognitive framework. Future studies should also examine the extent to which changes in self-efficacy mediate increases in physical activity that occur as a function of participation in a structured exercise intervention that facilitates mastery experiences. In terms of health outcomes, the role played by self-efficacy in understanding physical activity effects on cognitive function is not well understood. One potential approach might be to expand McAuley's global QOL model by including cognitive health status as well as physical and mental health status. Additionally, this model should be replicated in demographically diverse samples and alternative indicators of physical and mental health status should be explored. However, self-efficacy is a modifiable factor and should be a central component of physical activity programs designed for preventing and minimizing functional limitations and disability and improving QOL in older adults.

Concluding remarks

Self-efficacy remains one of the most consistent correlates and determinants of physical activity behavior (McAuley & Blissmer, 2000). In the decade following the McAuley and Blissmer review there has been a proliferation of studies in this area, many of which have moved away from the largely correlational, unidirectional early work dominating the literature. In this chapter, we have reviewed a considerable corpus of literature that has documented that self-efficacy plays an important role not only as a determinant and outcome of physical activity, but also as an explanatory mediator of the relationships between physical activity, well-being, quality of life, and functional performance and limitations. Some of the more recent work in these areas has used complex designs, contemporary statistical methods, and combined social cognitive and neuroscience approaches to understand physical activity patterns and consequences. We note, however, a dearth of studies that employ Bandura's (1997, 2004) full social cognitive model, examine differential efficacy responses and effects associated with sub-groups of participants within interventions, or specifically target self-efficacy as a modifiable construct and subsequently test how the intervention changed efficacy expectations, and the extent to which these changes are associated with changes in behavior. Relative to this last consideration, it should be noted that numerous studies state that interventions were guided by social cognitive theory, yet fail to effectively test the extent to which the intervention target was successfully changed or its effect on behavior. Nevertheless, we believe that the evidence continues to point to the importance of self-efficacy in human agency and look forward to another decade of innovative and significant application of this construct in the understanding of physical activity, health, and overall well-being.

Acknowledgments

Writing of this chapter was supported in part by a grant from the National Institute on Aging (2R01 AG020118) and a Shahid and Ann Carlson Khan Professorship.

References

Anderson, R. T., King, A., Stewart, A. L., Camacho, F., & Rejeski, W. J. (2005). Physical activity counseling in primary care and patient well-being: Do patients benefit? *Annals of Behavioral Medicine*, *30*(2), 146–154.

Ayotte, B. J., Margrett, J. A., & Hicks-Patrick, J. (2010). Physical activity in middle-aged and young-old adults: The roles of self-efficacy, barriers, outcome expectancies, self-regulatory behaviors and social support. *Journal of Health Psychology*, *15*(2), 173–185. doi:10.1177/1359105309342283

Bandura, A. (1989). Human agency in social cognitive theory. *American Psychologist*, *44*(9), 1175–1184.

Bandura, A. (1997). *Self-efficacy: The exercise of control*. New York: W.H. Freeman and Company.

Bandura, A. (2004). Health promotion by social cognitive means. *Health Education & Behavior*, *31*, 143–164. doi:10.1177/1090198104263660

Bennett, J. A., Young, H. M., Nail, L. M., Winters-Stone, K., & Hanson, G. (2008). A telephone-only motivational intervention to increase physical activity in rural adults: A randomized controlled trial. *Nursing Research, 57*(1), 24–32. doi:10.1097/01.NNR.0000280661.34502.c1

Blanchard, C. M., Fortier, M., Sweet, S., O'Sullivan, T., Hogg, W., Reid, R. D., et al. (2007). Explaining physical activity levels from a self-efficacy perspective: The physical activity counseling trial. *Annals of Behavioral Medicine, 34*(3), 323–328. doi:10.1007/BF02874557

Bock, B. C., Marcus, B. H., Pinto, B. M., & Forsyth, L. H. (2001). Maintenance of physical activity following an individualized motivationally tailored intervention. *Annals of Behavioral Medicine, 23*(2), 79–87. doi:10.1207/S15324796ABM2302_2

Caldwell, K., Harrison, M., Adams, M., & Travis Triplett, N. (2009). Effect of Pilates and taiji quan training on self-efficacy, sleep quality, mood, and physical performance of college students. *Journal of Bodywork & Movement Therapies, 13*(2), 155–163. doi:10.1016/j.jbmt.2007.12.001

Conn, V. S., Burks, K. J., Pomeroy, S., & Cochran, J. E. (2003). Are there different predictors of distinct exercise components? *Rehabilitation Nursing, 28*(3), 87–97.

D'Alonzo, K. T., Stevenson, J. S., & Davis, S. E. (2004). Outcomes of a program to enhance exercise self-efficacy and improve fitness in Black and Hispanic college-age women. *Research in Nursing & Health, 27*(5), 357–369. doi:10.1002/nur.20029

Diener, E., Scollon, C. N., & Lucas, R. E. (2003). The evolving concept of subjective well-being: The multi-faceted nature of happiness. In P. T. Costa & I. C. Siegler (Eds.), *Advances in cell aging and gerontology* (pp. 187–220). Amsterdam: Elsevier.

Dutton, G. R., Tan, F., Provost, B. C., Sorenson, J. L., Allen, B., & Smith, D. (2009). Relationship between self-efficacy and physical activity among patients with type 2 diabetes. *Journal of Behavioral Medicine, 32,* 270–277. doi:10.1007/s10865-009-9200-0

Elavsky, S., McAuley, E., Motl, R. W., Konopack, J. F., Marquez, D. X., Hu, L., . . . Diener, E. (2005). Physical activity enhances long-term quality of life in older adults: Efficacy, esteem, and affective influences. *Annals of Behavioral Medicine, 30*(2), 138–145. doi:10.1207/s15324796abm3002_6

Focht, B. C., Rejeski, W. J., Ambrosius, W. T., Katula, J. A., & Messier, S. P. (2005). Exercise, self-efficacy, and mobility performance in overweight and obese older adults with knee osteoarthritis. *Arthritis & Rheumatism, 53*(5), 659–665. doi:10.1002/art.21456

Fried, L. P., & Guralnik, J. M. (1997). Disability in older adults: Evidence regarding significance, etiology, and risk. *Journal of the American Geriatrics Society, 45*(1), 92–100.

Gyurcsik, N. C., Bray, S. R., & Brittain, D. R. (2004). Coping with barriers to vigorous physical activity during transition to university. *Family & Community Health, 27*(2), 130–142.

Hall, K. S., Crowley, G. M., McConnell, E. S., Bosworth, H. B., Sloane, R., Ekelund, C. C., & Morey, M. C. (2010). Change in goal ratings as a mediating variable between self-efficacy and physical activity in older men. *Annals of Behavioral Medicine, 39*(3), 267–273. doi:10.1007/s12160-010-9177-5

Hall, K. S., Sloane, R., Pieper, C. F., Peterson, M. J., Crowley, G. M., Cowper, P. A., & Morey, M. C. (2011). Long-term changes in physical activity following a one-year home-based physical activity counseling program in older adults with multiple morbidities. *Journal of Aging Research.* doi:10.4061/2011/308407

Hankonen, N., Absetz, P., Ghisletta, P., Renner, B., & Uutela, A. (2010). Gender differences in social cognitive determinants of exercise adoption. *Psychology and Health, 25*(1), 55–69. doi:10.1080/08870440902736972

Harris, T. J., Owen, C. G., Victor, C. R., Adams, R., & Cook, D. G. (2009). What factors are associated with physical activity in older people, assessed objectively by accelerometry? *British Journal of Sports Medicine, 43,* 442–450. doi:10.1136/bjsm.2008.048033

Huang, S.-J., Hung, W.-C., Chang, M., & Chang, J. (2009). The effect of an internet-based, stage-matched message intervention on young Taiwanese women's physical activity. *Journal of Health Communication, 14*(3), 210–227. doi:10.1080/10810730902805788

Hughes, S. L., Seymour, R. B., Campbell, R., Pollak, N., Huber, G., & Sharma, L. (2004). Impact of the fit and strong intervention on older adults with osteoarthritis. *Gerontologist, 44*(2), 217–228. doi:10.1093/geront/44.2.217

Irvine, A. B., Philips, L., Seeley, J., Wyant, S., Duncan, S., & Moore, R. W. (2011). Get moving: A web site that increases physical activity of sedentary employees. *American Journal of Health Promotion, 25*(3), 199–206. doi:10.4278/ajhp.04121736

Katula, J. A., Rejeski, W. J., & Marsh, A. P. (2008). Enhancing quality of life in older adults: A comparison of muscular strength and power training. *Health and Quality of Life Outcomes, 6*(1), 45. doi:10.1186/1477-7525-6-45

Katula, J. A., Sipe, M., Rejeski, W. J., & Focht, B. C. (2006). Strength training in older adults: An empowering intervention. *Medicine and Science in Sports and Exercise, 38*(1), 106–111. doi:10.1249/01.mss.0000183373.95206.2f

Keysor, J. J., & Jette, A. M. (2001). Have we oversold the benefit of late-life exercise? *Journal of Gerontology: Medical Sciences, 56A*(7), M412–M423.

Li, F., Harmer, P., McAuley, E., Fisher, K. J., Duncan, T. E., & Duncan, S. C. (2002). Tai chi, self-efficacy, and physical function in the elderly. *Prevention Science, 2*(4), 229–239. doi:10.1023/A:1013614200329

Li, F. Z., Fisher, K. J., Harmer, P., & McAuley, E. (2005). Falls self-efficacy as a mediator of fear of falling in an exercise intervention for older adults. *Journal of Gerontology: Psychological Sciences, 60*(1), P34–P40. doi:10.1093/geronb/60.1.P34

Linde, J. A., Rothman, A. J., Baldwin, A. S., & Jeffery, R. W. (2006). The impact of self-efficacy on behavior change and weight change among overweight participants in a weight loss trial. *Health Psychology, 25*(3), 282–291. doi:10.1037/0278-6133.25.3.282

Luszczynska, A., & Tryburcy, M. (2008). Effects of a self-efficacy intervention on exercise: The moderating role of diabetes and cardiovascular diseases. *Applied Psychology, 57*(4), 644–659. doi:10.1111/j.1464-0597.2008.00340.x

McAuley, E. (1993). Self-efficacy and the maintenance of exercise participation in older adults. *Journal of Behavioral Medicine, 16*(1), 103–113.

McAuley, E., & Blissmer, B. (2000). Self-efficacy determinants and consequences of physical activity. *Exercise and Sports Science Reviews, 28*(2), 85–88.

McAuley, E., Courneya, K. S., Rudolph, D. L., & Lox, C. L. (1994). Enhancing exercise adherence in middle-aged males and females. *Preventive Medicine, 23*(4), 498–506. doi:10.1006/pmed.1994.1068

McAuley, E., Doerksen, S. E., Morris, K. S., Motl, R. W., Hu, L., Wojcicki, T. R., . . . Rosengren, K. R. (2008). Pathways from physical activity to quality of life in older women. *Annals of Behavioral Medicine, 36*(1), 13–20. doi:10.1007/s12160-008-9036-9

McAuley, E., Jerome, G. J., Elavsky, S., Marquez, D. X., & Ramsey, S. N. (2003). Predicting long-term maintenance of physical activity in older adults. *Preventive Medicine, 37*(2), 110–118. doi:10.1016/s0091-7435(03)00089-6

McAuley, E., Jerome, G. J., Marquez, D. X., Elavsky, S., & Blissmer, B. (2003). Exercise self-efficacy in older adults: Social, affective, and behavioral influences. *Annals of Behavioral Medicine, 25*(1), 1–7. doi:10.1207/S15324796ABM2501_01

McAuley, E., Konopack, J. F., Morris, K. S., Motl, R. W., Hu, L. A., Doerksen, S. E., . . . Rosengren, K. R. (2006). Physical activity and functional limitations in older women: Influence of self-efficacy. *Journal of Gerontology: Psychological Sciences, 61*(5), P270–P277.

McAuley, E., Konopack, J. F., Motl, R. W., Morris, K. S., Doerksen, S. E., & Rosengren, K. R. (2006). Physical activity and quality of life in older adults: Influence of health status and self-efficacy. *Annals of Behavioral Medicine, 31*(1), 99–103. doi:10.1207/s15324796abm3101_14

McAuley, E., Mailey, E. L., Mullen, S. P., Szabo, A. N., Wójcicki, T. R., White, S. M., . . . Kramer, A. F. (2011). Growth trajectories of exercise self-efficacy in older adults: Influence of measures and initial status. *Health Psychology, 30*(1), 75–83. doi:10.1037/a0021567

McAuley, E., Morris, K. S., Doerksen, S. E., Motl, R. W., Liang, H., White, S. M., . . . Rosengren, K. (2007). Effects of change in physical activity on physical function limitations in older women: Mediating roles of physical function performance and self-efficacy. *Journal of the American Geriatrics Society, 55*(12), 1967–1973. doi:10.1111/j.1532-5415.2007.01469.x

McAuley, E., Morris, K. S., Motl, R. W., Hu, L., Konopack, J. F., & Elavsky, S. (2007). Long-term follow-up of physical activity behavior in older adults. *Health Psychology, 26*(3), 375–380. doi:10.1037/0278-6133.26.3.375

McAuley, E., Talbot, H. M., & Martinez, S. (1999). Manipulating self-efficacy in the exercise environment in women: Influences on affective responses. *Health Psychology, 18*(3), 288–294. doi:10.1037/0278-6133.18.3.288

Moore, S. M., Charvat, J. M., Gordon, N. H., Roberts, B. L., Pashkow, F., Ribisl, P., et al. (2006). Effects of a CHANGE intervention to increase exercise maintenance following cardiac events. *Annals of Behavioral Medicine, 31*(1), 53–62. doi:10.1207/s15324796abm3101_9

Netz, Y., Wu, M. J., Becker, B. J., & Tenenbaum, G. (2005). Physical activity and psychological well-being in advanced age: A meta-analysis of intervention studies. *Psychology and Aging, 20*(2), 272–284. doi:10.1037/0882-7974.20.2.272

Paterson, D. H., & Warburton, D. E. R. (2010). Physical activity and functional limitations in older adults: A systematic review related to Canada's Physical Activity Guidelines. *International Journal of Behavioral Nutrition and Physical Activity, 7*(1), 38. doi:10.1186/1479-5868-7-38

Paxton, R. J., Motl, R. W., Aylward, A., & Nigg, C. R. (2010). Physical activity and quality of life – The complementary influence of self-efficacy for physical activity and mental health difficulties. *International Journal of Behavioral Medicine, 17*(4), 255–263. doi:10.1007/s12529-010-9086-99

Plotnikoff, R. C., Brez, S., & Hotz, S. B. (2000). Exercise behavior in a community sample with diabetes: Understanding the determinants of exercise behavioral change. *Diabetes Educator, 26*(3), 450–459. doi:10.1177/014572170002600312

Rejeski, W. J., & Mihalko, S. L. (2001). Physical activity and quality of life in older adults. *Journals of Gerontology: Biological Sciences, 56A*, 23–35. doi:10.1093/gerona/56.suppl_2.23

Roesch, S. C., Norman, G. J., Villodas, F., Sallis, J. F., & Patrick, K. (2010). Intervention-mediated effects for adult physical activity: A latent growth curve analysis. *Social Science & Medicine, 71*, 494–501. doi:10.1016/j.socscimed.2010.04.032

Rovniak, L. S., Anderson, E. S., Winett, R. A., & Stephens, R. S. (2002). Social cognitive determinants of physical activity in young adults: A prospective structural equation analysis. *Annals of Behavioral Medicine, 24*(2), 149–156. doi:10.1207/S15324796ABM2402_12

Sacco, W. P., Wells, K. J., Friedman, A., Matthew, R., Perez, S., & Vaughan, C. A. (2007). Adherence, body mass index, and depression in adults with type 2 diabetes: The mediational role of diabetes symptoms and self-efficacy. *Health Psychology, 26*(6), 693–700. doi:10.1037/0278-6133.26.6.693

Strachan, S. M., Woodgate, J., Brawley, L. R., & Tse, A. (2005). The relationship of self-efficacy and self-identity to long-term maintenance of vigorous physical activity. *Journal of Applied Biobehavioral Research, 10*(2), 98–112. doi:10.1111/j.1751-9861.2005.tb00006.x

Sylvia-Bobiak, S., & Caldwell, L. L. (2006). Factors related to physically active leisure among college students. *Leisure Sciences, 28*(1), 73–89. doi:10.1080/01490400500332728

Van Dyck, D., Cardon, G., Deforche, B., Giles-Corti, B., Sallis, J. F., Owen, N., et al. (2010). Environmental and psychosocial correlates of accelerometer-assessed and self-reported physical activity in Belgian adults. *International Journal of Behavioral Medicine, 18*(3), 235–245. doi:10.1007/s12529-010-9127-4

White, S. M., Wójcicki, T. R., & McAuley, E. (2009). Physical activity and quality of life in community dwelling older adults. *Health and Quality of Life Outcomes, 7*(1), 10. doi:10.1186/1477-7525-7-10

White, S. M., Wójcicki, T. R., & McAuley, E. (2012). Social cognitive influences on physical activity behavior in middle-aged and older adults. *Journals of Gerontology, Series B: Psychological Sciences and Social Sciences, 67*(1), 18–26.

Wilbur, J., Miller, A. M., Chandler, P., & McDevitt, J. (2003). Determinants of physical activity and adherence to a 24-week home-based walking program in African American and Caucasian women. *Research in Nursing & Health, 26*(3), 213–224. doi:10.1002/nur.10083

Wilbur, J. E., Vassalo, A., Chandler, P., McDevitt, J., & Miller, A. M. (2005). Midlife women's adherence to home-based walking during maintenance. *Nursing Research, 54*(1), 33–40.

Williams, B. R., Bezner, J. R., Chesbro, S. B., & Leavitt, R. (2008). The relationship between achievement of walking goals and exercise self-efficacy in postmenopausal African American women. *Topics in Geriatric Rehabilitation, 24*(4), 305–314. doi:10.1097/TGR.0b013e31818ccfed

15

PHYSICAL ACTIVITY AND BODY IMAGE

Kathleen A. Martin Ginis, Desmond McEwan, and Rebecca L. Bassett-Gunter

The uptake of products, services, and informational resources devoted to helping men and women change and feel better about their bodies is staggering. For instance, the weight loss market in the United States alone is estimated to be over $60 billion per annum (Marketdata, 2011). Americans spend roughly $10 billion per year on cosmetic surgery (Fast facts, 2011). In addition, newsstands, grocery checkouts, and convenience stores are flooded with fitness and health magazines that are filled with stories and advertisements promoting strategies for physical self-improvement. Together, these examples attest to the importance—and fragility—of men's and women's body image within contemporary society.

Body image is defined as "the multifaceted psychological experience of embodiment, especially but not exclusively one's physical appearance" (Cash, 2004, p. 1), and reflects how people think, feel, see, and act toward their own bodies. Data derived from large-scale surveys indicate that rates of body image dissatisfaction are high among men and women living in westernized societies. For example, in 2006, an online survey (Frederick, Peplau, & Lever, 2006) of over 50,000 men and women revealed that only 54 percent of men and 41 percent of women felt "good" or "great" about their bodies. The remainder felt that their bodies were "just okay" or even unattractive.

These statistics are frequently cited as evidence of the prevalence of negative body image. However, it can be misleading to define "negative body image" solely in terms of body dissatisfaction. Such an approach fails to take into account the psychological significance and consequences of negative body image evaluations. Indeed, many people may be dissatisfied with their appearance, but their dissatisfaction does not necessarily impact their emotional well-being or daily functioning. In this chapter, we use the term "body image disorder" to refer to situations when body image concerns are persistent and result in some degree of impairment in psychosocial functioning, social activities, or occupational functioning (cf. Cash, Phillips, Santos, & Hrabosky, 2004). We interchangeably use "negative body image," "poor body image," and "body image disturbance" to capture the various multidimensional manifestations of a negative body image (e.g., body dissatisfaction, social physique anxiety, inaccurate perceptions of body shape or size).

We begin this chapter by discussing the role of body image in mental health. We then discuss both the positive and negative effects of exercise on body image. The chapter concludes with commentary regarding limitations of the extant research and some proposed future directions.

Body image and mental health

The mental health implications of a negative body image and body image disorders cannot be overstated. Poor body image has been linked to low self-esteem, is believed to be a cause of depression and anxiety, and plays a significant role in the etiology of psychiatric disorders such as eating disorders and muscle dysmorphia.

Self-esteem

Body image is an important contributor to global self-esteem such that people who feel better about their bodies tend to feel better about themselves overall. A positive relationship between body image and self-esteem has been demonstrated in studies of adolescents (Davison & McCabe, 2006) and adults (Davison & McCabe, 2005). However, because physical appearance is more central to the self-esteem of girls/women than to boys/men, body image tends to be a stronger predictor of global self-esteem in the former population than the latter (cf. Gentile et al., 2009). It is unclear whether a poor body image lowers self-esteem or if lowered self-esteem leads to poor body image. It is possible that the direction of the relationship varies at different points in development (Cash & Smolak, 2011).

Depression and anxiety

Depressed and anxious individuals view their appearance more negatively than do nondepressed and nonanxious individuals, even after controlling for actual differences in body weight and shape. The association between body image and emotional well-being has been demonstrated in both male (e.g., Olivardia, Pope, Borowiecki, & Cohane, 2004) and female (e.g., Cohen & Esther, 1993) samples. Although most studies have focused on adolescents, there is some evidence that this relationship persists into adulthood (e.g., Lichtenberger, Martin Ginis, MacKenzie, & McCartney, 2003). Preliminary data suggest that poor body image is a cause, rather than consequence, of increased depression (Paxton, Neumark-Sztainer, Hannan, & Eisenberg, 2006) and anxiety (Stice & Whitenton, 2002), such that having a poor body image may compromise emotional well-being.

Eating disorders

Body image disturbance is a risk factor for the development and relapse of eating disorders and is a key feature of eating disorder symptomatology (Polivy & Herman, 2002). For example, individuals diagnosed with anorexia nervosa or bulimia nervosa report greater body image dissatisfaction and more distorted body image perceptions than the general population (e.g., Cash & Deagle, 1997).

Muscle dysmorphia

Muscle dysmorphia (MD) is a psychiatric condition characterized by a preoccupation with, and inaccurate beliefs about, one's muscularity (Phillips, O'Sullivan, & Pope, 1997). Not surprisingly, given societal differences in the body image ideals for men versus women, MD is more prevalent among men (Olivardia, 2001). In addition to expressing greater body dissatisfaction, men with MD tend to be more preoccupied with their appearance (i.e., spend more time thinking about their muscularity), engage in more appearance checking behaviors, and are more likely to experience bodybuilding dependence (i.e., compulsive and excessive weight-lifting) than those without the condition (Cafri, Olivardia, & Thompson, 2008).

Using exercise to improve body image

Given the importance of body image to mental health, it is important to identify effective interventions to treat body image disorders and disturbances. Psychosocial interventions such as cognitive-behavioral therapy and experiential therapies (e.g., hypnotherapy, art therapy) are most commonly applied. However, there is evidence to suggest that exercise may be just as effective (Fisher & Thompson, 1994).

Three meta-analyses have examined the effects of exercise training interventions on body image (Campbell & Hausenblas, 2009; Hausenblas & Fallon, 2006; Reel et al., 2007). Overall, the average effect sizes were all statistically significant, and ranged from .29 in the largest and most rigorous meta-analysis to .47 in the smallest and methodologically weakest meta-analysis. Although the magnitude of these effects may not seem particularly impressive, the meta-analyses included studies that varied tremendously in overall methodological quality and rigor. Variability along these dimensions will impact the effects observed in individual studies and the average effect size across studies. Nevertheless, the results yield a consistent message: exercise has significant, positive effects on body image.

What remains unclear, however, is *how* exercise improves body image. An understanding of underlying mechanisms is crucial to the development of exercise programs that maximize improvements in body image. One possibility is that exercise alleviates the psychological comorbodities associated with a poor body image (e.g., depression, anxiety, low self-esteem) and, in turn, alleviates body dissatisfaction. Indeed, Fox (2000) has suggested that exercise improves body image by eliciting an undetermined psychophysiological mechanism that enhances mood and positive self-regard. To date, this hypothesis has been largely untested. Rather, most research has focused on three putative mechanisms: actual changes in physical fitness, perceived changes in fitness, and changes in self-efficacy.

Actual and perceived changes in physical fitness

Physical fitness encompasses body composition, cardiorespiratory endurance (aerobic fitness), muscular strength and endurance, flexibility, and the ability to perform functional activities such as those required for activities of daily living. It is often assumed that exercise improves body image through its effects on body composition—specifically through reductions in body fat and increases in muscle mass. Indeed, changes in body composition are the most frequently studied mechanism of exercise-induced body image change. However, a review of 11 exercise interventions that included measures of body composition change (Martin Ginis, Bassett, & Conlin, 2012) revealed that only six studies produced a statistically significant relationship between such changes and body image improvements. Furthermore, body composition change accounted for less than 15 percent of the variance in body image change, indicating that it plays a relatively minor role in body image improvements.

Changes in strength and cardiovascular fitness also seem to be minimally related to changes in body image. Martin Ginis and colleagues (2012) reported that only four published interventions examined the association between strength change and body image change, and only two yielded a significant association. Likewise, of six interventions that measured cardiovascular fitness change, only one found fitness changes to be associated with body image improvements. When significant relationships have emerged, changes in aerobic fitness and strength have accounted for only modest variance (typically less than 20 per cent).

One explanation for these findings is that absolute improvements in fitness are not as important as the exerciser's *interpretation* of those improvements. For instance, some people may experience large improvements in body image after losing relatively small amounts of fat and/or gaining minute amounts of muscle mass, while others may remain body dissatisfied despite losing considerable fat and/or significantly increasing their lean muscle mass. Body image responses to the physical changes will depend on whether the individual has moved closer to his/her body ideal. In short, *perceptions* of changes in fitness likely play a more important role than *actual* fitness changes when determining the effects of exercise on body image.

A recent exercise training study (Martin Ginis, McEwan, Josse, & Phillips, 2012) examined the relative importance of perceived versus actual fitness changes for body image change. Participants were 97 overweight and obese women involved in a 16-week diet, aerobic, and strength-training intervention. The investigators measured change in body image, and perceived and actual changes in aerobic fitness, strength, and body composition. Hierarchical regression analyses revealed that actual fitness changes accounted for just 9 percent of the variance in changes in body satisfaction while perceived fitness changes accounted for an additional 38 percent. In this sample of women, perceived fitness improvements were more relevant to body image change than actual improvements. Men's body image also seems to be more influenced by perceived than actual fitness improvements. Researchers (Martin Ginis, Eng, Arbour, Hartman, & Phillips, 2005) examined the extent to which perceived and actual changes in muscularity, strength, and body fat were related to men's body image improvements following a 5–day-per-week, 12-week strength training program. Changes in all three types of fitness perceptions—but none of the objective fitness measures—were significantly associated with changes in body image. Taken together, these results suggest that body image is most likely to improve when exercisers perceive a meaningful transformation in their physique and their physical capabilities.

Changes in self-efficacy

Self-efficacy refers to beliefs in one's capabilities to organize and execute the activities required to produce a given outcome (Bandura, 1997). Research has shown conclusively that exercise training programs increase physical self-efficacy (McAuley, Mailey, Szabo, & Gothe, Chapter 14, this volume). Such changes reflect an increased sense of personal control and mastery over one's body that, in turn, can bolster body image (Lindwall & Lindgren, 2005).

In their review, Martin Ginis, Bassett and colleagues (2012) identified three intervention studies that tested the relationship between self-efficacy change and body image change. Significant relationships emerged in all three studies and the predictive strength of self-efficacy was greater than the predictive strength of various objective measures of physical fitness such as body fat and aerobic fitness. More recently, Martin Ginis and colleagues (2012) found that although self-efficacy accounted for a significant 3 percent of the variance in body satisfaction change after controlling for actual fitness changes, perceived fitness improvements explained an additional 38 percent of the variance beyond self-efficacy.

Once again, the evidence suggests that when it comes to using exercise to improve body image, actual changes in physical abilities are not nearly as important as the experience and interpretation of those changes. However, an important caveat is that virtually all of this evidence is based on studies that measured changes in mechanism variables and changes in body image variables at the same time-point (i.e., at the end of the study). Such designs and analyses preclude any causal interpretations; prospective designs and meditational analyses are needed to establish firm conclusions regarding the mechanistic role of perceived fitness and self-efficacy for driving body image change.

Moderators of the effects of exercise on body image

The meta-analytic reviews have produced mixed evidence as to whether the effects of exercise on body image are moderated by characteristics of the exerciser (e.g., sex, age, gender-role orientation) and the exercise intervention (e.g., type, intensity, frequency). For instance, regarding a participant's sex as a moderator, the most recent meta-analysis found no significant differences in the effects of exercise on body image for men and women (Campbell & Hausenblas, 2009), whereas a previous meta-analysis found a larger effect for women (Hausenblas & Fallon, 2006). Similarly, regarding age as a moderator, the most recent meta-analysis yielded larger effects for older adults than youth (Campbell & Hausenblas), whereas a previous meta-analysis produced the opposite finding (Hausenblas & Fallon). With regard to exercise characteristics, the results of an intervention comparing aerobic and resistance exercise (Tucker & Mortell, 1993) produced superior body image effects for resistance training whereas the meta-analytic data (Campbell & Hausenblas) suggest the effects of the two modalities are equivalent.

Such equivocal findings suggest that other factors may be at play. Specifically, we propose that the exerciser's *body image ideals* supersede moderators such as age, sex, and exercise characteristics. For example, an individual with a body image goal of gaining muscle mass (typically produced through an intensive strength-training program) may experience little change in body image following a 6-week aerobic exercise program (typically resulting in little or no gain in muscle mass). Alternatively, an individual with a body image goal of losing body fat may experience significant improvements in body image following the same 6-week aerobic exercise program. Consistent with this perspective, preliminary data (Martin Ginis, McEwan et al. 2012) indicate that greater progress toward one's goals is associated with greater increases in body satisfaction.

We also propose that variables that have been considered moderators of the exercise–body image relationship may actually be moderators of *body image goals*. For instance, body image ideals are known to vary between the sexes, across cultures, and as a function of age and gender roles. Such variability may explain why the same exercise program can have a different effect on the body image for individuals drawn from different populations. Likewise, the explanation that body image goals are a key underlying moderator may help explain why different types (e.g., aerobic versus anaerobic), intensities, and amounts of exercise can differentially impact body image. Again, depending on the individual's body image goals, a given type and amount of exercise may be sufficient to improve body image for some, and insufficient for others.

Exercise and body image: the dark side

For some individuals, exercise may exacerbate body image concerns. For example, people who are motivated to exercise primarily for appearance-related reasons (e.g., weight control) are more likely to develop body image disturbance than those who exercise for other reasons (e.g., health, enjoyment; Strelan & Hargreaves, 2005). Likewise, attainment of personal fitness goals may generally lead to body image improvements (Martin Ginis, Bassett et al., 2012), but unrealistic expectations for body appearance change may exacerbate body image concerns in exercisers who do not perceive progress toward their goals. In addition, the pursuit of unrealistic body change goals can lead to excessive exercise.

Excessive exercise, also known as exercise dependence syndrome, is characterized by exercise that is uncontrollable, extreme, and obsessive and results in negative physiological and/or psychological symptoms (Hausenblas & Symons Downs, 2002). With primary exercise dependence, exercise is performed simply for the sake of exercising. With secondary dependence, exercise is used as a strategy to control body composition (Pierce, 1994). For individuals who are highly body dissatisfied, the compulsive need to exercise can control their lives. In some instances, self-regulatory behaviors that are normally considered positive and facilitative—such as scheduling exercise into one's day or setting exercise goals—can become obsessive and a concomitant of body image disturbance (e.g., Courtney, Munroe-Chandler, & Gammage, 2009).

Because men and women have different body ideals, excessive exercise behaviors typically differ between the sexes. For women, striving to achieve the societal ideal of a lean and thin body often involves calorie-burning activities (e.g., running). For men, striving to achieve the ideal of a muscular and lean body typically involves muscle-building activities (e.g., strength training). Regardless of exercise type, excessive activity can lead to physical (e.g., neuroendocrine system imbalances, suppression of the immune system; Fry, Morton, & Keast, 1991) and psychological problems (e.g., mood disturbances; Raglin, 1990).

The combination of body image disturbance and excessive exercise is particularly dangerous. This combination often presents itself in women with eating disorders such as anorexia nervosa—a disorder that can damage virtually every organ in the body and be fatal (Crow et al., 2009). Indeed, it is estimated that 40–80 percent of women with clinical eating disorders are also compulsive exercisers (Davis et al., 1997). In men, the combination of excessive exercise and body dissatisfaction is a risk factor for steroid use—a behavior linked to numerous physiological (e.g., increased risk for cardiovascular disease and liver disease) and psychological health problems (e.g., psychotic and manic episodes, depression; Cafri et al., 2005).

Interestingly, steroid use does not necessarily improve body image. Studies of recreational weightlifters have shown that those who use anabolic steroids tend to feel worse about their appearance than those who do not (Kanayama, Pope, Cohane, & Hudson, 2003). This finding raises the possibility that men with body image disturbance may be drawn to exercise-related activities that they believe will bring them closer to their body ideals. In support of this notion, Hildebrandt and colleagues (2006) found that over 70 percent of weightlifters had a body image disturbance and nearly 17 percent met the DSM-IV-TR criteria for body dysmorphic disorder (BDD)—a psychiatric disorder characterized by excessive preoccupation with a perceived defect of one's body. Given that only 1.4 percent of men in the general population meet the criteria for BDD (Rief, Buhlmann, Wilhelm, Borkenhagen, & Brahler, 2006), it seems that a disproportionately large number of men with BDD engage in weightlifting. Taken together, research on individuals with clinical body image disturbances (e.g., BDD) and related psychiatric disorder (e.g., anorexia nervosa) suggests that in these clinical populations, other forms of body image therapy (e.g., cognitive-behavioral and experiential therapies) may be more appropriate than exercise.

Limitations and future directions

In this section, we discuss key issues to be addressed in future research as well as some limitations of the existing research.

Theory development

As outlined in this chapter, there is still much to be learned about the mechanisms by which exercise exerts its effects, and the conditions when exercise is most versus least effective for eliciting body image improvements. A primary hindrance to the study of mediators and moderators has been the lack of an explicit model or framework to guide exercise and body image research. Currently, there are no frameworks explicitly designed to explain the effects of exercise on body image, although some investigators have couched their studies and hypotheses in complementary frameworks such as Bandura's (1997) Social Cognitive Theory and the Exercise and Self-Esteem Model (EXSEM; Sonstroem & Morgan, 1989). Recently, Martin Ginis, Bassett et al. (2012) developed a very basic model to help body image researchers select measures of putative mediator and moderator variables to be included in exercise training studies (see Figure 15.1). Testing relationships in this model will be vital to developing a theory to account for the effects of exercise on body image.

The dose–response relationship

Epidemiological data indicate that with larger volumes of exercise come greater improvements in health and larger reductions in disease risk (Warburton, Katzmarzyk, Rhodes, & Shephard, 2007). It is not known if a similar dose–response relationship exists between exercise and body image. To date, the relationship has been examined primarily through meta-analyses. Of the four exercise prescription components (frequency, intensity, type, time), only intensity has shown a positive relationship with body image change (Hausenblas & Fallon, 2006; Reel et al., 2007). The meta-analytic evidence indicates that body image benefits are greater for moderate-than mild-intensity exercise, but no additional benefits are incurred with heavy-intensity exercise (Campbell & Hausenblas, 2009; Hausenblas & Fallon, 2006). Within individual studies, the few investigations that have tested for a dose–response relationship have yielded mixed results. A couple of studies have shown greater participation leads to greater body image improvements, while other studies have found no such relationship (for a review, see Martin Ginis, Bassett et al., 2012). Clearly, there is a need to further examine dose–response effects to determine how much exercise is necessary to obtain short- and long-term body image improvements. Furthermore, given the potential risks associated with excessive exercise, there is merit in determining whether the exercise–body image relationship is truly linear or if it is curvilinear (i.e., an inverted U).

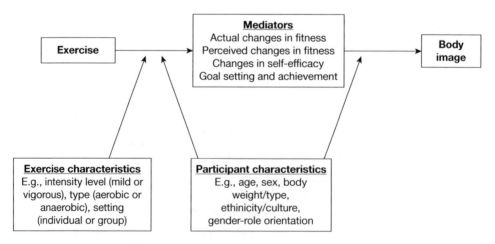

Figure 15.1 Basic model to guide research examining the effects of exercise interventions on body image (adapted from Martin Ginis, Bassett, & Conlin, 2012).

Determining the body image dimensions influenced by exercise

A limitation of the extant research is that most exercise studies have focused only on the cognitive and affective dimensions of body image (Martin Ginis, Bassett et al., 2012). Exercise may differentially affect thoughts, feelings, perceptions, and behaviors toward one's body. The four dimensions of body image are related but conceptually distinguishable constructs that require separate measurement approaches. To fully understand the effects of exercise on body image, researchers need to expand their scope to include appropriate measures of all dimensions. Having said that, exercise researchers are doing an excellent job of selecting the most valid and reliable body image measures available for their training studies. Ninety-five percent of the studies included in Campbell and Hausenblas's (2009) meta-analysis utilized psychometrically sound measures. Nevertheless, as researchers expand the measurement of body image dimensions in their studies, it will be important to consider the appropriateness of measures for different target populations, and to confirm the validity, reliability, and responsiveness of measures within study samples (see Bassett & Martin Ginis, 2009; Thompson, 2004).

The acute effects of exercise

Although most exercise studies have looked at the long-term effects of training on trait measures of body image, emerging research indicates that an acute bout of exercise can have a positive impact on state body image. For example, over a 10-day period, women's state body dissatisfaction was found to be lower immediately after exercise than at random points throughout the day (LePage & Crowther, 2010). Further research is needed to determine the mechanisms that underlie these improvements, the conditions when they are most likely to emerge, and how long the effects persist. There would also be merit in examining whether the accumulation of acute body image-enhancing bouts of exercise contributes to sustained improvements in trait body image. When addressing these issues, investigators will need to carefully consider the appropriateness of state and/or trait body image measures for their research questions. Trait measures may be insensitive to the effects of acute exercise manipulations (Martin Ginis, Murru, Conlin, & Strong, 2011). Hence, interpretation of some extant acute exercise studies has been limited because investigators have reported only the effects on trait (and not state) body image outcomes. The careful selection of state versus trait measures is integral to advancing knowledge regarding the acute and long-term effects of exercise on body image.

The effects of exercise on men's body image

Exercise and body image research has disproportionately focused on women. For example, in their meta-analysis of 57 exercise-training studies, Campbell and Hausenblas (2009) were able to extract 56 effect sizes for women and just 12 for men. Although they reported no differences in the effects of exercise for men versus women, with so relatively few studies of men to draw on, it is difficult to speak to the generalizability of this conclusion. Moreover, we know very little about mechanisms that drive exercise-induced body image change in men and variables that may moderate such changes. Given that men generally have a very different body ideal than women, it is likely that the mediators and moderators of body image change are also different. These issues require investigation.

A key limitation of the existing research on exercise and male body image is that many studies have utilized measures that do not fully capture men's body image concerns. Historically, the desire for a thin appearance has been equated with body image dissatisfaction (Thompson,

Heinberg, Altabe, & Tantleff-Dunn, 1999). Although measures that tap into concerns about not being sufficiently thin are appropriate for assessing women's body image, some men may be body dissatisfied because they believe they are too thin and not sufficiently muscular. Muscularity is a highly desirable trait for men (Cafri & Thompson, 2004), and a source of male body image concern. Measures of muscularity satisfaction, such as the Drive for Muscularity scale (McCreary & Sasse, 2000), can provide important information about the effects of exercise on men's body image. Measures of changes in muscularity concerns, coupled with measures that tap into men's concerns about body fatness, should be included in future studies of exercise and male body image.

Psychophysiological correlates of exercise-induced body image change

Preliminary data suggest that body image concerns may be related to biometric indicators of physiological stress. Putterman and Linden (2006) examined the relationship between body image and cortisol—a stress hormone that plays a critical role in regulating several bodily functions. They found that women's afternoon cortisol levels were negatively correlated with body image such that the highest levels of cortisol were present among women who felt worst about their bodies. On the one hand, the high levels of cortisol may have been due to a comorbid mood disorder, as people with anxiety and depressive disorders have elevated levels of cortisol secretion (McEwen, 1998). On the other hand, body image dissatisfaction may be a unique source of stress that increases cortisol secretion independent of mood disorders.

Exercise training has been shown to reduce cortisol secretion *vis-à-vis* re-regulation of the hypothalamic pituitary adrenal (HPA) axis (e.g., Foley et al., 2008). A question for future investigation is whether exercise-induced improvements in body image yield concomitant reductions in cortisol. Demonstrating such a relationship would attest to the potential for utilizing a biopsychosocial approach to better understand the effects of exercise on body image.

Conclusions

In general, exercise is an effective treatment for improving body image. Although the mechanisms underlying these effects are not fully understood, there is good evidence that perceived changes in physical fitness are a more potent determinant of body image improvements than are actual fitness improvements. A more complete understanding of the mechanisms underlying the effects of body image would contribute to the design of more effective exercise interventions. Furthermore, the effects of exercise on body image may depend on characteristics of the exerciser and the exercise intervention itself. The body image ideals of the exerciser, and the effects of the intervention on bringing the exerciser closer to his or her ideal, may be particularly important.

Under certain circumstances, exercise may exacerbate body image concerns, particularly when exercise is obsessive and compulsive. Future research should aim to determine the optimal exercise intervention characteristics to improve body image and the individuals who stand to benefit most from exercise as treatment for body image disturbance. A more complete understanding of the intricacies of the exercise–body image relationship could have important implications for improving mental health.

References

Bandura, A. (1997). *Self-efficacy: The exercise of control.* New York: W.H. Freeman.

Bassett, R. L., & Martin Ginis, K. A. (2009). Issues pertaining to body image measurement in exercise research. In S. B. Greene (Ed.), *Body image: Perceptions, interpretations, and attitudes* (pp. 245–254). New York: Nova Science.

Cafri, G., Olivardia, R., & Thompson, J. K. (2008). Symptom characteristics and psychiatric comorbidity among males with muscle dysmorphia. *Comprehensive Psychiatry*, *49*, 374–379.

Cafri, G., & Thompson, J. K. (2004). Measuring male body image: A review of the current methodology. *Psychology of Men and Muscularity*, *5*, 18–29.

Cafri, G., Thompson, J. K., Ricciardelli, L., McCabe, M., Smolak, L., & Yesalis, C. (2005). Pursuit of the muscular ideal: Physical and psychological consequences and putative risk factors. *Clinical Psychology Review*, *25*, 215–239.

Campbell, A., & Hausenblas, H. A. (2009). Effects of exercise interventions on body image: A meta-analysis. *Journal of Health Psychology*, *14*, 1–14.

Cash, T. F. (2004). Body image: Past, present, and future. *Body Image*, *1*, 1–5.

Cash, T. F., & Deagle, E. A. (1997). The nature and extent of body-image disturbances in anorexia nervosa and bulimia nervosa: A meta-analysis. *International Journal of Eating Disorders*, *22*, 107–125.

Cash, T. F., Phillips, K. A., Santos, M. T., & Hrabosky, J. I. (2004). Measuring "negative body image": Validation of the Body Image Disturbance Questionnaire in a nonclinical population. *Body Image*, *1*, 363–372.

Cash, T. F., & Smolak, L. (2011). *Body image: A handbook of science, practice, and prevention* (2nd ed.). New York: The Guilford Press.

Cohen, T., & Esther, M. (1993). Depressed mood and concern with weight and shape in normal young women. *International Journal of Eating Disorders*, *14*, 223–227.

Courtney, R. A., Munroe-Chandler, K. J., & Gammage, K. L. (2009). The relationship between the drive for muscularity and muscle dysmorphia in male and female weight trainers. *Journal of Strength and Conditioning Research*, *23*, 1656–1662.

Crow, S. J., Peterson, C. B., Swanson, S. A., Raymond, N. C., Specker, S., Eckert, E. D., & Mitchell, J. F. (2009). Increased mortality in bulimia nervosa and other eating disorders. *American Journal of Psychiatry*, *166*, 1342–1346.

Davis, C., Katzman, D. K., Kaptein, S., Kirsh, C., Brewer, H., Kalmbach, . . . Kaplan, A. S. (1997). The prevalence of high-level exercise in the eating disorders: Etiological implications. *Comprehensive Psychiatry*, *38*, 321–326.

Davison, T. E., & McCabe, M. P. (2005). Relationships between men's and women's body image and their psychological, social, and sexual functioning. *Sex Roles*, *52*, 463–475.

Davison, T. E., & McCabe, M. P. (2006). Adolescent body image and psychosocial functioning. *The Journal of Social Psychology*, *146*, 15–30.

Fast facts . . . fun facts . . . at your fingertips (2011). Retrieved August 18, 2011 from http://www.cosmetic surgery.com/articles/archive/an~82/

Fisher, E., & Thompson, J. K. (1994). A comparative evaluation of cognitive-behavioral therapy (CBT) versus exercise therapy (ET) for the treatment of body image disturbance: Preliminary findings. *Behavior Modification*, *18*, 171–185.

Foley, L. S., Prapavessis, H., Osuch, E. A., De Pace, J., Murphy, B. A., & Podolinsky, N. J. (2008). An examination of potential mechanisms for exercise as a treatment for depression: A pilot study. *Mental Health and Physical Activity*, *1*, 69–73.

Fox, K. R. (2000). The effects of exercise on self-perceptions and self-esteem. In S. J. H. Biddle, K. R. Fox, & S. H. Boutcher (Eds.), *Physical activity and psychological well-being* (pp. 88–118). London: Routhledge & Kegan Paul.

Frederick, D. A., Peplau, L. A., & Lever, J. (2006). The swimsuit issue: Correlates of body image in a sample of 52,677 heterosexual adults. *Body Image*, *3*, 413–419.

Fry, A. C., Morton, A. R., & Keast, D. (1991). Overtraining in athletes. An update. *Sports Medicine*, *12*, 32–65.

Gentile, B., Grabe, S., Dolan-Pascoe, B., Twenge, J. M., Wells, B. E., & Maitino, A. (2009). Gender differences in domain-specific self-esteem: A meta-analysis. *Review of General Psychology*, *13*, 34–45.

Hausenblas, H. A., & Fallon, E. A. (2006). Exercise and body image: A meta-analysis. *Psychology and Health*, *21*, 33–47.

Hausenblas, H. A., & Symons Downs, D. (2002). Exercise dependence: A systematic review. *Psychology of Sport and Exercise*, *3*, 89–123.

Hildebrandt, T., Schlundt, D., Langenbucher, J., & Chung, T. (2006). Presence of muscle dysmorphia symptomology among male weightlifters. *Comprehensive Psychiatry*, *47*, 127–135.

Kanayama, G., Pope, H. G., Cohane, G., & Hudson, J. I. (2003). Risk factors for anabolic-androgenic steroid use among weightlifters: A case-control study. *Drug and Alcohol Dependence*, *71*, 77–86.

LePage, M. L., & Crowther, J. H. (2010). The effects of exercise on body satisfaction and affect. *Body Image*, *7*, 124–130.

Lichtenberger, C. M., Martin Ginis, K. A., MacKenzie, C. L., & McCartney, N. (2003). Body image and depressive symptoms as correlates of self-reported versus clinician-reported physiologic function. *Journal of Cardiopulmonary Rehabilitation, 23*, 53–59.

Lindwall, M., & Lindgren, E. C. (2005). The effects of a 6-month exercise intervention programme on physical self-perceptions and social physique anxiety in non-physically active adolescent Swedish girls. *Psychology of Sport and Exercise, 6*, 643–658.

Marketdata Enterprises (2011). The U.S. weight loss and diet control market (11th ed.). Information retrieved August 18, 2011 from www.worldometers.info/weight-loss/

Martin Ginis, K. A., Bassett, R. L., & Conlin, C. (2012). Body image and exercise. In Edmund O. Acevedo (Ed.), *Oxford handbook of exercise psychology* (pp. 55–75). New York: Oxford University Press.

Martin Ginis, K. A., Eng, J. J., Arbour, K. P., Hartman, J. W., & Phillips, S. M. (2005). Mind over muscle? Sex differences in the relationship between body image change and subjective and objective physical changes following a 12-week strength-training program. *Body Image, 2*, 363–372.

Martin Ginis, K. A., McEwan, D., Josse, A., & Phillips, S. M. (2012). Body image change in obese and overweight women enrolled in a weight-loss intervention: The importance of perceived versus actual physical changes. *Body Image, 9*, 311–317.

Martin Ginis, K. A., Murru, E. C., Conlin, C., & Strong, H. (2011). Construct validation of a state version of the Social Physique Anxiety Scale. *Body Image, 8*, 52–57.

McCreary, D. R., & Sasse, D. K. (2000). An exploration of the drive for muscularity in adolescent boys and girls. *Journal of American College Health, 48*, 297–304.

McEwen, B. S. (1998). Stress, adaptation, and disease: Allostasis and allostatic load. *Annals of the New York Academy of Sciences, 840*, 33–44.

Olivardia, R. (2001). Mirror, mirror on the wall, who's the largest of them all? The features and phenomenology of muscle dysmorphia. *Harvard Review of Psychiatry, 9*, 254–259.

Olivardia, R., Pope, H. G. Jr., Borowiecki III, J. J., & Cohane, G. H. (2004). Biceps and body image: The relationship between muscularity and self-esteem, depression, and eating disorder symptoms. *Psychology of Men and Masculinity, 5*, 112–120.

Paxton, S. J., Neumark-Sztainer, D., Hannan, P. J., & Eisenberg, M. E. (2006). Body dissatisfaction prospectively predicts depressive mood and low self-esteem in adolescent girls and body. *Journal of Clinical Child and Adolescent Psychology, 35*, 539–549.

Phillips, K. A., O'Sullivan, R. L., & Pope, H. G. Jr. (1997). Muscle dysmorphia. *Journal of Clinical Psychiatry, 58*, 361.

Pierce, E. F. (1994). Exercise dependence syndrome in runners. *Sports Medicine, 18*, 149–155.

Polivy, J., & Herman, C. P. (2002). Causes of eating disorders. *Annual Review of Psychology, 53*, 187–213.

Putterman, E., & Linden, W. (2006). Cognitive dietary restraint and cortisol: Importance of pervasive concerns with appearance. *Appetite, 47*, 64–76.

Raglin, J. S. (1990). Exercise and mental health: Beneficial and detrimental effects. *Sports Medicine, 9*, 323–329.

Reel, J. J., Greenleaf, C., Baker, W. K., Aragon, S., Bishop, D., Cachaper, C., . . . Hattie, J. (2007). Relations of body concerns and exercise behaviour: A meta-analysis. *Psychological Reports, 101*, 927–942.

Rief, W., Buhlmann, U., Wilhelm, S., Borkenhagen, A., & Brahler, E. (2006). The prevalence of body dysmorphic disorder: A population-based survey. *Psychological Medicine, 36*, 877–885.

Sonstroem, R. J., & Morgan, W. P. (1989). Exercise and self-esteem: Rationale and model. *Medicine and Science in Sports and Exercise, 21*, 329–337.

Stice, E., & Whitenton, K. (2002). Risk factors for body dissatisfaction in adolescent girls: A longitudinal investigation. *Developmental Psychology, 38*, 669–678.

Strelan, P., & Hargreaves, D. (2005). Reasons for exercise and body esteem: Men's responses to self-objectification. *Sex Roles, 53*, 495–503.

Thompson, J. K. (2004). The (mis)measurement of body image: Ten strategies to improve assessment for applied and research purposes. *Body Image, 1*, 7–14.

Thompson, J. K., Heinberg, L., Altabe, M., & Tantleff-Dunn, S. (1999). *Exacting beauty*. Washington, DC: American Psychological Association.

Tucker, L. A., & Mortell, R. (1993). Comparison of the effects of walking and weight training programs on body image in middle-aged women: An experimental study. *American Journal of Health Promotion, 8*, 34–42.

Warburton, D. E. R., Katzmarzyk, P. T., Rhodes, R. E., & Shephard, R. J. (2007). Evidence-informed physical activity guidelines for Canadian adults. *Applied Physiology, Nutrition, and Metabolism, 32*, S16–S68.

PART 5

Cognitive function across the lifespan

Edited by
Jennifer L. Etnier

16

PHYSICAL ACTIVITY

Relations with children's cognitive and academic performance

Jennifer I. Gapin, Lisa A. Barella, and Jennifer L. Etnier

School-aged children in the United States are not performing well academically compared to children in other developed nations around the world (Organization for Economic Co-Operation and Development, 2004, 2007). The No Child Left Behind Elementary and Secondary Education Act was enacted in 2002 to address the concerns with the education system in the United States through a focus on accountability in important subject areas (Hardman, 2004). However, because this act did not include physical education (PE) or health as "important subject areas" and because of increased pressure for schools to meet state standards for academic performance, time and resources devoted to PE have declined in most schools (Hardman, 2004; Keyes, 2004).

The irony of these events is that there is evidence supporting the potentially beneficial role of physical activity (PA) for cognitive performance by children. This evidence comes in the form of studies demonstrating relationships between PA, physical fitness, or weight status and measures of academic achievement, cognitive performance, or cerebral structure and function. Although conclusions drawn in narrative reviews are mixed (Murray, Low, Hollis, Cross, & Davis, 2007; Taras, 2005), results from a meta-analytic review of the research with children suggest that PA has a small, yet significant effect on cognitive performance (Sibley & Etnier, 2003). The difficulty in bringing this literature to consensus is related to generally poor experimental designs. Most of the studies rely on correlational or quasi-experimental designs, and only a few studies have used true-experimental designs. Additional challenges of this literature relate to the various methods that have been used to assess PA and cognition. With regard to PA, the close relationship between the constructs of PA (the behavior), physical fitness (which is determined by PA and genetics), and weight status (which is determined by PA, diet, and genetics) means that all of these constructs have been used to make inferences about PA. With regard to cognition, both behavioral measures of cognitive performance and neuropsychological measures that provide indications of brain structure and function have been used. In this review of the literature, studies are organized by experimental design, by cognitive outcome, and by PA construct, and only studies that include a measure of PA or fitness are discussed.

Correlational studies

Academic achievement

Many researchers have used correlational designs to explore the relationship between PA and academic achievement in children. In these studies, PA has been assessed directly using accelerometers or self-report measures or has been inferred from measures of physical fitness or body mass index (BMI). Academic achievement has been measured using school-based measures of academic achievement (i.e., standardized tests), measures of cognitive performance in particular subject areas (i.e., grades), or self-reported academic performance (i.e., self-reported grades).

PA and academic achievement

Several researchers have explored relationships between PA and academic performance in elementary, middle-school, and high-school samples. The focus of these studies has primarily been on PA, but some have also included measures of sedentary behavior and/or BMI.

Wang and Veugelers (2008) investigated interrelationships between self-reported measures of PA, sedentary behavior, diet quality, and self-esteem; measures of height and weight; and standardized test performance in fifth-grade students (n = 4,945), ages 10–11. Results showed that PA was not predictive of test performance. Interestingly, however, more sedentary behavior was predictive of worse test performance and lower self-esteem. Results of this study may indicate that variability in PA is not as important as is the amount of time spent in sedentary activities.

Sigfusdottir, Kristjansson, and Allegrante (2007) were interested in the relationship between PA, BMI, diet, and academic performance. Self-reported data from a large sample of ninth- and tenth-grade students (n = 5,810) in Iceland were obtained. PA was assessed by asking students to self-report how often they participated in various levels of PA, while BMI was calculated from self-reported height and weight. Academic achievement was determined from self-reported average grades in four core subjects. Results indicated that higher levels of PA and lower BMI were significantly associated with better academic achievement.

Fox, Barr-Anderson, Neumark-Sztainer, and Wall (2010) attempted to disentangle effects of sport team participation from effects of PA. They examined the relationships among sports team participation, self-reported PA, and self-reported grade point average (GPA) in middle-school and high-school students (n = 4,746). Participants self-reported the two grades that they received most often and these were averaged (GPA). For middle-school boys, GPA was higher for those who participated on a sports team compared to those who did not. After controlling for socioeconomic variables and race/ethnicity, the independent associations of sports team participation and moderate-to-vigorous PA on academic achievement were assessed for the high-school students. Moderate-to-vigorous PA and sports team participation were both associated with better GPA in high-school girls; however, for high-school boys only sports team participation was associated with better GPA. Thus, in this study, sports team participation was a consistent predictor of better GPA, but PA itself was only predictive for high-school girls.

Only one study has used a longitudinal design to study the influence of PA on changes in academic achievement over time. Carlson et al. (2008) measured standardized test performance in students (n = 5,316) annually from kindergarten through fifth grade. PA was assessed as the teachers' report of the number of times/week and minutes/day the students participated in PE. Cross-sectional associations between PA and academic achievement showed no relationship for boys. For girls in kindergarten, first, and fifth grade, those with moderate and high levels of PA performed better in reading than those with low levels of PA. For girls in kindergarten and first grade, significant differences were also observed for math performance with students who participated in more PA performing better than those with less PA. When longitudinal associations were analyzed, no significant relationships were found for boys; however, for math and reading, girls in the high-PA category had significant gains in their mathematics and reading scores over time when compared to girls in the low-PA category. Thus, the results of this study indicated that PA is important to the cognitive gains experienced during elementary school by girls, but is not a significant predictor of cognitive gains for boys.

In summary, researchers generally report that greater PA or less sedentary behavior is predictive of better academic performance. Additionally, there is evidence that correlations are stronger for girls than for boys (Carlson et al., 2008; Fox et al., 2010). However, results from these studies must be interpreted cautiously because in addition to the limitations inherent in correlational designs, these studies also have limitations relative to the measures used – all of the studies rely on self-reported PA, one study used proxy measures of PA (Carlson et al., 2008), and two used self-reported measures of academic performance (Fox et al., 2010; Sigfusdottir et al., 2007).

Fitness and academic achievement

In studies assessing the relationship between physical fitness and academic achievement, physical fitness has typically been measured using the Fitnessgram. This is a standardized battery consisting of measures of aerobic fitness, muscular fitness, flexibility, and BMI. In some studies all of the tests have been used, while in others only the measure of aerobic fitness has been used. Academic achievement has been measured using mandatory standardized state examinations or by calculating a summary score from grades in courses.

In two studies, this relationship was tested in elementary-school children. Castelli, Hillman, Buck, and Erwin (2007) assessed the relationship in third- and fifth-grade students (n = 259). Results showed that aerobic fitness and muscular fitness were predictive of better performance on math, reading, and total academic achievement tests, and flexibility was predictive of better math and total academic achievement. Consistent with these findings, lower BMI was associated with better academic achievement for all three measures (total, math, reading). Eveland-Sayers, Farley, Fuller, Morgan, and Caputo (2009) assessed these same relationships in third-, fourth-, and fifth-grade children (n = 134). Results indicated that aerobic fitness and muscular fitness were predictive of better math performance. Interestingly, these relationships were stronger for girls than for boys. Thus, in elementary-school children, fitness was consistently predictive of math performance and was also reported to be predictive of reading and total scores.

Chomitz et al. (2009) explored the relationship between fitness and academic achievement in fourth-, fifth-, sixth-, and eighth-grade students (n = 1,841). The number of passing scores (according to criteria established by the Amateur Athletic Union and the Cooper Institute) for the fitness tests was summed and used to predict academic achievement. After controlling for gender, weight status, grade, ethnicity, and measures of socioeconomic status, the number of fitness tests passed predicted math and English test scores. This provides suggestive evidence regarding the importance of fitness for performance in particular academic achievement areas.

In a study including a similar age group of children (fifth, sixth, and ninth grades; n = 1,989), Roberts, Freed, and McCarthy (2010) found that scoring lower on the academic achievement tests for math, reading, and language was significantly related to having a BMI in the overweight or obese category. Additionally, regression models showed that for every additional minute it took to complete the 1-mile run, math performance was 1.9 points lower and reading performance was 1.1 points lower. Although not a causal design, the findings of this study suggest that improvements in fitness might result in improvements in math and reading performance.

Welk et al. (2010) looked at the relationship across students in grades 3–12. After controlling for school-level indicators of socioeconomic status, ethnicity, and school size, lower BMI and higher aerobic fitness were both associated with better academic achievement. When gender relationships were examined, stronger correlations were reported between BMI and academic achievement for girls across all grades; however, similar correlations were observed between aerobic fitness and academic achievement for boys and girls across all grades. Relative to grade, stronger relationships between aerobic fitness and academic achievement were found for middle-school children than for elementary-school children.

Davis and Cooper (2011) examined the relationships between measures of fitness and fatness with tests of cognition and measures of academic achievement in overweight sedentary 7–11-year-olds (n = 170). Partial correlations with academic achievement (reading and math) revealed significant negative relationships for body fat and significant positive relationships for fitness.

In summary, the results of studies exploring relationships between fitness and academic performance suggest that better fitness predicts better academic performance across all age groups. Additionally, several studies indicated that lower BMI was also associated with better academic performance. Lastly, there is some evidence that relationships between PA or BMI and academic achievement are stronger for girls than for boys (Eveland-Sayers et al., 2009; Welk et al., 2010). Given the limitations of correlational designs, it is important to note that these correlations remained after statistically controlling for important confounds (Chomitz et al., 2009; Welk et al., 2010).

PA, fitness, and academic achievement

There are two studies in which PA and fitness were assessed in the same sample and used to predict academic achievement. These studies allow for an examination of the unique variance in academic achievement predicted by these two related variables.

Kwak et al. (2009) tested the relationship between PA, physical fitness, and academic achievement (grades for 17 courses) in ninth-grade Swedish students (n = 232). In girls, vigorous PA was significantly associated with academic achievement but this relationship was not mediated by fitness. In boys, fitness was significantly associated with academic achievement. Clearly, these findings are somewhat perplexing as vigorous PA and fitness are themselves highly correlated.

Edwards, Mauch, and Winkelman (2011) investigated how self-reported PA and aerobic fitness were associated with the academic performance of sixth-grade students (n = 800). Aerobic fitness, sport participation, and self-reported vigorous PA were predictive of higher math performance and both moderate and vigorous PA were predictive of better reading performance.

Together these two studies suggest that PA and fitness may have independent effects on various measures of academic performance. Future research will be necessary to clarify our understanding of the complex relationship between PA, fitness, and academic outcomes.

Summary for academic achievement

Results from correlational studies generally support a link between PA, fitness, and academic performance. This provides foundational evidence to support research to further our understanding of the specific nature of the relationship with regard to academic measures (e.g., to focus on specific types of cognitive abilities), to explore potential underlying mechanisms (e.g., through the use of psychophysiological measures), and to develop randomized control trials (RCTs) to establish causal relationships.

Cognitive task performance, neuroelectric indices, and brain structure

A number of studies have been conducted using laboratory-based measures to assess particular types of cognitive abilities sensitive to PA and/or to include neuroelectric indices or measures of brain structure to explore potential mechanisms. In contrast to the focus on PA in the correlational studies, the focus in these studies has been on aerobic fitness. The premise underlying these studies is that aerobic fitness provides an indication of long-term regular PA participation.

Aerobic fitness and cognitive task performance

Buck, Hillman, and Castelli (2008) assessed the relationship between fitness and performance on the Stroop task in boys and girls aged 7–12 years (n = 74). The Stroop task was used to measure the ability to perform in various cognitive domains (i.e., speed of processing and inhibition) and was completed on a separate day from the fitness tests. Results showed that higher aerobic fitness predicted better task performance on all conditions of the Stroop task. The authors concluded that aerobic fitness may be related to cognitive performance on a more general, rather than selective level.

Neiderer et al. (2011) used a cross-sectional and longitudinal study to examine relationships between aerobic fitness and measures of spatial working memory and attention. Pre-school children in Switzerland (n = 245) were assessed at baseline and 9 months later. In cross-sectional analyses, aerobic fitness was positively associated with attention and working memory; however, after adjusting for confounding variables (age, sex, BMI, parental education, native language, and linguistic region), working memory was no longer significantly associated with aerobic fitness. The longitudinal analyses showed that baseline fitness was independently associated with improved attention over time suggesting that higher fitness in pre-school is predictive of attention in later years.

Wu et al. (2011) tested the relationship between aerobic fitness and both cognitive performance and cognitive variability in 48 preadolescent children (M age = 10.1 years). After performing a $\dot{V}O_2$ max test, children were categorized into either a higher fit or lower fit group. On a separate day, children performed cognitive tasks to assess reaction time, response variability, and response accuracy to incongruent and congruent trials. Results showed that higher fit children had less variable response time and were more accurate across conditions. This suggests that fitness may be important for cognitive control processes.

In sum, results from these studies support a positive relationship between fitness and cognitive task performance. These studies include a wide age range (5–19 years) and cognitive tasks focused predominantly on measures of executive function including the Stroop task, the Erikson Flankers task, attention, and working memory.

Aerobic fitness and neuroelectric indices

Researchers interested in testing the effects of fitness on brain function have typically used electroencephalographic (EEG) measures to record event-related potentials (ERPs) known to be influenced by chronic aerobic exercise. ERPs are time-locked to either a stimulus or a response and are indicative of brain activity relative to the processing of that event. Of particular interest are P3 amplitude and latency, which are linked to attentional allocation and memory. Increased P3 amplitude indicates that more attentional resources are being allocated to a task, whereas a shorter P3 latency represents decreased processing time.

Hillman, Castelli, and Buck (2005) examined P3 amplitude and latency in relation to aerobic fitness and cognitive task performance. Higher fit and lower fit children (n = 24; M age = 9.6) performed a visual oddball task during which P3 amplitude and latency were recorded. Results showed that there was greater P3 amplitude and faster P3 latency for the higher fit children compared to the lower fit children. Although behavioral measures of cognitive performance were not included, this finding suggests that fitness may be related to better cognitive performance in children, specifically on tasks related to attention and working memory.

Hillman, Buck, Themanson, Pontifex, and Castelli (2009) assessed N2 amplitude (an index of response inhibition), error-related negativity (ERN) (an index of control monitoring for errors), and P_e amplitude (resource allocation following errors). It was predicted that higher fit children would have greater N2 and P3 amplitude and smaller ERN, thus indicating greater cognitive control as a function of fitness level. Preadolescent children were identified as being higher fit (n = 24) or lower fit (n = 24) based on an aerobic capacity test. Results indicated that for higher fit children as compared to lower fit children, performance on measures requiring inhibitory control was better, P3 amplitude was greater for all conditions, and ERN amplitude was decreased and P_e was increased during error trials. Thus, more efficient resource allocation and better cognitive function were associated with higher physical fitness at young ages.

Pontifex et al. (2011) examined differences in P3 and ERN components in higher and lower fit preadolescents (M age = 10; n = 48) while performing a Flankers task modified to examine responses based on task difficulty. Consistent with previous studies, higher fit children had greater P3 amplitude and shorter P3 latency compared to lower fit children. Also, higher fit children were better at modulating their cognitive control processes to match task difficulty, as indicated by smaller ERN amplitudes for the compatible task than for the incompatible task. Smaller ERN amplitudes suggest greater efficiency in tasks requiring cognitive control. This adds an important element to the research as it suggests that higher fit children are more easily able to selectively control cognitive processes to successfully meet the demands of a task.

Collectively, these studies suggest that aerobic fitness is related to neuroelectric changes in the brain that are indicative of cognitive function. Specifically, higher fit children have more efficient cognitive control processes, perform better on tasks of attention and working memory, and better allocate attention to meet task demands. Thus, maintaining a higher level of fitness at a young age appears to have a positive relationship with cognitive health and may help children to reach a higher level of academic achievement.

Aerobic fitness and brain structure

Two recent studies assessed the relationship between fitness and cognitive performance by examining structural differences in the brain via magnetic resonance imaging (MRI) (Chaddock, Erickson, Prakash, Kim, et al., 2010; Chaddock, Erickson, Prakash, VanPatter, et al., 2010). Regions examined included prefrontal cortex (executive function), hippocampus (memory performance), and basal ganglia (attentional control).

Researchers identified children (ages 9–10) as higher fit or lower fit based on a $\dot{V}O_2$ max test (Chaddock, Erickson, Prakash, Kim, et al., 2010; Chaddock, Erickson, Prakash, VanPatter, et al., 2010). MRI was used to assess dorsal and ventral striatum volumes and hippocampal volume. Results indicated that compared to lower fit children, higher fit children performed better on a Flankers task, more accurately on a relational memory task, and had greater dorsal striatum volumes and greater hippocampal volume.

These studies suggest that better performance by higher fit children might be explained by structural differences in the brain. Clearly, more studies are needed to replicate these findings before firm conclusions can be drawn.

Summary for cognitive task performance, neuroelectric indices, and brain structure

Overall, this small body of literature supports a positive relationship between aerobic fitness and cognitive task performance in children. Evidence of potential underlying mechanisms is provided through findings regarding neuroelectric and cerebral structure differences relative to fitness. These results indirectly suggest that fitness may provide children with a cognitive advantage in school, thus leading to greater academic achievement (Hillman, Kamijo, & Scudder, 2011).

However, while these studies contribute to our understanding of the association between fitness and various types of cognitive performance, they are limited in a few important ways. First, all of these studies are cross-sectional in nature and thus do not allow for the establishment of causality. Second, by focusing on laboratory tasks, the generalizability of these results to real-world cognitive performance (including academic achievement) is unclear.

Interventions

The few intervention studies that have assessed the effects of PA on academic outcomes have generally implemented the PA program within the school day and have measured academic performance either directly through scores on school-based achievement tests or indirectly through cognitive tests designed to reflect academic potential. These interventions are dominated by quasi-experimental designs in which random assignment has not been used, but there are a few studies in which classrooms or schools have been randomly assigned to conditions.

Quasi-experimental designs

PA and academic achievement

Shephard, Lavallee, Volle, LaBarre, and Baucage (1994) assigned two successive cohorts of students in grades 1–6 to an experimental condition that received one extra hour of PE per day. Students in the cohorts immediately before and after the experimental cohorts were assigned to a control condition that received standard PE. Academic achievement was measured by classroom grades for French language, math, English, and science. Results showed that students in grades 2, 3, 5, and 6 receiving additional PE time had significantly higher grades than controls. Further, girls had a larger improvement in grades than boys. These results suggest that additional PE time has a positive effect on teacher-assigned grades. Also of importance is the fact that grades did not decline for the experimental group even though there was one hour less per day devoted to academics.

PA in multi-component programs and academic achievement

Recently, researchers have examined the impact of multi-component school-based programs on academic performance in children. These programs generally include nutrition, healthy lifestyle education, and PA components designed to prevent and/or decrease obesity in children.

Nansel, Huang, Rovner, and Sanders-Butler (2010) assessed school records over 11 years to retrospectively examine standardized test scores following implementation of the Healthy Kids, Smart Kids program at an elementary school. The sample consisted of approximately 1000 predominately low-income African American students (4–12 years). The program promoted nutrition and PA within the school. The PA changes included the addition of 40–60 minutes of daily PA, a weekly aerobic circuit training course, the distribution of pedometers and activity diaries, and the availability of fitness classes before and after school 3 days per week. Results showed that standardized scores on the Iowa Test of Basic Skills increased each year for the 6 years following program implementation.

Shilts, Lamp, Horowitz, and Townsend (2009) assessed English and math performance following participation in the EatFit program. The EatFit program is an educational prevention program that teaches health and behavioral skills to encourage PA and healthy eating. Sixth-grade, low-income students (n = 84) received the program for 5 weeks and then scores on an academic assessment test were compared to a 5-week period in which students did not participate in the EatFit program. English and math scores were higher after the EatFit program compared to when they were not participating in the EatFit program.

Rosas, Case, and Tholstrup (2009) utilized the coordinated school health program model (CSHP) to retrospectively examine school progress and performance ratings and specific academic performance for 158 schools. The CSHP focuses on improving school health by planning and organizing health activities. Results showed that schools that implemented the CSHP to a greater extent had higher performance scores (indicating improvement on composite scores for reading, math, science, and social studies) and progress ratings (meeting performance targets in various subject areas, improving scores for students performing below national standards, and better graduation rates).

Hollar et al. (2010) examined the effectiveness of a school-based obesity prevention program (Healthier Options for Public Schoolchildren) with nutritional, curricula, and PA components on academic achievement. Five elementary schools were non-randomly assigned to be an intervention school (n = 4) or a control school (n = 1). Children in the intervention schools added a 10–15-minute desk-side PA program (TAKE 10! or WISERCISE) during the academic curriculum. In addition, when possible, teachers added structured PA during recess. Over 2 years, children in the intervention schools (n = 3,032) scored significantly higher on math than children in the control school (n = 737).

Summary for quasi-experimental studies

Results from multi-component studies show positive effects on academic performance. However, it is impossible to determine which particular aspects of the program contribute to the enhanced performance. Further, in these studies PA was not measured and it remains unclear as to how much PA actually may have increased. In the only quasi-experimental study that examined PA in isolation, PA neither helped nor harmed academic performance. Thus, results from this group of studies are suggestive of beneficial effects, but these effects cannot be attributed to PA per se.

Experimental designs

Academic achievement

Dwyer, Coonan, Leitch, Hetzel, and Baghurst (1983) examined the effects of increased PE time on academic performance by 500 fifth-grade students from seven primary schools. At each school, three classes were randomly assigned to one of two experimental groups (fitness or skill groups) or a control group (30 minutes' PE). Both experimental groups received 75 minutes of PA. The fitness group focused on elevating heart rate, whereas the skill group focused on active games without an emphasis on intensity. Results showed that there were no significant differences between experimental and control groups on math or reading scores. Results indicate that there was no decrease in academic performance as a result of more time devoted to PE (and less to academics) during the school day.

Sallis et al. (1999) investigated the effects of Sport, Play, and Active Recreation for Kids (SPARK) on academic performance in seven K-5 schools. SPARK students engage in high levels of PA during a 30-minute PE class, with the goal of achieving health-related fitness. Schools were randomly assigned to one of three conditions: SPARK with trained teachers, SPARK with specialists, and regular PE (control). Over 2 years, SPARK groups received twice as many minutes of PE as the control group. In contrast to expectations, academic performance in all groups declined from baseline to post-test. However, there were differences between the groups at the post-test. Students in the SPARK program led by specialists scored higher on reading, but lower on language compared to controls. Students in the SPARK program led by teachers had higher language, reading, and composite scores than controls. Because performance scores decreased for all students, clearly PA did not lead to improvements in performance; however, it again appears that the provision of time for PA at the expense of academic time did not have a detrimental effect on cognitive performance.

Coe, Pivarnik, Womack, Reeves, and Malina (2006) explored the effects of PE on academic performance in 214 sixth-grade students. Students were randomly assigned to receive PE during the first semester or the second semester. When not in the PE course, students took an elective. No effects on academic achievement were evident for the PA intervention in general; however, specific findings support the potential of vigorous PA in particular. In the first semester, students who performed any vigorous PA achieved higher academic scores than those who performed no vigorous PA. In the second semester, students who self-reported PA that met or exceeded Healthy People 2010 guidelines for vigorous PA achieved higher academic scores compared with students in both semesters who did not meet the guidelines. Importantly, vigorous PA reported outside school was also associated with academic performance. Results from this study, therefore, suggest that vigorous PA is of particular relevance to academic performance.

Cognitive task performance

Tuckman and Hinkle (1986) randomly assigned 154 children in grades 4–6 to an experimental group (12-week running program) or a control group (PE class of non-aerobic activities only). Both groups met three times per week for 30 minutes/session. There were no effects in either experimental group for perceptual motor skill or visual motor coordination; however, there were beneficial effects on creativity for those children assigned to the experimental group.

In a similar study conducted by Hinkle, Tuckman, and Sampson (1993), children in eighth grade (n = 85) were randomly assigned to an experimental group (aerobic running program, 5 times/week for 8 weeks) or a PE class (only non-aerobic activities). Children in the aerobic running program performed better at post-test on measures of creative thinking (creative fluency, creative flexibility, and creative originality), lending support to the beneficial effects of regular exercise on cognitive performance.

Additional support for the benefits of PA comes from a recent RCT (Davis et al., 2007) looking at the effects of different doses of exercise on cognitive performance in 94 overweight children (7–11 years). Children were randomly assigned to one of three conditions: high exercise dose (40 minutes/session), low exercise dose (20 minutes/session), or no-exercise. Exercise occurred five times per week for 15 weeks. Results showed that exercise significantly improved scores on planning; however, the effect was only seen when examining differences between no-exercise and the high-dose exercise group. It appeared that 20 minutes was not long enough to elicit effects on cognition in this sample.

Recently, Kamijo et al. (2011) reported findings from a 9-month RCT in which 43 children (7–9 years) were randomly assigned to an after-school exercise program or a wait-list control. The exercise program was offered every day after school and included at least 70 minutes of moderate- to vigorous-intensity physical activity. The primary result of the study was that the exercise group improved working memory performance significantly while those in the wait-list group experienced no change in performance.

Academic achievement and cognitive task performance

The effects of PA on both academic achievement and cognitive task performance have only been examined in one study. Reed et al. (2010) tested the effects of PA on fluid intelligence and state achievement tests. A random sample of third-grade students from six classrooms (n = 155) were randomly assigned to an experimental group receiving PA for 30 minutes 3 days per week (n = 80) or a control group (n = 75) for a 3-month intervention. Although there were no differences between groups on the state achievement tests, those receiving PA performed significantly better than the control group on the fluid intelligence test. Fluid intelligence is an indirect assessment of academic performance in that it measures abstract reasoning ability and problem-solving and, hence, is not reliant on previously acquired knowledge. Thus, the results of this study suggest that PA may be important for children's cognitive and academic development.

Summary for experimental studies

In summary, there is not a consistently positive effect of PA on academic performance. That being said, there is evidence that academic performance is not hindered by the addition of PA, even though time was taken away from academic curricula. Additionally, benefits of PA were observed in studies in which performance was assessed in specific cognitive domains. Thus, it is possible that measures of academic performance are not sensitive to beneficial effects of PA over a relatively short period of time, but that task-specific cognitive benefits (e.g., for fluid intelligence, planning, creativity, and working memory) can accrue as a result of PA. Future research is necessary to determine if these ultimately can have an impact on academic performance with a stronger or longer PA stimulus.

Summary for interventions

The strengths of this literature include the use of large sample sizes, diverse samples, and the equal representation of genders. One of the major limitations is the lack of randomized assignment in the quasi-experimental studies and the failure to include well-designed control conditions in the experimental studies. The use of multiple measures of academic performance is also a limitation and may account for the variability in findings. More specifically, some studies used standardized achievement tests, whereas others used academic progress reports provided by teachers. Teacher reports and/or classroom grades may be a biased source of information and there is controversy over the validity of standardized tests as a valid measure of academic achievement. Another major limitation is that only three of thirteen studies (Davis et al., 2007; Mahar et al., 2006; Reed et al., 2010) measured PA to confirm the fidelity of the PA intervention and to inform the development of new intervention programs. Finally, since many of these interventions were school-based programs, they did not control for PA obtained outside the school day. Thus, the results of the studies might not be reflective only of the intervention, but rather of the effects of total accumulation of PA throughout the entire day. Future studies should control for PA accrued beyond school hours. Lastly, many studies are conducted within only one school district and are not random samples, thus limiting external validity.

Overall summary

As mentioned initially, synthesizing the results of this body of literature is challenging because of the diversity of designs, measurement approaches, and results. When correlational designs were used to assess relationships between PA and/or aerobic fitness and either academic achievement, cognitive task performance, neuroelectric indices, or brain structure, results fairly consistently supported a positive relationship. However, conclusions from these studies are limited by the reliance on correlational designs, which do not allow for causal conclusions. Studies using quasi-experimental designs to explore the benefits of PA also show consistently positive results, but are limited by a nearly exclusive use of multi-component programs, which do not allow for conclusions regarding the effects of PA per se. Studies using experimental designs that focus on academic achievement outcomes have consistently failed to show a positive effect of PA. However, authors of these studies emphasize that these results are encouraging because participants receiving PA in place of time in "academic" courses perform as well as those who do not receive PA. Certainly this is promising in suggesting that PA can be incorporated into the school day so that students can receive the health benefits of PA without a decline in academic performance. More promising results come from experimental studies that have shown that PA results in better performance on cognitive tasks assessing creativity, planning, working memory, and fluid intelligence. These results suggest the possibility that PA could be used to improve cognition in a way that may (over the long term) have implications for academic performance.

This review raises more questions than answers. It remains unclear as to what the ideal amount and type of exercise is to achieve benefits and no dose-response relationship has been established. It is also unclear as to what aspects of academic performance benefit the most, with some studies demonstrating effects for particular areas such as social studies (Reed et al., 2010), English/language arts (Hollar et al., 2010; Reed et al., 2010), and math (Hollar et al., 2010). Further, it is not clear if the benefits of PA for cognition differ depending upon whether it is integrated with academic lessons, is performed in a PE class, or is performed outside the school setting.

Future research should use strong experimental designs to improve our understanding of the relationship between PA and/or fitness and cognitive task performance, neuroelectric indices, brain structure, and academic achievement in the classroom. For example, longitudinal studies may lend insight as to the role PA plays throughout a child's cognitive development. Additionally, RCTs are necessary for the establishment of a causal relationship between PA and cognitive performance. Lastly, understanding mechanisms is critical so that we can move toward exercise prescription to benefit cognitive performance.

References

Buck, S. M., Hillman, C. H., & Castelli, D. M. (2008). The relation of aerobic fitness to Stroop task performance in preadolescent children. *Medicine & Science in Sports & Exercise, 40*(1), 166–172. doi:10.1249/mss.0b013e318159b035

Carlson, S. A., Fulton, J. E., Lee, S. M., Maynard, L. M., Brown, D. R., Kohl, H. W., 3rd, & Dietz, W. H. (2008). PE and academic achievement in elementary school: data from the early childhood longitudinal study. *American Journal of Public Health, 98*(4), 721–727. doi:AJPH.2007.117176

Castelli, D. M., Hillman, C. H., Buck, S. M., & Erwin, H. E. (2007). Physical fitness and academic achievement in third- and fifth-grade students. *Journal of Sport and Exercise Psychology, 29*(2), 239–252.

Chaddock, L., Erickson, K. I., Prakash, R. S., Kim, J. S., Voss, M. W., Vanpatter, M., . . . Kramer, A. F. (2010). A neuroimaging investigation of the association between aerobic fitness, hippocampal volume, and memory performance in preadolescent children. *Brain Research, 1358*, 172–183. doi:S0006-8993(10)01831-7

Chaddock, L., Erickson, K. I., Prakash, R. S., VanPatter, M., Voss, M. W., Pontifex, M. B., . . . Kramer, A. F. (2010). Basal ganglia volume is associated with aerobic fitness in preadolescent children. *Developmental Neuroscience, 32*(3), 249–256. doi:000316648

Chomitz, V. R., Slining, M. M., McGowan, R. J., Mitchell, S. E., Dawson, G. F., & Hacker, K. A. (2009). Is there a relationship between physical fitness and academic achievement? Positive results from public school children in the northeastern United States. *Journal of School Health, 79*(1), 30–37. doi:JOSH371

Coe, D. P., Pivarnik, J. M., Womack, C. J., Reeves, M. J., & Malina, R. M. (2006). Effect of PE and activity levels on academic achievement in children. *Medicine and Science in Sports and Exercise, 38*(8), 1515–1519. doi:10.1249/01.mss.0000227537.13175.1b

Davis, C. L., & Cooper, S. (2011). Fitness, fatness, cognition, behavior, and academic achievement among overweight children: do cross-sectional associations correspond to exercise trial outcomes? *Preventive Medicine, 52*(Suppl 1), S65–69. doi:S0091-7435(11)00048-X

Davis, C. L., Tomporowski, P. D., Boyle, C. A., Waller, J. L., Miller, P. H., Naglieri, J. A., & Gregoski, M. (2007). Effects of aerobic exercise on overweight children's cognitive functioning: a randomized controlled trial. *Research Quarterly for Exercise and Sport, 78*(5), 510–519.

Dwyer, T., Coonan, W. E., Leitch, D. R., Hetzel, B. S., & Baghurst, R. A. (1983). An investigation of the effects of daily physical activity on the health of primary school students in South Australia. *International Journal of Epidemiology, 12*(3), 308–313.

Edwards, J. U., Mauch, L., & Winkelman, M. R. (2011). Relationship of nutrition and physical activity behaviors and fitness measures to academic performance for sixth graders in a midwest city school district. *Journal of School Health, 81*(2), 65–73. doi:10.1111/j.1746-1561.2010.00562.x

Eveland-Sayers, B. M., Farley, R. S., Fuller, D. K., Morgan, D. W., & Caputo, J. L. (2009). Physical fitness and academic achievement in elementary school children. *Journal of Physical Activity and Health, 6*(1), 99–104.

Fox, C. K., Barr-Anderson, D., Neumark-Sztainer, D., & Wall, M. (2010). Physical activity and sports team participation: associations with academic outcomes in middle school and high school students. *Journal of School Health, 80*(1), 31–37. doi:JOSH454

Hardman, K. (2004). An up-date on the status of PE in schools worldwide: technical report for the World Health Organization: International Council for Sport Science and PE (ICSSPE).

Hillman, C. H., Buck, S. M., Themanson, J. R., Pontifex, M. B., & Castelli, D. M. (2009). Aerobic fitness and cognitive development: event-related brain potential and task performance indices of executive control in preadolescent children. *Developmental Psychology, 45*(1), 114–129. doi:2008-19282-003

Hillman, C. H., Castelli, D. M., & Buck, S. M. (2005). Aerobic fitness and neurocognitive function in healthy preadolescent children. *Medicine and Science in Sports and Exercise, 37*(11), 1967–1974. doi:00005768-200511000-00020

Hillman, C. H., Kamijo, K., & Scudder, M. (2011). A review of chronic and acute physical activity participation on neuroelectric measures of brain health and cognition during childhood. *Preventive Medicine, 52*(Suppl 1), S21–S28. doi:S0091-7435(11)00052-1

Hinkle, J. S., Tuckman, B. W., & Sampson, J. P. (1993). The psychology, physiology, and the creativity of middle school aerobic exercisers. *Elementary School Guidance & Counseling, 28*, 133–145.

Hollar, D., Messiah, S. E., Lopez-Mitnik, G., Hollar, T. L., Almon, M., & Agatston, A. S. (2010). Effect of a two-year obesity prevention intervention on percentile changes in body mass index and academic performance in low-income elementary school children. *American Journal of Public Health, 100*(4), 646–653. doi:AJPH.2009.165746

Kamijo, K., Pontifex, M. B., O'Leary, K. C., Scudder, M. R., Wu, C.-T., Castelli, D. M., & Hillman, C. H. (2011). The effects of an afterschool physical activity program on working memory in preadolescent children. *Developmental Science, 14*(5), 1046–1058.

Keyes, P. (2004). PE and health education professionals from across the country meet to address 'No Child Left Behind'. *NASPE*, Winter.

Kwak, L., Kremers, S. P., Bergman, P., Ruiz, J. R., Rizzo, N. S., & Sjostrom, M. (2009). Associations between physical activity, fitness, and academic achievement. *Journal of Pediatrics, 155*(6), 914–918. doi:S0022-3476(09)00573-3

Mahar, M. T., Murphy, S. K., Rowe, D. A., Golden, J., Shields, A. T., & Raedeke, T. D. (2006). Effects of a classroom-based program on physical activity and on-task behavior. *Medicine and Science in Sports and Exercise, 38*(12), 2086–2094. doi:10.1249/01.mss.0000235359.16685.a3

Murray, N. G., Low, B. J., Hollis, C., Cross, A. W., & Davis, S. M. (2007). Coordinated school health programs and academic achievement: a systematic review of the literature. *Journal of School Health, 77*(9), 589–600. doi:JOSH238

Nansel, T. R., Huang, T. T., Rovner, A. J., & Sanders-Butler, Y. (2010). Association of school performance indicators with implementation of the healthy kids, smart kids programme: case study. *Public Health Nutrition, 13*(1), 116–122. doi:S1368980009005898

Niederer, I., Kriemler, S., Gut, J., Hartmann, T., Schindler, C., Barral, J., & Puder, J. J. (2011). Relationship of aerobic fitness and motor skills with memory and attention in preschoolers (Ballabeina): a cross-sectional and longitudinal study. *BMC Pediatrics, 11*, 34. doi:1471-2431-11-34

Organization for Economic Co-operation and Development (2004). *Problem solving for tomorrow's world: First measures of cross-curricular competencies from PISA 2003*. Paris: Author.

Organization for Economic Co-operation and Development (2007). *PISA 2006: Science competencies for tomorrow's world*. Paris: Author.

Pontifex, M. B., Raine, L. B., Johnson, C. R., Chaddock, L., Voss, M. W., Cohen, N. J., . . . Hillman, C. H. (2011). Cardiorespiratory fitness and the flexible modulation of cognitive control in preadolescent children. *Journal of Cognitive Neuroscience, 23*(6), 1332–1345. doi:10.1162/jocn.2010.21528

Reed, J. A., Einstein, G., Hahn, E., Hooker, S. P., Gross, V. P., & Kravitz, J. (2010). Examining the impact of integrating physical activity on fluid intelligence and academic performance in an elementary school setting: a preliminary investigation. *Journal of Physical Activity and Health*, 7(3), 343–351.

Roberts, C. K., Freed, B., & McCarthy, W. J. (2010). Low aerobic fitness and obesity are associated with lower standardized test scores in children. *Journal of Pediatrics*, *156*(5), 711–718. doi:S0022-3476(09)01148-2

Rosas, S., Case, J., & Tholstrup, L. (2009). A retrospective examination of the relationship between implementation quality of the coordinated school health program model and school-level academic indicators over time. *Journal of School Health*, *79*(3), 108–115; quiz 144–106. doi:JOSH394

Sallis, J. F., McKenzie, T. L., Kolody, B., Lewis, M., Marshall, S., & Rosengard, P. (1999). Effects of health-related PE on academic achievement: project SPARK. *Research Quarterly for Exercise and Sport*, *70*(2), 127–134.

Shephard, R. J., Lavallee, H., Volle, M., LaBarre, R., & Beaucage, C. (1994). Academic skills and required PE: the Trois Rivieres experience. *Canadian Association for Health, Physical Education, and Recreation Research Supplement*, *1*(1), 1–12.

Shilts, M. K., Lamp, C., Horowitz, M., & Townsend, M. S. (2009). Pilot study: EatFit impacts sixth graders' academic performance on achievement of mathematics and English education standards. *Journal of Nutrition Education and Behavior*, *41*(2), 127–131. doi:S1499-4046(08)00692-1

Sibley, B. A., & Etnier, J. L. (2003). The relationship between physical activity and cognition in children: a meta-analysis. *Pediatric Exercise Science*, *15*(3), 243–256.

Sigfusdottir, I. D., Kristjansson, A. L., & Allegrante, J. P. (2007). Health behaviour and academic achievement in Icelandic school children. *Health Education Research*, *22*(1), 70–80. doi:cyl044

Taras, H. (2005). Physical activity and student performance at school. *Journal of School Health*, *75*(6), 214–218. doi:JOSH26

Tuckman, B. W., & Hinkle, J. S. (1986). An experimental study of the physical and psychological effects of aerobic exercise on schoolchildren. *Health Psychology*, *5*(3), 197–207.

Wang, F., & Veugelers, P. J. (2008). Self-esteem and cognitive development in the era of the childhood obesity epidemic. *Obesity Reviews*, *9*(6), 615–623. doi:OBR507

Welk, G. J., Jackson, A. W., Morrow, J. R., Jr., Haskell, W. H., Meredith, M. D., & Cooper, K. H. (2010). The association of health-related fitness with indicators of academic performance in Texas schools. *Research Quarterly for Exercise and Sport*, *81*(3 Suppl), S16–S23.

Wu, C. T., Pontifex, M. B., Raine, L. B., Chaddock, L., Voss, M. W., Kramer, A. F., & Hillman, C. H. (2011). Aerobic fitness and response variability in preadolescent children performing a cognitive control task. *Neuropsychology*, *25*(3), 333–341. doi:2011-06236-001

17

EXERCISE EFFECTS ON BRAIN AND COGNITION IN OLDER ADULTS

Michelle W. Voss and Kirk I. Erickson

The United States Census Bureau predicts that the percentage of people over the age of 65 will increase from approximately 11% of the population in 2000 to nearly 23% of the population by 2050 (US Census Bureau). Along with this increase comes an expected inflation in the prevalence of age-related diseases. For example, the number of persons with Alzheimer's disease (AD) is expected to increase from approximately 5.1 million in 2010 to nearly 13.5 million by 2050 (Alzheimer's Association, 2010). An increase in the prevalence of AD will be accompanied by elevated costs to treat and care for people with the disease. These costs are estimated to reach US$172 billion in 2010 and to increase to nearly US$1.078 trillion by 2050 (Alzheimer's Association, 2010).

Although not everyone develops AD, cognitive decline in late adulthood is quite common. For example, longitudinal studies in adults without dementia have found that there is often relative stability in cognitive function until about 55 years of age followed by a steady decline in several cognitive domains including inductive reasoning, perceptual speed, verbal ability, spatial orientation, numeric ability, and verbal memory (Hertzog, Kramer, Wilson, & Lindenberger, 2009). Preceding the decline in cognitive function is a decline in brain integrity as measured by both volumetric and functional measures. Several brain areas, such as the dorsolateral prefrontal cortex, begin to deteriorate at about the age of 30 and continue on a declining course throughout late life (Raz et al., 2005). On the other hand, regions like the hippocampus, a smaller structure located in the medial temporal lobe, remain relatively preserved until about the age of 50, and then decline in volume at about 1% per year in individuals without dementia; in adults with dementia there is an escalated rate of decline in volume of the hippocampus to over 3% annually (Jack et al., 1998). Coupled with age-related structural atrophy is alteration in the functional properties of many brain regions. Depending on the cognitive demands of the task, older adults have shown sometimes greater and sometimes less neural recruitment than younger adults. Therefore, unlike brain morphology, there is not always a straightforward translation between whether more or less neural recruitment reflects better or worse brain integrity. Thus, it is often necessary to interpret age-related differences in brain activation in the context of behavioral performance (Grady, 2008) and preferably following a targeted behavioral intervention or longitudinal assessment (Lustig, Shah, Seidler, & Reuter-Lorenz, 2009).

A measure of brain function that is a more consistent index of brain integrity than the magnitude of neural recruitment assesses the tendency for brain regions within distinct networks to co-activate during rest or task states. Co-activation is often termed functional connectivity, and studies have consistently found that older adults have decreased functional connectivity during the rest state in several brain networks. Three of these networks include the default network and two networks involved in cognitive control – a fronto-executive and fronto-parietal network (Andrews-Hanna et al., 2007; Voss, Prakash et al., 2010). While researchers have linked the functional connectivity of these cognitively relevant networks to the structural integrity of white matter tracts, there is also evidence that functional connectivity reflects unique variance associated with the functional interactions between brain regions (Van Dijk et al., 2010).

Despite the general age-related decline in brain integrity evidenced by volumetric and functional measures, there is significant individual variability in the rate and prevalence of decline, with some people showing more rapid decay and others aging quite successfully with minimal impairment. This suggests that cognitive and brain decay might not be ubiquitous and begs the following question: what factors explain variation in cognitive and brain function in late life? If factors can be identified that explain individual variability in the rate and prevalence of brain atrophy and dysfunction, could we develop interventions that prevent decline from occurring? In this chapter, we discuss the possibility that physical activity (PA), especially in the form of aerobic exercise, could act to not only prevent brain decay and dysfunction in late adulthood, but could also reverse atrophy and impairment already present.

Why aerobic exercise?

It may at first be surprising to hear that PA influences brain function. Indeed, usually when people think of methods that exercise the brain, they think of intellectual activities such as crossword puzzles, Sudoku, or reading. However, exercise appears to be an effective method for enhancing both the body and brain. Animal studies with rats and mice in which the intensity and duration of exercise can be monitored and manipulated allows for a controlled environment to assess the effect of exercise on brain morphology and function. From these studies, it has been found that a moderate amount of exercise increases the number of new neurons produced in the dentate gyrus of the hippocampus, even in aged animals (Kronenberg et al., 2006). With an increased number of new neurons comes an increased need for nutrients. Therefore, in concert with increased cell proliferation is an exercise-induced increase in blood flow and blood volume. Angiogenesis, or the proliferation of new vasculature, has been found in several brain regions including the cerebellum, hippocampus, motor cortex, frontal cortex, and basal ganglia (for reviews, see Cotman & Berchtold, 2002; Kramer, Erickson, & Colcombe, 2006). Exercise also increases the number of connections, or synapses, between neurons, and increases levels of neurotrophins in the brain that modulate processes of synaptic plasticity, which together lead to enhanced learning and memory (Christie et al., 2008; van Praag, Shubert, Zhao, & Gage, 2005; Vaynman, Ying, & Gomez-Pinilla, 2004). In sum, rodent studies have revealed some of the underlying molecular and cellular mechanisms by which exercise exerts its effects on the brain. These findings provide a biological foundation for examining the effects of exercise on brain integrity in humans.

Aerobic exercise, cognition, and brain morphology in humans

Early cross-sectional research found that older adult athletes outperformed their more sedentary peers on several cognitive tasks (Spirduso, 1975; for review, see Kramer, Erickson, & Colcombe, 2006). This cross-sectional work was followed by exercise interventions in which older adults were randomly assigned to a moderate-intensity exercise group or a control group (often consisting of stretching and toning exercises). Several of these interventions showed that aerobic exercise enhanced cognitive function. In a meta-analysis of 18 randomized clinical trials, exercise was found to have both general and specific effects on cognitive function (Colcombe & Kramer, 2003). The effects were general in the sense that most of cognition was enhanced with exercise, but specific in the sense that executive function (EF) was enhanced more than other cognitive domains. EF is an umbrella term that refers to several higher-level cognitive functions such as selective attention, task-coordination, planning, and maintaining items in working memory. EF is often found to be the most negatively affected with increasing age, yet appears to remain tractable, and exercise has the capacity to take advantage of this modifiability.

The results from intervention studies suggest that the brain regions supporting EF, such as the prefrontal and parietal cortex, are the ones most affected by exercise. To test this prediction, Colcombe and colleagues (2006) randomly assigned a group of older sedentary adults to a moderate-intensity aerobic exercise group that walked for 40 minutes 3 days per week or a non-aerobic stretching and toning control group that exercised in a group setting in the lab for the same amount of time as the walking group. A control group that experiences the same social setting as the experimental exercise group is important since social activity has also been linked to cognitive function in older adults (Bassuk, Glass, & Berkman, 1999; Lovden, Ghisletta, & Lindenberger, 2005). Both groups participated for 6 months. High-resolution brain scans from magnetic resonance imaging (MRI) were obtained before and after the intervention. Colcombe and colleagues reported that exercise was effective at increasing gray matter volume in the prefrontal, parietal, and lateral temporal regions and at increasing white matter volume in the genu of the corpus callosum. This study was important, as it was the first to suggest that age-related loss of brain volume might not be an inevitable consequence of getting older, and that moderate amounts of exercise could increase brain volume.

The hippocampus is of great interest in aging research because of its role in memory formation and because it shows considerable atrophy in late adulthood, which is hypothesized to contribute to AD and memory loss. Research in rodents has demonstrated that exercise unequivocally influences the hippocampus (Cotman & Berchtold, 2002; van Praag et al., 2005; Vaynman et al., 2004). This research led to the hypothesis in humans that higher fitness levels might be associated with less hippocampal atrophy and spared memory function. To test this, Erickson and colleagues (2009) examined cardiorespiratory fitness levels in a sample of 165 older adults without dementia and used MRI techniques to identify and measure the volume of the hippocampus. They found that after controlling for age, sex, and education, older adults who were more aerobically fit had larger hippocampal volumes than their less fit peers (see Figure 17.1). In addition, higher fit older adults performed better on a spatial memory task, and greater hippocampal volume partially mediated the fitness-memory association. These results directly linked for the first time cardiorespiratory fitness, age-related hippocampal atrophy, and memory function. There have now been other studies that have replicated this effect by showing that higher fitness levels are associated with greater hippocampal volumes across different populations (Chaddock et al., 2010; Honea et al., 2009).

Cross-sectional studies of cardiorespiratory fitness and hippocampal volume are provocative, but fail to demonstrate direct causal links between the variables. To address this, Erickson and colleagues (2011) conducted a 1-year randomized controlled trial (RCT) in which 120 sedentary older adults without dementia were assigned to a moderate-intensity exercise intervention or a stretching and toning control group. Similar to previous intervention studies, both groups received the same amount of social interaction and health instruction. Using MRI, they showed that 1 year of aerobic exercise was sufficient for increasing the size of the hippocampus. These findings support the claim that modest amounts of aerobic exercise can increase the size of some

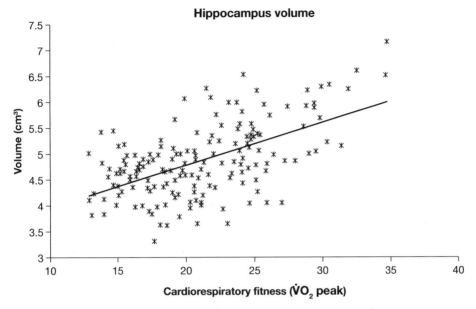

Figure 17.1 Aerobic fitness and hippocampal volume. Cardiorespiratory fitness (V̇O₂peak) is positively associated with hippocampal volume (data collapsed across left and right hemispheres) in 165 older adults (data adapted from Erickson et al., 2009).

brain regions that normally undergo deterioration and are involved in memory loss as we age. Furthermore, these results demonstrate that the brain remains modifiable well into late adulthood and that starting an exercise regimen in late adulthood is not futile; even those adults who have been sedentary can still benefit from starting to exercise.

The study by Erickson and colleagues (2011) supports the claim that relatively modest amounts of aerobic exercise are effective in augmenting the brain and cognition in late adulthood. However, how much and what intensity of exercise is necessary to observe effects on brain and cognition? Some epidemiological studies suggest that more strenuous activities are associated with a reduced risk of cognitive impairment (Barnes et al., 2003; Weuve et al., 2004), but dose–response studies in which the frequency, duration, or intensity of exercise is systematically manipulated have not yet been conducted to formally address this question (Chang & Etnier, 2009; Etnier, Nowell, Landers, & Sibley, 2006; Kramer & Erickson, 2007; Middelton et al., 2011).

To help address the question of the dose of PA needed to observe long-term effects on the brain, Erickson and colleagues (2010) conducted a 13-year longitudinal study of 299 adults over the age of 65. In this study, PA was assessed at baseline by asking participants how many blocks they walked on average in 1 week. Nine years later, MRI data were collected to examine whether PA was predictive of brain volume later in life. Erickson and colleagues (2010) found that more PA at baseline was predictive of greater gray matter volume in prefrontal, hippocampal, and occipital regions. However, they also found that this occurred in a dose-dependent fashion. That is, sparing of gray matter volume was only apparent in individuals reporting roughly 1 mile of walking per day. Those walking less than 1 mile daily had less brain volume than their more active peers. This finding suggested that there might be a threshold for the amount of activity needed to observe the benefits of exercise on brain morphology. Furthermore, a 4-year follow-up after the MRI assessment showed that those individuals with greater gray matter volume in the inferior frontal gyrus, hippocampus, and supplementary motor area had a two-fold reduced risk of developing cognitive impairment (Erickson et al., 2010).

In sum, recent research demonstrates that aerobic exercise is effective at augmenting brain and cognitive health in late adulthood and that even a modest amount of exercise is sufficient for increasing brain size in areas involved in memory and EF. At a time of life when memory impairment is prevalent, PA could be a low-cost and low-tech prevention and treatment that is accessible to most people. Although exercise will not cure AD, even if it delays the onset or reduces the risk for developing cognitive impairment, it may save millions of dollars in health care costs and reduce the emotional toll on caregivers and those afflicted with impairment.

Aerobic exercise and brain function

Some of the first studies to link aerobic fitness with better brain function in healthy elderly adults found that aerobic fitness was associated with electrophysiological markers of enhanced attention and processing speed (Bashore, 1989; Dustman et al., 1990). While electrophysiological techniques provide a glimpse of neural activity on a millisecond time-scale, they have poor spatial resolution, which prevents examination of where differences in brain activity originated. Offsetting this disadvantage, functional MRI (fMRI) is a neuroimaging technique that measures blood flow coupled to neural activity with millimeter spatial resolution. Broadly, two fMRI approaches have been used to study the effects of aerobic exercise on brain function. One approach examines how *much* individual brain regions activate during cognitive challenge, whereas a second approach examines how well individual brain regions activate *together* as part of brain networks known to support thoughts and behavior.

Given that previous research on the behavioral outcomes of aerobic training with elderly adults indicated that EF, attention, and processing speed are improved (Colcombe & Kramer, 2003; Smith, Blumenthal, et al., 2010), brain regions that support these processes, such as the frontal and parietal cortices, were hypothesized to be most sensitive to individual variation in aerobic fitness or to change following aerobic fitness training.

This prediction was first supported by a study by Colcombe and colleagues (2004) that examined changes in functional brain activation following a 6-month, thrice-weekly aerobic exercise program compared to a non-aerobic exercise control condition. Participants in both conditions performed a task involving speeded selective attention and EF at baseline and post-intervention. Following the intervention, the aerobic exercise group had increased brain activation during the more cognitively demanding condition of the task in regions that have been theorized to be involved in attentional control, including the right middle frontal gyrus in the prefrontal cortex and bilateral superior parietal lobule. In addition, brain activity in the anterior cingulate cortex decreased for the aerobic compared to the non-aerobic exercise group, which is a brain region theorized to help regulate attentional control enforced by the prefrontal cortices. Importantly, changes in brain activity were independent of local gray matter volume in activated regions, and changes in brain function were coupled with improved performance on the more demanding task condition for the aerobic exercise group only. This pattern of activation changes coupled with performance improvement suggested that aerobic training led to enhanced attentional control and EF via improved prefrontal cortex response to signals for increased attentional control from the anterior cingulate. Similar results have also been found with electrophysiological measures during speeded attention and EF performance (for review, see Hillman, Erickson, & Kramer, 2008). More generally, this study supports the hypothesis that aerobic fitness is not associated with a general increase in brain activity during cognitive challenge, but that specific brain regions such as the prefrontal and parietal cortices show the most benefit (see also Prakash et al., 2011).

The study by Colcombe and colleagues (2004) demonstrated that 6 months of moderate aerobic activity is enough to enhance brain function in regions typically affected by aging. But how might aerobic exercise continued over several years' impact brain function? One study examined this question by measuring brain function with fMRI following 3 years of a physically active lifestyle for 20 elderly adults compared to a group of 10 elderly adults who had been sedentary for the same amount of time (Rosano et al., 2010). All participants were originally part of a 1-year intervention that compared PA with health education treatment, and in this follow-up study, the active group was comprised of those who were in the PA group and stayed physically active for 2 additional years, whereas the control group were those who remained sedentary following their control treatment. Results demonstrated that being active for 3 years was related to greater improvements in a speeded task involving executive control and working memory (digit symbol substitution task), coupled with greater brain activity in the left and right prefrontal cortices during task performance, compared to the control group. Similar to Colcombe et al. (2004), changes in brain activation were independent of group differences in brain volume. This study also included participants who were on average 81 years of age during scanning, which is approximately 13 to 14 years older than participants in Colcombe et al. (2004), who were an average of 67 years of age. Together, these studies provide evidence to support the claim that the human brain remains responsive to benefits from both short- and long-term exercise well into the seventh decade of life.

Another important question regarding effects of exercise on brain function considers whether exercise is more beneficial for some individuals compared to others. The epidemiological literature has supported an association between PA and decreased incidence of AD (Larson et al., 2006), and there is some evidence that cognitive benefits of aerobic activity are stronger for carriers of the apolipoprotein E (APOE) e4 allele, a genetic risk factor for late-onset AD (Etnier et al., 2007; Schuit, Feskens, Launer, & Kromhout, 2001). Hence, a testable prediction for functional brain imaging studies is that the genetic risk for AD should moderate the association between fitness and brain activity associated with better performance in elderly adults. One study that found partial support for this prediction measured brain activity during a semantic memory task in older adults who varied by PA level (high active/low active) and presence of the APOE e4 allele (carrier/non-carrier) (Smith, Nielson, et al., 2010). The researchers found that only two of the 15 task-related activated regions were different between the high and low active groups for the non-carriers (low risk for AD), whereas a third of the regions differentiated high and low active groups for the carriers (high risk for AD), including the left angular gyrus, left middle frontal gyrus, right angular gyrus, left superior frontal gyrus, and right frontal insula. Further, five regions also differentiated risk among the high active people: left superior frontal gyrus, left medial frontal pole, left ventral medial frontal pole, right inferior parietal lobule, and the right frontal insula. Therefore, PA seemed to have a greater association with brain health for those at genetic risk for AD, and in general, these results provide preliminary support for the prediction that APOE moderates the association between PA and brain function.

In addition to studying how aerobic fitness and PA impact the level of activity in individual brain regions, important insights about exercise effects on brain function can also be gained by studying how well brain regions activate together, or synchronize their neural activity. This is particularly true for brain networks known to be involved in attention, processing speed, and EF. In the first study of this nature, Voss and colleagues examined whether functional connectivity in the default network was associated with aerobic fitness in a cross-sectional sample of 120 healthy older adults between the ages of 60 and 80 years (Voss, Erickson, et al., 2010). Brain regions in the default network encompass the frontal, parietal, occipital, and temporal cortex, including the posterior cingulate cortex, ventral and superior medial frontal cortex, and bilateral

lateral occipital, middle frontal, hippocampal and parahippocampal, and middle temporal cortices (see Figure 17.2; for review, see Buckner et al., 2008). Its function has been assessed either by measuring how much neural recruitment occurs in the network, or how synchronized different regions are with each other. The default network is thought to play a functional role in memory consolidation, self-referential thought, mind-wandering, and autobiographical memory, with an important role in executive control as well (Buckner et al., 2008). For instance, increased synchronization in the default network has been associated with better working memory performance in young adults (Hampson et al., 2006), and better EF performance in older adults (Andrews-Hanna et al., 2007; Damoiseaux et al., 2008). Thus, the default network is important for understanding determinants of healthy cognitive aging. Additionally, its dysfunction has been proposed as a biomarker for AD (Greicius, Srivastava, Reiss, & Menon, 2004).

To test if aerobic fitness was specifically associated with functional connectivity in the default network regions most negatively affected by age, Voss, Erickson, and colleagues (2010) first determined where age differences in functional connectivity were greatest. Almost all brain regions typically in the default network were more disconnected (i.e., out of sync) for the older adults compared to a college-age control group. Then, to test whether aerobic fitness was associated with less age-related network dysfunction, correlations were conducted between functional connectivity in region-to-region pairs disrupted with age and aerobic fitness. Results showed that connectivity between almost half of region-to-region connections disrupted with age was positively correlated with aerobic fitness among the older adults. Consistent with previous research, aerobic fitness was also most strongly associated with the function of the prefrontal cortex. For example, all region-to-region connections associated with fitness included a region in the frontal cortex. Additionally, results supported the hypothesis that default network connectivity is one route by which aerobic fitness benefits cognitive aging: mediation analysis showed that functional connectivity in the default network accounted for a statistically significant amount of variance in EF abilities including task-switching, spatial working memory, and "set shifting" or flexibility to changing rule sets. Therefore this study provided the first evidence that functional connectivity in brain networks may play an important role in how aerobic fitness benefits cognition.

However, it was still unknown if aerobic fitness would have an association with brain networks other than the default network and if aerobic training would lead to improved functional connectivity. To address these questions Voss and colleagues conducted an RCT with 65 healthy older adults (Voss, Prakash, et al., 2010), comprising a subset of the participants in the studies described above (Erickson et al., 2011; Voss, Erickson, et al., 2010). The study included an experimental walking group (n = 30) and a stretching and toning control group (n = 35). In addition to the default network, researchers also examined networks involved with EF, spatial attention, motor control, and audition. Overall, there were four region-to-region connections enhanced following 1 year of aerobic exercise. One of these connections was between the left and right prefrontal cortices in a network theorized to be involved in executive control and sustained attention. However, three out of four were in the default network. Also of interest, two of the three connections showing improved functional connectivity in the default network for the walking group included a region in the parahippocampus overlapping with the hippocampal dentate gyrus (see Figure 17.2). This is important since the finding makes a link to animal models of exercise effects on the brain, which have found that the dentate gyrus is particularly sensitive to the benefits of exercise, including the birth of new neurons and enhanced synaptic plasticity (Cotman et al., 2007). In addition, this study provides important evidence supporting the hypothesis that aerobic fitness training benefits not only task-related magnitude of brain activation, but also the coherence of brain networks important for cognition and neurological disease status.

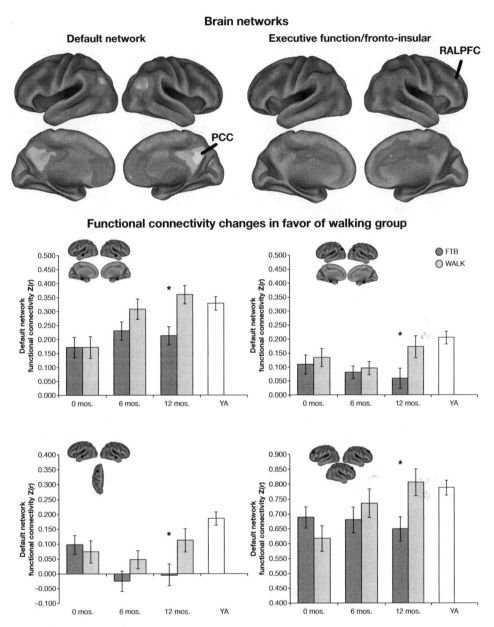

Figure 17.2 Aerobic exercise benefits brain networks. Top panel illustrates two brain networks that benefit from aerobic fitness training (WALK) compared to flexibility, toning, and balance (FTB) non-aerobic exercise training; PCC = posterior cingulate cortex, RALPFC = right anterior lateral prefrontal cortex, indicate regions that are prominent brain areas in the network, brain regions with activation that highly correlates with these regions are considered part of the respective networks. All brains shown in neurological orientation, R = R and L = L. ⋆$p < .05$ group difference in ANCOVA model, after controlling for group differences at baseline; YA = young adult control group for reference (data adapted from Voss, Prakash, et al., 2010).

Results of the study also showed increases in functional connectivity in favor of the stretching and toning group in the default network following 6 months of exercise. However, functional connectivity in these regions reverted to baseline levels at the end of the 1-year intervention. Since the stretching and toning intervention involved learning novel stretching and balance exercises and light yoga poses for the first 6 months, which were maintained and practiced for the second 6 months, it is possible that increases in functional connectivity for the stretching group reflect learning-related changes in default network connectivity. This would be consistent with the default network's association with cognitive abilities such as inward-focused thought and integrating an external world-view with your own, and suggest the possibility of an intervention based on these activities as a framework for combined exercise and cognitive training.

A third study that has examined the effects of aerobic exercise on brain function from a network perspective assessed whether aerobic exercise was associated with how connected *in parallel* the hippocampus was to all other brain regions (Burdette et al., 2010). Therefore positive results would indicate that not only does aerobic training impact specific inter-regional connections in the brain (Voss, Prakash, et al., 2010), but it also impacts how well connected the hippocampus is to all other brain regions. This could then affect the ease with which large networks simultaneously access the hippocampus during cognitive activity. This study included participants who had just completed a 4-month treatment in an RCT, as part of either an aerobic training group or a non-exercise control group (health education and light stretching). Results showed that aerobic exercisers had increased connectivity between the hippocampus and the rest of the brain compared to the control group, and follow-up analyses found the hippocampus and anterior cingulate were more functionally connected in the aerobic group compared to the control group. The aerobic group also had greater hippocampal blood flow compared to the control group, and increased hippocampal perfusion was positively correlated with increased anterior cingulate connectivity, providing preliminary evidence that increased hippocampal blood perfusion may be one factor associated with greater functional brain connectivity following aerobic exercise. Therefore this study makes an interesting link to the Colcombe et al. (2004) study, which found aerobic training resulted in decreased activity in the anterior cingulate cortex, coupled with improved task performance. Despite the overlap in regional changes, however, the interpretation for how these findings fit together is not straightforward at this time. Future research is needed to better understand how changes in the synchronization of brain regions interact with changes in the magnitude of brain activity, following aerobic exercise.

In sum, a growing number of studies support the claim that, in healthy elderly adults, aerobic fitness and aerobic training have a positive association with brain function. Enhanced brain function has been demonstrated through (a) the extent to which specific brain regions activate to support task-related cognitive processes and (b) how well brain regions coordinate with each other as part of brain networks known to support cognitive abilities affected by aging. In addition, the evidence from functional imaging studies is consistent with brain morphology studies finding that the prefrontal cortex and the hippocampus are two brain regions with high sensitivity to the benefits of aerobic exercise in late adulthood. Given that the prefrontal and hippocampal cortices are also areas that experience accelerated atrophy and dysfunction associated with aging and contribute to cognitive abilities important for everyday living such as EF and memory, evidence from functional neuroimaging studies provides converging evidence to the claim that aerobic exercise has great potential as a lifestyle intervention for improved quality of life.

Considerations for future research

We have outlined the evidence that modest amounts of aerobic exercise are sufficient for enhancing cognition and brain function. By using MRI technology, it has been consistently demonstrated that higher fit older adults have greater amounts of gray matter volume in several brain regions. Furthermore, exercise also increases brain activity and functional coordination in brain networks, which in some cases has been shown to parallel improvements in cognition. Overall, this evidence suggests that aerobic exercise can be envisioned as an effective method to prevent brain deterioration, maintain cognitive and brain function, and even increase the size of some brain areas. Despite these consistent and convincing findings, there remain important methodological issues to consider for future research and many unanswered and unexplored questions.

With regard to methodological issues, one over-arching issue is the generalizability of measures of cognitive function. While meta-analyses provide a means to systematically assess the consistency of exercise training benefits across overlapping cognitive domains (Colcombe & Kramer, 2003; Etnier, Nowell, Landers, & Sibley, 2006; Smith, Blumenthal, et al., 2010), when conceptual overlap among the task-specific cognitive outcomes is weak, the diversity of specialized laboratory paradigms for measuring cognitive benefits can lead to unreliable estimates of cognitive benefits. Therefore, it will be important for future research to strike a balance between innovative measures of specific cognitive mechanisms and standardized tests of cognitive function that permit straightforward comparison across a population of studies. Similarly, few studies of exercise effects on healthy older adults have assessed the transferability of improvements on laboratory tests of cognition to the real world, such as driving behavior or other tasks important for everyday living. However, this will be an important link to consider for understanding how exercise-related improvements in cognition impact everyday function and quality of life.

There are also many questions that are relatively unexplored. For example, one remaining question involves the dose-response relationship of exercise on brain and cognition. That is, as described above, there is relatively little information about how much exercise is necessary, what intensity should be achieved, and what types of exercises are best to enhance cognition. The answers to these questions are critically important if exercise is to be used in clinical contexts and be prescribed to patients as prevention or treatment for loss in cognitive function. There is also little known about the underlying mechanisms of aerobic exercise in humans. Is exercise working by influencing the creation of new vasculature or could exercise be directly affecting brain tissue? These are not mutually exclusive possibilities, and it will be important for future studies to consider the interactions between vasculature, neural, and extracellular changes in the brain as a function of exercise training. In addition to direct effects of exercise on the brain and its vasculature, could other mediating factors also be contributing to the effects of exercise on brain and cognition? For example, to what extent do improvements in sleep, reductions in stressor-evoked responses, improved peripheral vascular and metabolic function, or more consistent regulation of hypothalamic-pituitary-adrenal axis factors, contribute to the elevated brain and cognitive responses?

Also, the research described here has been largely limited to older adults free of cognitive impairment. There is little known as to the extent to which aerobic exercise prevents decay of the brain in those already experiencing cognitive impairment and there is a poor understanding of whether exercise could improve brain health in populations with multiple sclerosis, Parkinson's disease, schizophrenia, or other psychiatric or neurologic diseases. In short, more research is needed to understand the degree to which these conclusions can be generalized to other populations.

Finally, not everyone benefits equally from exercise. What are the factors that contribute to this individual variability? Could there be genetic factors that moderate the extent to which any single person would benefit from exercise? Are there other factors such as intellectual stimulation or dietary habits that either accentuate or attenuate the effects of exercise? For example, as briefly discussed in the review, preliminary evidence suggests that a genetic disposition for AD is an important factor in moderating the benefits of aerobic exercise on human brain function. However, larger studies that incorporate multiple perspectives on brain structure and function will be needed for a greater understanding of these factors and others that may impact the link between exercise and cognition.

Conclusion

Overall, we can argue that (a) the brains of older adults remain modifiable and that exercise can take advantage of this plasticity to increase the size of areas that frequently show atrophy in late life; (b) it is never too late to start exercising; even adults who have been sedentary most of their lives can reap the benefits of an exercise regimen; and (c) the effects of exercise are not global throughout the brain, but have some specificity to hippocampal and prefrontal brain areas. Together this research suggests that brain atrophy, dysfunction, and cognitive decline might not be as inevitable a consequence of aging as previously thought.

References

Alzheimer's Association (2010). 2010 Alzheimer's disease facts and figures. *Alzheimer's & Dementia, 6,* 158–194. doi:10.1016/j.jalz.2010.01.009

Andrews-Hanna, J. R., Snyder, A. Z., Vincent, J. L., Lustig, C., Head, D., Raichle, M. E., . . . Buckner, R. L. (2007). Disruption of large-scale brain systems in advanced aging. *Neuron, 56,* 924–935. doi:10.1016/j.neuron.2007.10.038

Barnes, D. E., Yaffe, K., Satariano, W. A., & Tager, I. B. (2003). A longitudinal study of cardiorespiratory fitness and cognitive function in healthy older adults. *Journal of the American Geriatrics Society, 51*(4), 459–465.

Bashore, T. R. (1989). Age, physical fitness, and mental processing speed. *Annual Review of Gerontology and Geriatrics, 9,* 120–144. Retrieved from http://www.springerpub.com/product/9780826106131

Bassuk, S. S., Glass, T. A., & Berkman, L. F. (1999). Social disengagement and incident cognitive decline in community-dwelling elderly persons. *Annals of Internal Medicine, 131,* 165–173.

Buckner, R. L., Andrews-Hanna, J. R., & Schacter, D. L. (2008). The brain's default network: Anatomy, function, and relevance to disease. *Annals of the New York Academy of Sciences, 1124*(1), 1–38. doi:10.1196/annals.1440.011

Burdette, J. H., Laurienti, P. J., Espeland, M. A., Morgan, A., Telesford, Q., Vechlekar, C. D., . . . Rejeski, W. J. (2010). Using network science to evaluate exercise-associated brain changes in older adults. *Frontiers in Aging Neuroscience, 2*(23), 1–10. doi:10.3389/fnagi.2010.00023

Chaddock, L., Erickson, K. I., Prakash, R. S., Kim, J. S., Voss, M. W., Vanpatter, M., . . . Kramer, A. F. (2010). A neuroimaging investigation of the association between aerobic fitness, hippocampal volume, and memory performance in preadolescent children. *Brain Research, 1358,* 172–183. doi:10.1016/j.brainres.2010.08.049

Chang, Y. K., & Etnier, J. L. (2009). Exploring the dose-response relationship between resistance exercise intensity and cognitive function. *Journal of Sport & Exercise Psychology, 31,* 640–656. Retrieved from http://journals.humankinetics.com/jsep

Christie, B. R., Eadie, B. D., Kannangara, T. S., Robillard, J. M., Shin, J., & Titterness, A. K. (2008). Exercising our brains: How physical activity impacts synaptic plasticity in the dentate gyrus. *NeuroMolecular Medicine, 10,* 47–58. doi:10.1007/s12017-008-8033-2

Colcombe, S., Erickson, K., Scalf, P., Kim, J., Prakash, R., Mcauley, E., . . . Kramer, A. F. (2006). Aerobic exercise training increases brain volume in aging humans. *Journals of Gerontology Series A: Biological and*

Medical Sciences, 61, 1166–1170. Retrieved from http://biomedgerontology.oxfordjournals.org/content/61/11/1166.full

Colcombe, S. J., & Kramer, A. F. (2003). Fitness effects on the cognitive function of older adults: A meta-analytic study. *Psychological Science: A Journal of the American Psychological Society/APS, 14,* 125–130. Retrieved from http://www.jstor.org/stable/40063782

Colcombe, S. J., Kramer, A. F., Erickson, K. I., Scalf, P., McAuley, E., Cohen, N. J., . . . Elavsky, S. (2004). Cardiovascular fitness, cortical plasticity, and aging. *Proceedings of the National Academy of Sciences of the United States of America, 101*(9), 3316–3321. doi:10.1073/pnas.0400266101

Cotman, C. W., & Berchtold, N. C. (2002). Exercise: A behavioral intervention to enhance brain health and plasticity. *Trends in Neurosciences, 25,* 295–301. doi:10.1016/S0166-2236(02)02143-4

Cotman, C. W., Berchtold, N. C., & Christie, L.-A. (2007). Exercise builds brain health: Key roles of growth factor cascades and inflammation. *Trends in Neurosciences, 30*(9), 464–472. doi:10.1016/j.tins.2007.06.011

Damoiseaux, J. S., Beckmann, C. F., Arigita, E. J. S., Barkhof, F., Scheltens, P., Stam, C. J., . . . Rombouts, S. A. (2008). Reduced resting-state brain activity in the "default network" in normal aging. *Cerebral Cortex, 18*(8), 1856–1864. doi:10.1093/cercor/bhm207

Dustman, R., Emmerson, R., Ruhling, R., Shearer, D. E., Steinhaus, L. A., Johnson, S. C., . . . Shigeoka, J. W. (1990). Age and fitness effects on EEG, ERPs, visual sensitivity, and cognition. *Neurobiology of Aging, 11,* 193–200. doi:10.1016/0197-4580(90)90545-B

Erickson, K., Prakash, R., Voss, M., Chaddock, L., Hu, L., Morris, K., . . . Kramer, A. F. (2009). Aerobic fitness is associated with hippocampal volume in elderly humans. *Hippocampus, 19,* 1030–1039. doi:10.1002/hipo.20547

Erickson, K. I., Raji, C. A., Lopez, O. L., Becker, J. T., Rosano, C., Newman, A. B., . . . Kuller, L. H. (2010). Physical activity predicts gray matter volume in late adulthood: The cardiovascular health study. *Neurology, 75,* 1415–1422. doi:10.1212/WNL.0b013e3181f88359

Erickson, K. I., Voss, M. W., Prakash, R. S., Basak, C., Szabo, A., Chaddock, L., . . . Kramer, A. F. (2011). Exercise training increases size of the hippocampus and improves memory. *Proceedings of the National Academy of Sciences, USA, 108,* 3017–3022. doi:10.1073/pnas.1015950108

Etnier, J., Nowell, P., Landers, D., & Sibley, B. (2006). A meta-regression to examine the relationship between aerobic fitness and cognitive performance. *Brain Research Reviews, 52,* 119–130. doi:10.1016/j.brainresrev.2006.01.002

Etnier, J. L., Caselli, R. J., Reiman, E. M., Alexander, G. E., Sibley, B. A., Tessier, D., . . . McLemore, E. C. (2007). Cognitive performance in older women relative to ApoE-epsilon4 genotype and aerobic fitness. *Medicine and Science in Sports and Exercise, 39,* 199–207. doi:10.1249/01.mss.0000239399.85955.5e

Grady, C. L. (2008). Cognitive neuroscience of aging. *Annals of the New York Academy of Sciences, 1124,* 127–144. doi:10.1196/annals.1440.009

Greicius, M., Srivastava, G., Reiss, A., & Menon, V. (2004). Default-mode network activity distinguishes Alzheimer's disease from healthy aging: Evidence from functional MRI. *Proceedings of the National Academy of Sciences, USA, 101,* 4637–4642. doi:10.1073/pnas.0308627101

Hampson, M., Driesen, N. R., Skudlarski, P., Gore, J. C., & Constable, R. T. (2006). Brain connectivity related to working memory performance. *The Journal of Neuroscience, 26*(51), 13338–13343. doi:10.1523/JNEUROSCI.3408-06.2006

Hertzog, C., Kramer, A. F., Wilson, R. S., & Lindenberger, U. (2009). Enrichment effects on adult cognitive development: Can the functional capacity of older adults be preserved and enhanced? *Psychological Science in the Public Interest, 9,* 1–65. doi:10.1111/j.1539-6053.2009.01034.x

Hillman, C. H., Erickson, K. I., & Kramer, A. F. (2008). Be smart, exercise your heart: Exercise effects on brain and cognition. *Nature Reviews Neuroscience, 9,* 58–65. doi:10.1038/nrn2298

Honea, R. A., Thomas, G. P., Harsha, A., Anderson, H. S., Donnelly, J. E., Brooks, W. M., . . . Burns, J. M. (2009). Cardiorespiratory fitness and preserved medial temporal lobe volume in Alzheimer disease. *Alzheimer Disease and Associated Disorders, 23,* 188–197. doi:10.1097/WAD.0b013e31819cb8a2

Jack, C. R., Petersen, R. C., Xu, Y., O'Brien, P. C., Smith, G. E., Ivnik, R. J., . . . Kokmen, E. (1998). Rate of medial temporal lobe atrophy in typical aging and Alzheimer's disease. *Neurology, 51,* 993–999. Retrieved from http://www.neurology.org/

Kramer, A. F., & Erickson, K. I. (2007). Capitalizing on cortical plasticity: Influence of physical activity on cognition and brain function. *Trends in Cognitive Sciences, 11,* 342–348. doi:10.1016/j.tics.2007.06.009

Kramer, A. F., Erickson, K. I., & Colcombe, S. J. (2006). Exercise, cognition, and the aging brain. *Journal of Applied Physiology, 101,* 1237–1242. doi:10.1152/japplphysiol.00500.2006

273

Kronenberg, G., Bick-Sander, A., Bunk, E., Wolf, C., Ehninger, D., & Kempermann, G. (2006). Physical exercise prevents age-related decline in precursor cell activity in the mouse dentate gyrus. *Neurobiology of Aging, 27*, 1505–1513. doi:10.1016/j.neurobiolaging.2005.09.016

Larson, E. B., Wang, L., Bowen, J. D., McCormick, W. C., Teri, L., Crane, P., . . . Kukull, W. (2006). Exercise is associated with reduced risk for incident dementia among persons 65 years of age and older. *Annals of Internal Medicine, 144*(2), 73–81. Retrieved from http://www.annals.org/

Lovden, M., Ghisletta, P., & Lindenberger, U. (2005). Social participation attenuates decline in perceptual speed in old and very old age. *Psychology and Aging,* 20, 423–434.

Lustig, C., Shah, P., Seidler, R., & Reuter-Lorenz, P. A. (2009). Aging, training, and the brain: A review and future directions. *Neuropsychology Review, 19*, 504–522. doi:10.1007/s11065-009-9119-9

Middleton, L. E., Manini, T. M., Simonsick, E. M., Harris, T. B., Barnes, D. E., Tylavsky, F., . . . Yaffe, K. (2011). Activity energy expenditure and incident cognitive impairment in older adults. *Archives of Internal Medicine, 171*(14), 1251–1257. doi:10.1001/archinternmed.2011.277

Prakash, R. S., Voss, M. W., Erickson, K. I., Lewis, J. M., Chaddock, L., Malkowski, E., . . . Kramer, A. F. (2011). Cardiorespiratory fitness and attentional control in the aging brain. *Frontiers in Human Neuroscience, 4*(229), 1–12. doi:10.3389/fnhum.2010.00229

Raz, N., Lindenberger, U., Rodrigue, K. M., Kennedy, K. M., Head, D., Williamson, A., . . . Acker, J. D. (2005). Regional brain changes in aging healthy adults: General trends, individual differences and modifiers. *Cerebral Cortex, 15*, 1676–1689. doi:10.1093/cercor/bhi044

Rosano, C., Venkatraman, V. K., Guralnik, J., Newman, A. B., Glynn, N. W., Launer, L., . . . Aizenstein, H. (2010). Psychomotor speed and functional brain MRI 2 years after completing a physical activity treatment. *Journals of Gerontology Series A: Biological and Medical Sciences, 65*, 639–647. doi:10.1093/gerona/glq038

Schuit, A. J., Feskens, E. J., Launer, L. J., & Kromhout, D. (2001). Physical activity and cognitive decline, the role of the apolipoprotein e4 allele. *Medicine & Science in Sports and Exercise, 33*, 772–777. Retrieved from http://journals.lww.com/acsm-msse/pages/default.aspx

Smith, J. C., Nielson, K. A., Woodard, J. L., Seidenberg, M., Durgerian, S., Antuono, P., . . . Rao, S. M. (2010). Interactive effects of physical activity and APOE-epsilon4 on BOLD semantic memory activation in healthy elders. *NeuroImage, 54*, 635–644. doi:10.1016/j.neuroimage.2010.07.070

Smith, P. J., Blumenthal, J. A., Hoffman, B. M., Cooper, H., Strauman, T. A., Welsh-Bohmer, K., . . . Sherwood, A. (2010). Aerobic exercise and neurocognitive performance: A meta-analytic review of randomized controlled trials. *Psychosomatic Medicine, 72*, 239–252. doi:10.1097/PSY.0b013e3181d14633

Spirduso, W. W. (1975). Reaction and movement time as a function of age and physical activity level. *Journals of Gerontology, 30*, 435–440. Retrieved from http://geronj.oxfordjournals.org/

US Census Bureau, http://www.census.gov/

Van Dijk, K. R. A., Hedden, T., Venkataraman, A., Evans, K. C., Lazar, S. W., & Buckner, R. L. (2010). Intrinsic functional connectivity as a tool for human connectomics: Theory, properties, and optimization. *Journal of Neurophysiology, 103*, 297–321. doi:10.1152/jn.00783.2009

Van Praag, H., Shubert, T., Zhao, C., & Gage, F. H. (2005). Exercise enhances learning and hippocampal neurogenesis in aged mice. *Journal of Neuroscience, 25*, 8680–8685. doi:10.1523/JNEUROSCI.1731-05.2005

Vaynman, S., Ying, Z., & Gomez-Pinilla, F. (2004). Hippocampal BDNF mediates the efficacy of exercise on synaptic plasticity and cognition. *European Journal of Neuroscience, 20*, 2580–2590. doi:10.1111/ejn.2004.20.issue-10

Voss, M. W., Erickson, K. I., Prakash, R. S., Chaddock, L., Malkowski, E., Alves, H., . . . Kramer, A. F. (2010). Functional connectivity: A source of variance in the association between cardiorespiratory fitness and cognition? *Neuropsychologia, 48*, 1394–1406. doi:10.1016/j.neuropsychologia.2010.01.005

Voss, M. W., Prakash, R. S., Erickson, K. I., Basak, C., Chaddock, L., Kim, J. S., . . . Kramer, A. F. (2010). Plasticity of brain networks in a randomized intervention trial of exercise training in older adults. *Frontiers in Aging Neuroscience, 2*(32), 1–17. doi:10.3389/fnagi.2010.00032

Weuve, J., Kang, J. H., Manson, J. E., Breteler, M. M. B., Ware, J. H., & Grodstein, F. (2004). Physical activity, including walking, and cognitive function in older women. *Journal of the American Medical Association, 292*(12), 1454–1461. doi:10.1001/jama.292.12.1454

18

PHYSICAL ACTIVITY, COGNITIVE IMPAIRMENT, AND DEMENTIA

Laura E. Middleton, Kristine Yaffe, and Deborah Barnes

Approximately 14% of adults over 70 years old in the United States have dementia (Plassman et al., 2007) and another 22% have milder cognitive impairment (Plassman et al., 2008). It is expected that the number of people who develop dementia worldwide will quadruple over the next 40 years due to the aging of the baby boomer generation and longer life expectancies (Brookmeyer, Johnson, Ziegler-Graham, & Arrighi, 2007). Current medications provide some symptomatic relief but do not cure or change the course of the disease. Therefore, there is tremendous interest in identifying strategies for preventing or delaying the onset of dementia. Physical activity (PA) has emerged as one of the most promising strategies for dementia prevention (Middleton & Yaffe, 2010). In this chapter we will provide a brief overview of cognitive function, cognitive impairment, and dementia and will then summarize the evidence from longitudinal studies and randomized controlled trials (RCTs) regarding the role of physical activity in the prevention of cognitive impairment and dementia.

Cognitive function, cognitive impairment, and dementia

Definitions and diagnosis

Cognitive function refers to mental abilities that enable us to receive, process, and act on information from the environment. Cognitive function is assessed using neuropsychological tests, and key cognitive domains include memory, speed of processing, language, visuospatial function, and executive function (the ability to plan and "execute" tasks). Although cognitive function generally declines with age, rates of decline vary widely, with some individuals experiencing substantial deterioration and others maintaining cognitive abilities until advanced old age (Barnes et al., 2007a).

Mild cognitive impairment (MCI) refers to a decline in one or more aspects of cognitive function that is greater than would be expected for an individual's age and education level but is not severe enough to affect their daily activities. Many different criteria have been developed, but the most commonly used are the Petersen criteria (Petersen et al., 1999). Individuals with MCI have an increased risk of developing dementia within 5 years (Bruscoli & Lovestone, 2004). Specific criteria have been developed to differentiate between MCI subtypes including "amnestic MCI," which primarily involves memory impairment, and "vascular MCI," which is more likely to be associated with executive dysfunction and linked with cerebrovascular disease (Marra, Ferraccioli, Vita, Quaranta, & Gainotti, 2004).

Dementia, in turn, is defined as a decline in memory and at least one other cognitive domain that is severe enough to affect an individual's daily activities such as eating, dressing, bathing, or toileting (American Psychiatric Association, 1994). While there are many types of dementia, Alzheimer's disease (AD) and vascular dementia are the most commonly diagnosed (Alzheimer's Association, 2010). AD is characterized by early symptoms of memory impairment and progressively worse cognitive impairment over the course of the disease. New diagnostic criteria for AD, MCI, and preclinical AD use biomarkers to increase the certainty of diagnosis (Albert et al., 2011; McKhann et al., 2011; Sperling et al., 2011) (Table 18.1). The symptoms and progression of vascular dementia are more variable across individuals compared to AD and are dictated by the location, severity, and progression of the underlying cerebrovascular disease. However, the neuropathogical features of AD and vascular dementia frequently occur concomitantly. As a result, mixed dementia, a combination of AD and vascular dementia, is likely the most common form of dementia.

Prevalence and prevention

Age is the greatest risk factor for dementia. After 65 years, the prevalence of dementia approximately doubles with every 5 years of age (Ziegler-Graham, Brookmeyer, Johnson, & Arrighi, 2008). Due to demographic changes and more people surviving to ages when dementia is common, the prevalence of dementia worldwide is expected to increase from 27 million in 2006 to 107 million in 2050 (Brookmeyer et al., 2007). Unfortunately, healthcare systems are largely unprepared for the expected rise in dementia prevalence in upcoming years. As a result, increasing attention is being paid to modifiable risk factors, particularly in high-risk populations such as those with more subtle symptoms of cognitive impairment.

Physical inactivity has recently been identified as one of the most important modifiable risk factors for dementia. Because physical inactivity is so common, Barnes and Yaffe (2011) estimated that as many as 13% of dementia cases worldwide and 21% of cases in the United States may be attributable to physical inactivity. A 25% reduction in the prevalence of physical activity could potentially prevent nearly 1 million cases worldwide and 232,000 in the United States. In the

Table 18.1 Overview of new diagnostic criteria proposed by the National Institute on Aging–Alzheimer's Association

Diagnosis	New proposed diagnostic criteria
Dementia	Cognitive impairment in at least two domains that reflects a decline from prior levels, is not explained by other factors such as delirium, and interferes with ability to perform usual activities.
Alzheimer's disease	**Probable:** Dementia with insidious onset, clear evidence of worsening over time, and lack of evidence for other causes (e.g., cerebrovascular disease, Parkinson's disease). Level of certainty increased with causative genetic mutation or biomarker evidence. **Possible:** Dementia with atypical course or etiologically mixed presentation.
Mild cognitive impairment	Concern regarding change in cognition, performance lower than expected for age and education in one or more domains, does not interfere with ability to perform usual activities, not caused by other factors. Level of certainty increased with biomarker evidence.
Preclinical Alzheimer's disease	Biomarker evidence of Alzheimer's disease with no or minimal evidence of cognitive change.

following sections, we will summarize the evidence from longitudinal studies and RCTs linking physical activity with a decreased risk of cognitive impairment and dementia.

Longitudinal studies of physical activity, cognitive impairment, and dementia

Longitudinal studies of physical activity and cognitive impairment in late life

In numerous studies in different populations and using various definitions of physical activity, people who are more physically active in late life have been found to have less chance of being diagnosed with dementia over the next 3 to 10 years than people who are sedentary (Rockwood & Middleton, 2007). A recent meta-analysis examined the association between PA and several neurodegenerative diseases including all-cause dementia and AD (Hamer & Chida, 2009). A total of 16 studies (total n = 163,797 participants) were identified; of these, 11 studies (n = 23,168) examined dementia as an outcome and six studies (n = 13,771) examined AD. Most individual studies (Abbott et al., 2004; Ho, Wood, Shame, Chan, & Yu 2001; Larson et al., 2006; Laurin, Verreault, Lindsay, Macpherson, & Rockwood 2001; Podewils et al., 2005; Rovio et al., 2005; Scarmeas et al., 2009; Sumic, Michael, Carlson, Howieson, & Kaye, 2007; Yoshitake et al., 1995), though not all (Fabrigoule et al., 1995; Verghese et al., 2003; Wang, van Belle, Kukull, & Larson, 2002; Wang et al., 2006; Wilson et al., 2002), found a significant protective association between greater PA and reduced risk of dementia (Figure 18.1) or AD (Figure 18.2). The combined results suggested that individuals in the highest PA group had a 28% lower risk of developing dementia (relative risk [RR], 0.72; 95% confidence interval [CI]: 0.60, 0.86) and a 45% lower risk of developing AD (RR, 0.55; 95% CI: 0.36, 0.84) as compared to those in the lowest PA group (Hamer & Chida, 2009).

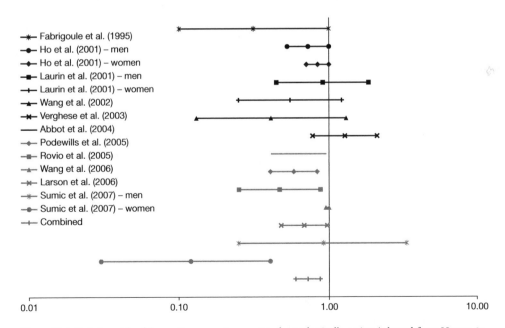

Figure 18.1 Relative risk of dementia comparing most to least physically active (adapted from Hamer & Chida, 2009).

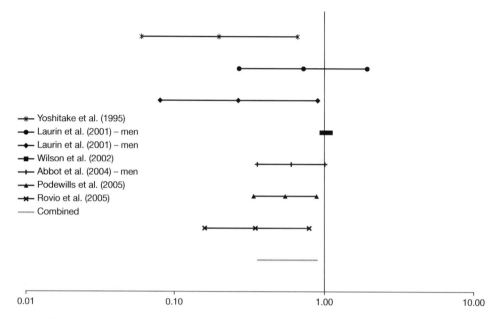

Figure 18.2 Relative risk of Alzheimer's disease comparing most to least physically active (adapted from Hamer & Chida, 2009).

The association between PA and risk of vascular dementia was examined in another recent meta-analysis (Aarsland, Sardahee, Anderssen, & Ballard, 2010). Of the five studies identified (Abbott et al., 2004; Laurin et al., 2001; Podewils et al., 2005; Ravaglia et al., 2008; Yoshitake et al., 1995), only one found a significant association between PA and reduced risk of vascular dementia (Ravaglia et al., 2008). However, the point estimates for vascular dementia were consistently lower in individuals who were physically active, and the combined results from the meta-analysis suggested that people who were more physically active had a 38% lower risk of developing vascular dementia than those who were less physically active (RR, 0.62; 95% CI: 0.42, 0.92). The lack of statistical significance in individual studies was likely due to small sample size because, until recently, vascular dementia has been diagnosed much less often than AD.

Fewer longitudinal studies have examined the association between PA and the risk of developing MCI (Verghese et al., 2006; Middleton, Kirkland, & Rockwood, 2008a; Lee et al., 2011). One study found that PA was more strongly associated with the risk of vascular-type MCI than amnestic-type MCI (Middleton et al., 2008a). However, another study found that cognitive activity, but not PA, was associated with reduced risk of amnestic-type MCI (Verghese et al., 2006). A third study found that PA was associated with reduced risk of all-cause MCI in women but not men (Lee et al., 2011). Additional studies are needed to clarify the association between PA and MCI and to determine whether there are differences in the association based on variables such as MCI type or sex.

Many studies have examined the association between PA and risk of cognitive decline or cognitive impairment based on changes in neuropsychological test performance rather than diagnostic criteria (Etgen et al., 2010; Flicker et al., 2005; Ho et al., 2001; Laurin et al., 2001; Lytle, Vander Bilt, Pandav, Dodge, & Ganguli, 2004; Middleton et al., 2008a; Middleton, Mitnitski, Fallah, Kirkland, & Rockwood, 2008b; Schuit, Feskens, Launer, & Kromhout, 2001; Stewart, Richards, Brayne, & Mann, 2001; Sturman et al., 2005; Weuve et al., 2004; Yaffe,

Barnes, Nevitt, Lui, & Covinsky, 2001). Most of these studies suggest that PA is associated with a reduced likelihood of cognitive decline and cognitive impairment in late life. There also is evidence that PA may not simply lower the risk of experiencing cognitive decline, cognitive impairment, or dementia, but that it may also increase the likelihood of maintaining normal cognitive function in late life. Indeed, one longitudinal study concluded that PA is associated with increased likelihood of stable or improved cognition with aging and not just slower decline (Middleton et al., 2008b).

Evidence for dose response

The presence of a dose-response relationship is often used to support the hypothesis that a relationship in an observational study is causal. Several studies have examined the association between the dose of PA and cognitive outcomes and the results are generally supportive of a dose-response relationship. One analysis from the Nurses' Health Study yielded a significant dose-response relationship between PA and decline in cognitive function 8 to 15 years later (Weuve et al., 2004). PA levels were reported using questionnaires by 18,766 women in 1986 and were used to divide the women into PA quintiles. Cognition was then assessed among the women in 1995–2001 when the women were 70–81 years old and again 2 years later to evaluate their rate of cognitive decline. A significant dose-response relationship was observed such that those who reported the most PA at baseline had the least cognitive decline over the following 2 years. Other studies also confirm a dose response by overall PA level (Laurin et al. 2001), PA intensity (Flicker et al., 2005; van Gelder et al., 2004; Weuve et al., 2004), daily PA duration (Schuit et al., 2001), and blocks walked per week (Yaffe et al., 2001).

Other studies, however, suggest that there may be a threshold effect such that moderate and high levels of PA are associated with similar cognitive benefits. One study followed 1,146 persons at least 65 years old at baseline and recorded self-reported exercise levels and scores on the Mini Mental State Examination (MMSE) (Lytle et al., 2004). Participants were divided into three groups: no exercise, low exercise, and high exercise. The high exercise group was initially defined as those participating in at least 30 minutes of aerobic exercise at least three times per week. Using this criterion, people in the high exercise group had significantly lower odds of cognitive decline (OR = 0.39; 95% CI: 0.19, 0.78). However, when the threshold for high exercise was increased to 5 days per week, the low and high exercise groups had similar risks of cognitive decline, suggesting that threshold for maximum benefits is realized at 3 days per week of activity and that 5 days per week of activity was no more beneficial (Lytle et al., 2004). It is unclear whether there are similar thresholds for intensity or duration of PA with regard to attaining maximum cognitive effects.

Early and mid-life PA, MCI, and dementia

Although longitudinal studies provide consistent evidence that people who are more physically active in late life have lower risk of dementia, cognitive impairment, and dementia, the length of these studies (generally less than 10 years) may be insufficient to rule out the presence of sub-clinical cognitive impairment and neuropathological features of dementia at baseline. Those with subtle cognitive deficits at baseline may also be less likely to be physically active, confounding the findings of these studies. By examining the relationship between PA earlier in life and the subsequent risk of cognitive impairment and dementia, the possibility of pre-clinical cognitive impairment at baseline influencing PA levels is reduced.

Evidence to date suggests that mid-life PA is beneficial to late life cognitive function. One study conducted in Finland examined cognitive function in 1,449 older adults (aged 65 to 79 years) who had previously reported PA levels during mid-life, approximately 21 years earlier (Rovio et al., 2005). Adjusted analyses revealed that people who participated in leisure time PA during mid-life had significantly lower odds of dementia (OR = 0.47, 95% CI: 0.25, 0.90) or AD (OR = 0.35; 95% CI: 0.16, 0.80) as compared with sedentary persons. This odds reduction is at least comparable to the odds reduction reported in studies of PA in late life. Interestingly, another study in this cohort found no association between work-related PA and risk of dementia or AD (Rovio et al., 2007). Although not entirely clear, this lack of relationship may be due to residual confounding factors such as socioeconomic status or level of cognitive stimulation at work. However, more recent studies also report inconsistent results with some (Andel et al., 2008; Middleton, Barnes, Lui & Yaffe, 2010) but not all (Carlson et al., 2008; Yamada et al., 2003) finding a significant association between mid-life PA and reduced rates of cognitive impairment 20 to 40 years later.

A few studies have also examined the relationship between early life (teenage to 30s) PA and late life cognition and found that early life PA is associated with lower rates of cognitive impairment, better information processing speed, and slower memory decline in late life (Dik, Deeg, Visser, & Jonker, 2003; Middleton et al., 2010; Richards, Hardy, & Wadsworth, 2003). Thus, the question arises: is PA more important at one age than another? To answer this question, a recent study examined the rates of late life cognitive impairment in 9,344 women who self-reported PA levels as teenagers, at age 30 years, at age 50 years, and during late life (Middleton et al., 2010). Although PA at any age was associated with reduced likelihood of cognitive impairment, PA during the teenage years was associated with the largest reduction in risk.

Objective measures of PA, MCI, and dementia

A limitation of most observational studies is their reliance on subjective self-reports of PA, which usually focus on moderate or vigorous exercise-related PA but do not adequately capture low-intensity PA, such as chores and movement around the house, which accounts for the majority of activity energy expenditure in people who do not regularly exercise (Donahoo, Levine, & Melanson, 2004). Such activity may be important to health outcomes such as cognitive impairment. In addition, since people with even subtle cognitive deficits may be more likely to misreport PA, there could be systematic misclassification of PA in studies relying on self-reports. Consequently, objective measures of PA are needed to confirm results from studies using self-reports.

Only a few studies have used objective measures of PA to examine the relationship between PA and cognitive function in late life. One early study measured cardiorespiratory fitness, which is primarily determined by PA as well as genetic predisposition, using maximum oxygen consumption ($\dot{V}O_2$ max) in 349 adults aged 55 years or older (Barnes, Yaffe, Satariano, & Tager, 2003). A modified MMSE was administered to each participant at baseline and 6 years later. Analyses revealed a strong dose-response relationship between cardiorespiratory fitness and cognitive decline such that people with better cardiorespiratory fitness at baseline had slower cognitive decline over the 6-year follow-up period.

In a second study, energy expended on activity was measured in 197 older adults using doubly-labeled water methods, arguably the gold-standard of PA measurement (Middleton et al., 2011). Cognitive function was assessed at baseline and 5 to 8 years later. In adjusted analyses, those in the highest tertile of activity at baseline had much lower rates of incident cognitive impairment (OR = 0.19; 95% CI: 0.01, 0.79) at the subsequent measurement, and there was evidence for dose response where increasing levels of activity energy expenditure were associated with decreasing risk of cognitive impairment. The decrease in the odds of cognitive impairment by tertile of activity energy expenditure was at least as great as those from published studies using self-reported PA. This suggests that total daily PA may be as or even more important than purposeful exercise, which is more readily captured by self-reports.

Strengths and limitations of longitudinal studies

Taken together, longitudinal studies of PA across the life course provide evidence that people who are more physically active have lower risk of dementia, cognitive impairment, and cognitive decline. The findings are reasonably consistent across different study populations, measures of PA, definitions of cognitive decline and dementia, sample sizes, and follow-up times. The evidence is further strengthened by studies suggesting that there is a dose–response relationship, that PA earlier in life is beneficial, and that objective measures of PA yield similar results to those found with subjective measures of PA. However, there are also several limitations. First, few studies examined whether one type of PA is better than another. As a result, the relative merits of different exercise regimens, such as those incorporating different levels of resistance, cardiovascular, and flexibility training, are unclear. One study that examined the rates of cognitive impairment by activity types concluded that ballroom dancing may offer the best protection against incident cognitive impairment (Verghese et al., 2003). Second, most studies assess PA only at study baseline and so our understanding of how PA patterns over time are associated with the development of cognitive impairment is poor. However, two studies provide preliminary data suggesting that rates of cognitive decline are faster in those who decrease their PA levels compared to those who maintain or increase their PA levels (Barnes et al., 2009; Van Gelder et al., 2004). Finally, arguably the most important weakness of observational studies is that people are self-selected to PA levels and not randomly assigned. Consequently, even in analyses that are adjusted for relevant covariates, there may be important residual differences between PA groups that are associated with the risk of cognitive impairment. Thus, it is imperative that RCTs examine the relationship between PA and cognitive function to complement the results from longitudinal, observational studies. The results from RCTs are discussed in the following section as well as in Chapter 17 in this volume.

RCTS of PA, cognitive impairment, and dementia

Most RCTs performed to date have examined the effects of exercise on cognitive change over a period of weeks or months in study populations ranging from healthy elders to individuals with MCI or dementia. Although findings have varied across studies, most have found that exercise—particularly aerobic exercise—results in improvements in some aspects of cognitive function—particularly executive function, motor speed, and attention. However, to date, RCTs have not directly measured whether PA can reduce the risk of or delay the onset of cognitive impairment, AD, or dementia.

Healthy elders

An early meta-analysis identified 18 RCTs of exercise interventions in healthy older adults (Colcombe & Kramer, 2003). Most studies used relatively small samples, with a total of 197 subjects included in the 18 studies. Nonetheless, the meta-analysis found significantly greater improvements in cognitive function over time in the exercise intervention participants (effect size [ES] = 0.48 standard deviations) compared to control participants (ES = 0.16). Improvements were observed for multiple cognitive domains including executive function (ES = 0.68), controlled processing (ES = 0.46), visuospatial function (ES = 0.43), and speed (ES = 0.27). Effect sizes (the difference between the intervention and control groups in standard deviation units) were slightly larger for combined aerobic and strength training interventions (ES = 0.59) than aerobic-only interventions (ES = 0.41) and for interventions with moderate (31–45 minutes, ES = 0.61) or long (46–60 minutes, ES = 0.47) rather than short (15–30 minutes, ES = 0.18) session durations. In addition, there was evidence that effect sizes were larger for studies with more female participants (ES = 0.60) than for studies with more male (ES = 0.15) participants and for middle-aged (66–70 years, ES = 0.69) and older (71–80 years, ES = 0.55) than younger (55–65, ES = 0.30) participants.

However, a more recent Cochrane systematic review that focused on the effects of aerobic exercise was less conclusive (Angevaren, Aufdemkampe, Verhaar, Aleman, & Vanhees, 2008). This review included fewer studies with a total of 11 RCTs with 625 subjects, most of which had non-significant results. When the RCTs were combined, significant effect sizes were observed for cognitive speed (ES = 0.24) and visual attention (ES = 0.26) when aerobic exercise was compared to any control group. Significant effects were observed for motor function (ES = 1.17) and auditory attention (ES = 0.50) only in studies where aerobic exercise was compared to a no-intervention control group. The question of the most appropriate control group remains controversial and options include a stretching and toning group, an educational group, or a no-contact group, each with its own advantages and disadvantages. The most conservative option, a stretching and control group, enables participant blinding but may induce non-trivial cognitive benefits as two studies have shown that resistance training (toning) is associated with positive cognitive changes (Cassilhas et al., 2007; Liu-Ambrose et al., 2010).

A major limitation of the exercise RCTs conducted to date in healthy elders is that they have focused on cognitive change on standardized cognitive tests as their primary outcome. RCTs with cognitively normal older adults that examine whether PA interventions reduce the incidence of MCI and dementia are critically needed (Barnes et al., 2007b). In addition, the lack of standardization in exercise interventions, control group activities, and outcome measures makes comparisons across studies and combination of findings difficult.

Cognitive impairment and dementia

Several recent studies have examined the impact of exercise interventions on cognitive decline in individuals diagnosed with cognitive impairment or dementia. Some studies were conducted in the community and others in residential care. In 2004, a meta-analysis combined the results of RCTs in which the subjects had evidence of cognitive impairment, defined as having a mean MMSE score of less than 26 or a diagnosis of cognitive impairment or dementia (Heyn, Beatriz, & Ottenbacher, 2004). This meta-analysis identified 10 trials including 820 subjects with cognitive impairment and found that those in the exercise groups improved significantly more than controls on measures of cognitive function (ES = 0.57; 95% CI: 0.43, 1.117). Although a more recent Cochrane review with more strict recruitment criteria (only two studies were included) was inconclusive, the results of the 2004 meta-analysis are sufficient to suggest that PA may improve cognitive outcomes even among those already exhibiting symptoms of impairment.

Two recent RCTs provide additional evidence that PA can improve cognitive function in individuals with MCI. In one study, 170 individuals who reported memory problems but did not have dementia were randomized to participate in a 24-week PA intervention or a usual care control group. The exercise group experienced significantly better cognitive outcomes than the control group both over the course of the intervention and after an additional 12-month follow-up (Lautenschlager et al., 2008). Another RCT of 33 individuals with MCI found that aerobic exercise had sex-specific effects in which the benefits on executive function were larger for women (Baker et al., 2010). Several additional studies that will provide further evidence regarding the cognitive effects of various exercise regimens in elders with MCI or dementia are currently underway, including Fitness for the Aging Brain II (FABS II) (Australia New Zealand Clinical Trials Registry: ACTRN12609000755235); Promotion of the Mind Through Exercise (PROMoTE) (ClinicalTrials.gov Protocol Registration System: NCT01027858); and Preventing Loss of Independence through Exercise (PLIÉ) (ClinicalTrials.gov Protocol Registration System: NCT01371214).

Summary and limitations

Numerous RCTs have examined the effects of exercise interventions on cognitive outcomes in healthy elders with a smaller number testing the effects in elders with MCI or dementia. Most trials have been limited by small sample sizes. In addition, the lack of consistency in intervention, control, and outcome measures makes combining results difficult. As alluded to earlier, the choice of control group is of particular concern and likely affects the magnitude of observed responses. For example, a control intervention that included social engagement would only detect differences based solely on physical movement and would omit effects based on the social aspects of PA. Despite these limitations, studies to date suggest that exercise results in small improvements in cognitive function across all cognitive classifications. Larger, well-controlled RCTs are needed to provide definitive evidence that engaging in PA can lead to a reduced risk of cognitive impairment and dementia and can benefit the cognitive performance of those already experiencing cognitive impairment.

Conclusions and future directions

Robust and consistent results from longitudinal studies provide evidence that PA is associated with reduced risk of cognitive impairment and dementia in late life. Preliminary evidence from RCTs generally provides supportive evidence. However, RCTs that examined the cognitive benefits of PA interventions in people with cognitive impairment are more limited in both sample size and quality. Larger RCTs are needed to investigate the role of PA in relation to cognitive performance and the incidence of dementia. Such trials are underway relative to cognitive performance—for example, the lifestyle interventions and independence for elders (LIFE) study began in 2010 and is randomizing 1,600 healthy older adults to either exercise or control groups for an average of 2.7 years. The PA intervention is comprised of three phases: adoption (8 weeks), transition (12 weeks), and maintenance (to end of trial). Although there will be no clinical cognitive diagnosis, the LIFE study includes cognitive function as a secondary outcome and should provide more definitive data to support or oppose a causal relationship between PA and reduced cognitive decline.

At this time, it is not known whether increased participation in PA will reduce the overall prevalence of cognitive impairment and dementia. No RCTs have followed people long enough to capture the transition from normal cognition to cognitive impairment. However, PA has many other beneficial effects on cardiovascular and metabolic outcomes, and there is no evidence to suggest that it might be harmful. Therefore, while we wait for results from ongoing studies and for future long-term trials, PA can be recommended as a strategy that has many known health benefits, may improve cognitive performance, and may lower risk or delay onset of cognitive impairment and dementia.

References

Aarsland, D., Sardahaee, F. S., Anderssen, S., & Ballard, C. (2010). Is physical activity a potential preventive factor for vascular dementia? A systematic review. *Aging & Mental Health, 14,* 386–395.

Abbott, R. D., White, L. R., Ross, G. W., Masaki, K. H., Curb, J. D., & Petrovitch, H. (2004). Walking and dementia in physically capable elderly men. *Journal of the American Medical Association, 292,* 1447–1453.

Albert, M. S., DeKosky, S. T., Dickson, D., Dubois, B., Feldman, H. H., Fox, N. C., . . . Phelps, C. H. (2011). The diagnosis of mild cognitive impairment due to Alzheimer's disease: Recommendations from the National Institute on Aging–Alzheimer's Association workgroups on Diagnostic Guidelines for Alzheimer's disease. *Alzheimer's & Dementia, 7,* 270–279.

Alzheimer's Association. (2010). *2010 Alzheimer's Disease Facts & Figures.* http://www.alz.org/documents_custom/report_alzfactsfigures2010.pdf. Accessed March 13, 2011.

American Psychiatric Association. (1994). *Diagnostic and Statistical Manual of Mental Disorders* (4th ed.). Arlington, VA: American Psychological Association.

Andel, R., Crowe, M., Pedersen, N. L., Fratiglioni, L., Johansson, B., & Gatz, M. (2008). Physical exercise at midlife and risk of dementia three decades later: A population-based study of Swedish twins. *Journals of Gerontology Series A-Biological Sciences and Medical Sciences, 63,* 62–66.

Angevaren, M., Aufdemkampe, G., Verhaar, H. J. J., Aleman, A., & Vanhees, L. (2008). Physical activity and enhanced fitness to improve cognitive function in older people without known cognitive impairment. *Cochrane Database Systematic Review, 3* (CD005381). doi:10.1002/14651858.CD005381.pub3

Baker, L. D., Frank, L. L., Foster-Schubert, K., Green, P. S., Wilkinson, C. W., McTiernan, A., . . . Craft, S. (2010). Effects of aerobic exercise on mild cognitive impairment: A controlled trial. *Archives of Neurology, 67,* 71–79.

Barnes, D. E., Yaffe, K., Satariano, W. A., & Tager, I. B. (2003). A longitudinal study of cardiorespiratory fitness and cognitive function in healthy older adults. *Journal of the American Geriatrics Society, 51,* 459–465.

Barnes, D. E., Cauley, J. A., Lui, L. Y., Fink, H. A., McCulloch, C., Stone, K. L., & Yaffe, K. (2007a). Women who maintain optimal cognitive function into old age. *Journal of the American Geriatrics Society, 55,* 259–264.

Barnes, D. E., Whitmer, R. A., & Yaffe, K. (2007b). Physical activity and dementia: The need for prevention trials. *Exercise & Sport Sciences Reviews, 35,* 24–29.

Barnes, D. E., Simonsick, E., Harris, T., Brach, J., Pope, S., Rosano, C., & Yaffe, K. (2009). The impact of changes in physical activity levels on rate of cognitive decline. Presented at the International Conference on Alzheimer's Disease, July 2009, Vienna, Austria.

Barnes, D. E., & Yaffe, K. (2011). The projected effect of risk factor reduction on Alzheimer's disease prevalence. *Lancet Neurology, 10,* 819–828.

Brookmeyer, R., Johnson, E., Ziegler-Graham, K., & Arrighi, H. M. (2007). Forecasting the global burden of Alzheimer's disease. *Alzheimer's & Dementia, 3,* 186–191.

Bruscoli, M., & Lovestone, S. (2004). Is MCI really just early dementia? A systematic review of conversion studies. *International Psychogeriatrics, 16,* 129–140.

Carlson, M. C., Helms, M. J., Steffens, D. C., Burke, J. R., Potter, G. G., & Plassman, B. L. (2008). Midlife activity predicts risk of dementia in older male twin pairs. *Alzheimer's & Dementia, 4,* 324–331.

Cassilhas, R. C., Viana, V. A., Grassmann, V., Santos, R. T., Santos, R. F., Tufik, S., & Mello, M. T. (2007). The impact of resistance exercise on the cognitive function of the elderly. *Medicine & Science in Sports & Exercise, 39,* 1401–1407.

Colcombe, S., & Kramer, A. F. (2003). Fitness effects on the cognitive function of older adults: A meta-analytic study. *Psychological Science, 14,* 125–130.

Dik, M., Deeg, D. J., Visser, M., & Jonker, C. (2003). Early life physical activity and cognition at old age. *Journal of Clinical & Experimental Neuropsychology, 25,* 643–653.

Donahoo, W. T., Levine, J. A., & Melanson, E. L. (2004). Variability in energy expenditure and its components. *Current Opinion in Clinical Nutrition & Metabolic Care, 7,* 599–605.

Etgen, T., Sander, D., Huntgeburth, U., Poppert, H., Forstl, H., & Bickel, H. (2010). Physical activity and incident cognitive impairment in elderly persons: The INVADE study. *Archives of Internal Medicine, 170,* 186–193.

Fabrigoule, C., Letenneur, L., Dartigues, J. F., Zarrouk, M., Commenges, D., & Barberger-Gateau, P. (1995). Social and leisure activities and risk of dementia: A prospective longitudinal study. *Journal of the American Geriatrics Society, 43,* 485–490.

Flicker, L., Almeida, O. P., Acres, J., Le, M. T., Tuohy, R. J., Jamrozik, K., . . . Norman, P. (2005). Predictors of impaired cognitive function in men over the age of 80 years: Results from the Health in Men Study. *Age and Ageing, 34*, 77–80.

Hamer, M., & Chida, Y. (2009). Physical activity and risk of neurodegenerative disease: A systematic review of prospective evidence. *Psychological Medicine, 39*, 3–11.

Heyn, P., Beatriz, C. A., & Ottenbacher, K. J. (2004). The effects of exercise training on elderly persons with cognitive impairment and dementia: A meta-analysis. *Archives of Physical Medicine & Rehabilitation, 85*, 1694–1704.

Ho, S. C., Woo, J., Sham, A., Chan, S. G., & Yu, A. L. (2001). A 3-year follow-up study of social, lifestyle and health predictors of cognitive impairment in a Chinese older cohort. *International Journal of Epidemiology, 30*, 1389–1396.

Larson, E. B., Wang, L., Bowen, J. D., McCormick, W. C., Teri, L., Crane, P., & Kukull, W. (2006). Exercise is associated with reduced risk for incident dementia among persons 65 years of age and older. *Annals of Internal Medicine, 144*, 73–81.

Laurin, D., Verreault, R., Lindsay, J., MacPherson, K., & Rockwood, K. (2001). Physical activity and risk of cognitive impairment and dementia in elderly persons. *Archives of Neurology, 58*, 498–504.

Lautenschlager, N. T., Cox, K. L., Flicker, L., Foster, J. K., Van Bockxmeer, F., Xiao, J., . . . Almeida, O. P. (2008). Effects of physical activity on cognitive function in older adults at risk for Alzheimer disease. *Journal of the American Medical Association, 300*, 1027–1037.

Lee, L. K., Shahar, S., Chin, A. V., Mohd Yusoff, N. A., Rajab, N., & Aziz, S. A. (2011). Prevalence of gender disparities and predictors affecting the occurrence of mild cognitive impairment (MCI). *Archives of Gerontology and Geriatrics* [Epub ahead of print].

Liu-Ambrose, T., Nagamatsu, L. S., Graf, P., Beattie, B. L., Ashe, M. C., & Handy, T. C. (2010). Resistance training and executive functions: A 12-month randomized controlled trial. *Archives of Internal Medicine, 170*, 170–178.

Lytle, M. E., Vander Bilt, J., Pandav, R. S., Dodge, H. H., & Ganguli, M. (2004). Exercise level and cognitive decline: The MoVIES project. *Alzheimer Disease & Associated Disorders, 18*, 57–64.

Marra, C., Ferraccioli, M., Vita, M. G., Quaranta, D., & Gainotti, G. (2011). Patterns of cognitive decline and rates of conversion to dementia in patients with degenerative and vascular forms of MCI. *Current Alzheimer Research, 8*, 24–31.

McKhann, G. M., Knopman, D. S., Chertkow, H., Hyman, B. T., Jack, C. R., Jr., Kawas, C. H., . . . Phelps, C. H. (2011). The diagnosis of dementia due to Alzheimer's disease: Recommendations from the National Institute on Aging–Alzheimer's Association workgroups on Diagnostic Guidelines for Alzheimer's Disease. *Alzheimer's & Dementia, 7*, 263–269.

Middleton, L., Kirkland, S., & Rockwood, K. (2008a). Prevention of CIND by physical activity: Different impact on VCI-ND compared with MCI. *Journal of the Neurological Sciences, 269*, 80–84.

Middleton, L. E., Mitnitski, A., Fallah, N., Kirkland, S. A., & Rockwood, K. (2008b). Changes in cognition and mortality in relation to exercise in late life: A population based study. *PLoS ONE, 3*, e3124.

Middleton, L. E., & Yaffe, K. (2010). Targets for the prevention of dementia. *Journal of Alzheimer's Disease, 20*, 915–924.

Middleton, L. E., Barnes, D. E., Lui, L. Y., & Yaffe, K. (2010). Physical activity over the life course and its association with cognitive performance and impairment in old age. *Journal of the American Geriatrics Society, 58*, 1322–1326.

Middleton, L. E., Manini, T. M., Simonsick, E. M., Harris, T. B., Barnes, D. E., Tylavsky, F., . . . Yaffe, K. (2011). Activity energy expenditure and incident cognitive impairment in older adults. *Archives of Internal Medicine, 171*, 1251–1257.

Petersen, R. C., Smith, G. E., Waring, S. C., Ivnik, R. J., Tangalos, E. G., & Kokmen, E. (1999). Mild cognitive impairment: Clinical characterization and outcome. *Archives of Neurology, 56*, 303–308.

Plassman, B. L., Langa, K. M., Fisher, G. G., Heeringa, S. G., Weir, D. R., Ofstedal, M. B., . . . Wallace, R. B. (2007). Prevalence of dementia in the United States: The Aging, Demographics, and Memory Study. *Neuroepidemiology, 29*, 125–132.

Plassman, B. L., Langa, K. M., Fisher, G. G., Heeringa, S. G., Weir, D. R., Ofstedal, M. B., . . . Wallace, R. B. (2008). Prevalence of cognitive impairment without dementia in the United States. *Annals of Internal Medicine, 148*, 427–434.

Podewils, L. J., Guallar, E., Kuller, L. H., Fried, L. P., Lopez, O. L., Carlson, M., & Lyketsos, C. G. (2005). Physical activity, APOE genotype, and dementia risk: Findings from the cardiovascular health cognition study. *American Journal of Epidemiology, 161*, 639–651.

Ravaglia, G., Forti, P., Lucicesare, A., Pisacane, N., Rietti, E., Bianchin, M., & Dalmonte, E. (2008).

Physical activity and dementia risk in the elderly: Findings from a prospective Italian study. *Neurology*, 70, 1786–1794.

Richards, M., Hardy, R., & Wadsworth, M. E. (2003). Does active leisure protect cognition? Evidence from a national birth cohort. *Social Science & Medicine*, 56, 785–792.

Rockwood, K., & Middleton, L. (2007). Physical activity and the maintenance of cognitive function. *Alzheimer's & Dementia*, 3, S38–S44.

Rovio, S., Kareholt, I., Helkala, E. L., Viitanen, M., Winblad, B., Tuomilehto, J., . . . Kivipelto, M. (2005). Leisure-time physical activity at midlife and the risk of dementia and Alzheimer's disease. *Lancet Neurology*, 4, 705–711.

Rovio, S., Kareholt, I., Viitanen, M., Winblad, B., Tuomilehto, J., Soininen, H., . . . Kivipelto, M. (2007). Work-related physical activity and the risk of dementia and Alzheimer's disease. *International Journal of Geriatric Psychiatry*, 22, 874–882.

Scarmeas, N., Luchsinger, J. A., Schupf, N., Brickman, A. M., Cosentino, S., Tang, M. X., & Stern, Y. (2009). Physical activity, diet, and risk of Alzheimer disease. *Journal of the American Medical Association*, 302, 627–637.

Schuit, A. J., Feskens, E. J., Launer, L. J., & Kromhout, D. (2001). Physical activity and cognitive decline, the role of the apolipoprotein e4 allele. *Medicine & Science in Sports & Exercise*, 33, 772–777.

Sperling, R. A., Aisen, P. S., Beckett, L. A., Bennett, D. A., Craft, S., Fagan, A. M., . . . Phelps, C. H. (2011). Toward defining the preclinical stages of Alzheimer's disease: Recommendations from the National Institute on Aging–Alzheimer's Association workgroups on Diagnostic Guidelines for Alzheimer's disease. *Alzheimer's & Dementia*, 7, 280–292.

Stewart, R., Richards, M., Brayne, C., & Mann, A. (2001). Vascular risk and cognitive impairment in an older, British, African-Caribbean population. *Journal of the American Geriatrics Society*, 49, 263–269.

Sturman, M. T., Morris, M. C., Mendes de Leon, C. F., Bienias, J. L., Wilson, R. S., & Evans, D. A. (2005). Physical activity, cognitive activity, and cognitive decline in a biracial community population. *Archives of Neurology*, 62, 1750–1754.

Sumic, A., Michael, Y. L., Carlson, N. E., Howieson, D. B., & Kaye, J. A. (2007). Physical activity and the risk of dementia in oldest old. *Journal of Aging & Health*, 19, 242–259.

van Gelder, B. M., Tijhuis, M. A., Kalmijn, S., Giampaoli, S., Nissinen, A., & Kromhout, D. (2004). Physical activity in relation to cognitive decline in elderly men: The FINE Study. *Neurology*, 63, 2316–2321.

Verghese, J., Lipton, R. B., Katz, M. J., Hall, C. B., Derby, C. A., Kuslansky, G., . . . Buschke, H. (2003). Leisure activities and the risk of dementia in the elderly. *New England Journal of Medicine*, 348, 2508–2516.

Verghese, J., LeValley, A., Derby, C., Kuslansky, G., Katz, M., Hall, C., . . . Lipton, R. B. (2006). Leisure activities and the risk of amnestic mild cognitive impairment in the elderly. *Neurology*, 66, 821–827.

Wang, J. Y., Zhou, D. H., Li, J., Zhang, M., Deng, J., Tang, M., . . . Chen, M. (2006). Leisure activity and risk of cognitive impairment: The Chongqing aging study. *Neurology*, 66, 911–913.

Wang, L., van Belle, G., Kukull, W. B., & Larson, E. B. (2002). Predictors of functional change: A longitudinal study of nondemented people aged 65 and older. *Journal of the American Geriatrics Society*, 50, 1525–1534.

Weuve, J., Kang, J. H., Manson, J. E., Breteler, M. M., Ware, J. H., & Grodstein, F. (2004). Physical activity, including walking, and cognitive function in older women. *Journal of the American Medical Association*, 292, 1454–1461.

Wilson, R. S., Bennett, D. A., Bienias, J. L., Aggarwal, N. T., Mendes De Leon, C. F., Morris, M. C., . . . Evans, D. A. (2002). Cognitive activity and incident AD in a population-based sample of older persons. *Neurology*, 59, 1910–1914.

Yaffe, K., Barnes, D., Nevitt, M., Lui, L. Y., & Covinsky, K. (2001). A prospective study of physical activity and cognitive decline in elderly women: Women who walk. *Archives of Internal Medicine*, 161, 1703–1708.

Yamada, M., Kasagi, F., Sasaki, H., Masunari, N., Mimori, Y., & Suzuki, G. (2003). Association between dementia and midlife risk factors: The Radiation Effects Research Foundation Adult Health Study. *Journal of the American Geriatrics Society*, 51, 410–414.

Yoshitake, T., Kiyohara, Y., Kato, I., Ohmura, T., Iwamoto, H., Nakayama, K., . . . Fujishima, M. (1995). Incidence and risk factors of vascular dementia and Alzheimer's disease in a defined elderly Japanese population: The Hisayama Study. *Neurology*, 45, 1161–1168.

Ziegler-Graham, K., Brookmeyer, R., Johnson, E., & Arrighi, H. M. (2008). Worldwide variation in the doubling time of Alzheimer's disease incidence rates. *Alzheimer's & Dementia*, 4, 316–323.

19

EXERCISE AND COGNITIVE FUNCTION

Neurobiological mechanisms

Nicole C. Berchtold and Carl W. Cotman

The concept that lifestyle factors such as exercise, diet, and intellectual activity affect the health and function of the brain has gained increasing traction over the past decade. In particular, exercise participation has emerged as a powerful strategy to improve learning and memory, delay age-related cognitive decline, and reduce the risk of neurodegeneration. In humans, the benefits of exercise have been most clearly demonstrated in elderly populations, where sustained exercise participation improves a wide range of cognitive processes. The most robust benefits emerge for the brain's frontal lobes (responsible for executive function), as well as the hippocampus (critical for learning and memory), and the anterior cingulate (involved in both executive function and aspects of memory). Essentially, the cognitive capacities that are most susceptible to functional decline with age are those that are most benefited by exercise, suggesting that exercise slows brain aging. Research aimed at understanding the underlying mechanisms that mediate benefits of physical activity on brain health and cognitive function is an area of intense activity, with many exciting findings discovered in the past two decades. In addition, an emerging field that builds on the benefits of exercise reveals that lifestyle factors such as cognitive stimulation ("enrichment") and diet interact with exercise to further benefit brain health and function. This chapter focuses on the neurobiological mechanisms that have been identified as key factors mediating benefits of exercise on cognitive health, and will briefly review recent findings on interactive effects of exercise, diet, and enrichment on brain health and function.

Human studies

Human research using neuroimaging has revealed a number of striking effects of exercise on brain structure, connectivity, blood perfusion, and function. Techniques such as magnetic resonance imaging (MRI) and diffusion tensor imaging can visualize features of the brain in a living individual, and have been used to compare the brains in elderly individuals who have participated in lifelong exercise versus age-matched individuals who have been generally sedentary. Imaging studies reveal exercise and improved cardiovascular fitness affect the brain on multiple levels. For example, fitness training counteracts the declines in gray matter density and white matter integrity that occur with aging (for review, see Ahlskog, Geda, Graff-Radford, & Petersen, 2011) and elicits positive changes in brain function and connectivity (Burdette et al., 2010), notably in brain regions critical for higher cognitive function, such as the hippocampus, anterior cingulate, and prefrontal region. The increased interconnectivity between these regions indicates that information can be more readily transmitted throughout the brain to support more efficient communication. Importantly, exercise improves the cognitive functions that often decline with age, such as the capacity for learning, memory, and executive function (important for selective attention, multi-tasking, and shifting between different tasks), suggesting that exercise slows brain aging.

Animal studies

Animal studies have provided much insight as to the physiological response of the brain to exercise. Converging evidence implicates the hippocampus as a crucial brain region for exercise benefits to cognitive function, and the vast majority of exercise studies in animals have focused on exercise effects on this brain structure. Consistent with research in humans, rodent studies demonstrate that exercise improves cognitive function, facilitating both learning and memory in young and aged animals, in various hippocampus-dependent tasks (Cotman & Berchtold, 2002). Animal models of exercise have indicated several key mechanisms through which aerobic training may enhance brain function. These pathways include improvement in the structural integrity of the brain (synaptogenesis, neurogenesis, and angiogenesis), increased production of key growth factors that promote synaptic plasticity among other effects, improved energy metabolism, and modulation of the brain's immune response to a healthier profile, particularly in aging. Animal models are shedding light on how aging interacts with these molecular and cellular effects of exercise on brain and cognition.

Plasticity and synaptic complexity in the hippocampus

Synaptic plasticity, or the capacity of the brain to undergo changes in synaptic connections and synaptic strength, provides the foundation for learning and memory. One mechanism by which exercise is thought to facilitate learning and memory is by enhancing synaptic plasticity in the hippocampus. Changes in synaptic efficacy can be assessed at the electrophysiological level by measuring short-term potentiation (STP) and long-term potentiation (LTP), which are synaptic analogues of learning. Exercise enhances both STP and LTP in the hippocampus (Farmer et al., 2004; van Praag, Christie, Sejnowski, & Gage, 1999), revealing that the strength of hippocampal synaptic communication is increased with exercise exposure. In addition, exercise reduces the threshold of stimulation required for LTP (Farmer et al., 2004), indicating that hippocampal synapses are more responsive to encoding new information. The enhanced responsiveness of the hippocampus is paralleled by increased length and complexity of dendrites, increased dendritic spine density, and increased number of newly generated neurons, or neurogenesis (Eadie, Redila, & Christie, 2005). Such increased structural complexity is also observed in many regions of the cortex in response to exercise (Cotman & Berchtold, 2002), revealing that exercise effects extend beyond the hippocampus. At a molecular level, exercise facilitates synaptic plasticity by increasing levels of many synaptic proteins, neurotransmitter receptors, and growth factors. Some examples include synapsin I, synaptophysin, glutamate receptors (NR2b, GluR5), brain-derived neurotrophic factor (BDNF), insulin-like growth factor 1 (IGF-1), and vascular endothelial-derived growth factor (VEGF).

Growth factors

An exciting discovery in the mid-1990s was the finding that exercise is a potent stimulus that increases the availability of several classes of growth factors in the brain. One of the most exciting aspects of this discovery was that the growth factor response was most prominent in highly plastic brain regions important for higher cognitive function, notably the hippocampus and regions of the cortex, regions not normally associated with motor function. This discovery was the catalyst for an explosive interest in elucidating potential benefits of exercise on cognition as well as on overall brain health and function. It has become clear that the increased availability of the various growth factors is central to many of the benefits of exercise on the brain (for reviews, see Cotman & Berchtold, 2002; Cotman, Berchtold, & Christie, 2007; Voss, Nagamatsu, Liu-Ambrose, & Kramer, 2011). The growth factors that are the principal ones known to mediate the effects of exercise on the hippocampus and other brain regions are BDNF, IGF-1, and VEGF. These growth factors work in concert to produce complementary effects, modulating both overlapping and unique aspects of exercise-related benefits in brain plasticity, function, and health.

BDNF

Extensive evidence supports the idea that BDNF is essential for hippocampal function, synaptic plasticity, learning, and modulation of depression, all endpoints that are improved with exercise (Cotman et al., 2007). In animal studies, exercise rapidly increases BDNF in several brain regions, with the most robust and enduring response in the hippocampus. BDNF gene and protein expression are increased in neurons throughout the hippocampus after a few days of exercise, and protein levels continue to rise with sustained exercise for several weeks (Berchtold, Chinn, Chou, Kesslak, & Cotman, 2005). Induction of BDNF in the hippocampus is regulated by effects of exercise on neuroendocrine systems, other growth factors such as IGF-1, and neurotransmitter systems. With respect to the neurotransmitter system, glutamate signaling by neurons in the hippocampus ultimately drives BDNF regulation with exercise, with input by the noradrenergic system important for exercise-induction of BDNF (Garcia, Chen, Garza, Cotman, & Russo-Neustadt, 2003). BDNF binding to its receptor trkB activates many downstream molecular effects, including many pathways that are involved in learning and memory. Indeed, recent studies demonstrate that BDNF signaling (by binding to its receptor) is a crucial mechanism underlying improved learning in response to exercise. If BDNF signaling is blocked in the hippocampus (by infusing an antibody that blocks BDNF activation of its receptor), the beneficial effects of exercise on hippocampal-dependent learning are blocked, specifically blocking improvements in both acquisition and retention (Vaynman, Ying, Yin, & Gomez-Pinilla, 2006). These findings demonstrate that BDNF signaling must be active in the hippocampus for the effects of exercise on hippocampal plasticity to manifest.

IGF-1

IGF-1 is another growth factor that is increased in response to exercise, and IGF-1 signaling is another crucial mechanism underlying cognitive improvements in response to exercise. Like BDNF, IGF-1 gene expression is increased in hippocampal neurons in response to exercise, occurring several days after exercise onset (Q. Ding, Vaynman, Akhavan, Ying, & Gomez-Pinilla, 2006). In addition to the increased IGF-1 gene activity in neurons in the brain, levels of IGF-1 increase outside the brain, with peripheral circulating levels of IGF-1 increasing within 1 hour after exercise. IGF-1 produced in the periphery can enter the brain through the circulating blood, and interestingly, this peripheral IGF-1 appears to be essential for some of the effects of exercise on the hippocampus. For example, if peripheral IGF-1 is prevented from entering the CNS, many benefits of exercise do not occur in the brain, including enhanced neurogenesis (Trejo, Carro, & Torres-Aleman, 2001), vessel remodeling (angiogenesis) (Lopez-Lopez, LeRoith, & Torres-Aleman, 2004), and improved memory. Further, if function of IGF-1 is blocked specifically in the hippocampus, many of the benefits of exercise on hippocampal function are diminished, such as improved recall in a hippocampal-dependent task and exercise induction of synaptic molecules including synapsin I, calmodulin-kinase II (CamKII), mitogen-activated protein kinase II (MAPKII), and BDNF. Overall, IGF-1 and BDNF systems are both intricately involved in mediating effects of exercise, with convergence on BDNF signaling appearing to be a final common downstream mechanism important for exercise benefits to hippocampal function (described in more detail in Cotman et al., 2007).

VEGF

Like IGF-1, VEGF is increased in the peripheral circulation in response to exercise, and crosses the blood-brain barrier to enter the CNS. In further parallel to IGF-1, peripheral VEGF contributes to exercise-dependent stimulation of neurogenesis and angiogenesis in the brain, as demonstrated by studies using antibodies that block entry of peripheral VEGF into the brain (Fabel et al., 2003). IGF-1 and VEGF signaling appear to mediate overlapping aspects of exercise effects on hippocampal function, but likely have unique functionality as well. The role of VEGF in mediating exercise effects has not been extensively studied and warrants further investigation.

Other growth factors

In addition to the effects of exercise on BDNF, IGF, and VEGF, exercise modulates availability of several other growth factors in the brain as well. These include increases in nerve growth factor (NGF) and fibroblast-growth factor-2 (FGF-2), and decreases in bone morphogenetic protein (BMP). The responses of FGF-2 and NGF appear to be transitory and less robust than the responses of BDNF, IGF, and VEGF, and current data suggest that FGF-2, NGF, and BMP have relatively minor roles in modulating effects of exercise on the brain. However, a recent study indicated that exercise-dependent declines in hippocampal BMP protein appear to contribute to the effects of exercise on neurogenesis and cognition (Gobeske et al., 2009), an interesting finding that merits further study.

Summary

Currently, there is strong evidence that BDNF, IGF, and VEGF have essential roles in mediating various effects of exercise on the CNS. Growth factor levels can come directly from production locally in the brain, as well as entering the CNS after being increased in the periphery, with both sources emerging as important for modulating brain function with exercise. Altogether, the various growth factors work in concert to produce complementary effects, modulating both overlapping and unique aspects of exercise-related benefits in brain plasticity, function, and health. IGF-1 and BDNF signaling are important in promoting neural plasticity and behavioral improvements with exercise, while IGF-1 and VEGF signaling appear to orchestrate the effects of exercise on neurogenesis and angiogenesis.

Neurogenesis

One effect of exercise that has garnered intense interest is the stimulation of neurogenesis and the generation of new neurons in the hippocampus. While it was long believed that no new neurons were generated in the brain after birth, this dogma has been overturned with the discovery that specific brain regions contain neural progenitor cells that generate new brain cells throughout the lifespan, most notably in the hippocampus and around the ventricles of the brain (Lazarov, Mattson, Peterson, Pimplikar, & van Praag, 2010). These neural progenitor cells divide and differentiate to become neurons and glia, and the proliferation, differentiation, and survival are sensitive to a variety of factors including exercise exposure. Hippocampal neurogenesis, particularly the generation of new neurons, is an important component of hippocampal-dependent learning (Castilla-Ortega, Pedraza, Estivill-Torrus, & Santin, 2011), with the role of neurogenesis becoming increasingly important with increasing task difficulty (Drew, Denny, & Hen, 2010). The rate of proliferation, differentiation into neurons or glia, and eventual survival is regulated by the chemical environment of the neurogenic regions, including changes in levels of hormones and growth factors. As described above, exercise changes the chemical environment present in the hippocampus, notably increasing availability of growth factors that modulate neurogenesis, particularly IGF-1, VEGF, and BDNF. Increased peripheral IGF-1 and VEGF mediate the exercise-induced proliferation of neural progenitors, and IGF-1 also promotes neuronal survival following exercise (Fabel et al., 2003; Trejo et al., 2001). The role of BDNF signaling in exercise-dependent neurogenesis has not been directly tested; however, BDNF regulates baseline levels of hippocampal neurogenesis, suggesting that this growth factor may also contribute to exercise effects.

New neurons become functionally integrated into the hippocampal architecture (van Praag et al., 2002) and have unusual electrophysiological properties that give them heightened synaptic plasticity. More specifically, new neurons have a lower threshold of excitability than mature hippocampal granule cells (Schmidt-Hieber, Jonas, & Bischofberger, 2004). This reduced threshold for excitability is an important feature underlying hippocampal plasticity. In addition, it makes the new neurons good candidates for mediating enhanced plasticity in response to exercise, such as facilitated LTP, described earlier. Accumulating evidence indicates that integration of the new, young neurons leads to a lasting modification in the hippocampal network, and appears to be particularly important for the role of the hippocampus in "pattern separation" (Aimone, Deng, & Gage, 2011), a key step in the ability to form distinct memories despite potential contextual similarities (e.g., the process of discriminating subtle differences in similar information). Exercise enhances pattern separation ability, potentially through stimulation of neurogenesis (Creer, Romberg, Saksida, van Praag, & Bussey, 2010). Recent findings indicate that hippocampal neurogenesis is also critical for buffering the response to stress and protects from developing depressive behavior in response to stress. Interestingly, emerging evidence from both human and animal studies suggests that exercise increases the tolerance for stress and may provide a margin of protection from development of depression (see Cotman et al., 2007), an effect that may potentially involve neurogenesis (Snyder, Soumier, Brewer, Pickel, & Cameron, 2011). As a side note, the effect of stress on brain health and risk of depression is described by a bell-shaped curve, with stressors perceived as mild generally having beneficial effects, while stronger sustained stressors tending to induce depressive-like behaviors. Interestingly, exercise appears to shift the valence of a stressor to make it milder, and can interact with a mild stressor to benefit brain health and function (Adlard, Engesser-Cesar, & Cotman, 2011), potentially via stimulatory effects on neurogenesis.

Overall, enhanced hippocampal neurogenesis with exercise may be a key mechanism mediating the effect of exercise on facilitating plasticity, improving learning and memory, and providing a margin of protection from harmful effects of excessive stress. It is important to note that while hippocampal neurogenesis declines with advanced age, exercise stimulates neurogenesis in both young and aged animals, albeit the capacity of exercise to counteract age-related declines appears to be dramatically reduced in very old animals (Creer et al., 2010).

Angiogenesis

To sustain the multitude of changes that occur in the brain in response to exercise (e.g., enhanced plasticity, growth of new synaptic connections, neurogenesis, increased production of growth factors and synaptic proteins), increased energy and nutrient supply to the responding brain regions is required. One way in which the brain meets the increased regional demand is by stimulating angiogenesis, or the sprouting of new capillaries from existing blood vessels. With exercise, angiogenesis occurs in various brain regions including the hippocampus, cortex, and cerebellum, in both young and aged animals (Black, Isaacs, Anderson, Alcantara, & Greenough, 1990; Y. H. Ding, Li, et al., 2006). Data from human and animal studies support the concept that angiogenesis and increased blood flow are important components underlying exercise benefits to hippocampal-dependent learning (Kerr, Steuer, Pochtarev, & Swain, 2010).

Angiogenesis is largely regulated by growth factors, notably IGF-1 and VEGF, which undergo increased availability with exercise. In particular, IGF-1 produced in the periphery that enters the CNS via the circulation appears to be critical for exercise-induced vessel remodeling in the brain (Lopez-Lopez et al., 2004). In addition, increased VEGF is likely to be an important regulator of exercise-induced angiogenesis, as this growth factor has potent mitotic activity specific to vascular endothelial cells, affecting proliferation, survival, adhesion, migration, and capillary tube formation.

Overall, exercise stimulation of angiogenesis is likely to be an important component of cognitive health and function, particularly in aging. Indeed, with aging, the human brain undergoes reduced blood perfusion for a variety of reasons, and the decline in blood flow (and associated nutrient and energy supply) is thought to be a central factor relating to declining cognitive function with age (Ahlskog et al., 2011). Age-related declines in cerebral perfusion arise in part from an accumulation of mild, microscopic ischemic events that often go undetected. Exercise conditioning provides the brain with some ischemic tolerance, reducing the extent of neural deficits associated with ischemia and reducing the development of brain infarction. These benefits of exercise are likely mediated in large part by stimulating angiogenesis.

Bioenergetic adaptations in the brain

The various exercise-induced brain changes are coupled to mechanisms beyond angiogenesis in order to meet increased regional energy demands. Notably, bioenergetic adaptations occur in mitochondria, the cellular organelles responsible for oxidative energy transformation and generation of energy in the form of adenosine triphosphate (ATP). In muscle, mitochondrial activity and number are increased in response to the high metabolic demand during exercise (Irrcher, Adhihetty, Joseph, Ljubicic, & Hood, 2003). Recent findings demonstrate that similar changes occur in the brain. In hippocampal neurons, exercise increases mitochondrial respiration, mitochondrial number (Dietrich, Andrews, & Horvath, 2008), and levels of several mitochondrial proteins important in energy metabolism (Navarro, Gomez, Lopez-Cepero, & Boveris, 2004).

Exercise also induces adaptive changes to offset oxidative stress. Oxidative stress is generated by mitochondria as a by-product of energy generation and increases in the brain with age. Free radicals generated during oxidative respiration can harm cellular health and function by damaging proteins and other cell components, including the mitochondria themselves. Animal studies demonstrate that exercise decreases oxidative damage in the brain, particularly in aging, with notably reduced oxidative damage to mitochondria. Decreased oxidative damage with exercise comes about in part by increases in the activity of protective enzymes that counteract oxidative stress (Navarro et al., 2004). In addition, exercise increases hippocampal levels of uncoupling protein 2 (UCP2), a mitochondrial protein that regulates free radical production during oxidative respiration and that is emerging as having an important role in neuroprotection from brain pathologies associated with energy deficits (Parkinson's disease, epilepsy, stroke) as well as in normal brain function (Dietrich et al., 2008). Induction of UCP2 in the brain increases the overall production of ATP, while also decreasing superoxide production and associated damage from this free radical (Bechmann et al., 2002). UCP2 gene expression increases in the hippocampus following several days of exercise. Recent findings reveal that UCP2 may be a key element mediating the effects of exercise on mitochondrial adaptations as well as several aspects of hippocampal synaptic plasticity. Indeed, the effects of exercise on mitochondrial respiration, mitochondrial number, synaptogenesis, and BDNF in the hippocampus are all dependent on upregulation of UCP2 (Dietrich et al., 2008; Vaynman, Ying, Wu, & Gomez-Pinilla, 2006).

These data reveal that exercise prompts extensive bioenergetic adaptations in the brain, and that the effects of exercise on synaptic plasticity are tightly coupled to mitochondrial function and plasticity. The effects of exercise to increase energy production, anti-oxidant capacity, and overall mitochondrial function in the brain are particularly important in aging, where all of these capacities are compromised.

Exercise as an anti-inflammatory

While it has long been known that exercise modulates immune function and has anti-inflammatory effects in the peripheral body, this concept has recently evolved to recognize that exercise also affects the immune health of the brain. Inflammation is a component of many health conditions that accrue with aging, including obesity, diabetes, and cardiovascular disease, among others (Gleeson et al., 2011), and it is known that persistent inflammation is a risk factor for cognitive decline. It has been proposed that reduction of inflammation by exercise is a common means by which exercise reduces both peripheral and CNS risk factors for cognitive decline and neurodegeneration (Cotman et al., 2007).

There is accumulating evidence that immune activation, such as occurs with infection and inflammation (both acute and chronic), impairs cognition in humans and animals (Gorelick, 2010), with the aged being particularly vulnerable. For example, following a brief peripheral bacterial infection, aged rats show prolonged long-term memory impairments on hippocampal-related tasks (Barrientos, Watkins, Rudy, & Maier, 2009), while cognition in young animals returns to normal shortly following recovery from the infection. The immune response to infection is thought to be to blame for the prolonged impairment in hippocampal function in aged animals. Specifically, immune signals that enter the brain result in production of pro-inflammatory molecules in the brain, called cytokines, which disrupt normal cognitive function, particularly in the hippocampus. One pro-inflammatory cytokine that appears to be central to the harmful effects of peripheral infection on hippocampal function is interleukin-1 beta (IL-1b) (Frank et al., 2010). In aged animals, the CNS shows an amplified inflammatory response to peripheral infection, with greater and more prolonged presence of IL-1b than in young animals (Godbout et al., 2005). The exaggerated neuroinflammatory response produces a dramatic and specific deficit in BDNF-dependent synaptic plasticity, suppresses hippocampal neurogenesis, and impairs hippocampal-dependent memory (Chapman, Barrientos, Ahrendsen, Maier, & Patterson, 2010; Wu et al., 2007). Intriguingly, exercise prior to the peripheral infection prevents all of the detrimental responses to infection in the aged animals, including the age-related microglial sensitization, exaggerated neuroinflammatory response, suppression of neurogenesis, and blunted BDNF induction.

The mechanisms by which exercise counteracts the harmful effects of inflammation on brain function are not yet well understood. However, it is known that in response to exercise, expression of a wide variety of immune molecules is increased in the CNS of aged mice (Parachikova, Nichol, & Cotman, 2008). One beneficial molecule that may be a critical factor in blocking the harmful effects of infection on hippocampus-dependent long-term memory is a molecule that blocks the action of IL-1b (e.g., IL-1b receptor antagonist, IL-1RA). Blocking IL-1b signaling with IL-1RA eliminated the infection-associated memory impairment, protected against failure of long-lasting synaptic plasticity, and prevented hippocampal BDNF reductions in aged rats following infection (Chapman et al., 2010; Frank et al., 2010). Thus, IL-1RA appears to be a key molecule protecting the aged brain from the cognitive impairing effects of peripheral infection, and might be involved in protective effects of exercise. Indeed, it is known that exercise increases levels of IL-1RA and other anti-inflammatory molecules in the periphery, initiated by IL-6 release from contracting muscles (which is triggered by reduced glycogen) (Steensberg, Fischer, Keller, Moller, & Pedersen, 2003). A similar anti-inflammatory mechanism may be active in the brain, where exercise increases IL-6 release. It is important to consider that peripheral circulating immune/inflammation factors likely contribute to modulating brain health and function (Perry, 2004), even in the absence of overt infection, an idea that has been scantily addressed in the current literature.

Overall, exercise is a highly effective anti-inflammatory therapeutic that decreases the general state of inflammation in the periphery by targeting multiple tissue types and pathways (Gleeson et al., 2011). The effect of exercise on immune health and peripheral and central inflammation is likely to be an important contributor to preserved brain health and function in aging.

Synergistic effects with lifestyle

The literature summarized above demonstrates that exercise participation provides many beneficial effects to the brain. Building on these findings, a new field has emerged addressing how other lifestyle factors, such as cognitive stimulation ("environmental enrichment") and diet, can interact with exercise to modulate brain health and function.

Exercise with environmental enrichment

In animal studies of enriched environment (EE), animals are exposed to cognitive, physical, and social stimulation, in that they are housed in big cages with several animals (generally 4–10 per cage) along with a variety of different objects that can be climbed on, played with, and explored by the animals. Exposure to EE provides animals with an opportunity for various learning experiences including spatial learning as they acquire information on the location of water, food, and other items in the cages, and social learning as they interact with cage-mates. Most EE paradigms include one or more running wheels, providing animals with access to exercise stimulation. EE has been studied for many decades, and it has been firmly established to have profound effects on the brain and CNS at the molecular, anatomical, and functional levels throughout life (for a recent review, see Baroncelli et al., 2010). Many of the effects of EE overlap with the beneficial effects of exercise alone, including benefits to learning and memory, neurogenesis, induction of growth factors, and improved recovery from brain injury. Because most EE studies have included an exercise component, the specific gains derived from exercise versus other aspects of enrichment (social, cognitive) have not been well defined. However, a few studies have compared the various enrichment paradigms (i.e., exercise alone, EE alone, and EE with exercise (EEX)), and have revealed that the effects of exercise and cognitive/social enrichment can be additive. For example, the stimulation of hippocampal neurogenesis with exercise, thought to translate to a greater reserve for plasticity, is amplified when exercise is combined with EE (Kempermann et al., 2010). With respect to neurogenesis, exercise appears to be the key component of EE, and it has been proposed that exercise brings the brain into a "state of readiness" allowing it to better respond to environmental factors (Fabel et al., 2009). Future studies are needed to elucidate the extent to which exercise benefits can be augmented with cognitive/social enrichment, and to define the optimal dosing of the various components of EE (e.g., exercise, cognitive stimulation, social stimulation) to maximize benefits to the brain.

Exercise and diet

Another lifestyle factor that can affect brain function is nutrition. Recent studies have begun to investigate the idea that an interactive relationship may exist between dietary factors, exercise, and brain function. These have taken the perspectives of investigating the harmful effects of consuming a diet rich in saturated fats and sugar (similar in content to "junk food") and how exercise can counteract these effects, as well as investigating the beneficial effects of dietary supplementation and whether benefits can be augmented with exercise. Animal studies reveal that unhealthy diets impair cognitive performance, reduce hippocampal neurogenesis, decrease availability of synaptic proteins (IGF-1, BDNF, synapsin I, CREB), increase oxidative stress, and decrease recovery from brain injury (Dietrich et al., 2007; Gomez-Pinilla & Gomez, 2011). Exercise can compensate for some of the harmful effects of diet, with concurrent exposure to exercise restoring cognitive performance, growth factor, and synaptic protein availability, and reducing the oxidative stress induced by the diet (Gomez-Pinilla & Gomez, 2011). In turn, exercise can boost the benefits of a healthy diet on neuroplasticity. While research on this topic is still sparse, current findings suggest that the effects of exercise on the brain can be enhanced by consumption of natural products such as omega fatty acids or plant polyphenols, specifically enhancing exercise effects on spatial learning, synaptic plasticity, neurogenesis, and BDNF protein (van Praag et al., 2007; Wu, Ying, & Gomez-Pinilla, 2008). Overall, these data suggest that the combination of diet and exercise can deliver more beneficial effects than either intervention alone, and appear to act via effects on BDNF-mediated plasticity. The extent to which use of dietary supplements can enhance exercise benefits will need to be studied in further detail, in particular to evaluate (1) the types of supplements that are effective, (2) if a particular supplement is effective in isolation or if supplements need to be combined, (3) the relative effectiveness of synthetic or natural supplements, and (4) if sustained supplementation has greater long-term benefits to brain function than exercise alone, particularly in the course of aging.

Exercise, EE, and diet

This section reviews findings on interactive benefits of diet and exercise in the context of the EE paradigm, where exercise is further supplemented with cognitive and social stimulation. These studies are perhaps of greatest relevance to human lifestyle, where dietary factors, physical activity, and cognitive and social stimulation tend to all be present. Further, these studies have been undertaken in aged canines (rather than rodents), which represent a higher animal model of aging, and which undergo many similar aging-related changes as occur in humans. For example, like humans, the canine naturally develops cognitive dysfunction with age, and the brain undergoes selective neuron loss, decreased hippocampal neurogenesis, decreased bioenergetic capacity, declines in BDNF, and accumulation of oxidative damage and neuropathologies such as beta-amyloid (Aβ), a characteristic pathology of Alzheimer's disease (Cotman & Head, 2008). In these studies, the impacts of enrichment (with exercise, social, and cognitive stimulation), dietary supplementation (with antioxidants and mitochondrial cofactors), and the combined treatment were investigated in aged canines. The interventions were long term, over the course of 2+ years, and the effects on various parameters of brain health and function that decline with aging were assessed (Cotman & Head, 2008).

These studies have revealed that long-term dietary or EE interventions each benefit brain health and cognitive function, and that the effects of the combined intervention are superior to either treatment alone on nearly every parameter investigated. These benefits were seen for visual discrimination learning and spatial memory, which show pronounced decline with age, as well as for age-related declines in BDNF, and age-related accumulation of oxidative damage, (Aβ) pathology, and activation of harmful proteases (such as caspases) that can provoke degeneration. In addition, some parameters were found to be specifically improved by only one intervention. For example, preservation of hippocampal neuron number occurred specifically with EE but not with the antioxidant diet, while the antioxidant diet (but not EE) improved mitochondrial function (Head et al., 2009). These data suggest that there may be independent pathways engaged by each treatment that can improve neuronal function. Thus, the combination treatment may result in further improvements in neural function due to additive effects of independent molecular cascades (Cotman & Head, 2008).

We hypothesize that a significant mechanism underlying the additive benefits from dietary supplementation and EE revolves around improved mitochondrial function with the antioxidant diet. The improved mitochondrial function allows the aged brain to respond better to EE than when mitochondria are partially dysfunctional. In other words, neurons with healthy mito-chondria are more able to benefit from EE conditions. In parallel, our findings suggest that the antioxidant and behavioral interventions engage molecular mechanisms, such as BDNF signaling, that enhance "cognitive reserve," and allow the canine brain to maintain healthy function despite the continued presence of (Aβ) and other pathologies in the brain.

Future directions

Tremendous advances have been made in the past two decades in understanding the benefits provided by exercise to brain health and function, and these have in turn revealed many additional future directions. Of practical interest are the questions of exercise type, intensity, frequency, and dosing, in order to obtain optimal benefits. Mechanistically, this translates to the idea that a molecular memory for exercise exists after exercise has ended. Animal studies suggest that benefits of exercise endure for several weeks after exercise has ceased and that cognitive benefits continue to evolve during this "down time" (Berchtold, Castello, & Cotman, 2010; Berchtold et al., 2005). A better understanding of (1) how the molecular mechanisms activated by exercise mature over time and (2) the optimal exercise interval for reactivation of these mechanisms will help guide optimization of exercise intervention strategies. Another future direction focuses on the role of genetics in modifying benefits that can be derived from exercise, and how genetics may differentially affect the mechanisms activated by exercise in the brain. For example, recent evidence suggests that some genotypes may reap greater benefits from exercise, notably those with ApoE4 genotype (Deeny et al., 2008), an effect that may be mediated by genetic influences on neural plasticity (Pearson-Fuhrhop & Cramer, 2010). Finally, given the recent awareness of the involvement of peripheral inflammation and peripherally derived growth factors in mediating benefits of exercise on the brain, it will be important to further define how peripheral factors that influence brain health and function respond to exercise. A better understanding of how peripheral dysfunction impacts CNS function, and the effects of exercise on ameliorating peripheral health, will expand our understanding of the global mechanisms by which exercise modulates brain health and cognitive function.

References

Adlard, P. A., Engesser-Cesar, C., & Cotman, C. W. (2011). Mild stress facilitates learning and exercise improves retention in aged mice. *Experimental Gerontology, 46*(1), 53–59. doi:10.1016/j.exger.2010.10.001

Ahlskog, J. E., Geda, Y. E., Graff-Radford, N. R., & Petersen, R. C. (2011). Physical exercise as a preventive or disease-modifying treatment of dementia and brain aging. *Mayo Clinical Proceedings, 86*(9), 876–884. doi:86/9/876

Aimone, J. B., Deng, W., & Gage, F. H. (2011). Resolving new memories: A critical look at the dentate gyrus, adult neurogenesis, and pattern separation. *Neuron, 70*(4), 589–596. doi:S0896-6273(11)00391-6

Baroncelli, L., Braschi, C., Spolidoro, M., Begenisic, T., Sale, A., & Maffei, L. (2010). Nurturing brain plasticity: Impact of environmental enrichment. *Cell Death & Differentiation, 17*(7), 1092–1103. doi:cdd2009193

Barrientos, R. M., Watkins, L. R., Rudy, J. W., & Maier, S. F. (2009). Characterization of the sickness response in young and aging rats following E. coli infection. *Brain Behavior and Immunity, 23*(4), 450–454. doi:S0889-1591(09)00043-9

Bechmann, I., Diano, S., Warden, C. H., Bartfai, T., Nitsch, R., & Horvath, T. L. (2002). Brain mitochondrial uncoupling protein 2 (UCP2): A protective stress signal in neuronal injury. *Biochemical Pharmacology, 64*(3), 363–367. doi:S0006295202011668

Berchtold, N. C., Castello, N., & Cotman, C. W. (2010). Exercise and time-dependent benefits to learning and memory. *Neuroscience, 167*(3), 588–597. doi:S0306-4522(10)00278-2

Berchtold, N. C., Chinn, G., Chou, M., Kesslak, J. P., & Cotman, C. W. (2005). Exercise primes a molecular memory for brain-derived neurotrophic factor protein induction in the rat hippocampus. *Neuroscience, 133*(3), 853–861.

Black, J. E., Isaacs, K. R., Anderson, B. J., Alcantara, A. A., & Greenough, W. T. (1990). Learning causes synaptogenesis, whereas motor activity causes angiogenesis, in cerebellar cortex of adult rats. *Proceedings of the National Academy of Science USA, 87*(14), 5568–5572.

Burdette, J. H., Laurienti, P. J., Espeland, M. A., Morgan, A., Telesford, Q., Vechlekar, C. D., . . . Rejeski, W. J. (2010). Using network science to evaluate exercise-associated brain changes in older adults. *Frontiers in Aging Neuroscience, 2*, 23 doi:10.3389/fnagi.2010.00023

Castilla-Ortega, E., Pedraza, C., Estivill-Torrus, G., & Santin, L. J. (2011). When is adult hippocampal neurogenesis necessary for learning? Evidence from animal research. *Reviews in Neuroscience, 22*(3), 267–283. doi:10.1515/RNS.2011.027

Chapman, T. R., Barrientos, R. M., Ahrendsen, J. T., Maier, S. F., & Patterson, S. L. (2010). Synaptic correlates of increased cognitive vulnerability with aging: Peripheral immune challenge and aging interact to disrupt theta-burst late-phase long-term potentiation in hippocampal area CA1. *Journal of Neuroscience, 30*(22), 7598–7603. doi:30/22/7598

Cotman, C. W., & Berchtold, N. C. (2002). Exercise: A behavioral intervention to enhance brain health and plasticity. *Trends in Neuroscience, 25*(6), 292–298.

Cotman, C. W., Berchtold, N. C., & Christie, L. A. (2007). Exercise builds brain health: An interplay of central and peripheral factors. *Trends in Neurosciences, 30*(9), 464–472.

Cotman, C. W., & Head, E. (2008). The canine (dog) model of human aging and disease: Dietary, environmental and immunotherapy approaches. *Journal of Alzheimer's Disease, 15*(4), 685–707.

Creer, D. J., Romberg, C., Saksida, L. M., van Praag, H., & Bussey, T. J. (2010). Running enhances spatial pattern separation in mice. *Proceedings of the National Academy of Science USA, 107*(5), 2367–2372. doi:0911725107

Deeny, S. P., Poeppel, D., Zimmerman, J. B., Roth, S. M., Brandauer, J., Witkowski, S., . . . Hatfield, B. D. (2008). Exercise, APOE, and working memory: MEG and behavioral evidence for benefit of exercise in epsilon4 carriers. *Biological Psychology, 78*(2), 179–187.

Dietrich, M. O., Andrews, Z. B., & Horvath, T. L. (2008). Exercise-induced synaptogenesis in the hippocampus is dependent on UCP2-regulated mitochondrial adaptation. *Journal of Neuroscience, 28*(42), 10766–10771. doi:28/42/10766

Dietrich, M. O., Muller, A., Bolos, M., Carro, E., Perry, M. L., Portela, L. V., . . . Torres-Aleman, I. (2007). Western style diet impairs entrance of blood-borne insulin-like growth factor-1 into the brain. *Neuromolecular Medicine, 9*(4), 324–330. doi:10.1007/s12017-007-8011-0

Ding, Q., Vaynman, S., Akhavan, M., Ying, Z., & Gomez-Pinilla, F. (2006). Insulin-like growth factor I interfaces with brain-derived neurotrophic factor-mediated synaptic plasticity to modulate aspects of exercise-induced cognitive function. *Neuroscience, 140*(3), 823–833.

Ding, Y. H., Li, J., Zhou, Y., Rafols, J. A., Clark, J. C., & Ding, Y. (2006). Cerebral angiogenesis and expression of angiogenic factors in aging rats after exercise. *Current Neurovascular Research, 3*(1), 15–23.

Drew, M. R., Denny, C. A., & Hen, R. (2010). Arrest of adult hippocampal neurogenesis in mice impairs single- but not multiple-trial contextual fear conditioning. *Behavioral Neuroscience, 124*(4), 446–454. doi:2010-16138-002

Eadie, B. D., Redila, V. A., & Christie, B. R. (2005). Voluntary exercise alters the cytoarchitecture of the adult dentate gyrus by increasing cellular proliferation, dendritic complexity, and spine density. *The Journal of Comparative Neurology, 486*(1), 39–47.

Fabel, K., Tam, B., Kaufer, D., Baiker, A., Simmons, N., Kuo, C. J., & Palmer, T. D. (2003). VEGF is necessary for exercise-induced adult hippocampal neurogenesis. *European Journal of Neuroscience, 18*(10), 2803–2812.

Fabel, K., Wolf, S. A., Ehninger, D., Babu, H., Leal-Galicia, P., & Kempermann, G. (2009). Additive effects of physical exercise and environmental enrichment on adult hippocampal neurogenesis in mice. *Frontiers in Neuroscience, 3*, 50. doi:10.3389/neuro.22.002.2009

Farmer, J., Zhao, X., van Praag, H., Wodtke, K., Gage, F. H., & Christie, B. R. (2004). Effects of voluntary exercise on synaptic plasticity and gene expression in the dentate gyrus of adult male Sprague-Dawley rats in vivo. *Neuroscience, 124*(1), 71–79.

Frank, M. G., Barrientos, R. M., Hein, A. M., Biedenkapp, J. C., Watkins, L. R., & Maier, S. F. (2010). IL-1RA blocks E. coli-induced suppression of Arc and long-term memory in aged F344xBN F1 rats. *Brain Behavior and Immunity, 24*(2), 254–262. doi:S0889-1591(09)00469-3

Garcia, C., Chen, M. J., Garza, A. A., Cotman, C. W., & Russo-Neustadt, A. (2003). The influence of specific noradrenergic and serotonergic lesions on the expression of hippocampal brain-derived neurotrophic factor transcripts following voluntary physical activity. *Neuroscience, 119*(3), 721–732.

Gleeson, M., Bishop, N. C., Stensel, D. J., Lindley, M. R., Mastana, S. S., & Nimmo, M. A. (2011). The anti-inflammatory effects of exercise: Mechanisms and implications for the prevention and treatment of disease. *Nature Reviews in Immunology, 11*(9), 607–615. doi:nri3041

Gobeske, K. T., Das, S., Bonaguidi, M. A., Weiss, C., Radulovic, J., Disterhoft, J. F., & Kessler, J. A. (2009). BMP signaling mediates effects of exercise on hippocampal neurogenesis and cognition in mice. *PLoS ONE, 4*(10), e7506. doi:10.1371/journal.pone.0007506

Godbout, J. P., Chen, J., Abraham, J., Richwine, A. F., Berg, B. M., Kelley, K. W., & Johnson, R. W. (2005). Exaggerated neuroinflammation and sickness behavior in aged mice following activation of the peripheral innate immune system. *Faseb Journal, 19*(10), 1329–1331. doi:05-3776fje

Gomez-Pinilla, F., & Gomez, A. G. (2011). The influence of dietary factors in central nervous system plasticity and injury recovery. *PM & R, 3*(6 Suppl 1), S111–S116. doi:S1934-1482(11)00142-0

Gorelick, P. B. (2010). Role of inflammation in cognitive impairment: Results of observational epidemiological studies and clinical trials. *Annals of the New York Academy of Science, 1207*, 155–162. doi:10.1111/j.1749-6632.2010.05726.x

Head, E., Nukala, V. N., Fenoglio, K. A., Muggenburg, B. A., Cotman, C. W., & Sullivan, P. G. (2009). Effects of age, dietary, and behavioral enrichment on brain mitochondria in a canine model of human aging. *Experimental Neurology, 220*(1), 171–176. doi:S0014-4886(09)00337-9

Irrcher, I., Adhihetty, P. J., Joseph, A. M., Ljubicic, V., & Hood, D. A. (2003). Regulation of mitochondrial biogenesis in muscle by endurance exercise. *Sports Medicine, 33*(11), 783–793. doi:33111

Kempermann, G., Fabel, K., Ehninger, D., Babu, H., Leal-Galicia, P., Garthe, A., & Wolf, S. A. (2010). Why and how physical activity promotes experience-induced brain plasticity. *Frontiers in Neuroscience, 4*, 189. doi:10.3389/fnins.2010.00189

Kerr, A. L., Steuer, E. L., Pochtarev, V., & Swain, R. A. (2010). Angiogenesis but not neurogenesis is critical for normal learning and memory acquisition. *Neuroscience, 171*(1), 214–226. doi:S0306-4522(10)01075-4

Lazarov, O., Mattson, M. P., Peterson, D. A., Pimplikar, S. W., & van Praag, H. (2010). When neurogenesis encounters aging and disease. *Trends in Neuroscience, 33*(12), 569–579. doi:S0166-2236(10)00134-7

Lopez-Lopez, C., LeRoith, D., & Torres-Aleman, I. (2004). Insulin-like growth factor I is required for vessel remodeling in the adult brain. *Proceedings of the National Academy of Science USA, 101*(26), 9833–9838. doi:10.1073/pnas.0400337101

Navarro, A., Gomez, C., Lopez-Cepero, J. M., & Boveris, A. (2004). Beneficial effects of moderate exercise on mice aging: Survival, behavior, oxidative stress, and mitochondrial electron transfer. *American Journal of Physiology, 286*(3), R505–R511.

Parachikova, A., Nichol, K. E., & Cotman, C. W. (2008). Short-term exercise in aged Tg2576 mice alters neuroinflammation and improves cognition. *Neurobiology of Disease, 30*(1), 121–129.

Pearson-Fuhrhop, K. M., & Cramer, S. C. (2010). Genetic influences on neural plasticity. *PM & R, 2*(12 Suppl 2), S227–S240. doi:S1934-1482(10)01189-5

Perry, V. H. (2004). The influence of systemic inflammation on inflammation in the brain: Implications for chronic neurodegenerative disease. *Brain Behavior and Immunity, 18*(5), 407–413. doi:10.1016/j.bbi.2004.01.004

Schmidt-Hieber, C., Jonas, P., & Bischofberger, J. (2004). Enhanced synaptic plasticity in newly generated granule cells of the adult hippocampus. *Nature, 429*(6988), 184–187. Epub 2004 Apr 2025.

Snyder, J. S., Soumier, A., Brewer, M., Pickel, J., & Cameron, H. A. (2011). Adult hippocampal neurogenesis buffers stress responses and depressive behaviour. *Nature, 476*(7361), 458–461. doi:nature10287

Steensberg, A., Fischer, C. P., Keller, C., Moller, K., & Pedersen, B. K. (2003). IL-6 enhances plasma IL-1ra, IL-10, and cortisol in humans. *American Journal of Physiology – Endocrinology and Metabolism, 285*(2), E433–E437. doi:10.1152/ajpendo.00074.2003

Trejo, J. L., Carro, E., & Torres-Aleman, I. (2001). Circulating insulin-like growth factor I mediates exercise-induced increases in the number of new neurons in the adult hippocampus. *Journal of Neuroscience, 21*(5), 1628–1634.

van Praag, H., Christie, B. R., Sejnowski, T. J., & Gage, F. H. (1999). Running enhances neurogenesis, learning, and long-term potentiation in mice. *Proceedings of the National Academy of Science USA, 96*(23), 13427–13431.

van Praag, H., Lucero, M. J., Yeo, G. W., Stecker, K., Heivand, N., Zhao, C., . . . Gage, F. H. (2007). Plant-derived flavanol (-)epicatechin enhances angiogenesis and retention of spatial memory in mice. *Journal of Neuroscience, 27*(22), 5869–5878. doi:27/22/5869

van Praag, H., Schinder, A. F., Christie, B. R., Toni, N., Palmer, T. D., & Gage, F. H. (2002). Functional neurogenesis in the adult hippocampus. *Nature, 415*(6875), 1030–1034.

Vaynman, S., Ying, Z., Wu, A., & Gomez-Pinilla, F. (2006). Coupling energy metabolism with a mechanism to support brain-derived neurotrophic factor-mediated synaptic plasticity. *Neuroscience, 139*(4), 1221–1234.

Vaynman, S. S., Ying, Z., Yin, D., & Gomez-Pinilla, F. (2006). Exercise differentially regulates synaptic proteins associated to the function of BDNF. *Brain Research, 1070*(1), 124–130.

Voss, M. W., Nagamatsu, L. S., Liu-Ambrose, T., & Kramer, A. F. (2011). Exercise, brain, and cognition across the lifespan. *Journal of Applied Physiology, 111*(5), 1505–1513. doi:japplphysiol.00210.2011

Wu, A., Ying, Z., & Gomez-Pinilla, F. (2008). Docosahexaenoic acid dietary supplementation enhances the effects of exercise on synaptic plasticity and cognition. *Neuroscience, 155*(3), 751–759.

Wu, C. W., Chen, Y. C., Yu, L., Chen, H. I., Jen, C. J., Huang, A. M., . . . Kuo, Y. M. (2007). Treadmill exercise counteracts the suppressive effects of peripheral lipopolysaccharide on hippocampal neurogenesis and learning and memory. *Journal of Neurochemistry, 103*(6), 2471–2481. doi:JNC4987

PART 6

Psychosocial stress

Edited by
Mark Hamer

20

PHYSICAL ACTIVITY, STRESS REACTIVITY, AND STRESS-MEDIATED PATHOPHYSIOLOGY

Mark Hamer and Andrew Steptoe

Stress refers to the consequences of the failure of a human or animal to respond appropriately to emotional or physical threats to the organism, whether actual or imagined (Seyle, 1965), resulting in disruption of homeostasis. In particular, the causes or consequences of stress in modern-day life include interpersonal, social, familial, societal, and social psychological factors. Evidence from population cohort studies suggests that psychosocial stress is a risk factor for cardiovascular diseases (CVD) (Kivimaki et al., 2012; Brotman, Golden, & Wittstein, 2007; Rosengren et al., 2004). An important way of investigating the mechanisms underlying these associations is acute psychophysiological stress testing, involving measurement of cardiovascular and biological responses to laboratory-induced behavioural stressors (Steptoe, 2007). Psychophysiological stress testing allows individual differences in responses to standardised stress tasks to be evaluated and related to psychosocial factors (Chida & Hamer, 2008) and future risk of CVD (Chida & Steptoe, 2010). Behaviourally evoked psychophysiological responses are relatively stable individual characteristics, consistent across time and stressor type. The magnitude or pattern of an individual's stress response is largely mediated by the immediate actions of the autonomic nervous system and delayed response of the hypothalamic pituitary adrenal (HPA) axis, which releases various hormones (i.e., catecholamines, cortisol, etc.) into the circulation. These systems drive specific responses that include an increase in blood pressure (BP) and heart rate, changes in cardiac sympatho-vagal balance, skeletal muscle vasodilatation, the stimulation of haemostatic and inflammatory responses, and activation of various immune cells, all of which might be relevant to CVD risk. Individual differences in patterns of stress responding are accounted for by factors such as race and ethnicity, genetics, background stress, and lifestyle habits. In particular, exercise has been studied for its stress buffering effects. Physical exercise and mental stress have similar acute physiological effects in that both result in cardiovascular activation and release of catecholamines and cortisol, although paradoxically they have different chronic effects on health – regular exercise is associated with protective effects whilst chronic mental stress has been linked with health risks, in particular CVD. This paradox is poorly understood, and might prevent some health professionals from acknowledging the true importance of physical activity in treating stress-related illnesses. The goal of this chapter is to focus on the effects of exercise on psycho-physiological stress responses, with reference to pathophysiological mechanisms in health and disease.

Stress mediated pathophysiology

Much of the evidence linking psychosocial stress with disease risk has come from epidemiological studies that follow cohorts of individuals over time and are able to assess the association between chronic stress exposure and long-term health outcomes such as death and clinical CVD events. Some examples of epidemiological findings include the association between work stress and an increased risk of CVD (Kivimaki et al., 2012) and a body of evidence showing higher risks of premature death in caregivers under emotional strain (Schulz & Beach, 1999). Further epidemiological evidence suggests that factors such as depression, hostility, loneliness, and social networks are related to a greater risk of future CVD and mortality in initially healthy individuals (Van der Kooy et al., 2007; Chida & Steptoe, 2009; Heffner, Waring, Roberts, Eaton, & Gramling, 2011). It is problematic to experimentally induce chronic stress in humans although some studies have assessed the effects of stress reduction interventions on health outcomes. Results from recent intervention trials that have examined the effects of various stress reduction and anti-depressant treatments on future risk of CVD events and mortality have been inconsistent (Blumenthal et al., 2005; Burg et al., 2005; Glassman, Bigger, & Gaffney, 2009), even when psychological symptoms are resolved, which has therefore raised some doubts about the direct role of stress in CVD. Nevertheless, none of this work has been performed in the context of primary prevention since the aforementioned studies have all been undertaken in patient groups.

The pathways linking stress and CVD are poorly understood but both behavioural pathways and direct pathophysiological processes appear to be involved. Behavioural pathways might include reduced physical activity, smoking, alcohol, and diet. In particular, physical activity levels are lower in participants that report depression or psychological distress, which has been shown to partly explain their increased risk of CVD (Hamer, Molloy, & Stamatakis, 2008; Whooley et al., 2008). Similarly, acute life events, social networks, and various types of chronic adversity such as work stress are associated with unhealthy diets and with smoking (Heikkilä et al., 2012; Christakis & Fowler, 2008; Steptoe et al., 1998). Pathophysiological processes might include sympathetic nervous system hyperactivity, inflammation, haemostasis, and altered metabolic and cardiac autonomic control. The existing evidence suggests that these pathways explain a modest amount of the association between stress and CVD. For example, in a recent study adiposity appeared to partly mediate the association between depression and coronary atherosclerosis in women (Greco et al., 2009). Disturbed sympathetic activity is a plausible mechanism in explaining the stress–CVD association, and the increased prevalence of carotid plaque found in chronically stressed spousal caregivers of people with Alzheimers disease was partly explained by prolonged sympathoadrenal arousal to acute stress (Roepke et al., 2011). Inflammatory markers [C-reactive protein (CRP) and interleukin-6] and the metabolic syndrome explained approximately 17% and 7%, respectively, of the association between depression and CVD events in women with suspected coronary ischemia (Vaccarino et al., 2007). Autonomic dysfunction and inflammation contributed 12.7% to the increased cardiovascular mortality risk associated with depression in the Cardiovascular Health Study (Kop et al., 2010). In other studies, various inflammatory markers did not, however, explain any of the association between depressive symptoms/stress and risk of CVD (Surtees et al., 2008; Nabi et al., 2008); thus there is clearly a need for further research in this area.

A clear limitation of the existing work in this area is that most studies are unable to provide a robust test of mediation because the potential mediating variables are usually measured at the same point in time as the markers of stress exposure, thus making it difficult to determine the temporal nature of the association. Indeed, the association of stress with intermediate risk factors for CVD might be bi-directional in that stress not only causes disturbances in behaviour and pathophysiological markers but also vice versa. For example, there appears to be a bi-directional association between depressive symptoms and inflammatory markers (Gimeno et al., 2009). As discussed elsewhere in this *Handbook*, physical activity appears to be protective against the development of depression and stress-related illness, although individuals with mental illness are less likely to undertake any activity.

Psychophysiological stress testing can also be used to better understand the mechanisms underlying the association between stress and CVD. Although acute psychophysiological responses are not clinically meaningful in themselves, they represent the way in which individuals respond to daily stressors in their normal lives, and if elicited regularly might have clinical relevance. A body of work has examined the association between psychophysiological stress reactivity and cardiovascular risk (Chida & Steptoe, 2010). Much of the work in humans has been based upon seminal work in primates, which demonstrated significantly greater coronary artery atherosclerosis in monkeys with exaggerated heart rate responses to behaviourally induced stressors (Manuck, Kaplan, Adams, & Clarkson, 1989). The research in humans to date has largely focused on the associations between cardiovascular (BP, heart rate) stress responses and future risk using various markers of sub-clinical CVD, such as carotid intima-media thickness (IMT) and coronary artery calcification (CAC). These measures are important since they are associated with risk of future CVD events. Additionally, assessment of sub-clinical atherosclerosis before clinical events occur helps delineate the temporal relationship between stress and CVD. In studies that have included healthy participants at baseline, BP reactivity to standardised stressors has been most consistently related to risk of sub-clinical atherosclerosis. For example, in 756 men from the Kuopio Ischemic Heart Disease study, systolic BP reactivity at the baseline assessment was related to carotid IMT after 7 years' follow-up and also to the progression of IMT, independently of established risk factors including smoking, cholesterol, fasting glucose, and resting BP (Jennings et al., 2004). Two separate studies in healthy women showed that greater pulse pressure and systolic BP reactivity were respectively associated with greater carotid IMT (Matthews et al., 1998) and the presence of CAC (Matthews, Zhu, Tucker, & Whooley, 2006). In both of these studies, however, measures of atherosclerosis were not available at baseline, thus the possibility of reverse causality cannot be ruled out. A recent study of cardiovascular risk in young Finns showed that higher heart rate, respiratory sinus arrhythmia, and pre-ejection period reactivity were associated with lower IMT values (Heponiemi et al., 2007), which is in contrast to data in US women that showed a greater response in heart rate variability was related to higher CAC (Gianaros et al., 2005).

The existing evidence therefore suggests that vascular stress reactivity (indexed by BP responses) more consistently predicts the progression of atherosclerosis than do cardiac autonomic responses. From a mechanistic standpoint, stress-induced BP surges that contribute to increased shear stress in the arteries could promote endothelial damage and inflammatory responses that are thought to play a role in atherogenesis (Kher & Marsh, 2004). Endothelial dysfunction plays a key role in the initiation of atherosclerosis because nitric oxide production from healthy endothelial cells has an anti-atherogenic effect by inhibiting cellular adhesion, migration, and proliferation responses (Ross, 1999). Heightened cardiovascular stress reactions have also been shown to predict future hypertension (Flaa, Eide, Kjeldsen, & Rostrup, 2008), increases in lipid levels and adiposity (Steptoe & Brydon, 2005; Steptoe & Wardle, 2005), and development of insulin resistance (Flaa, Aksnes, Kjeldsen, Eide, & Rostrup, 2008), which may represent key mechanisms in relation to stress and CVD risk. Chida and Steptoe's (2010) meta-analysis concluded that the strength of the association between stress reactivity and CVD risk is modest but consistent. Rate of recovery following stress exposure may also be important, although the evidence is limited at present. For example, prolonged recovery of systolic BP after stressors was associated with carotid IMT in various studies after accounting for conventional risk factors (Chida & Steptoe, 2010).

Exercise and cardiovascular stress buffering effects

Similarities between central and peripheral responses to exercise and psychological stressors have led to the theory of "cross-stressor adaptation", where adaptations resulting from regular exercise lead to both improved physiological control during exercise, and also lower cardiovascular responses to psychological stressors. Since exaggerated responses to mental stress can have detrimental effects on health, the potential stress buffering effects of exercise are of importance. Much of the existing psychophysiological work relating to physical activity has focused on cardiovascular responses, and several types of study have been carried out. These include experiments testing the impact of single bouts of exercise, the aim of which is to test whether stress reactivity or rate of recovery is modified after physical activity; comparisons of stress responses in physically fit and unfit individuals; and training studies in which psychophysiological stress responses are compared before and after exercise training.

The most consistent evidence is from the acute studies, where a single bout of acute exercise has been repeatedly associated with buffering BP and cardiac responses to standardised behavioural challenges in the laboratory (Hamer, Taylor, & Steptoe, 2006). Studies that have examined psychophysiological responses in relation to physical fitness (an indicator of training status) and exercise training have produced more mixed results. In an early meta-analytic review of 34 studies, aerobic fitness was associated with nearly half a standard deviation reduction in BP stress reactivity (Crews & Landers, 1987), but more recent updated reviews suggested both positive and inverse associations between fitness and heart rate reactivity (Dishman & Jackson, 2006; Forcier et al., 2006). Dishman and Jackson (2006) reported that fitness was related to greater heart rate reactivity but better recovery from mental challenge in 73 studies, although these effects were diminished when only randomised controlled exercise training studies were included and when fitness was measured as peak oxygen uptake. In contrast, Forcier and colleagues (2006) demonstrated an inverse association between fitness and heart rate reactivity in an analysis containing only studies with evidence of an exercise training effect. One of the difficulties in interpreting data from short-term (often 8–12 weeks) exercise trials is that individual changes in fitness are usually modest, which suggests a short period of exercise training may not be sufficient to induce the types of chronic adaptations required to observe stress buffering effects. Another common problem in this area is limited sample size, which can often lead to studies with insufficient statistical power. This issue was, however, addressed in a recent large randomised trial consisting of 149 healthy, young sedentary participants who were randomised to a 12-week exercise programme followed by a further 4 weeks of sedentary de-conditioning (Sloan et al., 2011). Participants performed various stressors before and after the intervention, including a public speaking task, mental arithmetic, and the Stroop Color-Word task, although there was no indication of any stress buffering effects following exercise training. In addition, a recent trial that examined the effects of 8 weeks' exercise training on muscle sympathetic nervous activity measured directly from the peroneal nerve found no evidence of sympatho-inhibition (Ray & Carter, 2010). Another study examined exercise training in the context of weight loss in obese children, and found that weight loss through 4 months of exercise training and diet, but not diet alone, improved vasodilatation responses to the Stroop mental challenge. This suggests that exercise in combination with weight loss might be important (Ribeiro et al., 2005).

From the present evidence it is difficult to conclude whether physical fitness per se or habitual physical activity underlies possible stress buffering effects. Much of the research in this field has relied on self-report measures of physical activity, and the problems with these are well known. We therefore conducted a study to examine the association between objectively measured habitual physical activity levels and psychophysiological responses in women (Poole et al., 2011). Participants wore an accelerometer device during waking hours for 1 week, and in addition recorded their daily moods and took part in psychophysiological testing. We observed robust associations between objectively assessed physical activity and daily mood, which is displayed in Figure 20.1, where physical activity groups reflect tertile of average daily minutes active recorded by accelerometry. However, we found no associations with cardiovascular reactivity to behavioural stressors administered in the laboratory. Further work is required to examine whether habitual physical activity is more closely linked with physiological reactivity to naturalistic stressors. Taken together, inconsistencies in this area may be due, in part, to small sample sizes, insufficient exercise training effects, inconsistencies in methodology (i.e., design, types of stressors, types of stress response measures), failure to account for the after-effects of a recent bout of acute exercise, and other confounding factors. Furthermore, based on the law of initial values, it is likely that exercise will have the greatest effects in those individuals with heightened responses from the outset or some degree of underlying disease pathology. For example, exercise has been strongly associated with stress buffering effects in participants with parental history of hypertension (Hamer, Boutcher, & Boutcher, 2002) and chronically stressed individuals, such as caregivers (King, Baumann, O'Sullivan, Wilcox, & Castro, 2002) compared with healthy low-risk individuals. It should also be noted that previous studies have generally tended to measure BP intermittently with conventional arm cuffs, which may not capture the full contour of the response that can be obtained using beat-to-beat devices such as the Finometer.

The potential stress buffering benefits of regular exercise may be largely accounted for by the fact that exercisers are more often in the post-exercise window when they encounter daily stressors. The attenuation in BP reactivity immediately following a single bout of acute exercise is thought to be best explained by a reduction in regional vascular resistance mediated by sympathetic nervous inhibition (Halliwill, 2001). West, Brownley, and Light (1998) observed a significant reduction in vascular resistance during mental challenge following acute exercise. Brownley et al. (2003) also showed that reduced noradrenaline response to a behavioural stress task was the best single predictor of the attenuation in post-exercise BP stress responses. Furthermore, significant increases in post-exercise $\beta 1$- and $\beta 2$-receptor responsiveness were

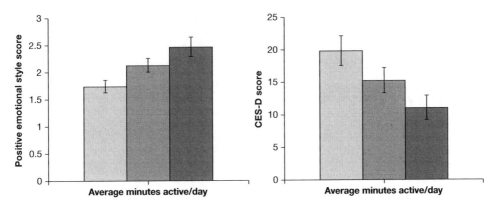

Figure 20.1 The association between physical activity and (a) daily positive mood and (b) depressive mood measured from the Centre Epidemiological Studies Depression (CES-D) scale. Physical activity groups reflect tertile of average daily minutes active recorded by accelerometry (≤213.88 minutes/day, 213.89–262.33 minutes/day and ≥262.34 minutes/day).

observed, indicating that the BP response was primarily blunted by enhancing β2-mediated vasodilatation (Brownley et al., 2003). Taken together, improvements in haemodynamic function during mental stress may be an important mechanism contributing to the stress buffering effects of acute exercise in relation to CVD risk. Consistent with this, studies in cardiac patients have demonstrated that exercise training reduces mental stress-induced ischaemia and results in fewer adverse cardiac events compared with controls over 5 years of follow-up (Blumenthal et al., 2002).

Exercise and psychobiology

A number of biological processes may explain the association between mental stress and physical disease, although far less work has focused upon neuroendocrine, inflammatory, and haemostatic processes. The HPA axis, for example, plays an important role in the stress response by releasing cortisol into the circulation. Abnormalities in HPA function have been described in several chronic inflammatory disorders, and it is thought to be one of the possible mechanisms through which psychosocial stress may influence the risk of CVD (Nijm & Jonasson, 2009). Several population studies have demonstrated associations between disturbances in diurnal cortisol profiles and sub-clinical atherosclerosis (Dekker et al., 2008; Matthews, Schwartz, Cohen, & Seeman, 2006). In a sample of 514 healthy British civil servants taken from the Whitehall II cohort we recently demonstrated an association between cortisol responses to laboratory-induced mental stress and sub-clinical coronary disease (Hamer, O'Donnell, Lahiri, & Steptoe, 2010). Those participants with a notable (>1nmol/l) rise in cortisol following two mental stress tasks were over two times more likely to have clinically relevant levels of coronary artery calcium after accounting for conventional risk factors such as cholesterol, smoking, and blood pressure.

Recent studies have consistently demonstrated blunted HPA responses to mental stressors in physically trained individuals (Traustadottir, Bosch, & Matt, 2005; Rimmele et al., 2009). For example, in a sample of elderly women, those defined as physically fit demonstrated plasma cortisol stress responses that were comparable with those of younger sedentary participants, but were blunted in comparison to elderly unfit counterparts (Traustadottir et al., 2005). Interestingly, physical fitness levels were not associated with cardiovascular responses to mental stress in these elderly women. In young men a blunted HPA stress response was only apparent in highly trained sportsmen, but amateur sportsmen had similar responses to the untrained men (Rimmele et al., 2009). This suggests that a certain threshold of exercise training is required to achieve adaptations in HPA stress responses. Paradoxically, recent data have demonstrated higher levels of cortisol in the hair of trained athletes compared with controls, suggesting greater chronic exposure to cortisol in trained individuals (Skoluda, Dettenborn, Stalder, & Kirschbaum, 2012).

There has been a large amount of interest in studying inflammatory responses to stress, since these mechanisms might be important in CVD (Steptoe, Hamer, & Chida, 2007). The specific nature of inflammatory responses to different types of stressors is, however, poorly understood. There is strong animal and in vitro evidence that the autonomic nervous system and neuroendocrine pathways are involved in the stimulation of interleukin (IL)-1β, IL-6, and tumor necrosis factor (TNF)-α production (Sanders & Kavelaars, 2007). Since these pathways are activated during acute mental stress and exercise, they could be responsible for increased circulating levels of inflammatory factors. Bierhaus and colleagues (2003) elegantly demonstrated that nuclear factor-κB (NF-κB) in peripheral blood mononuclear cells (PBMC) is rapidly induced during acute mental stress exposure in parallel with catecholamine and cortisol responses. This might represent a key mechanism given that NF-κB is a redox-sensitive and oxidant-activated transcription factor that regulates inflammation-related gene expression. In animal models, the activation of NF-κB is stimulated by norepinephrine-dependent pathways. Parasympathetic stimulation has the reverse effect, inhibiting NF-κB activation (Pavlov & Tracey 2005). However, direct evidence for sympathoadrenal processes in acute inflammatory stress responses in humans is limited at present. In a randomised controlled trial, von Känel et al. (2008) showed that 5 days' administration of aspirin but not propranolol attenuated the stress-induced increase in plasma IL-6 levels. In contrast, intravenous infusion of epinephrine rapidly increased plasma IL-6 in rats and this response could be blocked by propranolol (DeRijk, Boelen, Tilders, & Berkenbosch, 1994), but prolonged β-adrenergic stimulation at physiologic levels in humans induces local IL-1β, IL-6, and TNF-α expression in the myocardium without altering circulating levels (Murray, Prabhu, & Chandrasekar, 2000). Other data indicate that sympathoadrenal pathways play only a limited role in IL-6 responses to physical exercise (Febbraio & Pedersen, 2002), and intramuscular IL-6 expression appears to be regulated instead by a network of signalling cascades that are likely to involve the CA^{2+}/NFAT and glycogen/p38 MAPK pathways (Pedersen, 2011).

The precise mechanisms through which cytokine release is stimulated acutely therefore remain unclear. Controversially, it has been argued that the increases in circulating IL-6 that are observed after exercise promote an anti-inflammatory environment by increasing IL-1 receptor antagonist and IL-10 synthesis, while inhibiting pro-inflammatory markers such as TNF-α (Febbraio & Pedersen 2002). Indeed, the cytokines released during exercise are thought to originate from exercising skeletal muscle, and work in a hormone-like fashion exerting specific endocrine effects on various organs and signalling pathways. This hypothesis might explain why a large number of observational studies have demonstrated an inverse association between regular physical activity and various pro-inflammatory markers in humans (Hamer, 2007). In contrast, the release in IL-6 that is consistently observed following acute mental stress probably originates from a different source and is thought to be pro-inflammatory, which has been linked with indicators of CVD risk (Ellins et al., 2008). In addition, data from epidemiological studies also demonstrate positive associations between chronic psychosocial stress (indicated by low social economic status, chronic work stress, caregiver strain, early life adversity, hostility, and social isolation) and circulating levels of C-reactive protein, IL-6, and TNF-α. In one of the only studies to date, Hamer and Steptoe (2007) examined the association between physical fitness and inflammatory cytokine (IL-6 and TNF-α) responses to mental stress in a sample of 207 healthy, older adults. Physical fitness was assessed using a sub-maximal exercise test, and participants in the lowest tertile of fitness demonstrated the highest inflammatory responses to mental stress, independently of age, gender, social position, smoking, alcohol consumption, and basal levels of inflammatory markers, which is shown in Figure 20.2. Thus, there appears to be a unique cross-over effect of exercise in terms of stress-induced inflammatory responses.

In a further study we experimentally manipulated physical activity levels by asking a group of habitual exercisers to withdraw from their regular training for 2 weeks (Endrighi, Steptoe, & Hamer, 2011). The adherence to exercise withdrawal was mixed, as indicated by objective physical activity records, but in participants with greater mood disturbances (assessed using the 28-item General Health Questionnaire) following 2 weeks' withdrawal we observed significantly higher inflammatory responses to mental stress compared to those with low or no mood disturbance. These findings are presented in Figure 20.3, which shows that participants in the highest tertile of mood disturbance demonstrated the greatest inflammatory responses to mental stress after statistical adjustments for age, gender, body mass index, and pre-intervention inflammatory stress response. These results largely support our previous cross-sectional findings showing an inverse association between fitness and inflammatory stress responses, although it is difficult to conclude whether exercise withdrawal or mood disturbance per se is mainly driving the observed disturbances in inflammatory responses. One important aspect might be the ability

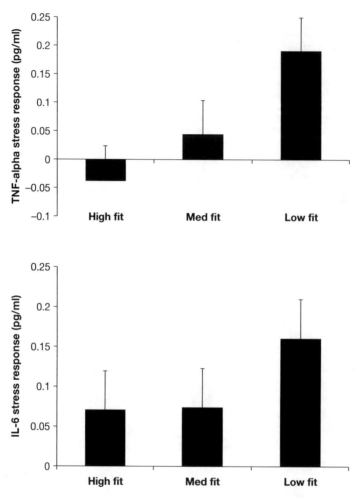

Figure 20.2 The association between physical fitness and the inflammatory response to mental stress [TNF-α (upper panel) and IL-6 (lower panel)]. Participants were 207 men and women drawn from the Whitehall II epidemiological cohort. Data are presented as mean ± SEM, adjusted for age, gender, body mass index, employment grade, smoking, alcohol, and basal levels of inflammatory cytokines. Physical fitness tertiles are based on heart rate response to cycling ergometry exercise at a standardised workload.

of the neuroendocrine system to suppress inflammatory responses. Following stress, the sensitivity of the immune system to dexamethasone (a synthetic version of the hormone cortisol that has potent anti-inflammatory properties) inhibition is reduced, as manifest by a reduction in this hormone's capacity to suppress the production of inflammatory cytokines (Rohleder, Schommer, Hellhammer, Engel, & Kirschbaum, 2001). In endurance-trained individuals, however, an acute bout of exercise has been shown to increase tissue sensitivity to glucocorticoids, which is thought to act as a mechanism to prevent an excessive muscle inflammatory reaction (Duclos, Gouarne, & Bonnemaison, 2003).

It is likely that the immune system interacts with the HPA axis and sympathetic nervous system in orchestrating an overall stress response. Previous research has indicated an intriguing link between efferent cholinergic activity of the vagus nerve (the parasympathetic arm of the

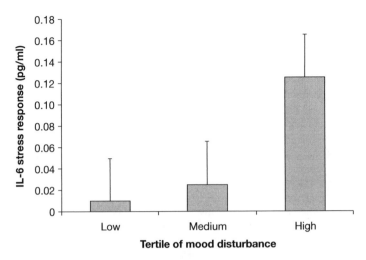

Figure 20.3 The association between mood disturbance following 2 weeks' exercise withdrawal and IL-6 responses to mental stress. Participants were 41 healthy men and women regularly engaged in exercise. Mood disturbance was assessed using the 28-item General Health questionnaire. Data are presented as mean ± SEM, adjusted for age, gender, body mass index, and pre-intervention inflammatory stress response.

autonomic nervous system) and inhibition of inflammatory processes (Tracy, 2002). Our findings indicated that fitter individuals maintained greater parasympathetic control during mental stress and also demonstrated the lowest inflammatory stress responses (Hamer & Steptoe 2007). The decline in parasympathetic control with ageing is attenuated with regular exercise training (Carter, Banister, & Blaber, 2003). Thus it is feasible that fitness-related improvements in parasympathetic activity may play a role in mediating the inhibition of stress-induced inflammatory processes. Other mechanisms are also likely to be important. For example, exercise has a favourable impact on insulin sensitivity and recent research has shown that the highest inflammatory cytokine responses to stress were in participants with the greatest levels of insulin resistance (Suarez, Boyle, Lewis, Hall, & Young, 2006). Other potential mediating effects may involve high-density lipoprotein cholesterol, adiponectin, and reduced reactive oxygen species—all of which demonstrate anti-inflammatory actions and are influenced by exercise training (Greenburg & Obin, 2006).

Conclusion

Interventions that reduce the magnitude of psychophysiological responses are justified, at least in part, by the notion that exaggerated responses to mental stress can have detrimental effects on health. Regular exercise is known to be an effective lifestyle intervention in the primary prevention of CVD, and this could be partly mediated through the buffering of haemodynamic, neuroendocrine, inflammatory, and haemostatic responses to daily mental stressors. There is reasonably strong evidence to suggest that a single bout of acute exercise can blunt cardiovascular stress responses although data from chronic training intervention studies are less consistent. Inconsistencies in this area may be due, in part, to small sample sizes, insufficient exercise training effects, inconsistencies in methodology (i.e., design, types of stressors, types of stress response measures), failure to account for the after-effects of a recent bout of acute exercise, and other confounding factors. At present there is some limited evidence to suggest that exercise might also modify biological stress responses (cortisol, inflammatory markers), although further experimental work is needed to extend the current findings.

Acknowledgements

The authors are funded by the British Heart Foundation, UK.

References

Bierhaus, A., Wolf, J., Andrassy, M., Rohleder, N., Humpert, P.M., Petrov, D., . . . Nawroth, P.P. 2003. A mechanism converting psychosocial stress into mononuclear cell activation. *Proceedings of the National Academy Science USA, 100*, 1920–1925.

Blumenthal, J.A., Babyak, M., Wei, J., O'Connor, C., Waugh, R., Eisenstein, E., . . . Reed, G. 2002. Usefulness of psychosocial treatment of mental stress-induced myocardial ischemia in men. *American Journal of Cardiology, 89*, 164–168.

Blumenthal, J.A., Sherwood, A., Babyak, M.A., Watkins, L.L., Waugh, R., Georgiades, A., . . . Hinderliter, A. 2005. Effects of exercise and stress management training on markers of cardiovascular risk in patients with ischemic heart disease: A randomized controlled trial. *Journal of the American Medical Association, 293*, 1626–1634.

Brotman, D.J., Golden, S.H., & Wittstein, I.S. 2007. The cardiovascular toll of stress. *Lancet, 370*, 1089–1100.

Brownley, K.A., Hinderliter, A.L., West, S.G., Girdler, S.S., Sherwood, A., & Light, K.A. 2003. Sympathoadrenergic mechanisms in reduced hemodynamic stress responses after exercise. *Medicine & Science in Sports & Exercise, 35*, 978–986.

Burg, M.M., Barefoot, J., Berkman, L., Catellier, D.J., Czajkowski, S., Saab, P., . . . Taylor, C.B.; ENRICHD Investigators. 2005. Low perceived social support and post-myocardial infarction prognosis in the enhancing recovery in coronary heart disease clinical trial: The effects of treatment. *Psychosomatic Medicine, 67*, 879–888.

Carter, J.B., Banister, E.W., & Blaber, A.P. 2003. Effect of endurance exercise on autonomic control of heart rate. *Sports Medicine, 33*, 33–46.

Chida, Y., & Hamer, M. 2008. Chronic psychosocial factors and acute physiological responses to laboratory-induced stress in healthy populations: A quantitative review of 30 years of investigations. *Psychological Bulletin, 134*, 829–885.

Chida, Y., & Steptoe, A. 2009. The association of anger and hostility with future coronary heart disease: A meta-analytic review of prospective evidence. *Journal of the American College of Cardiology, 53*, 936–946.

Chida, Y., & Steptoe, A. 2010. Greater cardiovascular responses to laboratory mental stress are associated with poor subsequent cardiovascular risk status: A meta-analysis of prospective evidence. *Hypertension, 55*, 1026–1032.

Christakis, N.A., & Fowler, J.H. 2008. The collective dynamics of smoking in a large social network. *New England Journal of Medicine, 358*, 2249–2258.

Crews, D.J., & Landers, D.M. 1987. A meta-analytic review of aerobic fitness and reactivity to psychosocial stressors. *Medicine & Science in Sports & Exercise, 19*, S114–S120.

Dekker, M.J., Koper, J.W., van Aken, M.O., Pols, H.A., Hofman, A., de Jong, F.H., . . . Tiemeier, H. 2008. Salivary cortisol is related to atherosclerosis of carotid arteries. *Journal of Clinical Endocrinology and Metabolism, 93*, 3741–3747.

DeRijk, R.H., Boelen, A., Tilders, F.J., & Berkenbosch, F. 1994. Induction of plasma interleukin-6 by circulating adrenaline in the rat. *Psychoneuroendocrinology, 19*, 155–163.

Dishman, R.K., & Jackson, E.M. 2006. Cardiorespiratory fitness and laboratory stress: A meta-regression analysis. *Psychophysiology, 43*, 57–72.

Duclos, M., Gouarne, C., & Bonnemaison, D. 2003. Acute and chronic effects of exercise on tissue sensitivity to glucocorticoids. *Journal of Applied Physiology, 94*, 869–875.

Ellins, E., Halcox, J., Donald, A., Field, B., Brydon, L., Deanfield, J., & Steptoe, A. 2008. Arterial stiffness and inflammatory response to psychophysiological stress. *Brain Behavior and Immunity, 22*, 941–948.

Endrighi, R., Steptoe, A., & Hamer, M. 2011. Mood disturbance following exercise withdrawal is associated with greater inflammatory responses to stress. *Psychosomatic Medicine, 73*, A110.

Febbraio, M.A., & Pedersen, B.K. 2002. Muscle-derived interleukin-6: Mechanisms for activation and possible biological roles. *FASEB Journal*, 16, 1335–1347.

Flaa, A., Aksnes, T.A., Kjeldsen, S.E., Eide, I., & Rostrup, M. 2008. Increased sympathetic reactivity may predict insulin resistance: An 18-year follow-up study. *Metabolism*, 57, 1422–1427.

Flaa, A., Eide, I.K., Kjeldsen, S.E., & Rostrup, M. 2008. Sympathoadrenal stress reactivity is a predictor of future blood pressure: An 18-year follow-up study. *Hypertension*, 52, 336–341.

Forcier, K., Stroud, L.R., Papandonatos, G.D., Hitsman, B., Reiches, M., Krishnamoorthy, J., & Niaura, R. 2006. Links between physical fitness and cardiovascular reactivity and recovery to psychological stressors: A meta-analysis. *Health Psychology*, 25, 723–739.

Gianaros, P.J., Salomon, K., Zhou, F., Owens, J.F., Edmundowicz, D., Kuller, L.H., & Matthews, K.A. 2005. A greater reduction in high-frequency heart rate variability to a psychological stressor is associated with subclinical coronary and aortic calcification in postmenopausal women. *Psychosomatic Medicine*, 67, 553–560.

Gimeno, D., Kivimäki, M., Brunner, E.J., Elovainio, M., De Vogli, R., Steptoe, A., . . . Ferrie, J.E. 2009. Associations of C-reactive protein and interleukin-6 with cognitive symptoms of depression: 12-year follow-up of the Whitehall II study. *Psychological Medicine*, 39, 413–423.

Glassman, A.H., Bigger, J.T., Jr, & Gaffney, M. 2009. Psychiatric characteristics associated with long-term mortality among 361 patients having an acute coronary syndrome and major depression: Seven-year follow-up of SADHART participants. *Archives of General Psychiatry*, 66, 1022–1029.

Greco, C.M., Kao, A.H., Sattar, A., Danchenko, N., Maksimowicz-McKinnon, K.M., Edmundowicz, D., . . . Manzi, S. 2009. Association between depression and coronary artery calcification in women with systemic lupus erythematosus. *Rheumatology (Oxford)*, 48, 576–581.

Greenberg, A.S., & Obin, M.S. 2006. Obesity and the role of adipose tissue in inflammation and metabolism. *American Journal of Clinical Nutrition*, 83, 461S–465S.

Halliwill, J.R. 2001. Mechanisms and clinical implications of post-exercise hypotension in humans. *Exercise and Sport Science Reviews*, 29, 65–70.

Hamer, M. 2007. The relative influences of fitness and fatness on inflammatory factors. *Preventive Medicine*, 44, 3–11.

Hamer, M., Boutcher, Y., & Boutcher, S.H. 2002. Cardiovascular and renal responses to mental challenge in highly and moderately active males with a family history of hypertension. *Journal of Human Hypertension*, 16, 319–326.

Hamer, M., O'Donnell, K., Lahiri, A., & Steptoe, A. 2010. Salivary cortisol responses to mental stress are associated with coronary artery calcification in healthy men and women. *European Heart Journal*, 31, 424–429.

Hamer, M., Molloy, G.J., & Stamatakis, E. 2008. Psychological distress as a risk factor for cardiovascular events: Pathophysiological and behavioral mechanisms. *Journal of the American College of Cardiology*, 52, 2156–2162.

Hamer, M., & Steptoe, A. 2007. Association between physical fitness, parasympathetic control, and proinflammatory responses to mental stress. *Psychosomatic Medicine*, 69, 660–666.

Hamer, M., Taylor, A., & Steptoe, A. 2006. The effect of acute aerobic exercise on stress related blood pressure responses: A systematic review and meta-analysis. *Biological Psychology*, 71, 183–190.

Heffner, K.L., Waring, M.E., Roberts, M.B., Eaton, C.B., & Gramling, R. 2011. Social isolation, C-reactive protein, and coronary heart disease mortality among community-dwelling adults. *Social Science and Medicine*, 72, 1482–1488.

Heikkilä, K., Nyberg, S.T., Fransson, E.I., Alfredsson, L., De Bacquer, D., Bjorner, J.B., . . . Kivimäki, M.; IPD-Work Consortium. 2012. Job strain and tobacco smoking: An individual-participant data meta-analysis of 166,130 adults in 15 European studies. *PLoS One*, 7, e35463.

Heponiemi, T., Elovainio, M., Pulkki, L., Puttonen, S., Raitakari, O., & Keltikangas-Järvinen, L. 2007. Cardiac autonomic reactivity and recovery in predicting carotid atherosclerosis: The cardiovascular risk in young Finns study. *Health Psychology*, 26, 13–21.

Jennings, J.R., Kamarck, T.W., Everson-Rose, S.A., Kaplan, G.A., Manuck, S.B., & Salonen, J.T. 2004. Exaggerated blood pressure responses during mental stress are prospectively related to enhanced carotid atherosclerosis in middle-aged Finnish men. *Circulation*, 110, 2198–2203.

Kher, N., & Marsh, J.D. 2004. Pathobiology of atherosclerosis—A brief review. *Seminars in Thrombosis and Hemostasis*, 30, 665–672.

King, A.C., Baumann, K., O'Sullivan, P., Wilcox, S., & Castro, C. 2002. Effects of moderate-intensity exercise on physiological, behavioral, and emotional responses to family caregiving: A randomized controlled trial. *Journals of Gerontology A: Biological Sciences and Medical Sciences*, 57, M26–M36.

Kivimäki, M., Nyberg, S.T., Batty, G.D., Fransson, E.I., Heikkilä, K., Alfredsson, L., . . . Theorell, T.; IPD-Work Consortium. 2012. Job strain as a risk factor for coronary heart disease: A collaborative meta-analysis of individual participant data. *Lancet, 380*, 1491–1497.

Kop, W.J., Stein, P.K., Tracy, R.P., Barzilay, J.I., Schulz, R., & Gottdiener, J.S. 2010. Autonomic nervous system dysfunction and inflammation contribute to the increased cardiovascular mortality risk associated with depression. *Psychosomatic Medicine, 72*, 626–635.

Manuck, S.B., Kaplan, J.R., Adams, M.R., & Clarkson, T.B. 1989. Behaviorally elicited heart rate reactivity and atherosclerosis in female cynomolgus monkeys (Macaca fascicularis). *Psychosomatic Medicine, 51*, 306–318.

Matthews, K.A., Schwartz, J., Cohen, S., & Seeman, T. 2006. Diurnal cortisol decline is related to coronary calcification: CARDIA study. *Psychosomatic Medicine, 68*, 657–661.

Matthews, K.A., Zhu, S., Tucker, D.C., & Whooley, M.A. 2006. Blood pressure reactivity to psychological stress and coronary calcification in the Coronary Artery Risk Development in Young Adults Study. *Hypertension, 47*, 391–395.

Matthews, K.A., Owens, J.F., Kuller, L.H., Sutton-Tyrrell, K., Lassila, H.C., & Wolfson, S.K. 1998. Stress-induced pulse pressure change predicts women's carotid atherosclerosis. *Stroke, 29*, 1525–1530.

Murray, D.R., Prabhu, S.D., & Chandrasekar, B. 2000. Chronic beta-adrenergic stimulation induces myocardial proinflammatory cytokine expression. *Circulation, 101*, 2338–2341.

Nabi, H., Singh-Manoux, A., Shipley, M., Gimeno, D., Marmot, M.G., & Kivimaki, M. 2008. Do psychological factors affect inflammation and incident coronary heart disease. The Whitehall II Study. *Arteriosclerosis, Thrombosis and Vascular Biology, 28*, 1398–1406.

Nijm, J., & Jonasson, L. 2009. Inflammation and cortisol response in coronary artery disease. *Annals of Medicine, 41*, 224–233.

Pavlov, V.A., & Tracey, K.J. 2005. The cholinergic anti-inflammatory pathway. *Brain, Behavior and Immunity, 19*, 493–499.

Pedersen, B.K. 2011. Exercise-induced myokines and their role in chronic diseases. *Brain, Behavior and Immunity, 25*, 811–816.

Poole, L., Steptoe, A., Wawrzyniak, A.J., Bostock, S., Mitchell, E.S., & Hamer, M. 2011. Associations of objectively measured physical activity with daily mood ratings and psychophysiological stress responses in women. *Psychophysiology, 48*(8), 1165–1172. doi: 10.1111/j.1469-8986.2011.01184.x.

Ray, C.A., & Carter, J.R. 2010. Effects of aerobic exercise training on sympathetic and renal responses to mental stress in humans. *American Journal of Physiology – Heart and Circulation Physiology, 298*, H229–H234.

Ribeiro, M.M., Silva, A.G., Santos, N.S., Guazzelle, I., Matos, L.N., Trombetta, I.C., . . . Villares, S.M. 2005. Diet and exercise training restore blood pressure and vasodilatory responses during physiological maneuvers in obese children. *Circulation, 111*, 1915–1923.

Rimmele, U., Seiler, R., Marti, B., Wirtz, P.H., Ehlert, U., & Heinrichs, M. 2009. The level of physical activity affects adrenal and cardiovascular reactivity to psychosocial stress. *Psychoneuroendocrinology, 34*, 190–198.

Roepke, S.K., Chattillion, E.A., von Kanel, R., Allison, M., Ziegler, M.G., Dimsdale, J.E., . . . Grant, I. 2011. Carotid plaque in Alzheimer caregivers and the role of sympathoadrenal arousal. *Psychosomatic Medicine, 73*, 206–213.

Rohleder, N., Schommer, N.C., Hellhammer, D.H., Engel, R., & Kirschbaum, C. 2001. Sex differences in glucocorticoid sensitivity of proinflammatory cytokine production after psychosocial stress. *Psychosomatic Medicine, 63*, 966–972.

Rosengren, A., Hawken, S., Ounpuu, S., Sliwa, K., Zubaid, M., Almahmeed, W.A., . . . Yusuf, S.; INTERHEART investigators. 2004. Association of psychosocial risk factors with risk of acute myocardial infarction in 11119 cases and 13648 controls from 52 countries (the INTERHEART study): Case-control study. *Lancet, 364*, 953–962.

Ross, R. 1999. Atherosclerosis—An inflammatory disease. *New England Journal Medicine, 340*, 115–126.

Sanders, V.M., & Kavelaars, A. 2007. Adrenergic regulation of immunity. In R. Ader (Ed.), *Psychoneuroimmunology* (4th ed., pp. 63–83). San Diego: Academic Press.

Schulz, R., & Beach, S.R. 1999. Caregiving as a risk factor for mortality: The Caregiver Health Effects Study. *Journal of the American Medical Association, 282*, 2215–2219.

Seyle, H. 1965. *The stress of life*. New York: McGraw-Hill.

Skoluda, N., Dettenborn, L., Stalder, T., & Kirschbaum, C. 2012. Elevated hair cortisol concentrations in endurance athletes. *Psychoneuroendocrinology, 37*, 611–617.

Sloan, R.P., Shapiro, P.A., Demeersman, R.E., Bagiella, E., Brondolo, E.N., McKinley, P.S., . . . Myers, M.M. 2011. Impact of aerobic training on cardiovascular reactivity to and recovery from challenge. *Psychosomatic Medicine, 73*, 134–141.

Steptoe, A. 2007. Psychophysiological contributions to behavioural medicine and psychosomatics. In J.T. Cacioppo, L.G. Tassinary, & G. Bernston (Eds.), *Handbook of psychophysiology* (3rd ed.). New York: Cambridge University Press.

Steptoe, A., & Brydon, L. 2005. Associations between acute lipid stress responses and fasting lipid levels 3 years later. *Health Psychology, 24*, 601–607.

Steptoe, A., Hamer, M., & Chida, Y. 2007. The effects of acute psychological stress on circulating inflammatory factors in humans: A review and meta-analysis. *Brain, Behavior and Immunity, 21*, 901–912.

Steptoe, A., & Wardle, J. 2005. Cardiovascular stress responsivity, body mass and abdominal adiposity. *International Journal of Obesity, 29*, 1329–1337.

Steptoe, A., Wardle, J., Lipsey, Z., Mills, R., Oliver, G., Jarvis, M., & Kirschbaum, C. 1998. A longitudinal study of work load and variations in psychological well-being, cortisol, smoking, and alcohol consumption. *Annals of Behavioral Medicine, 20*, 84–91.

Suarez, E.C., Boyle, S.H., Lewis, J.G., Hall, R.P., & Young, K.H. 2006. Increases in stimulated secretion of proinflammatory cytokines by blood monocytes following arousal of negative affect: The role of insulin resistance as moderator. *Brain, Behavior and Immunity, 20*, 331–338.

Surtees, P.G., Wainwright, N.W., Boekholdt, S.M., Luben, R.N., Wareham, N.J., & Khaw, K.T. 2008. Major depression, C-reactive protein, and incident ischemic heart disease in healthy men and women. *Psychosomatic Medicine, 70*, 850–855.

Tracey, K.J. 2002. The inflammatory reflex. *Nature, 420*, 853–859.

Traustadóttir, T., Bosch, P.R., & Matt, K.S. 2005. The HPA axis response to stress in women: Effects of aging and fitness. *Psychoneuroendocrinology, 30*(4), 392–402.

Vaccarino, V., Johnson, B.D., Sheps, D.S., Reis, S.E., Kelsey, S.F., Bittner, V., et al; National Heart, Lung, and Blood Institute. 2007. Depression, inflammation, and incident cardiovascular disease in women with suspected coronary ischemia: The National Heart, Lung, and Blood Institute-sponsored WISE study. *Journal of the American College of Cardiology, 50*, 2044–2050.

Van der Kooy, K., van Hout, H., Marwijk, H., Marten, H., Stehouwer, C., & Beekman, A. 2007. Depression and the risk for cardiovascular diseases: Systematic review and meta analysis. *International Journal of Geriatric Psychiatry, 22*, 613–626.

von Känel, R., Kudielka, B.M., Metzenthin, P., Helfricht, S., Preckel, D., Haeberli, A., Stutz, M., Fischer, J.E. 2008. Aspirin, but not propranolol, attenuates the acute stress-induced increase in circulating levels of interleukin-6: A randomized, double-blind, placebo-controlled study. *Brain, Behavior and Immunity, 22*, 150–157.

West, S.G., Brownley, K.A., & Light, K.C. 1998. Post-exercise vasodilatation reduces diastolic blood pressure responses to stress. *Annals of Behavioral Medicine, 20*, 77–83.

Whooley, M.A., de Jonge, P., Vittinghoff, E., Otte, C., Moos, R., & Carney, R.M. 2008. Depressive symptoms, health behaviours, and risk of cardiovascular events in patients with coronary heart disease. *Journal of the American Medical Association, 300*, 2379–2388.

21

IMPACT OF PHYSICAL ACTIVITY ON DIURNAL RHYTHMS

A potential mechanism for exercise-induced stress resistance and stress resilience

*Monika Fleshner, Robert S. Thompson,
and Benjamin N. Greenwood*

Individuals vary in their susceptibility to the negative consequences of stressor exposure. The mechanisms for these differences include many factors that are beyond our control including genetic differences, age, or gender. Results from our work and others', however, suggest that maintaining a physically active lifestyle, a behavioral choice that is within our control, can reduce stress vulnerability and increase stress resistance and stress resilience.

There is clear evidence in the human literature that people who regularly exercise have a reduction in their risk for developing stress-exacerbated disorders (see Gerber & Puhse, 2009 for review) including cardiovascular disease (Lavie, Milani, O'Keefe, & Lavie, 2011; Mosca et al., 2011; Soderman, Lisspers, & Sundin, 2007), obesity (Brumby et al., 2011), mood disorders (e.g., anxiety and depression; Dinas, Koutedakis, & Flouris, 2011; Lincoln, Shepherd, Johnson, & Castaneda-Sceppa, 2011; Mata et al., 2011; Mehnert et al., 2011), attention deficit disorder (Archer & Kostrzewa, 2011), inflammatory bowel disease (Packer, Hoffman-Goetz, & Ward, 2010), communicable illness (Brown & Siegel, 1988), and sleep disorders (Elder et al., 2011). Most of these studies not only report improvements in these disease states, but also either directly assess or strongly suggest that reductions in the negative impact of stressor exposure may be an important mediator for the positive effects of exercise. We propose, therefore, that regular, moderate physical activity reduces the negative effects of stress on mental and physical health by increasing both stress resistance and stress resilience.

What are stress resistance and stress resilience?

The acute stress response is a highly adaptive cascade of physiological reactions that work in concert to facilitate successful fight/flight responses and increase an organism's chances of survival. Why then would stress resistance be a good thing? It is important to recognize that stress resistance does not imply the absence of the stress response. Rather it has been suggested that increased stress resistance allows an organism to experience greater stressor intensities and/or longer stressor duration before stress consequences cross over from adaptive to maladaptive (Fleshner, Maier, Lyons, & Raskind, 2011). In contrast, stress resilience is directed at recovery. Resilience, by definition, is having or showing power of recovery (Williams, 1979). Thus, changes in stress resilience are only realized after an organism has suffered negative consequences of stress. Stress resilient organisms, therefore, require less time and/or treatment to recover after crossing the tipping point from adaptive to maladaptive effects (Fleshner et al., 2011).

Using a well-established animal model of stress (learned helplessness), we have evidence that 6 weeks of wheel running, but not treadmill training (Moraska, Deak, Spencer, Roth, & Fleshner, 2000), improves both stress resistance and stress resilience in rats. Specifically, physically active, compared to sedentary, rats are protected against stress-induced immunosuppression (Moraska & Fleshner, 2001), mood disruptions (i.e., learned helplessness behavior, depression and anxiety (Greenwood & Fleshner, 2011; Greenwood, Foley, et al., 2003; Moraska & Fleshner, 2001), and improve their recovery after suffering negative stress effects (Greenwood, Strong, Dorey, & Fleshner, 2007; Moraska & Fleshner, 2001).

Mechanisms for stress-buffering effects of exercise

Six weeks of wheel running constrains activation of stress-responsive neurocircuitry

There are several ways that the central neurocircuitry of the stress response is changed in physically active rats, and such adaptations can be mechanistically linked to stress resistance effects. For example, 6 weeks, but not 3 weeks, of wheel running constrains activation of the serotonin (5-HT) neurons in the dorsal raphe nucleus (DRN) during exposure to uncontrollable stress (Greenwood, Foley, Burhans, Maier, & Fleshner, 2005). This constraint is evidenced by a reduction in c-Fos expression in 5-HT neurons and upregulation of $5HT_{1A}$ inhibitory auto-receptors (Greenwood, Foley, Burhans, et al., 2005; Greenwood, Foley, Day, et al., 2005). Given that the exaggerated DRN 5-HT neuronal response produced by uncontrollable stress is both necessary and sufficient to produce learned helplessness behaviors (Maier & Watkins, 2005), constraint in this response is likely a critical mechanism responsible for exercise-evoked protection against uncontrollable stress effects on mood and anxiety (see Greenwood & Fleshner, 2011 for a recent review). In addition, we have equally compelling evidence that 6 weeks of wheel running constrains central autonomic neurocircuitry responsible for activating the peripheral sympathetic nervous system (SNS) response to stress (M. Fleshner, 2000). Rats that ran for 6 weeks on running wheels have reduced c-Fos expression in primary central autonomic regulatory centers (Greenwood, Kennedy, et al., 2003), including a rostral ventral lateral medulla, A5 noradrenergic neurons, and locus coeruleus (LC). The beneficial consequences of constraint over stress-evoked autonomic responses include protection against immunosuppression and inflammatory protein increases (i.e., interleukin-1beta), both of which are mediated by excessive SNS responses (Fleshner, 2006; Johnson et al., 2005; Kennedy et al., 2005).

It is important to note that exercise does not eliminate the stress response; rather it constrains it, thus preventing an excessive response. Uncontrollable tail shock is a potent stressor, designed to reveal maladaptive consequences of the stress response. It drives the stress response to exhaustion, as evidenced by desensitization of DRN inhibitory $5HT_{1A}$ autoreceptors (Rozeske et al., 2011) and LC and splenic catecholamine depletion (Greenwood, Kennedy, et al., 2003). In animals that are allowed to habitually voluntarily run in wheels for 6 weeks, this extreme response is prevented. Interestingly, the changes produced by 6 weeks of wheel running, which help buffer against the maladaptive effects of stress, persist after wheel running has ceased. Greenwood, Loughridge, Sadaoui, Christianson, and Fleshner (2012) reported that exercise-evoked protection against stress-induced deficits in shuttle box escape learning persists for 15 days, but was lost 25 days, after forced exercise cessation. The results to date are therefore consistent with the idea that persistent adaptations in specific neurotransmitters, neuropeptides, and/or growth factors in physically active organisms likely contribute to reductions in stress vulnerability.

Voluntary wheel running is rewarding

The mesolimbic reward pathway includes a major dopaminergic projection from the ventral tegmental area (VTA) to the nucleus accumbens (Acb). Activation of this pathway has been implicated in the treatment of depression (Nestler & Carlezon, 2006; Yadid & Friedman, 2008) and anxiety (Pezze & Feldon, 2004; Talalaenko et al., 1994), and may play an etiological role in stress resistance produced by exercise. Physical activity is a powerful natural reward as evidenced by spontaneous wheel running behavior in many animal species. In addition, rats will work (learn to press a lever) to gain access to a running wheel (Belke, 2000a, 2000b; Iversen, 1993). We have recently reported that rats display (1) a conditioned place preference for wheel running, (2) an increase in the reward-related plasticity marker FosB/ΔFosB and Δ-opioid receptor mRNA in Acb, and (3) increased levels of tyrosine hydroxylase (TH) mRNA in the VTA (Greenwood et al., 2011). These observations support the idea that wheel running elicits plasticity in the mesolimbic reward pathway. Future work is required to determine whether such changes contribute to exercise-evoked increases in stress resistance and resilience.

Controllability of wheel running is not necessary for stress resistance

Research in humans and animals indicates that the experience of choice can itself improve mental health and produce stress resistance. A series of recently completed studies in our laboratory began to explore if controllability of wheel running behavior is critical for stress-buffering effects. Rats were housed for 6 weeks with either (1) a locked wheel, (2) a voluntary running wheel, (3) a yoked motorized wheel, or (4) were trained daily on a treadmill. The motorized wheel was programmed to rotate at a speed, pattern, and duration that mimicked voluntary wheel running. Rats in the motorized wheel thus ran a similar distance, pattern, and duration as the voluntary running animals; however, they had no control over their running behavior. In other words, the physical activity patterns between the groups were equal, and only the choice to run was different. After 6 weeks, rats were exposed to uncontrollable tail shock and tested for negative behavioral consequences (shuttle box escape learning, social exploration, and exaggerated fear conditioning). Results indicated that choosing to run is not critical to reveal stress-buffering effects. Rats that were forced to run in wheels and rats that voluntarily ran in wheels were equally protected against the behavioral consequences of uncontrollable stress. This result was surprising to us given the fact that forced treadmill training, despite producing significant fitness benefits, failed to produce any stress-buffering effects. The critical difference between treadmill training and forced wheel running could lie in the pattern of the behavior or the ability of the behavior to influence diurnal/circadian rhythms. Rats forced to run in treadmills are typically made to run continuously for a brief period. In contrast, rats that run voluntarily in wheels (and the rats forced to run in motorized wheels in the study described above) run in a markedly different pattern. These rats run in brief, repeated bursts throughout the active cycle. It is possible that this pattern of exercise is particularly able to influence diurnal/circadian physiology. Wheel running may therefore be producing stress resistance and resilience by influencing diurnal/circadian rhythms.

New ideas: diurnal/circadian effects of exercise contribute to exercise-induced stress resistance and resilience

Diurnal rhythms of physiology and behavior are driven by both circadian and non-circadian mechanism. Those effects that are circadian occur in the absence of photic or non-photic diurnal cues and are generated by a core set of clock genes that regulate their own expression in an approximately 24-hour transcriptional-translational feedback loop. It is clear from the stress literature that disruptions in diurnal/circadian rhythms are ubiquitous in people suffering from negative mental and physical consequences of stress, including metabolic disease (Arble, Ramsey, Bass, & Turek, 2010; Cagampang, Poore, & Hanson, 2011), cardiovascular disease (Portaluppi et al., 2012; Takeda & Maemura, 2011), and depression/anxiety (Bunney & Potkin, 2008; McClung, 2007). Interestingly, many of the biological rhythm changes are normalized in patients who are successfully treated with antidepressants, including SSRIs (Bunney & Potkin, 2008) and desipramine (Jiang et al., 2011). It remains unclear if changes found in diurnal/circadian rhythms are symptomatic of the disease state or etiologically linked to these negative outcomes. With recent advances in animal models that allow direct genetic manipulations, however, evidence is accumulating that disrupting rhythms by genetically knocking out components of the clock genes may indeed directly contribute to disease development. Circadian locomotor output kaput (CLOCK) and Brain and Muscle ARNT-Like protein (BMAL) gene knockout mice, for example, develop hyperinsulinemia and diabetes (Marcheva et al., 2010), Cryptochorme (Cry1/Cry2)-deleted mice develop hypertension (Okamura, Doi, Yamaguchi, & Fustin, 2011), and CLOCKΔ19 mice express anxiety behavior (Coque et al., 2011).

The impact of stress on biological rhythms has been reported many times, but the precise nature of the disruption remains an active area of research. The most consistent observation reported in the literature is that exposure to intense, repeated, or chronic stressors dampens rhythms and flattens amplitudes such that the peak-to-trough, but not the period or frequency, of the physiological or behavioral rhythm is impacted. The types of diurnal rhythms dampened by exposure to a variety of stressors include rhythms of mean arterial pressure (Thompson, Strong, & Fleshner, 2012), heart rate (Meerlo, Sgoifo, & Turek, 2002; Thompson, Strong, & Fleshner, 2012), core body temperature (Kant et al., 1991; Meerlo et al., 2002; Sgoifo et al., 2002; Thompson et al., 2012), glucocorticoids (Fleshner, Deak, et al., 1995; Ushijima, Morikawa, To, Higuchi, & Ohdo, 2006), and wheel running or spontaneous activity behavior (Meerlo et al., 2002; Moraska & Fleshner, 2001; Sgoifo et al., 2002; Solberg, Horton, & Turek, 1999).

Figure 21.1 is an example our recent data revealing the impact of exposure to acute uncontrollable tail shock stress (100, 1.5mA, 5-s tail shocks) on diurnal rhythms. Adult male F344 rats were instrumented with biotelemetric devices that allow automated moment-to-moment recording of spontaneous activity, core body temperature, heart rate, and EEG. After 2 weeks of recovery, rats (8/group) were exposed to tail shock stress or remained in their home cages. Figure 21.1 reveals that stress produced an expected stress-induced hyperthermic (SIH) response. SIH is a well-characterized phenomenon in humans (Oka, Oka, & Hori, 2001) and animals (Lkhagvasuren, Nakamura, Oka, Sudo, & Nakamura, 2011). Telemetry data were collected after all rats were returned to their home cages and remained undisturbed for 6 days. Figure 21.1 reveals that rats not exposed to stress have clear diurnal rhythms in core body temperature. In stark contrast, rats exposed to stress have a dampened diurnal rhythm due to an elevation in the trough body temperature during light. Using a diurnal rhythm, non-linear, least squares, dual harmonic analysis (Gronfier, Wright, Kronauer, Jewett, & Czeisler, 2004), we concluded that the amplitude was reliably flattened for 72 hours. We did not find a reliable change in the phase of the rhythm.

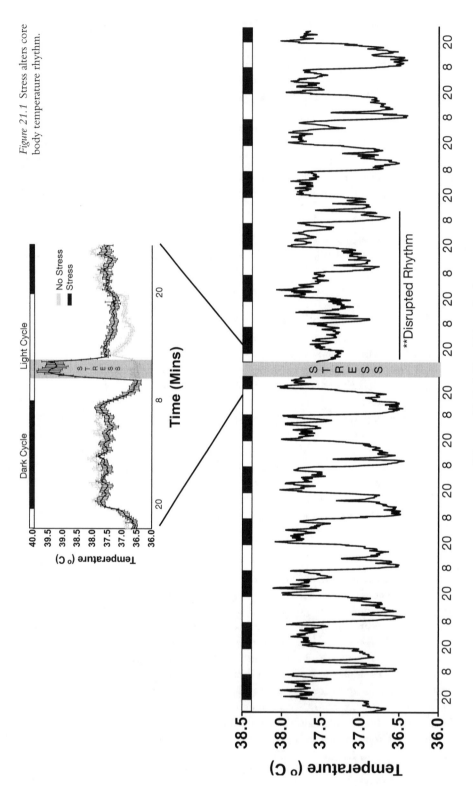

Figure 21.1 Stress alters core body temperature rhythm.

The mechanisms for stress–induced amplitude flattening of diurnal behavioral and biological rhythms are unknown. Amplitude flattening could be produced by dyssynchrony in circadian clocks. It has been reported, for example, that exposure to chronic unpredictable stress reduces the amplitude of rhythmic expression of period 2 (Per2) protein in the brain's "master clock," the suprachiasmatic nucleus. Diurnal/circadian rhythms and clock gene expression are synchronized to the environment. The most important synchronizing (entraining) environmental stimulus is light (Morin & Allen, 2006; Pickard, 1985). In addition, there are several other very powerful non–photic entrainment cues as well, including feeding schedules (Girotti et al., 2006; Mendoza, 2007), behavioral patterns (Edgar & Dement, 1991), temperature (Buhr, Yoo, & Takahashi, 2010), and adrenal hormones (Amir & Stewart, 2009; Segall, Perrin, Walker, Stewart, & Amir, 2006).

Treatment of stress-related mood disorders often includes clock "resetting"

Restoring circadian rhythms may be a new way to successfully manage depression (Gorwood, 2010). In fact, many therapeutic strategies currently in use target the circadian system. These include both pharmaceutical strategies such as agomelatine (melatonin receptor agonist and a $5HT_{2c}$ antagonist, (Gorwood, 2010) and adenosine A_{2a} receptor antagonists (Batalha et al., 2012), and non-pharmacological entrainment strategies such as bright light (Ashkenazy, Einat, & Kronfeld-Schor, 2009; McClung, 2007), sleep deprivation (Bunney & Potkin, 2008), temperature (Lowry, Lightman, & Nutt, 2009), and scheduled activity/exercise (Barr-Anderson, AuYoung, Whitt-Glover, Glenn, & Yancey, 2011). Thus there is interest in exploiting the restoration of circadian/diurnal rhythms for effective therapeutic strategies to treat stress-related mood disorders.

We hypothesize that just as regular exercise can be used therapeutically to perhaps restore circadian disruptions, it may also function to increase central and peripheral clock synchrony, thus resulting in greater rhythm amplitudes and hence increased resistance to stress-induced amplitude flattening. In fact, there is recent evidence that through a daily rhythm of endogenous dopamine release in multiple brain regions, exercise can directly modulate clock gene expression in the brain (Hood et al., 2010). In addition, exercise has been reported to coordinate clock gene regulation in muscle of humans (Zambon et al., 2003). Thus it is feasible to propose that habitual exercise synchronizes clock genes across specific brain neurocircuitry and peripheral tissues, and that this robust synchronization would increase the amplitude of physiological and behavioral rhythms, making it more difficult to disrupt them with stress. This new hypothesis and our evidence to support it is preliminary but promising.

Figure 21.2 shows core body temperature diurnal rhythms in sedentary and wheel running rats measured with biotelemetry (4/group). Rats that run in a wheel for 6 weeks, but not 1 or 3 weeks, have higher peak levels of core body temperature, leading to a greater amplitude of the rhythm of core body temperature compared to rats that remain sedentary for 6 weeks. This is intriguing because this time course is mirrored for the impact of wheel running on stress resistance as well. Rats are protected against stress-evoked increases in anxiety/depression if they run for 6 weeks, but not 3 weeks (Greenwood, Foley, Burhans, et al., 2005).

Exposure to uncontrollable tail shock additionally produces flattened diurnal rhythms of corticosterone (Fleshner, Deak, et al., 1995). This is due primarily to an elevation in trough corticosterone concentrations. As depicted in Figure 21.3, sedentary male F344 rats (8/group) exposed to uncontrollable tail shock have elevated trough levels of corticosterone measured 24 hours after stress, at 0900, when low trough levels of corticosterone should be found. In contrast, this effect of stress on elevating trough levels of corticosterone is reduced in rats that ran for 6 weeks prior to stress.

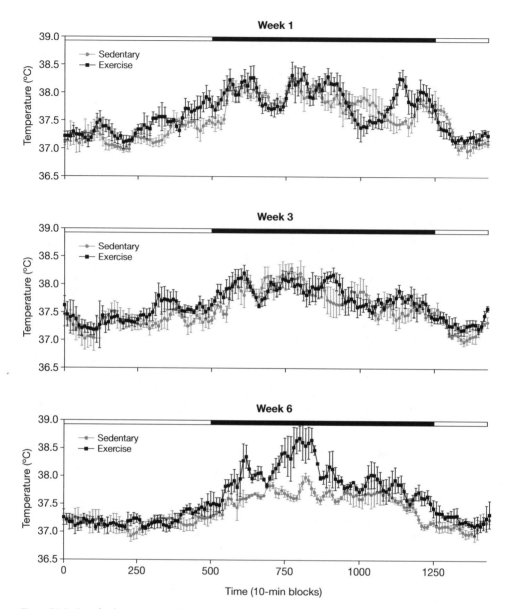

Figure 21.2 Core body temperature has greater peak amplitude after 6 weeks of wheel running.

Finally, Figure 21.4 shows that exposure to uncontrollable tail shock stress can disrupt the normal expression of clock genes, and exercise may prevent this effect. Male F344 rats (7–16/group) were allowed to run on wheels for 6 weeks (exercise) or remained sedentary. Rats were then exposed to either uncontrollable tail shock stress or no stress and were sacrificed immediately after stressor termination between Zeitgeber Time (ZT) 5–7. Using *in situ* hybridization, we measured the expression of period 1 (Per1) clock gene mRNA in the dentate gyrus (DG) of the hippocampus. DG was assessed because it is known to be activated by wheel running (Clark, Bhattacharya, Miller, & Rhodes, 2011) and is linked to stress-related mood

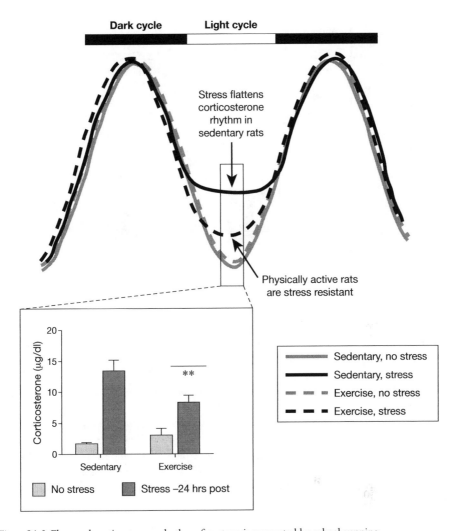

Figure 21.3 Flattened corticosterone rhythm after stress is prevented by wheel running.

disorders and corticosterone regulation (de Kloet, Karst, & Joels, 2008; Joels, 2007). Exposure to stress reduced levels of Per1 mRNA in the DG of sedentary rats. Exercise not only altered basal expression of Per1 mRNA in the DG at this clock time, it prevented the ability of stress to suppress Per1 mRNA in the DG. These data provide intriguing preliminary evidence that exercise can affect expression of clock genes in specific brain regions and can prevent shifts in clock gene expression produced by stress; thus providing a potential mechanism for how exercise might impact diurnal/circadian rhythms of behavior and physiology.

Conclusions and future directions

Individuals vary in their vulnerability to experience the negative consequences of stressor exposure. Maintaining a physically active lifestyle, a behavioral choice that is within our control, can reduce stress vulnerability and increase stress resistance and resilience. The fact that regular

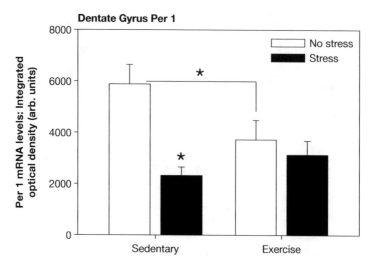

Figure 21.4 Hippocampal clock genes are disrupted by stress and protected by wheel running.

habitual exercise produces global protections against the negative consequences of stress that range from immunosuppression and learning deficits, to depression and anxiety, suggests that the mechanisms could be many and/or biologically fundamental. We have identified a variety of specific neurobiological changes in the brain that function to confer protection, and may be important as future pharmaceutical targets for treatment. In addition, our recent work suggests that there is something special about the habitual pattern of exercise that promotes broad stress resistance and stress resilience. In this chapter we propose the novel hypothesis that regular, habitual exercise in the active part of the diurnal cycle is a powerful non-photic entrainment cue that may function to synchronize both central and peripheral tissue clocks such that the synchronized output results in greater amplitude rhythms that are resistant to stress-evoked flattening. Future work should explore the mechanisms for this effect, and whether synchrony of diurnal/circadian rhythms is mechanistically linked to the increase in stress resistance and resilience produced by exercise.

References

Amir, S., & Stewart, J. (2009). Behavioral and hormonal regulation of expression of the clock protein, PER2, in the central extended amygdala. *Progress in Neuro-psychopharmacology & Biological Psychiatry, 33*(8), 1321–1328. doi:10.1016/j.pnpbp.2009.04.003

Arble, D. M., Ramsey, K. M., Bass, J., & Turek, F. W. (2010). Circadian disruption and metabolic disease: Findings from animal models. *Best Practice & Research. Clinical Endocrinology & Metabolism, 24*(5), 785–800. doi:10.1016/j.beem.2010.08.003

Archer, T., & Kostrzewa, R. M. (2011). Physical exercise alleviates ADHD symptoms: Regional deficits and development trajectory. *Neurotoxicity Research*. doi:10.1007/s12640-011-9260-0

Ashkenazy, T., Einat, H., & Kronfeld-Schor, N. (2009). Effects of bright light treatment on depression- and anxiety-like behaviors of diurnal rodents maintained on a short daylight schedule. *Behavioural Brain Research, 201*(2), 343–346. doi:10.1016/j.bbr.2009.03.005

Barr-Anderson, D. J., AuYoung, M., Whitt-Glover, M. C., Glenn, B. A., & Yancey, A. K. (2011). Integration of short bouts of physical activity into organizational routine: A systematic review of the literature. *American Journal of Preventive Medicine, 40*(1), 76–93. doi:10.1016/j.amepre.2010.09.033

Batalha, V. L., Pego, J. M., Fontinha, B. M., Costenla, A. R., Valadas, J. S., Baqi, Y., . . . Lopes, L. V.

(2012). Adenosine A(2A) receptor blockade reverts hippocampal stress-induced deficits and restores corticosterone circadian oscillation. *Molecular Psychiatry.* doi:10.1038/mp.2012.8

Belke, T. W. (2000a). Studies of wheel-running reinforcement: Parameters of Herrnstein's (1970) response-strength equation vary with schedule order. *Journal of the Experimental Analysis of Behavior, 73*(3), 319–331. doi:10.1901/jeab.2000.73-319

Belke, T. W. (2000b). Varying wheel-running reinforcer duration within a session: Effect on the revolution-postreinforcement pause relation. *Journal of the Experimental Analysis of Behavior, 73*(2), 225–239. doi:10.1901/jeab.2000.73-225

Brown, J. D., & Siegel, J. M. (1988). Exercise as a buffer of life stress: A prospective study of adolescent health. *Health Psychology, 7*(4), 341–353.

Brumby, S., Chandrasekara, A., McCoombe, S., Torres, S., Kremer, P., & Lewandowski, P. (2011). Reducing psychological distress and obesity in Australian farmers by promoting physical activity. *BMC Public Health, 11*, 362. doi:10.1186/1471-2458-11-362

Buhr, E. D., Yoo, S. H., & Takahashi, J. S. (2010). Temperature as a universal resetting cue for mammalian circadian oscillators. *Science, 330*(6002), 379–385. doi:10.1126/science.1195262

Bunney, J. N., & Potkin, S. G. (2008). Circadian abnormalities, molecular clock genes and chronobiological treatments in depression. *British Medical Bulletin, 86*, 23–32. doi:10.1093/bmb/ldn019

Cagampang, F. R., Poore, K. R., & Hanson, M. A. (2011). Developmental origins of the metabolic syndrome: Body clocks and stress responses. *Brain, Behavior, and Immunity, 25*(2), 214–220. doi:10.1016/j.bbi.2010.09.005

Clark, P. J., Bhattacharya, T. K., Miller, D. S., & Rhodes, J. S. (2011). Induction of c-Fos, Zif268, and Arc from acute bouts of voluntary wheel running in new and pre-existing adult mouse hippocampal granule neurons. *Neuroscience, 184*, 16–27. doi:10.1016/j.neuroscience.2011.03.072

Coque, L., Mukherjee, S., Cao, J. L., Spencer, S., Marvin, M., Falcon, E., . . . McClung, C. A. (2011). Specific role of VTA dopamine neuronal firing rates and morphology in the reversal of anxiety-related, but not depression-related behavior in the ClockDelta19 mouse model of mania. *Neuropsychopharmacology, 36*(7), 1478–1488. doi:10.1038/npp.2011.33

de Kloet, E. R., Karst, H., & Joels, M. (2008). Corticosteroid hormones in the central stress response: Quick-and-slow. *Frontiers in Neuroendocrinology, 29*(2), 268–272. doi:10.1016/j.yfrne.2007.10.002

Dinas, P. C., Koutedakis, Y., & Flouris, A. D. (2011). Effects of exercise and physical activity on depression. *Irish Journal of Medical Science, 180*(2), 319–325. doi:10.1007/s11845-010-0633-9

Edgar, D. M., & Dement, W. C. (1991). Regularly scheduled voluntary exercise synchronizes the mouse circadian clock. *American Journal of Physiology, 261*(4 Pt 2), R928–R933.

Elder, C. R., Gullion, C. M., Funk, K. L., Debar, L. L., Lindberg, N. M., & Stevens, V. J. (2011). Impact of sleep, screen time, depression and stress on weight change in the intensive weight loss phase of the LIFE study. *International Journal of Obesity.* doi:10.1038/ijo.2011.60

Fleshner, M. (2000). Exercise and neuroendocrine regulation of antibody production: Protective effect of physical activity on stress-induced suppression of the specific antibody response. *International Journal of Sports Medicine, 21* (Suppl 1), S14–S19.

Fleshner, M. (Ed.). (2006). *Stress-induced sympathetic nervous system activation contributes to both suppressed acquired immunity and potentiated innate immunity: The role of splenic NE depletion and extracellular Hsp72.* New York: Springer.

Fleshner, M., Deak, T., Spencer, R.L., Laudenslauger, M.L., Watkins, L.R., & Maier, S.F. (1995). A long term increase in basal levels of corticosterone and a decrease in corticosteroid-binding globulin after acute stressor exposure. *Endocrinology, 136*(12), 5336–5342.

Fleshner, M., Maier, S. F., Lyons, D. M., & Raskind, M. A. (2011). The neurobiology of the stress-resistant brain. *Stress.* doi:10.3109/10253890.2011.596865

Gerber, M., & Puhse, U. (2009). Review article: Do exercise and fitness protect against stress-induced health complaints? A review of the literature. *Scandinavian Journal of Public Health, 37*(8), 801–819. doi:10.1177/1403494809350522

Girotti, M., Pace, T. W., Gaylord, R. I., Rubin, B. A., Herman, J. P., & Spencer, R. L. (2006). Habituation to repeated restraint stress is associated with lack of stress-induced c-fos expression in primary sensory processing areas of the rat brain. *Neuroscience, 138*(4), 1067–1081. doi:10.1016/j.neuroscience.2005.12.002

Gorwood, P. (2010). Restoring circadian rhythms: A new way to successfully manage depression. *Journal of Psychopharmacology, 24* (Suppl 2), 15–19. doi:10.1177/1359786810372981

Greenwood, B. N., & Fleshner, M. (2011). Exercise, stress resistance, and central serotonergic systems. *Exercise and Sport Sciences Reviews, 39*(3), 140–149. doi:10.1097/JES.0b013e31821f7e45

Greenwood, B. N., Foley, T. E., Burhans, D., Maier, S. F., & Fleshner, M. (2005). The consequences of uncontrollable stress are sensitive to duration of prior wheel running. *Brain Research, 1033*(2), 164–178.

Greenwood, B. N., Foley, T. E., Day, H. E., Burhans, D., Brooks, L., Campeau, S., & Fleshner, M. (2005). Wheel running alters serotonin (5-HT) transporter, 5-HT1A, 5-HT1B, and alpha 1b-adrenergic receptor mRNA in the rat raphe nuclei. *Biological Psychiatry, 57*(5), 559–568.

Greenwood, B. N., Foley, T. E., Day, H. E., Campisi, J., Hammack, S. H., Campeau, S., . . . Fleshner, M. (2003). Freewheel running prevents learned helplessness/behavioral depression: Role of dorsal raphe serotonergic neurons. *Journal of Neuroscience, 23*(7), 2889–2898.

Greenwood, B. N., Foley, T. E., Le, T. V., Strong, P. V., Loughridge, A. B., Day, H. E., & Fleshner, M. (2011). Long-term voluntary wheel running is rewarding and produces plasticity in the mesolimbic reward pathway. *Behavioural Brain Research, 217*(2), 354–362. doi:10.1016/j.bbr.2010.11.005

Greenwood, B. N., Kennedy, S., Smith, T. P., Campeau, S., Day, H. E., & Fleshner, M. (2003). Voluntary freewheel running selectively modulates catecholamine content in peripheral tissue and c-Fos expression in the central sympathetic circuit following exposure to uncontrollable stress in rats. *Neuroscience, 120*(1), 269–281.

Greenwood, B. N., Loughridge, A. B., Sadaoui, N., Christianson, J. P., & Fleshner, M. (2012). The protective effects of voluntary exercise against the behavioral consequences of uncontrollable stress persist despite an increase in anxiety following forced cessation of exercise. *Behavioural Brain Research.* doi:10.1016/j.bbr.2012.05.017

Greenwood, B. N., Strong, P. V., Dorey, A. A., & Fleshner, M. (2007). Therapeutic effects of exercise: Wheel running reverses stress-induced interference with shuttle box escape. *Behavioral Neuroscience, 121*(5), 992–1000.

Gronfier, C., Wright, K. P., Jr., Kronauer, R. E., Jewett, M. E., & Czeisler, C. A. (2004). Efficacy of a single sequence of intermittent bright light pulses for delaying circadian phase in humans. *American Journal of Physiology. Endocrinology and Metabolism, 287*(1), E174–E181. doi:10.1152/ajpendo.00385.2003

Hood, S., Cassidy, P., Cossette, M. P., Weigl, Y., Verwey, M., Robinson, B., . . . Amir, S. (2010). Endogenous dopamine regulates the rhythm of expression of the clock protein PER2 in the rat dorsal striatum via daily activation of D2 dopamine receptors. *Journal of Neuroscience, 30*(42), 14046–14058. doi:10.1523/JNEUROSCI.2128-10.2010

Iversen, I. H. (1993). Techniques for establishing schedules with wheel running as reinforcement in rats. *Journal of the Experimental Analysis of Behavior, 60*(1), 219–238. doi:10.1901/jeab.1993.60-219

Jiang, W. G., Li, S. X., Zhou, S. J., Sun, Y., Shi, J., & Lu, L. (2011). Chronic unpredictable stress induces a reversible change of PER2 rhythm in the suprachiasmatic nucleus. *Brain Research, 1399*, 25–32. doi:10.1016/j.brainres.2011.05.001

Joels, M. (2007). Role of corticosteroid hormones in the dentate gyrus. *Progress in Brain Research, 163*, 355–370. doi:10.1016/S0079-6123(07)63021-0

Johnson, J. D., Campisi, J., Sharkey, C. M., Kennedy, S. L., Nickerson, M., Greenwood, B. N., & Fleshner, M. (2005). Catecholamines mediate stress-induced increases in peripheral and central inflammatory cytokines. *Neuroscience, 135*(4), 1295–1307.

Kant, G. J., Bauman, R. A., Pastel, R. H., Myatt, C. A., Closser-Gomez, E., & D'Angelo, C. P. (1991). Effects of controllable vs. uncontrollable stress on circadian temperature rhythms. *Physiology & Behavior, 49*(3), 625–630.

Kennedy, S. L., Nickerson, M., Campisi, J., Johnson, J. D., Smith, T. P., Sharkey, C., & Fleshner, M. (2005). Splenic norepinephrine depletion following acute stress suppresses in vivo antibody response. *Journal of Neuroimmunology, 165*(1–2), 150–160.

Lavie, C. J., Milani, R. V., O'Keefe, J. H., & Lavie, T. J. (2011). Impact of exercise training on psychological risk factors. *Progress in Cardiovascular Diseases, 53*(6), 464–470. doi:10.1016/j.pcad.2011.03.007

Lincoln, A. K., Shepherd, A., Johnson, P. L., & Castaneda-Sceppa, C. (2011). The impact of resistance exercise training on the mental health of older Puerto Rican adults with type 2 diabetes. *The Journals of Gerontology. Series B, Psychological Sciences and Social Sciences, 66*(5), 567–570. doi:10.1093/geronb/gbr034

Lkhagvasuren, B., Nakamura, Y., Oka, T., Sudo, N., & Nakamura, K. (2011). Social defeat stress induces hyperthermia through activation of thermoregulatory sympathetic premotor neurons in the medullary raphe region. *European Journal of Neuroscience, 34*(9), 1442–1452. doi:10.1111/j.1460-9568.2011.07863.x

Lowry, C. A., Lightman, S. L., & Nutt, D. J. (2009). That warm fuzzy feeling: Brain serotonergic neurons and the regulation of emotion. *Journal of Psychopharmacology, 23*(4), 392–400. doi:10.1177/0269881 108099956

Maier, S. F., & Watkins, L. R. (2005). Stressor controllability and learned helplessness: The roles of the dorsal raphe nucleus, serotonin, and corticotropin-releasing factor. *Neuroscience and Biobehavioral Reviews*, *29*(4–5), 829–841. doi:10.1016/j.neubiorev.2005.03.021

Marcheva, B., Ramsey, K. M., Buhr, E. D., Kobayashi, Y., Su, H., Ko, C. H., . . . Bass, J. (2010). Disruption of the clock components CLOCK and BMAL1 leads to hypoinsulinaemia and diabetes. *Nature*, *466*(7306), 627–631. doi:10.1038/nature09253

Mata, J., Thompson, R. J., Jaeggi, S. M., Buschkuehl, M., Jonides, J., & Gotlib, I. H. (2011). Walk on the bright side: Physical activity and affect in major depressive disorder. *Journal of Abnormal Psychology*. doi:10.1037/a0023533

McClung, C. A. (2007). Circadian genes, rhythms and the biology of mood disorders. *Pharmacology & Therapeutics*, *114*(2), 222–232. doi:10.1016/j.pharmthera.2007.02.003

Meerlo, P., Sgoifo, A., & Turek, F. W. (2002). The effects of social defeat and other stressors on the expression of circadian rhythms. *Stress*, *5*(1), 15–22. doi:10.1080/102538902900012323

Mehnert, A., Veers, S., Howaldt, D., Braumann, K. M., Koch, U., & Schulz, K. H. (2011). Effects of a physical exercise rehabilitation group program on anxiety, depression, body image, and health-related quality of life among breast cancer patients. *Onkologie*, *34*(5), 248–253. doi:10.1159/000327813

Mendoza, J. (2007). Circadian clocks: Setting time by food. *Journal of Neuroendocrinology*, *19*(2), 127–137. doi:10.1111/j.1365-2826.2006.01510.x

Moraska, A., Deak, T., Spencer, R. L., Roth, D., & Fleshner, M. (2000). Treadmill running produces both positive and negative physiological adaptations in Sprague-Dawley rats. *American Journal of Physiolology Regulatory, Integrative, and Comparative Physiology*, *279*(4), R1321–R1329.

Moraska, A., & Fleshner, M. (2001). Voluntary physical activity prevents stress-induced behavioral depression and anti-KLH antibody suppression. *American Journal of Physiolology Regulatory, Integrative, and Comparative Physiology*, *281*(2), R484–R489.

Morin, L. P., & Allen, C. N. (2006). The circadian visual system, 2005. *Brain Research Reviews*, *51*(1), 1–60. doi:10.1016/j.brainresrev.2005.08.003

Mosca, L., Benjamin, E. J., Berra, K., Bezanson, J. L., Dolor, R. J., Lloyd-Jones, D. M., . . . Wenger, N. K. (2011). Effectiveness-based guidelines for the prevention of cardiovascular disease in women—2011 update: A guideline from the American Heart Association. *Journal of the American College of Cardiology*, *57*(12), 1404–1423. doi:10.1016/j.jacc.2011.02.005

Nestler, E. J., & Carlezon, W. A., Jr. (2006). The mesolimbic dopamine reward circuit in depression. *Biological Psychiatry*, *59*(12), 1151–1159. doi:10.1016/j.biopsych.2005.09.018

Oka, T., Oka, K., & Hori, T. (2001). Mechanisms and mediators of psychological stress-induced rise in core temperature. *Psychosomatic Medicine*, *63*(3), 476–486.

Okamura, H., Doi, M., Yamaguchi, Y., & Fustin, J. M. (2011). Hypertension due to loss of clock: Novel insight from the molecular analysis of Cry1/Cry2-deleted mice. *Current Hypertension Reports*, *13*(2), 103–108. doi:10.1007/s11906-011-0181-3

Packer, N., Hoffman-Goetz, L., & Ward, G. (2010). Does physical activity affect quality of life, disease symptoms and immune measures in patients with inflammatory bowel disease? A systematic review. *Journal of Sports Medicine and Physical Fitness*, *50*(1), 1–18.

Pezze, M. A., & Feldon, J. (2004). Mesolimbic dopaminergic pathways in fear conditioning. *Progress in Neurobiology*, *74*(5), 301–320. doi:10.1016/j.pneurobio.2004.09.004

Pickard, G. E. (1985). Bifurcating axons of retinal ganglion cells terminate in the hypothalamic suprachiasmatic nucleus and the intergeniculate leaflet of the thalamus. *Neuroscience Letters*, *55*(2), 211–217.

Portaluppi, F., Tiseo, R., Smolensky, M. H., Hermida, R. C., Ayala, D. E., & Fabbian, F. (2012). Circadian rhythms and cardiovascular health. *Sleep Medicine Reviews*, *16*(2), 151–166. doi:10.1016/j.smrv.2011. 04.003

Rozeske, R. R., Evans, A. K., Frank, M. G., Watkins, L. R., Lowry, C. A., & Maier, S. F. (2011). Uncontrollable, but not controllable, stress desensitizes 5-HT1A receptors in the dorsal raphe nucleus. *Journal of Neuroscience*, *31*(40), 14107–14115. doi:10.1523/JNEUROSCI.3095-11.2011

Segall, L. A., Perrin, J. S., Walker, C. D., Stewart, J., & Amir, S. (2006). Glucocorticoid rhythms control the rhythm of expression of the clock protein, Period2, in oval nucleus of the bed nucleus of the stria terminalis and central nucleus of the amygdala in rats. *Neuroscience*, *140*(3), 753–757. doi:10.1016/j.neuroscience.2006.03.037

Sgoifo, A., Pozzato, C., Meerlo, P., Costoli, T., Manghi, M., Stilli, D., . . . Musso, E. (2002). Intermittent exposure to social defeat and open-field test in rats: Acute and long-term effects on ECG, body temperature and physical activity. *Stress*, *5*(1), 23–35. doi:10.1080/102538902900012387

Soderman, E., Lisspers, J., & Sundin, O. (2007). Impact of depressive mood on lifestyle changes in patients with coronary artery disease. *Journal of Rehabilitation Medicine*, *39*(5), 412–417. doi:10.2340/16501977-0064

Solberg, L. C., Horton, T. H., and Turek, F. W. (1999). Circadian rhythms and depression: Effect of exercise in an animal model. *American Journal of Physiology*, *276*, R152–R161.

Takeda, N., & Maemura, K. (2011). Circadian clock and cardiovascular disease. *Journal of Cardiology*, *57*(3), 249–256. doi:10.1016/j.jjcc.2011.02.006

Talalaenko, A. N., Abramets, I. A., Stakhovskii Yu, V., Shekhovtsov, A. A., Chernikov, A. V., & Shevchenko, S. L. (1994). The role of dopaminergic mechanisms on the brain in various models of anxious states. *Neuroscience and Behavioral Physiology*, *24*(3), 284–288.

Thompson, R. S., Strong, P. V., & Fleshner, M. (2012). Physiological consequences of repeated exposures to conditioned fear. *Behavioral Sciences*, *2*(2), 57–78. doi: 10.3390/bs2020057

Ushijima, K., Morikawa, T., To, H., Higuchi, S., & Ohdo, S. (2006). Chronobiological disturbances with hyperthermia and hypercortisolism induced by chronic mild stress in rats.. *Behavioural Brain Research*, *173*(2), 326–330. doi:10.1016/j.bbr.2006.06.038

Williams, E. B. (Ed.) (1979). *The Scribner-Bantam English dictionary* (revised Bantam edition). New York: Bantam Books.

Yadid, G., & Friedman, A. (2008). Dynamics of the dopaminergic system as a key component to the understanding of depression. *Progress in Brain Research*, *172*, 265–286. doi:10.1016/S0079-6123(08)00913-8

Zambon, A. C., McDearmon, E. L., Salomonis, N., Vranizan, K. M., Johansen, K. L., Adey, D., . . . Conklin, B. R. (2003). Time- and exercise-dependent gene regulation in human skeletal muscle. *Genome Biology*, *4*(10), R61. doi:10.1186/gb-2003-4-10-r61

22

PHYSICAL ACTIVITY AND STRESS

Peripheral physiological adaptations

Jacqueline L. Beaudry, Anna D'souza, and Michael C. Riddell

Stress constitutes a sophisticated physiological response coordinated by the activation of the hypothalamic pituitary adrenal (HPA) axis and sympathetic nervous system (SNS). These primary mediators of the stress response act on peripheral tissues (liver, muscle, and adipose tissue) to mobilize energy stores and prepare the body for a "fight or flight" action. In today's society, stressors are more likely to be psychological than physical in nature, and are comprised of a variety of adverse forces including emotional, social, or professional. Psychological stress is viewed as a prolonged or chronic type of stress as the origin and termination of the stressor is most likely unclear. On the other hand, physical activity, a stressor in and of itself, provides beneficial adaptations rather than deleterious effects to the body in animals (Campbell et al., 2010) and in humans (Luger et al., 1987). Activation of both the HPA axis and SNS has profound effects on metabolism, cardiovascular function, immune function, and reproduction. Chronic stress is associated with a number of metabolic disturbances including heart disease, insulin resistance, and central obesity (De Kloet, Vreugdenhil, Oitzl, & Joels, 1998; Habib, Gold, & Chrousos, 2001; Miller & O'Callaghan, 2002; Seckl, Morton, Chapman, & Walker, 2004). In contrast, physical activity also increases mobilization of energy but reverses undesirable metabolic effects associated with chronic stress (Schmidt, Wijga, Von Zur Muhlen, Brabant, & Wagner, 1997). This chapter will highlight the dynamic physiological adaptations that occur in peripheral tissues in response to both physical activity and chronic psychological stress.

Glucocorticoid activation during stress

Central stress response: activation of the HPA axis and SNS

The stress response first begins by recognition of a threat and excitatory signals stimulate the parvocellular neurons of the paraventricular nucleus (PVN) of the hypothalamus to secrete corticotrophin releasing hormone (CRH) and arginine vasopressin (AVP) into hypophyseal portal circulation. In brief, both CRH and AVP travel to the anterior pituitary to secrete adrenocorticotrophic hormone (ACTH) and its precursor proopiomelancortin (POMC) (Tsigos & Chrousos, 2002). AVP is secreted along with CRH as it functions to exaggerate the stimulatory effect of CRH and binds to similar receptors on the pituitary to facilitate the entry of calcium into the cells. However, alone AVP does not affect ACTH levels as it does not induce POMC transcription (Antoni, 1993). ACTH, released from the pituitary gland, binds to the melanocortin 2 receptors localized within the zona fasciculate of the adrenal cortex (Gallo-Payet, Cote, Chorvatova, Guillon, & Payet, 1999). This process is critical as it stimulates the release of glucocorticoids (GCs) into circulation from the adrenal in the active form of either cortisol or corticosterone in humans or rodents, respectively. Secretion of GCs occurs in response to stressful stimuli and as a result of a regular diurnal pattern of release. GCs that are released in the systemic circulation bind to GC receptors (GRs), which are ubiquitously expressed throughout the body and brain.

Overexposure of stress hormones in the tissues is prevented by a negative feedback system in which GCs bind to their respective receptors in the hypothalamus and anterior pituitary to decrease HPA activation and GC production (Reul & de Kloet, 1985). As lipid-soluble hormones, GCs are capable of freely diffusing through the blood–brain barrier to bind to mineralocorticoid receptors (MRs) or GRs located in the hippocampus, anterior pituitary, or PVN of the hypothalamus. In the hippocampus, GCs have a 10-fold higher binding affinity for MRs in the brain, thus at lower concentrations GCs primarily bind to MRs (Yao & Denver, 2007). Therefore, MRs are involved in the maintenance of basal HPA activity, while GRs are responsible for shutting off HPA activity when GCs increase (i.e., during the peak of the diurnal rhythm or during a stress response). The negative feedback effects of GCs are exerted directly on the anterior pituitary to inhibit the synthesis and secretion of ACTH and centrally to block CRH production. Activation of the PVN neurons occurs in combination with the central catecholaminergic neurons in the brainstem. Both the HPA axis and SNS work together to coordinate a stress response that is initiated in the CNS but is concluded in peripheral target tissues.

Peripheral stress response: activation of GR and 11βHSD1

The peripheral actions of GCs are mediated primarily via their binding to their receptor, although non–receptor–mediated, non–genomic actions have recently been described. As such, the tissue-specific response is determined by the concentration of hormone, the expression and activity of the enzymes responsible for pre-receptor metabolism, and the density of GR (Seckl et al., 2004). GCs are known for their transcriptional control and are capable of up-regulating or inhibiting transcription of hundreds of diverse genes (Revollo & Cidlowski, 2009).

GC action in peripheral tissues is further regulated by the pre-receptor enzyme activity of 11 β hydroxysteroid dehyodrogenase (11βHSD). These intracellular NADPH-dependent enzymes regulate pre-receptor metabolism of GCs (Albiston, Obeyesekere, Smith, & Krozowski, 1994). They exist in two isoforms: 11βHSD1 and 11βHSD2. The predominant isoform outside of the kidney, 11βHSD1, is distributed in adipose, liver, and muscle tissue and is involved in the inter-conversion of inert GCs (e.g., cortisone) into their active form (e.g., cortisol), thus enabling increased GC action. 11βHSD1 activity/expression can amplify levels of active GCs by 10- to 15-fold over that found in plasma, thereby potentially contributing to a host of deleterious metabolic consequences (Masuzaki et al., 2001).

Types of stress

The term "stressor" may be considered any threat to homeostasis. This may be difficult to define any further since the perception of stress differs from organism to organism. In rodent models, stress research incorporates a number of modalities including exercise, physical restraint, electric shock, near drowning, exposure to cold, and an introduction of a socially dominant member of the same species (Rosmond, 2005). In humans, the definition of a stressor becomes even more complex and may include adversity endured in a number of social and emotional situations and remains difficult to simulate within the laboratory setting. In a laboratory or clinical setting, a stress response in humans is often provoked by manipulation of the environment (cold temperature), perceived uncontrollability, and through a social-evaluative threat typically referred to as the Trier Social Stress Test. This test may be the most useful and appropriate standardized protocol for studies of stress hormone reactivity as the test combines a social component of a psychological stress where task performance could be negatively judged by others and uncontrollability of the immediate situation (Birkett, 2011).

Chronic stress

A tight regulation of GC release via the circadian rhythm and negative feedback of the HPA axis is required to protect against the deleterious effects of chronically elevated GC levels. These deleterious effects are highlighted in spontaneous conditions of excess GC production, as occurs in Cushing's syndrome, in which patients experience central adiposity, impaired glucose tolerance, and attenuated muscle mass. Similarly, individuals with type 2 diabetes mellitus (T2DM) or insulin resistance and cardiometabolic disease often have elevated basal plasma GC levels, suggesting a link between altered GC concentrations and development of metabolic disease (Andrews & Walker, 1999). Altered GC release may also occur in response to chronic psychological stress that includes emotional, social, or professional stress, which can negatively impact the rhythmic release of GCs.

Tissue actions of glucocorticoids

Whole body metabolism

GCs facilitate the delivery of substrates to specific tissues (e.g., muscle, heart), ideally in situations of increased metabolic rate. Within adipose tissue, elevations in GCs are associated with increased lipolysis, liberating free fatty acids into circulation where they may be taken up and oxidized by other tissues, although the acute lipolytic effect of GCs on adipose tissue has recently been challenged (Peckett, Wright, & Riddell, 2011). Evidence is emerging that the hormone may actually inhibit lipolysis through non-genomic mechanisms (Campbell, Peckett, D'souza, Hawke, & Riddell, 2011), although further clarification is needed. In the liver, GCs drive the increase in glucose production from non-glucose substrates (i.e., gluconeogenesis), by escalating the expression of the rate-limiting enzymes phosphoenopyruvate carboxykinase (PEPCK) and glucose 6 phosphatase (G6Pase). Other sources of non-glucose substrates may be derived from other tissues including skeletal muscle, in which GCs promote liberation of amino acids. The negative consequences of elevated GCs are demonstrated in transgenic mice with 11βHSD1 adipocyte over-expression, which causes hyperglycemia, insulin resistance, dyslipidemia, and hypertension (Masuzaki et al., 2001; Rask et al., 2001). 11βHSD1 knockout mice have much healthier fat partitioning, which helps to protect against the development of the metabolic syndrome (Wamil et al., 2011).

Visceral adiposity

Numerous epidemiological studies have linked elevated stress levels with the development of cardiac and metabolic conditions, which may be driven by the potent adipogenic effects of these hormones, particularly in central adipose depots (Bjorntorp, 2001). GCs regulate adipose tissue differentiation and distribution, and in excess clearly induce visceral obesity (Peckett et al., 2011; van Raalte, Ouwens, & Diamant, 2009). The location of excess adiposity is extremely important as visceral adiposity is particularly associated with development of insulin resistance, T2DM, and other metabolic conditions (Kahn, Hull, & Utzschneider, 2006). Clinical studies have demonstrated a positive correlation between hypercortisolemia, as seen in Cushing's syndrome patients, and visceral fat accumulation (Chandola, Brunner, & Marmot, 2006). The mechanism behind this increased central adiposity is believed to be due to the elevated concentration of GR and 11βHSD1 in adipose depots, indicating increased sensitivity to GC action. Moreover, in male Sprague-Dawley rats elevated exogenous GC treatment (400mg corticosterone pellets for 14 days) (Shpilberg et al., 2012) significantly increased mRNA expressions of 11βHSD1 and GR compared to placebo animals (those administered wax pellets) in both epididymal and subcutaneous adipose depots. As well, GC treated animals had significantly more epididymal fat depots representing visceral adiposity than placebo animals. These findings suggest that a high level of GCs, perhaps indicative of chronic stress, promotes increases in GR and 11βHSD1 expression that lead to increased adipogenesis rather than elevated lipolysis, at least in the central adipose depots. Moreover, in the presence of insulin, cortisol has a greater stimulatory effect on lipoprotein lipase activity, which hydrolyzes triglycerides from the lipid droplet in human adipose tissue *in vitro*, resulting in increased lipolysis of adipose tissue. It is likely due to the elevated insulin levels as well as other factors associated with obesity that contribute to the accumulation of visceral adiposity (Peckett et al., 2011). However, these mechanisms still remain unclear and further investigations are required.

Insulin sensitivity

T2DM is caused by a combination of insulin deficiency and insulin resistance. GCs and catecholamines (also released from the adrenals) are known to oppose the effects of insulin. Elevated cortisol secretion or a decrease in diurnal variability is associated with glucose intolerance and insulin resistance (Buren & Eriksson, 2005). GCs *in vivo* appear to impair insulin-dependent glucose uptake in peripheral tissues (Shpilberg et al., 2012) and stimulate gluconeogenesis in the liver (D'souza et al., 2012; Rizza, Mandarino, & Gerich, 1982). In skeletal muscle, GCs decrease GLUT4 translocation and inhibit glycogen synthesis, thus increasing glucose availability for the brain (Dimitriadis et al., 1997; Nielsen et al., 2004).

Elevated GC levels are a hallmark feature of experimental models of diabetes (Chan, Inouye, Riddell, Vranic, & Matthews, 2003). Zucker Diabetic Fatty (ZDF) rats gradually develop hypercortisolemia after 5 weeks of age as well as hyperinsulinemia (Campbell et al., 2010). These elevated GC levels may also mediate the observed hyperglycemia that occurs in this and other models of obesity/T2DM (Shimomura, Bray, & Lee, 1987). Moreover, clinical studies have also provided compelling evidence of a relationship between chronic stress or elevated GC levels and impaired glucose tolerance (Hoes et al., 2011; van Raalte et al., 2010; van Raalte et al., 2011).

Physical inactivity: the exercise-deficient phenotype

Currently, there is considerable research available that draws the association between sedentary individuals and the prevalence of "cardiometabolic-based diseases" (LaMonte & Blair, 2006). Unfortunately, increasing psychological stress is associated with a decline in physical activity – a behavior that protects against disease (Geulayov, Goral, Muhsen, Lipsitz, & Gross, 2010).

Adaptive effects of exercise

Exercise as a "stressor"

In the general sense, a "stress" implies a disturbance to the "normal" physiological equilibrium, and thus is often associated with a negative connotation. However, not all "stressors" have adverse effects. Physical activity and exercise have the capacity to disturb the normal homeostasis, and can be considered a "stressor" by definition (Hackney, 2006; Steadman & Sharkey, 1969). Exercise in this context is considered to be a period of purposeful physical activity in which the metabolic rate significantly rises above rest for a period of time. Exercise can be acute (30 minutes of brisk walking at a significantly elevated heart rate) or chronic (e.g., several weeks of an exercise training program). Selye (1976) was the first to acknowledge the systemic effects of physical exercise as being different from those produced by other stress stimuli – he termed exercise a "eustressor." These differences are related to the fact that training, or repeated bouts of the same exercise, results in an attenuated HPA axis response. However, it should be noted that the type and duration of training are critical determinants of whether or not there is an attenuated stress response (Garcia, Mari, Valles, Dal-Zotto, & Armario, 2000).

Forms of exercise stress

Exercise training and the adaptations to the initial stress of exercise are unique compared to chronic psychological stress in that exercise promotes an adaptive response that reduces the stress response over time. Resting or basal levels of GCs have been found to rise initially but eventually return to pre-training levels during the course of exercise training, at least in rodents (Coutinho, Campbell, Fediuc, & Riddell, 2006; Park et al., 2005). Paradoxically, non-exercise forms of acute stress may also be advantageous to the body as well. Exposure to intermittent restraint stress or swimming stress in a rodent model of T2DM (ZDF rats) delayed development of hyperglycemia due to adaptation of feedback sensitivity of the HPA axis and adaptation to pancreatic β-cells (Bates et al., 2007; Bates, Sirek, Kiraly, Yue, Goche Montes et al., 2008; Bates, Sirek, Kiraly, Yue, Riddell, et al., 2008). ZDF rats that were subjected to intermittent stress (restraint) had lower baseline GC levels as well as higher insulin levels and better glucose control. Moreover, other forms of strenuous stress such as forced swimming have been investigated on diabetes development. Kiraly et al. (2007) examined male ZDF rats after a series of non-volitional exercise bouts and showed improved glycemic control compared to sedentary controls in just 5 weeks of daily forced swimming exercise.

Benefits of exercise – peripheral adaptations

The central stress response can cause debilitating effects to the brain that can induce hippocampal remodeling, suppression of gonadal and growth hormones, as well as lead to other comorbidities such as hypertension, cardiovascular disease, and diabetes. On the other hand, regular exercise alters tissue sensitivity to stress not only through the central system but through peripheral tissue adaptations such as the adrenal glands, adipose, and skeletal muscle (Campbell, Fediuc, Hawke, & Riddell, 2009). These benefits include improvements in metabolic function, insulin sensitivity, and increasing fuel supplies for oxidation rather than for storage. Therefore, it is now well established that in the presence of chronic social stress, regular exercise is imperative (Tsatsoulis & Fountoulakis, 2006).

Glucocorticoid sensitivity

Adaptations in GC sensitivity as a result of exercise training are tissue specific and are largely due to altered expression of GR and 11βHSD1. For example, endurance swim training in rodents results in decreases in hepatic and thymus GR content (Peijie, Zicai, Haowen, & Renbao, 2004). This lowering of GR content has also been demonstrated in rodent muscle and liver following 4 weeks of voluntary wheel running in hamsters (Coutinho et al., 2006). Normal sedentary males who undergo 6 weeks of training experienced reduced basal cortisol levels, significant reductions in mRNA levels of GR, and reduced pro-inflammatory cytokine expression including NFKB1 and IkB kinase A levels (Sousa e Silva et al., 2010). Another study demonstrated that exercise training led to a decrease in GR in human peripheral blood cells and cultured monocytes of trained male adult athletes (Peijie et al., 2004). This down-regulation of monocyte GC sensitivity suggests an adaptation of the HPA axis to repeated, prolonged exercise that induces increases in GC secretion to protect the body from detrimental effects of chronic stress (Duclos, Gouarne, & Bonnemaison, 2003). Even low-grade exercise in obese youth (ages 9–15) has been shown to induce reductions in GC sensitivity after 3 months (Faria et al., 2010).

Skeletal muscle

Evidence shows that exercise training improves glucose transport via an insulin-independent mechanism within skeletal muscle. Training results in a rapid increase in the expression of GLUT4 content translocation to the plasma membrane in skeletal muscle (Kraniou, Cameron-Smith, & Hargreaves, 2006). Other mechanisms of improved skeletal muscle insulin sensitivity may include modulations to peripheral GC action. Following 4 weeks of voluntary wheel running, rodents had decreased GR and 11βHSD1 content in skeletal muscle, which would be expected to improve insulin sensitivity (Coutinho et al., 2006). At the very least, regular exercise should help offset the insulin resistance in skeletal muscle caused by elevated GCs, although surprisingly few studies have investigated this in human or animal models of Cushing's Syndrome.

Visceral adiposity and body composition

Voluntary wheel running in rodents promotes a reduction in body weight and improves body composition (Narath, Skalicky, & Viidik, 2001). In contrast to what is observed in liver and muscle tissue, GR and 11βHSD1 content in adipose tissue increase in animals undergoing voluntary training (Campbell, Rakhshani, Fediuc, Bruni, & Riddell, 2009). This increase in GC activity and content is believed to facilitate increased lipolysis when insulin levels are low, but may set the stage for adiposity rebound if the animal stops exercising and insulin levels rise. These findings suggest that GC-mediated central obesity is avoided with training because training lowers circulating insulin levels and increases adipose tissue lipase activity (Campbell et al., 2010). A summary of the abovementioned peripheral adaptations to GC secretion and exercise training can be found in Figure 22.1.

Exercise type influences adaptations to GC sensitivity

Changes to GC sensitivity occur after a single bout of exercise and are tissue specific. For example, GR expression in peripheral blood cells is down-regulated in response to a single bout of exercise (Smits, Grunberg, Derijk, Sterk, & Hiemstra, 1998) while GR expression paradoxically increases in muscle following a single exercise bout of strenuous eccentric exercise (Willoughby, Taylor,

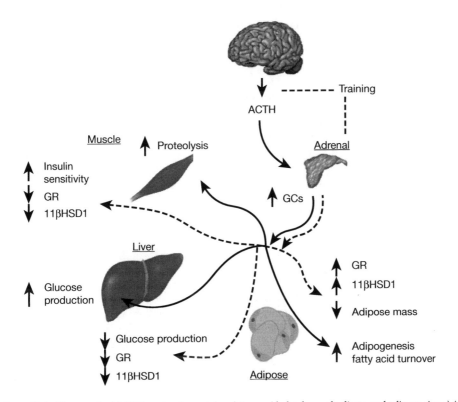

Figure 22.1 Glucocorticoid (GC) action in peripheral tissues (skeletal muscle, liver, and adipose tissue) in the presence and absence of exercise training. Perceived stress activates ACTH release from the pituitary gland in the brain, which stimulates GC release from the adrenal gland. Solid black lines indicate GCs actions. Dashed lines indicate inhibitory actions of training. GCs stimulate adipogenesis and increased fatty acid turnover in the adipose tissue. In the liver, GCs increase glucose production through mechanisms of gluconeogenesis and glycogenolysis. In skeletal muscle, GCs up-regulate proteolysis. In the presence of exercise training, the brain adapts to exercise as a stress and decreases ACTH release into circulation. This lowers GC release from the adrenal gland and contributes to reduced amounts of GC in the plasma. Dashed line indicates GC action as a result of exercise training in peripheral tissues. Overall, regular exercise lowers basal (resting) GC levels in the circulation. With regular exercise, GR and 11βHSD1 mRNA expression may be decreased in skeletal muscle and liver, while expression in adipose tissue increases. Adipose mass decreases and insulin sensitivity increases in liver and muscle. The functional significance of increased GC exposure in adipose tissue with training, via increased GR and 11βHSD1 expression, is unclear but may help to promote lipolysis and adiposity rebound if regular exercise ceases.

& Taylor, 2003). Elevations in GC levels typically return to normal within 24 hours after a single bout of exercise (Duclos, Corcuff, Rashedi, Fougere, & Manier, 1997). However, men undergoing a single bout of rowing exercise have a decrease in peripheral blood lymphocyte GC sensitivity and GC–induced cytokine (IL–6, TNF–alpha) release (DeRijk, Petrides, Deuster, Gold, & Sternberg, 1996; Smits et al., 1998). These findings demonstrate that even acute physical activity has the potential to temporarily alter the sensitivity to stress hormones in peripheral tissues.

A number of animal studies have demonstrated that basal (i.e., resting, unstimulated) GCs are lowered with regular exercise, after a period of brief elevation. In one study, obese ZDF rats that were exercise trained 5 days per week for 14 weeks demonstrated lower basal GC levels after exercise training (Martin-Cordero, Garcia, Hinchado, & Ortega, 2011). However, after a single bout of exercise, the obese ZDF animals had higher GC levels than untrained animals in the post-exercise period. These data suggest exercise training adapts to chronic stimulation of the HPA axis; however, a single bout of exercise still can promote increases in GC levels, perhaps to increase fuel utilization and recovery.

Research methodology: issues worth considering

Challenges in the investigation of the physiological adaptations that occur with exercise and stress include the variability of the stressors used, difficulty in quantifying the stress response, and a lack of uniformity in techniques employed to assess the stress response. Physical activity involves a number of variables that regulate the amount of energy expenditure or rate of energy expenditure that occurs, including the type, intensity, regularity, and duration of the activity. In addition to the variability in the types of activity performed are the ways in which stress is quantified to reflect adaptations by the stress system.

Models of exercise

Animal models of exercise are commonly used to study the stress response to exercise as these experimental designs provide a controlled dose and timing of exercise, but at a cost. Forced exercise models are considered a form of anticipatory stress because they elicit a physiological and psychological response (e.g., anxiety) (Pacak & Palkovits, 2001). Animal models employ the use of foot shock and cold water stimulus, and despite providing beneficial effects to metabolism by increasing mitochondrial capacity and reducing weight gain, they also result in adverse effects, including adrenal hypertrophy and suppressed immune function, which make them difficult to relate to human models of exercise (Moraska, Deak, Spencer, Roth, & Fleshner, 2000). Also, these forms of exercise are typically employed during daylight hours—the normal sleep period for rodents. Alternatively, the use of voluntary wheel running in rodent models of stress and exercise is regarded as the most "natural" model of exercise training, as it generates a stress response similar to human exercise (Stranahan, Lee, & Mattson, 2008). However, voluntary exercise is not without its own limitations. Of primary concern is the inability to regulate exercise quantity, quality, timing, and intensity among individual animals. For example, young hamsters may run 17–20 kilometers per night, while rats typically will run between 2 and 15 kilometers. Similarly, the age of rodents used may also influence the exercise outcome. Older C57BL/6J mice (19–22 months) experienced a decline in the number of wheel revolutions per day and decrease in activity duration in comparison to adult (6–9 months) mice (Valentinuzzi, Scarbrough, Takahashi, & Turek, 1997). These studies demonstrate the variability of exercise response that occurs as a result of the strain and age of animals, and suggest that a more streamlined methodology should be employed to allow for an easier comparison between exercise studies examining the stress response.

Measuring the peripheral response

Methods employed to assess the peripheral stress response usually involve quantification of hormone levels released during the stressor/exercise. These methods range from salivary, urine, fecal material and/or plasma samples for cortisol, corticosterone, or their metabolites. The testing of hormones from saliva offers a non-invasive, stress-free alternative to serum that is commonly employed in human studies of stress and exercise. Measurements of cortisol in saliva are a useful tool to analyze stress response; however, the concentrations in the saliva differ from those in serum as salivary glands have the capacity to metabolize steroids into their inactive forms (Shimojo et al., 1997). The uniformity with which salivary hormone samples are collected must also be taken into consideration as confounders including type of exercise, time of day, and method of collecting sample can all influence hormone values (Gatti & De Palo, 2011). Similarly, cortisol sampling via urine collection has a wide variation in the response to stress. As recently reported, a case study in healthy women for 65 days in 12-hour intervals provided evidence that the appearance of cortisol in the urine was extremely dependent on the perceived stress that was either categorized as positive or negative, as well as the emotional level of the stressful event (Schubert et al., 2012).

Future directions

The field of stress physiology has grown tremendously since Dr. Selye first acknowledged the stress response in the late 1930s. However, there still remains a great deal of refinement of techniques and additional information that is required to better understand the peripheral physiological adaptations to stress and exercise. Topics requiring further research include (a) examining the intermediate to long-term benefits of exercise on the stress system by conducting extended term follow up studies; (b) utilizing both animal and human models of various ages of development and use of disease models to determine the influence of stress adaptations that occur with exercise; (c) characterizing features of physical activity to distinguish between the effects of voluntary and involuntary exercise, intensity, duration, and frequency on the peripheral stress system; and (d) streamlining physiological measures, which will help determine the appropriate method of stress hormone measurement (salivary GCs, plasma GCs) that provides the most accurate reflection of the stress response and ensure little technical variability in data collection.

Conclusion

It has long been established that exercise has a positive influence on energy balance and other aspects of fitness. However, additional benefits to exercise exist with respect to its influence on stress hormone levels, behavior, mood, and immune function. The study of the physiological adaptations that occur with regular physical activity is important to determine how it can be utilized to mitigate the effects of chronic stress. The mechanisms behind these protective and adaptive effects are multiple and tissue specific. Understanding the integrative response of the stress system to physical activity will lead to valuable clues about the potential benefits of exercise in protecting against development of chronic diseases including obesity, diabetes, and cardiovascular disease.

References

Albiston, A. L., Obeyesekere, V. R., Smith, R. E., & Krozowski, Z. S. (1994). Cloning and tissue distribution of the human 11 beta-hydroxysteroid dehydrogenase type 2 enzyme. *Molecular and Cellular Endocrinology*, *105*(2), R11–R17.

Andrews, R. C., & Walker, B. R. (1999). Glucocorticoids and insulin resistance: Old hormones, new targets. *Clinical Science (London, England: 1979)*, *96*(5), 513–523.

Antoni, F. A. (1993). Vasopressinergic control of pituitary adrenocorticotropin secretion comes of age. *Frontiers in Neuroendocrinology*, *14*(2), 76–122. doi:10.1006/frne.1993.1004

Bates, H. E., Kiraly, M. A., Yue, J. T., Goche Montes, D., Elliott, M. E., Riddell, M. C., et al. (2007). Recurrent intermittent restraint delays fed and fasting hyperglycemia and improves glucose return to baseline levels during glucose tolerance tests in the Zucker diabetic fatty rat—Role of food intake and corticosterone. *Metabolism: Clinical and Experimental*, *56*(8), 1065–1075. doi:10.1016/j.metabol. 2007.03.015

Bates, H. E., Sirek, A. S., Kiraly, M. A., Yue, J. T., Goche Montes, D., Matthews, S. G., et al. (2008). Adaptation to mild, intermittent stress delays development of hyperglycemia in the Zucker diabetic fatty rat independent of food intake: Role of habituation of the hypothalamic-pituitary-adrenal axis. *Endocrinology, 149*(6), 2990–3001. doi:10.1210/en.2007-1473

Bates, H. E., Sirek, A., Kiraly, M. A., Yue, J. T., Riddell, M. C., Matthews, S. G., et al. (2008). Adaptation to intermittent stress promotes maintenance of beta-cell compensation: Comparison with food restriction. *American Journal of Physiology: Endocrinology and Metabolism, 295*(4), E947–58. doi:10.1152/ajpendo. 90378.2008

Birkett, M. A. (2011). The trier social stress test protocol for inducing psychological stress. *Journal of Visualized Experiments, (56)*. doi:10.3791/3238; 10.3791/3238

Bjorntorp, P. (2001). Do stress reactions cause abdominal obesity and comorbidities? *Obesity Reviews, 2*(2), 73–86.

Buren, J., & Eriksson, J. W. (2005). Is insulin resistance caused by defects in insulin's target cells or by a stressed mind? *Diabetes/Metabolism Research and Reviews, 21*(6), 487–494. doi:10.1002/dmrr.567

Campbell, J. E., Fediuc, S., Hawke, T. J., & Riddell, M. C. (2009). Endurance exercise training increases adipose tissue glucocorticoid exposure: Adaptations that facilitate lipolysis. *Metabolism: Clinical and Experimental, 58*(5), 651–660.

Campbell, J. E., Kiraly, M. A., Atkinson, D. J., D'souza, A. M., Vranic, M., & Riddell, M. C. (2010). Regular exercise prevents the development of hyperglucocorticoidemia via adaptations in the brain and adrenal glands in male Zucker diabetic fatty rats. *American Journal of Physiology: Regulatory, Integrative and Comparative Physiology, 299*(1), R168–R176.

Campbell, J. E., Peckett, A. J., D'souza, A. M., Hawke, T. J., & Riddell, M. C. (2011). Adipogenic and lipolytic effects of chronic glucocorticoid exposure. *American Journal of Physiology: Cell Physiology, 300*(1), C198–209. doi:10.1152/ajpcell.00045.2010

Campbell, J. E., Rakhshani, N., Fediuc, S., Bruni, S., & Riddell, M. C. (2009). Voluntary wheel running initially increases adrenal sensitivity to adrenocorticotrophic hormone, which is attenuated with long-term training. *Journal of Applied Physiology (Bethesda, MD: 1985), 106*(1), 66–72. doi:10.1152/japplphysiol.91128.2008

Chan, O., Inouye, K., Riddell, M. C., Vranic, M., & Matthews, S. G. (2003). Diabetes and the hypothalamo–pituitary–adrenal (HPA) axis. *Minerva Endocrinologica, 28*(2), 87–102.

Chandola, T., Brunner, E., & Marmot, M. (2006). Chronic stress at work and the metabolic syndrome: Prospective study. *BMJ (Clinical Research Ed.), 332*(7540), 521–525. doi:10.1136/bmj.38693.435301.80

Coutinho, A. E., Campbell, J. E., Fediuc, S., & Riddell, M. C. (2006). Effect of voluntary exercise on peripheral tissue glucocorticoid receptor content and the expression and activity of 11beta-HSD1 in the Syrian hamster. *Journal of Applied Physiology (Bethesda, MD: 1985), 100*(5), 1483–1488. doi:10.1152/japplphysiol.01236.2005

De Kloet, E. R., Vreugdenhil, E., Oitzl, M. S., & Joels, M. (1998). Brain corticosteroid receptor balance in health and disease. *Endocrine Reviews, 19*(3), 269–301.

DeRijk, R. H., Petrides, J., Deuster, P., Gold, P. W., & Sternberg, E. M. (1996). Changes in corticosteroid sensitivity of peripheral blood lymphocytes after strenuous exercise in humans. *Journal of Clinical Endocrinology and Metabolism, 81*(1), 228–235.

Dimitriadis, G., Leighton, B., Parry-Billings, M., Sasson, S., Young, M., Krause, U., et al. (1997). Effects of glucocorticoid excess on the sensitivity of glucose transport and metabolism to insulin in rat skeletal muscle. *Biochemical Journal, 321*(Pt 3), 707–712.

D'souza, A. M., Beaudry, J. L., Szigiato, A. A., Trumble, S. J., Snook, L. A., Bonen, A., et al. (2012). Consumption of a high fat diet rapidly exacerbates the development of fatty liver disease that occurs with chronically elevated glucocorticoids. *American Journal of Physiology: Gastrointestinal and Liver Physiology*, Jan 19. [Epub ahead of print] doi:10.1152/ajpgi.00378.2011

Duclos, M., Corcuff, J. B., Rashedi, M., Fougere, V., & Manier, G. (1997). Trained versus untrained men: Different immediate post-exercise responses of pituitary adrenal axis. A preliminary study. *European Journal of Applied Physiology and Occupational Physiology, 75*(4), 343–350.

Duclos, M., Gouarne, C., & Bonnemaison, D. (2003). Acute and chronic effects of exercise on tissue sensitivity to glucocorticoids. *Journal of Applied Physiology (Bethesda, MD: 1985), 94*(3), 869–875.

Faria, C. D., Castro, R. B., Longui, C. A., Kochi, C., Barbosa, V. L., Sousa E Silva, T., et al. (2010). Impact of prolonged low-grade physical training on the in vivo glucocorticoid sensitivity and on glucocorticoid receptor-alpha mRNA levels of obese adolescents. *Hormone Research in Paediatrics, 73*(6), 458–464. doi:10.1159/000313591

Gallo-Payet, N., Cote, M., Chorvatova, A., Guillon, G., & Payet, M. D. (1999). Cyclic AMP-independent effects of ACTH on glomerulosa cells of the rat adrenal cortex. *Journal of Steroid Biochemistry and Molecular Biology, 69*(1–6), 335–342.

Garcia, A., Marti, O., Valles, A., Dal-Zotto, S., & Armario, A. (2000). Recovery of the hypothalamic-pituitary-adrenal response to stress. Effect of stress intensity, stress duration and previous stress exposure. *Neuroendocrinology, 72*(2), 114–125.

Gatti, R., & De Palo, E. F. (2011). An update: Salivary hormones and physical exercise. *Scandinavian Journal of Medicine & Science in Sports, 21*(2), 157–169. doi:10.1111/j.1600-0838.2010.01252.x

Geulayov, G., Goral, A., Muhsen, K., Lipsitz, J., & Gross, R. (2010). Physical inactivity among adults with diabetes mellitus and depressive symptoms: Results from two independent national health surveys. *General Hospital Psychiatry, 32*(6), 570–576. doi:10.1016/j.genhosppsych.2010.09.004

Habib, K. E., Gold, P. W., & Chrousos, G. P. (2001). Neuroendocrinology of stress. *Endocrinology and Metabolism Clinics of North America, 30*(3), 695–728; vii–viii.

Hackney, A. C. (2006). Stress and the neuroendocrine system: The role of exercise as a stressor and modifier of stress. *Expert Review of Endocrinology & Metabolism, 1*(6), 783–792. doi:10.1586/17446651.1.6.783

Hoes, J. N., van der Goes, M. C., van Raalte, D. H., van der Zijl, N. J., den Uyl, D., Lems, W. F., et al. (2011). Glucose tolerance, insulin sensitivity and beta-cell function in patients with rheumatoid arthritis treated with or without low- to medium-dose glucocorticoids. *Annals of the Rheumatic Diseases, 70*(11), 1887–1894. doi:10.1136/ard.2011.151464

Kahn, S. E., Hull, R. L., & Utzschneider, K. M. (2006). Mechanisms linking obesity to insulin resistance and type 2 diabetes. *Nature, 444*(7121), 840–846. doi:10.1038/nature05482

Kiraly, M. A., Bates, H. E., Yue, J. T., Goche-Montes, D., Fediuc, S., Park, E., et al. (2007). Attenuation of type 2 diabetes mellitus in the male Zucker diabetic fatty rat: The effects of stress and non-volitional exercise. *Metabolism: Clinical and Experimental, 56*(6), 732–744. doi:10.1016/j.metabol.2006.12.022

Kraniou, G. N., Cameron-Smith, D., & Hargreaves, M. (2006). Acute exercise and GLUT4 expression in human skeletal muscle: Influence of exercise intensity. *Journal of Applied Physiology (Bethesda, MD: 1985), 101*(3), 934–937. doi:10.1152/japplphysiol.01489.2005

LaMonte, M. J., & Blair, S. N. (2006). Physical activity, cardiorespiratory fitness, and adiposity: Contributions to disease risk. *Current Opinion in Clinical Nutrition and Metabolic Care, 9*(5), 540–546. doi:10.1097/01.mco.0000241662.92642.08

Luger, A., Deuster, P. A., Kyle, S. B., Gallucci, W. T., Montgomery, L. C., Gold, P. W., et al. (1987). Acute hypothalamic-pituitary-adrenal responses to the stress of treadmill exercise. Physiologic adaptations to physical training. *New England Journal of Medicine, 316*(21), 1309–1315. doi:10.1056/NEJM198705213162105

Martin-Cordero, L., Garcia, J. J., Hinchado, M. D., & Ortega, E. (2011). The interleukin-6 and noradrenaline mediated inflammation-stress feedback mechanism is dysregulated in metabolic syndrome: Effect of exercise. *Cardiovascular Diabetology, 10*, 42. doi:10.1186/1475-2840-10-42

Masuzaki, H., Paterson, J., Shinyama, H., Morton, N. M., Mullins, J. J., Seckl, J. R., et al. (2001). A transgenic model of visceral obesity and the metabolic syndrome. *Science (New York, NY), 294*(5549), 2166–2170.

Miller, D. B., & O'Callaghan, J. P. (2002). Neuroendocrine aspects of the response to stress. *Metabolism: Clinical and Experimental, 51*(6 Suppl 1), 5–10.

Moraska, A., Deak, T., Spencer, R. L., Roth, D., & Fleshner, M. (2000). Treadmill running produces both positive and negative physiological adaptations in Sprague-Dawley rats. *American Journal of Physiology. Regulatory, Integrative and Comparative Physiology, 279*(4), R1321–R1329.

Narath, E., Skalicky, M., & Viidik, A. (2001). Voluntary and forced exercise influence the survival and body composition of ageing male rats differently. *Experimental Gerontology, 36*(10), 1699–1711.

Nielsen, M. F., Caumo, A., Chandramouli, V., Schumann, W. C., Cobelli, C., Landau, B. R., et al. (2004). Impaired basal glucose effectiveness but unaltered fasting glucose release and gluconeogenesis during short-term hypercortisolemia in healthy subjects. *American Journal of Physiology. Endocrinology and Metabolism, 286*(1), E102–E110.

Pacak, K., & Palkovits, M. (2001). Stressor specificity of central neuroendocrine responses: Implications for stress-related disorders. *Endocrine Reviews, 22*(4), 502–548.

Park, E., Chan, O., Li, Q., Kiraly, M., Matthews, S. G., Vranic, M., et al. (2005). Changes in basal hypothalamo-pituitary-adrenal activity during exercise training are centrally mediated. *American Journal of Physiology. Regulatory, Integrative and Comparative Physiology, 289*(5), R1360–R1371.

Peckett, A. J., Wright, D. C., & Riddell, M. C. (2011). The effects of glucocorticoids on adipose tissue lipid metabolism. *Metabolism: Clinical and Experimental, 60*(11), 1500–1510. doi:10.1016/j.metabol.2011.06.012

Peijie, C., Zicai, D., Haowen, X., & Renbao, X. (2004). Effects of chronic and acute training on glucocorticoid receptors concentrations in rats. *Life Sciences, 75*(11), 1303–1311.

Rask, E., Olsson, T., Soderberg, S., Andrew, R., Livingstone, D. E., Johnson, O., et al. (2001). Tissue-specific dysregulation of cortisol metabolism in human obesity. *Journal of Clinical Endocrinology and Metabolism, 86*(3), 1418–1421.

Reul, J. M., & de Kloet, E. R. (1985). Two receptor systems for corticosterone in rat brain: Microdistribution and differential occupation. *Endocrinology, 117*(6), 2505–2511.

Revollo, J. R., & Cidlowski, J. A. (2009). Mechanisms generating diversity in glucocorticoid receptor signaling. *Annals of the New York Academy of Sciences, 1179*, 167–178. doi:10.1111/j.1749-6632.2009. 04986.x

Rizza, R. A., Mandarino, L. J., & Gerich, J. E. (1982). Effects of growth hormone on insulin action in man. Mechanisms of insulin resistance, impaired suppression of glucose production, and impaired stimulation of glucose utilization. *Diabetes, 31*(8 Pt 1), 663–669.

Rosmond, R. (2005). Role of stress in the pathogenesis of the metabolic syndrome. *Psychoneuroendocrinology, 30*(1), 1–10.

Schmidt, T., Wijga, A., Von Zur Muhlen, A., Brabant, G., & Wagner, T. O. (1997). Changes in cardiovascular risk factors and hormones during a comprehensive residential three month kriya yoga training and vegetarian nutrition. *Acta Physiologica Scandinavica. Supplementum, 640*, 158–162.

Schubert, C., Geser, W., Noisternig, B., Fuchs, D., Welzenbach, N., Konig, P., et al. (2012). Stress system dynamics during "life as it is lived": An integrative single-case study on a healthy woman. *PloS One, 7*(3), e29415. doi:10.1371/journal.pone.0029415

Seckl, J. R., Morton, N. M., Chapman, K. E., & Walker, B. R. (2004). Glucocorticoids and 11beta-hydroxysteroid dehydrogenase in adipose tissue. *Recent Progress in Hormone Research, 59*, 359–393.

Selye, H. (1976). The stress concept. *Canadian Medical Association Journal, 115*(8), 718.

Shimojo, M., Ricketts, M. L., Petrelli, M. D., Moradi, P., Johnson, G. D., Bradwell, A. R., et al. (1997). Immunodetection of 11 beta-hydroxysteroid dehydrogenase type 2 in human mineralocorticoid target tissues: Evidence for nuclear localization. *Endocrinology, 138*(3), 1305–1311.

Shimomura, Y., Bray, G. A., & Lee, M. (1987). Adrenalectomy and steroid treatment in obese (ob/ob) and diabetic (db/db) mice. *Hormone and Metabolic Research, 19*(7), 295–299. doi:10.1055/s-2007-1011804

Shpilberg, Y., Beaudry, J. L., D'Souza, A., Campbell, J. E., Peckett, A., & Riddell, M. C. (2012). A rodent model of rapid-onset diabetes induced by glucocorticoids and high-fat feeding. *Disease Models & Mechanisms, 5*(5):671–680. doi:10.1242/dmm.008912

Smits, H. H., Grunberg, K., Derijk, R. H., Sterk, P. J., & Hiemstra, P. S. (1998). Cytokine release and its modulation by dexamethasone in whole blood following exercise. *Clinical and Experimental Immunology, 111*(2), 463–468.

Sousa e Silva, T., Longui, C. A., Rocha, M. N., Faria, C. D., Melo, M. R., Faria, T. G., et al. (2010). Prolonged physical training decreases mRNA levels of glucocorticoid receptor and inflammatory genes. *Hormone Research in Paediatrics, 74*(1), 6–14. doi:10.1159/000313586

Steadman, R. T., & Sharkey, B. J. (1969). Exercise as a stressor. *Journal of Sports Medicine and Physical Fitness, 9*(4), 230–235.

Stranahan, A. M., Lee, K., & Mattson, M. P. (2008). Central mechanisms of HPA axis regulation by voluntary exercise. *Neuromolecular Medicine, 10*(2), 118–127.

Tsatsoulis, A., & Fountoulakis, S. (2006). The protective role of exercise on stress system dysregulation and comorbidities. *Annals of the New York Academy of Sciences, 1083*, 196–213.

Tsigos, C., & Chrousos, G. P. (2002). Hypothalamic-pituitary-adrenal axis, neuroendocrine factors and stress. *Journal of Psychosomatic Research, 53*(4), 865–871.

Valentinuzzi, V. S., Scarbrough, K., Takahashi, J. S., & Turek, F. W. (1997). Effects of aging on the circadian rhythm of wheel-running activity in C57BL/6 mice. *American Journal of Physiology, 273*(6 Pt 2), R1957–R1964.

van Raalte, D. H., Brands, M., van der Zijl, N. J., Muskiet, M. H., Pouwels, P. J., Ackermans, M. T., et al. (2011). Low-dose glucocorticoid treatment affects multiple aspects of intermediary metabolism in healthy humans: A randomised controlled trial. *Diabetologia, 54*(8), 2103–2112. doi:10.1007/s00125-011-2174-9

van Raalte, D. H., Nofrate, V., Bunck, M. C., van Iersel, T., Elassaiss Schaap, J., Nassander, U. K., et al. (2010). Acute and 2-week exposure to prednisolone impair different aspects of beta-cell function in healthy men. *European Journal of Endocrinology/European Federation of Endocrine Societies, 162*(4), 729–735. doi:10.1530/EJE-09-1034 van Raalte, D. H., Ouwens, D. M., & Diamant, M. (2009). Novel insights into glucocorticoid-mediated diabetogenic effects: Towards expansion of therapeutic options? *European Journal of Clinical Investigation*, *39*(2), 81–93. doi:10.1111/j.1365-2362.2008.02067.x

Wamil, M., Battle, J. H., Turban, S., Kipari, T., Seguret, D., de Sousa Peixoto, R., et al. (2011). Novel fat depot-specific mechanisms underlie resistance to visceral obesity and inflammation in 11 beta-hydroxysteroid dehydrogenase type 1-deficient mice. *Diabetes*, *60*(4), 1158–1167. doi:10.2337/db10-0830

Willoughby, D. S., Taylor, M., & Taylor, L. (2003). Glucocorticoid receptor and ubiquitin expression after repeated eccentric exercise. *Medicine and Science in Sports and Exercise*, *35*(12), 2023–2031.

Yao, M., & Denver, R. J. (2007). Regulation of vertebrate corticotropin-releasing factor genes. *General and Comparative Endocrinology*, *153*(1–3), 200–216. doi:10.1016/j.ygcen.2007.01.046

23

PHYSICAL ACTIVITY, STRESS, AND IMMUNE FUNCTION

Kate M. Edwards and Paul J. Mills

The mind–body connection links many psychological processes and physiological systems. While connections between the mind and the immune system specifically have been recognized for well over a century, the mechanisms involved are only more recently being elucidated, and ways that we can utilize this interaction for clinical benefit are still being explored.

Examining the functions of the immune system can take several forms. The enumerative method simply records the numbers of cells, separating different cell types (e.g., monocytes, neutrophils, natural killer cells, T cells, B cells), differentiation stages (e.g., naïve, cytotoxic), and homing potential (e.g., chemokine receptor expression, adhesion molecule expression). Changes in cell numbers across short- or long-term situations/experiences give us a limited amount of information about cell mobilization, and differentiation. *In vitro* tests such as natural killer cell cytotoxicity and T-cell cytokine production are often combined with enumerative methods to provide information on the functioning capacity of cells during the time of study. Finally, *in vivo* tests such as wound healing and vaccination allow us to examine the function of the system as a whole rather than in separate portions. In and of themselves these latter tests lack the ability to provide detail on mechanisms of change but are the most clinically relevant assessment of the capacity of the immune system to respond to a challenge.

It is critical to understand that an *in vivo* immune response involves much more than just immune cells. The interactions of the autonomic nervous system and the endocrine system, in particular the hypothalamic-pituitary-adrenal axis, with immune function are well known, but the complexity of the interaction means they are less well understood. In discussion of behavioral influences on immune function we must recognize the impacts of such behaviors on these intricately linked systems. Stimuli such as stress and exercise activate and alter the functioning of these regulatory systems and thus alter control of immune responses, but the precise mechanisms of action remain to be firmly established.

In this chapter we will describe the use of the vaccination response as an *in vivo* method of assessing immune function. Vaccination is a fascinating tool for understanding the impact of stress and behavior on the function of the immune system, but also in the wider context of its clinical implications. Arguably the greatest medical intervention, alterations in vaccine responses, have enormous public health importance. We begin with a brief discussion of the immunological steps that together form the vaccine response, and the different ways it is possible to quantify this response. Then we review evidence for the negative effects of psychological stress on vaccination responses and finally detail various behavioral interventions that have been investigated as methods of boosting the vaccination response.

Vaccination response

Vaccination is a complex process that includes many possible points that may be susceptible to alteration by stress or physical activity. The first step of the immune response is antigen encounter, internalization and presentation performed by specialized antigen-presenting cells, including macrophages and the highly efficient dendritic cells. Antigens are presented on the cell membrane by the major histocompatibility complex (MHC) and are recognized and bound to by the rare naïve antigen-specific CD4+ T lymphocytes. After activation comes proliferation and maturation into T-helper (T_H) cells, which help direct the response. Antigen-specific naïve B cells, similarly recognize native antigen, internalize, and, using MHC molecules, present it for cognate interaction with T-helper cells, providing activation and co-stimulatory signals. Activated B lymphocytes mature and differentiate into plasma cells, the antibody secreting cells, or to long-lived memory B cells. In the case of a response to a polysaccharide antigen (called T-independent, compared to the T-dependent response to a protein antigen), the antibody response is not dependent on the cognate interaction between T_H lymphocytes and the B lymphocyte. In this situation, co-stimulation is provided by direct interaction with the native antigen; however, for efficient B-cell proliferation to plasma and memory cells and antibody (Ig) class switching, T_H-derived cytokines are needed. The maintenance of the response to vaccination is dependent on the memory lymphocyte pools and antibody production by plasma cells, which continues without a secondary antigen exposure, but slowly declines over time (for further details of the generation of the immune response, see Goldsby, Kindt, & Osborne, 2000).

The quantification of the response to an antigen through vaccination can be achieved in two main ways: antibody production and memory lymphocyte response. The plasma cells' production of antibody is quantifiable simply by measurement of serum IgG (antibody titre) change from pre-vaccination antibody titre to a point post-vaccination, most often 4–8 weeks post for peak responses and 6–12 months for sustained responses. The memory lymphocyte response can be measured *ex vivo*, without re-exposing the participant to the antigen. *In vitro* stimulation of peripheral blood mononucleocytes with the antigen causes stimulation of the memory T lymphocytes; subsequent quantification of cytokine released can therefore measure the cell-mediated capacity of the immune response to vaccination.

Measuring the response to vaccination through antibody production or cell-mediated response allows the quantification of the response, but, given the overarching aims of vaccination, it is important to consider the clinical implications of these outcomes. In fact, there is strong evidence that the size of the antibody response is related to protection against infection (Hannoun, Megas, & Piercy, 2004; Schuerman, Prymula, Henckaerts, & Poolman, 2007). Indeed, a 4-fold increase in antibody titre is the consensus for 'seroconversion', deemed protective, after vaccination. Thus, these measures of response strength have direct clinical implications.

Effects of chronic psychological stress on vaccination responses

The detrimental effects of chronic psychological stress on the body are well established. The vaccination model provides us with many examples that immune function is negatively affected in situations of chronic stress. Studies have primarily taken two different approaches to characterize stress, either comparing 'stressed' and 'non-stressed' groups (particular situations of chronic psychological stress such as caregiving for a relative with Alzheimer's disease or a child with disabilities, or patients with post-traumatic stress (PTSD) compared with age and sex-matched control groups), or cross-sectional analyses determining numbers of life-events and perceived stress. While many different populations have been examined, the two most commonly studied have been the elderly and young, healthy adults.

The strong justification for a focus on elderly patients is found in immunosenescence, the detrimental effects on immune function of age. The reduction in functional capacity through dysregulation of the immune system is seen in the increased rates of infectious disease and associated mortality in the elderly (Bender, 2003). Indeed, the public health impact of immunosenescence is compounded by the double hit, that vaccination, our most effective tool for preventing infectious disease, is less effective in the aged population, the response affected by the same immunosenescent changes.

Several extensive reviews have concluded that chronic psychological stress can impair the immune response to immunization (Burns, Carroll, Ring, & Drayson, 2003; Cohen, Miller, & Rabin, 2001; Glaser, Kiecolt-Glaser, Malarkey, & Sheridan, 1998). Glaser et al. (1998) concluded that the elderly or other at-risk populations show the greatest stress-related immunological impairment and, as such, suffer the most potent adverse health consequences of infection, disease, and mortality. Cohen et al. (2001) agreed with this conclusion and suggested that the small to medium effects of stress are seen most easily when the immune response has the greatest variability. Therefore, stress-related effects are most likely to emerge in populations with poor immune function, such as the elderly, or in responses to antigens that do not elicit robust responses. Burns et al. (2003) extended the discussion and highlighted that the most convincing evidence for stress-induced immunosuppression emerges from secondary, rather than primary, responses to T-dependent vaccinations, and that these effects are most apparent some time after the vaccination (6–12 months), rather than during the peak immune response 4–6 weeks later. These reviews suggest that both the type of vaccine and the time scale of the immune response should be considered when investigating stress-related effects.

In 2009 a meta-analysis reviewed 15 studies to assess the overall reported effect of chronic psychosocial stress on influenza vaccination responses (the most commonly used vaccine). A significant adverse effect of stress was confirmed, and using a 4-fold increase in antibody titre to signify protection, the size of the effect was 41% protected and 59% unprotected in stressed individuals, and 59% protected, 41% unprotected in unstressed individuals. Interestingly, the effect of immunosenescence (reduction of immune function with age) did appear to interact with stress, with the association of stress with reduced vaccination responses greater in older adults (over 43 years counted as 'older'; 37.5% protected older stressed, 62.5% protected older unstressed; Pedersen, Zachariae, & Bovbjerg, 2009).

Most recently, Powell, Allen, Hufnagle, Sheridan, and Bailey (2011) reviewed evidence for psychosocial stress effects on vaccination responses, including examination of potential mechanisms. Given the paucity of human studies, they included animal studies and concluded that the primary mediator is likely to be cortisol (product of hypothalamic-pituitary-adrenal (HPA) activation) in particular through its effects on dendritic cell functions of processing and presenting antigen (Powell et al., 2011).

Interventions

The loss of immune function capacity through disease, age, or chronic stress has great implications for population morbidity and mortality. Unsurprisingly then, identifying factors and interventions that promote stronger responses are of great interest and public health importance. Traditionally this has involved the search for exogenous adjuvants to add to vaccine formulations and development of vaccines with greater immunogenicity, a search that pharmaceutical companies are continuously engaged in. The use of behavioral interventions, however, has many advantages over this exogenous approach and has shown good success. Thus, these interventions are of potential clinical interest as well as academic interest in terms of how immune function is modulated in response to such interventions. In this section, summarized in Figure 23.1, we will describe the studies that are advancing our understanding of modulation of immune function through behavior and thus enhancement of vaccine responses.

Psychological component interventions: meditation and stress management

There are now several examples of intervention studies based around psychological components such as meditation and stress management. For example, a group of healthy adults who were randomized to receive mindfulness meditation training for 8 weeks showed greater antibody responses to influenza vaccination compared with a waitlist control group (Davidson et al., 2003). Similarly an 8-week cognitive behavioral stress management intervention in elderly caregivers was associated with better protection rates after influenza vaccination compared to non-intervention caregivers (Vedhara et al., 2003).

The traditional Chinese wellness practices of Tai Chi (also called Taiji) and Qigong involve a combination of 'three regulations': body focus, breath focus, and mind focus. Both involve physical movements (slow, meditative, dance-like movements), meditation postures, and gentle or vigorous body shaking (Jahnke, Larkey, Rogers, Etnier, & Lin, 2010). The practice of Tai Chi or Qigong has been associated with many health benefits, and although there is an exercise portion to the practice, the emphasis on meditation has led to inclusion in this section. There are two randomized controlled trials examining the effects of Tai Chi or Qigong on response to vaccination, with both reporting benefits for immune function. Yang et al. (2007) conducted a

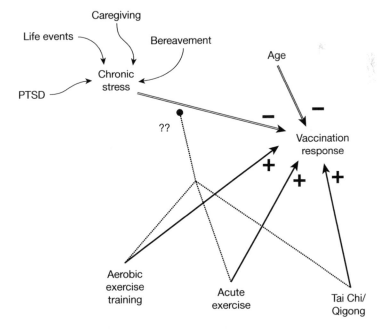

Figure 23.1 The effects of behaviors and stressors on vaccination responses.

5-month training of combined Taiji and Qigong practice in older adults, with three sessions per week (N = 27), and a parallel waitlist control group (N = 23). All subjects received the influenza vaccine and antibody responses were assessed at 3, 6, and 20 weeks post-vaccination. The Taiji and Qigong group showed a significant increase in magnitude and duration of antibody response compared to control group participants, and when analyzed for seroconversion, the percentage of participants showing a protective antibody titre post-vaccination was greater in the Taiji and Qigong group. In a larger (N = 112) study, Irwin and colleagues found that after a 16-week Tai Chi intervention, compared to health education control training, elderly adults similarly showed improved responses to Varicella zoster virus vaccination (Irwin, Olmstead, & Oxman, 2007).

Effects of chronic physical activity on vaccination responses

The effects of chronic physical activity, or exercise training, on vaccination response have been investigated primarily in elderly populations. Several cross-sectional studies as well as recent longitudinal studies have addressed the question of the impact of chronic physical activity or exercise training on vaccine responses. Kohut and colleagues (Kohut, Cooper, Nickolaus, Russell, & Cunnick, 2002) categorized older adults according to habitual physical activity. They found that those who participated in vigorous exercise three or more times per week had a higher influenza antibody titre than those who exercised at a lower intensity or not at all. Similar results were found by Smith, Kennedy, and Fleshner (2004) who compared physically active and sedentary older and young adults in their response to vaccination with a novel antigen KLH (keyhole-limpit hemocyanin, a benign protein). Again, the positive effects of physical activity were found in the older group, with greater antibody responses. However, in the younger cohort, all of whom showed the expected stronger responses compared to the elderly cohort, the effects of chronic physical activity were not apparent in antibody responses. Finally, Keylock et al. (2007) in a small study compared high- and low-fit older adults' responses to influenza and tetanus vaccine responses, but found very few differences among groups.

In addition to these cross-sectional studies, there are now several examples of well-designed randomized controlled trials that examined exercise training effects on vaccine responses. The first and smallest of these studies was by Kohut et al. (2004), who conducted a 10-month, three sessions per week, aerobic training program in 14 older adults, while a control group of 13 older adults continued their usual activities of low-level exercise or no exercise. All participants received the annual influenza vaccine prior to commencing the intervention, and showed similar responses, with marginally smaller responses in the exercise group. After the 10-month intervention, participants received the influenza vaccine for the following annual vaccine. In the post-intervention data, the exercise group showed significantly stronger responses to two of the three strains contained in the vaccine, with no difference in the third strain. This initial study has been followed by two further examinations, both of which show confirmatory results. Grant et al. (2008) compared an 8-month aerobic exercise program with a flexibility and balance program and assessed immunization with keyhole-limpit hemocyanin. In the primary response to this novel antigen, the aerobic training group showed greater antibody responses than the flexibility group. Finally, Woods et al. (2009), in the largest study to date (N = 144), compared the response to influenza vaccine in elderly adults after a 4-month cardiovascular aerobic training program (3 days per week) with a flexibility and balance control group. The cardiovascular training group showed a longer-lasting seroprotective response in a greater percentage of participants than the flexibility group, extending the protection afforded by vaccination.

In contrast to the beneficial effects of moderate exercise training, intensive exercise training has been associated with increased risk of upper respiratory tract infections and suppression of various immune parameters (e.g., Heath, Macera, & Nieman, 1992; Brenner, Shek, & Shephard, 1994). However, in a study comparing the antibody responses to the polysaccharide pneumococcal vaccine in elite swimmers at the end of an intensive 12-week training program, at 14 days post-vaccination no differences in antibody responses were found between swimmers and age-matched controls (Gleeson et al., 1996).

In sum, there is good evidence that moderate chronic levels of physical activity or exercise training lead to better immune function as measured by response to vaccination. The effect is apparent after relatively short periods of training (4–10 months) and is indicated to have the largest and thus most beneficial effects in the elderly.

Effects of acute exercise on vaccination responses

It is reasonably intuitive that chronic stress might harm immune function, while moderate chronic exercise would benefit it, but to understand how acute exercise has come to be considered a way to boost immune function we must first think about the immune responses elicited by a single acute exercise bout. One of the best-known effects of acute exercise (indeed, or psychological stress) is lymphocytosis, a rapid increase in the numbers of circulating immune cells (Benschop, Rodriguez-Feuerhahn, & Schedlowski, 1996). This increase is roughly proportional to the length and intensity of the exercise bout and is controlled by the neuroendocrine response to stress, i.e., the rapid release of epinephrine along with the increased shear stress of blood flow causing a mobilization of cells into the circulation. At the cessation of acute exercise the number of circulating lymphocytes decreases, and often is seen to reduce to below pre-exercise levels. This reduction represents the next stage of the response – the distribution of cells to sites of potential need. Dhabhar and McEwen elegantly demonstrated this effect by measurement of lymphocyte influx to an implanted surgical sponge in the skin, and found that the number of cells infiltrating the 'wound' was increased after acute stress (Viswanathan & Dhabhar, 2005). Subsequently, they used military metaphors to describe the meaning of the response (Dhabhar & McEwen, 1997). At rest, cells are found in the 'barracks', such as the spleen. On a signal for action (exercise or stress), they enter the circulation, the 'boulevards' to patrol, and from there they traffic towards sites of danger or potential danger, the skin or gut endothelial tissue, the 'battle stations' (Dhabhar & McEwen, 2001). This mobilization to 'patrol for danger' and move to 'sites of battle' has been identified as a possible method to enhance immune responses; if the system has been primed by exercise, its readiness to respond might result in better responses to challenge at this time compared to at rest. Figure 23.2 illustrates the response using the same metaphors described by Dhabhar and McEwen, including the suggestion of vaccination timed with exercise to harness the effects of the redistribution of cells.

In fact the lymphocytosis of exercise is only part of the hypothesis of how exercise might help the immune system respond to a vaccine. Other variables such as increased blood flow, greater capillary permeability, cytokine and chemokine release from exercising muscles, and increased lymph flow might all be involved in changing the response. These will all be described in more detail in the later mechanisms section.

Although we will not describe them here, there are many examples in the animal literature that show enhancing effects of acute stress on the immune response to antigen (Millan et al., 1996; Persoons, Berkenbosch, Schornagel, Thepen, & Kraal, 1995; Silberman, Wald, & Genaro, 2003); our focus is to describe the evidence in humans. Historically there are two papers that seem to address the question of acute exercise effects on vaccine response. In fact they were designed according to the 'open window hypothesis' that suggested a period of immune suppression and vulnerability to infection after a single bout of strenuous and prolonged exercise.

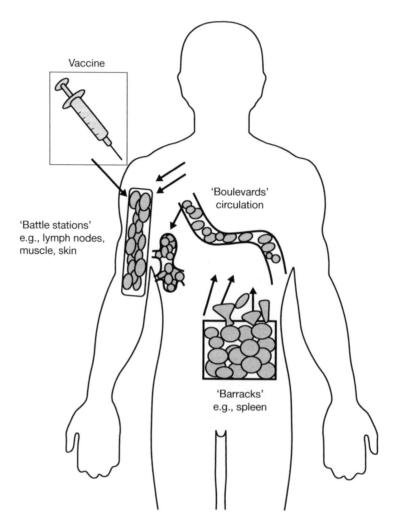

Vaccine

'Boulevards'
circulation

'Battle stations'
e.g., lymph nodes,
muscle, skin

'Barracks'
e.g., spleen

Figure 23.2 Military metaphors model of acute stress-induced redistribution of lymphocytes.

In contrast to the open window hypothesis, but in keeping with the acute stress-induced enhancement hypothesis, Eskola and colleagues found that the antibody response to tetanus toxoid vaccination was higher in a group who had completed a marathon prior to inoculation, compared with a non-runner control group (Eskola et al., 1978). A similar study by Bruunsgaard and colleagues did not, however, find differences in antibody responses to diphtheria, tetanus toxoid, and six pneumococcal serotypes between triathletes who had just completed a half-ironman competition prior to vaccination compared with either resting triathletes or sedentary controls (Bruunsgaard et al., 1997). The design of these studies used extreme bouts of prolonged, intense exercise, the sample sizes were relatively small, and neither controlled for the exact duration and relative intensity of exercise in each participant. Despite these limitations in both investigations, it is important to note that neither study supported the hypothesis that exercise suppresses antibody response to vaccination; indeed, they provide pilot data for the acute stress-induced immunoenhancement hypothesis.

Recently, several studies have begun to examine the acute stress-induced immunoenhancement hypothesis in humans in more detail, and show good evidence for a beneficial effect on vaccination response. In the first of these studies, the effects of either resting control, acute dynamic (cycling) exercise, or psychological stress on the response to two vaccines (influenza and meningococcal A+C) were assessed (Edwards et al., 2008, 2006). Two vaccines were used to represent thymus-dependent (influenza) and thymus-independent (meningococcal) vaccines, and thus discern the importance of the role played by T cells in altering the response. Sixty young adult participants all completed one 45-minute task; the exercise group completed a moderate-intensity cycling task, those in the psychological stress group completed a time-pressured mental arithmetic test, and those in a non-stress control group rested quietly. Immediately following their allotted task, participants received the two vaccines into contralateral arms. Results indicated task-induced immune response enhancements to both vaccines, but only in the situation of a weaker control response. For the influenza vaccine, women in both the exercise group and psychological stress groups showed enhanced antibody responses to the A/Panama influenza strain at 4 and 20 weeks post-vaccination, in comparison to the resting control group (Edwards et al., 2006). This strain elicited particularly poor antibody responses in the female control group, while in contrast, men displayed robust responses to all strains, and no effects of exercise or stress were observed. In response to the meningococcal vaccine, both exercise and psychological stress groups improved the antibody response to meningococcal A in men compared with controls (Edwards et al., 2008). In agreement with influenza findings, augmentation was observed where the control group response was poor; on this occasion, men, rather than women, in the control group had weaker responses to this particular strain. These results confirmed that the adjuvant effects of exercise and psychological stress are not limited to thymus-dependent (e.g., influenza) or thymus-independent (e.g., meningococcal) vaccines, and thus do not seem to be dependent on T-cell interactions.

The follow-up study was very similar in design, but changed the task used based on the hypothesis of potential mechanisms (Edwards et al., 2007). A resistance-based, eccentric exercise protocol was developed, designed to initiate a local inflammatory response in the biceps brachialis and deltoid muscles of the arm into which the influenza vaccine would be injected. The hypothesis described a response initiated in the tissue where the vaccine would be received to provide the most efficient way of stimulating the immune response. Sixty healthy young adults were randomly allocated to either an exercise group or a control group. The 25-minute exercise task involved the eccentric portion of exercise only; 50 repetitions each of the bicep curl and lateral raise exercises being performed with the non-dominant arm using a weight 85% of the single repetition maximum (1RM). The control group rested quietly for the same time. A 6-hour delay was included prior to vaccination (to allow for the cytokine response to the exercise to develop) after which participants received an influenza vaccine into the non-dominant (exercised) arm. Results indicated that women in the exercise group showed greater antibody responses to two of the influenza strains at 6 and 20 weeks post-vaccination. Again, an enhancement effect was found in strains with a weaker control response. The two strains producing relatively weak antibody responses in women in the control group were enhanced by exercise; however, men showed more robust responses to all strains and no effects of exercise were found.

These two initial studies provided evidence that acute exercise might benefit responses to vaccination in a setting of less robust control responses. There followed two larger studies, which provide somewhat mixed findings, but taken together, extended the evidence for the acute stress-induced immunoenhancement hypothesis. These two studies investigated the effects of exercise timing and intensity, with a view to elucidating the most efficacious protocol, and were again in a population of young, healthy adults. Interestingly, in the timing study (Campbell et al., 2010) a full-dose influenza vaccine was used, while the intensity study (Edwards et al., 2010) used a reduced dose (0.5 of recommended dose) influenza vaccine, examining the importance of strength of response to the enhancing capacity of exercise.

Campbell, Edwards, and colleagues first examined the timing of exercise (Campbell et al., 2010) in 156 healthy young adults. Three timings were compared to a purely resting control, with all three exercise groups completing the same eccentric exercise task as previously described (85% 1RM) (Edwards et al., 2007). In keeping with the first eccentric exercise study, a time point 6 hours prior to vaccination was employed based on reported kinetics of the cytokine interleukin-6 (IL-6) response to eccentric exercise (Edwards et al., 2007; MacIntyre, Sorichter, Mair, Berg, & McKenzie, 2001). However, the first study had employed a task immediately prior to vaccination according to the observation that many of the exercise-induced physiological and immunological changes peak at exercise cessation and return to baseline, thus a group was including exercising immediately before vaccination. Finally, a group performed the task 48 hours prior to vaccination. This time point was included to capture the peak of the muscle damage response, which at 48 hours post-exercise is shown to include a peak in accumulated inflammatory infiltrate, including neutrophils, mononuclear cells, cytokines, and heat shock proteins (Fielding et al., 1993; J. M. Peake et al., 2005). A full-dose influenza vaccine was administered and all three strains produced robust responses in both men and women (23-, 10-, and 14-fold changes from baseline to 28 days), which were not different between exercise and control groups, nor among exercise groups. Physiological indices demonstrated that exercise timing did alter the profiles of muscle damage (pain and plasma creatine kinase) among the groups at the time of vaccination, but contrary to expectation IL-6 was highest in the 48-hour and immediately prior exercise groups, indicating that the kinetics did not follow the same inflammatory response as previously reported (MacIntyre et al., 2001; Paulsen et al., 2005). Although this null finding was unexpected, it was not entirely surprising given the strong responses to all strains of virus contained in the seasonal influenza vaccine.

Edwards, Campbell, and colleagues also set out to examine the influence of exercise intensity (Edwards et al., 2010). In a similar design, the effects of three different exercise intensities were compared with a resting control group. This, the largest of the studies in the literature, included 160 healthy young adults randomized to one of four groups. Exercise intensities of 60%, 85% (as had been used in prior studies), and 110% of 1RM were used. The importance of intensity on the adjuvant effect is of particular interest, not only to determine a task with maximum efficacy, but also for clinical application, i.e., if intensity shows no effect, a modest bout of exercise could still be prescribed for a beneficial effect on protection afforded by vaccination. In this cohort, a reduced-dose (50% of recommended dose) influenza vaccination was used, based on the previous finding that, in a similar population, a full-dose seasonal influenza vaccine produced robust responses in all three strains, without any exercise-induced enhancement. Administering a reduced dose modeled poorer responses, which might be elicited by a less immunogenic antigen exposure or an immune-compromised population. As expected, smaller-fold changes were seen, with two strains showing responses of 5- and 6-fold changes, while the final strain still showed a robust 19-fold response. As hypothesized, exercise enhanced the antibody response in both of the strains that demonstrated a weaker response in the control group. There were no differences among the three exercise groups in antibody responses, despite physiological differences such as dose-dependent changes in arm circumference and reported pain, and the creatine kinase response.

Most recently, the speculation that exercise elicits enhancing effects on weaker, but not stronger, responses was directly addressed (Edwards et al., 2012). In a study of 133 healthy young adults, the effects of a 15-minute resistance band-based exercise task versus resting control prior to receiving the pneumococcal vaccine was evaluated, with half of the cohort receiving the full dose of vaccine and half receiving a reduced dose (50%) of vaccine. The findings demonstrated an overall effect of exercise groups showing stronger responses than control groups to the 11 pneumococcal strains measured. Importantly, when examining the effect of dose, within groups receiving the full dose there was no significant difference between exercise and control participants' responses. However, in the groups that received the reduced dose, the exercise group showed significantly stronger responses than the control group. These data add to the hypothesis that acute exercise enhances poorer responses and encourages investigation of the potential to use adjuvant vaccine responses in populations known to suffer vaccine failure and poor response rates.

Potential mechanisms

We began this section describing the lymphocytosis response to acute stress and illustrating how this might relate to enhanced immune responses to challenge at the time of acute stress. This is one likely potential mechanism of acute stress-induced enhancement. The rapid increase in cell numbers observed in the circulation includes increases in monocytes and dendritic cells (Ho et al., 2001; Hong & Mills, 2008), which are responsible for antigen recognition, uptake, and presentation. Thus, acute exercise initiates leukocyte mobilization and subsequent extravasation into tissues, guided by chemoattractants of the transient inflammatory response in the exercised muscles. In this way, acute exercise would induce leukocyte mobilization and localization in exercised muscles, the intra-muscular administration of antigen further attracts leukocytes, and the immune response develops, theoretically enhanced by the exercise-induced magnification of accumulation of leukocytes.

There are also several other related and linked mechanisms that may also contribute to acute stress-induced immunoenhancement, which are summarized in Figure 23.3. Firstly, the 'danger signal' response of cells to stress such as exercise. This response is especially true in exercise that includes eccentric (muscle applies force as it lengthens) components, which causes damage to the internal structure of the muscle fibers, and results in oedema, muscle pain, muscle weakness, leakage of muscle and cellular proteins, and cellular infiltration (Peake, Nosaka, & Suzuki, 2005; Peake et al., 2005). This damage is greater than that observed with concentric (shortening) muscle contractions (Sorichter, Puschendorf, & Mair, 1999) and is greatest when the exercise is unaccustomed (Sorichter et al., 2006). The range of danger signals released includes IL-6, uric acid, Heat Shock Protein (HSP) 60, and HSP70, which are thought to play a role in orchestrating inflammation and repair of the surrounding tissues (Hirose et al., 2004; Matzinger, 2002). They may also result in increased leukocyte homing to the site of vaccine administration and/or enhanced antigen uptake and processing, making the initial phase of the immune response more efficient and subsequently enhancing the antibody response. In support of this hypothesis, the extent of the self-reported pain and the change in upper arm limb circumference following eccentric exercise, both indirect indicators of muscle damage, have been significantly positively correlated with the subsequent cell-mediated immune response to the vaccination (Edwards et al., 2007).

Within the danger signals described, we must in particular describe the role of cytokines, such as IL-6, which have been specifically implicated in enhancing vaccine responses (Krakauer, 1995; Lee, Youn, Seong, & Sung, 1999). For example, higher levels of circulating IL-6 have been found in patients with good antibody responses than in patients who do not respond to vaccination (Krakauer, 1995). Further, the co-administration of IL-6 gene with vaccine completely protects mice from a lethal challenge with influenza virus (Lee et al., 1999). Given these findings,

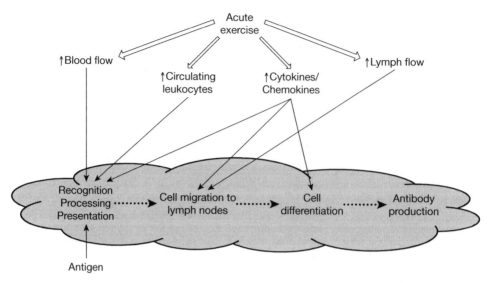

Figure 23.3 Potential pathways for acute stress-induced responses involvement in vaccination response.

it has been hypothesized that increased levels of IL-6 in the systemic circulation as part of the acute stress response may play a role in augmenting the immune response to vaccination. Indeed, the extent of the IL-6 response to a bout of acute exercise has been associated with the antibody response at 6 weeks post-vaccination (Edwards et al., 2006). However, no associations have been observed between the IL-6 response 24 hours post-exercise and the antibody response to vaccination (Campbell et al., 2010; Edwards et al., 2010). Given differences in task and timing of measurements, it is difficult to discern the true role of the IL-6 exercise response and the enhancement of vaccine responses, especially as circulating levels of IL-6 do not always accurately represent intra-muscular signaling following eccentric exercise (Tomiya, Aizawa, Nagatomi, Sensui, & Kokubun, 2004). Thus, it is likely that local milieu rather than systemic measurements are needed for mechanistic understanding.

A final mechanistic pathway to be considered is the increase in lymph drainage. There is evidence to suggest that muscular contractions are associated with a temporary increase in lymph drainage around the site of exercised muscle tissue (Havas et al., 1997). Thus, exercise contractions would lead to enhanced immune cell transport from the site of antigen administration into exercised muscles via the altered lymph fluid dynamics. Therefore, it is be hypothesized that performing exercise could enhance antigenic transport to the lymph nodes where recognition by lymphocytes takes place and thus make the response more efficient. However, this is yet to be directly measured in vaccination studies and thus remains speculation.

Summary: stress and exercise effects on immune function

It is widely acknowledged that chronic psychological stress has a negative impact on immune function while, conversely, exercise training and physical activity confer benefits to immune function over sedentary behavior. Both of these findings mirror much of the literature regarding health risks and therefore emphasize the importance of prescription of moderate exercise, perhaps especially in the setting of immunocompromise such as advanced age. The recent evidence that acute exercise enhances vaccination responses might seem less intuitive, but offers an opportunity to understand acute physiological changes and their impact on immune response to challenge.

In addition, the public health relevance of both acute and chronic exercise in improving the response to, and thus protection afforded by, vaccination indicates that this line of research may lead to clinical benefit. It is not clear how behavioral interventions including acute and chronic exercise or meditative practices like Tai Chi will interact with the immune dysregulation effects of chronic stress, age, or even disease, although it appears that positive effects may be most pronounced in these settings. These answers will help inform the best practice for maintaining or improving immune function when impacted by deleterious factors.

References

Bender, B. S. (2003). Infectious disease risk in the elderly. *Immunology and Allergy Clinincs of North America*, *23*(1), 57–64.

Benschop, R. J., Rodriguez-Feuerhahn, M., & Schedlowski, M. (1996). Catecholamine-induced leukocytosis: Early observations, current research, and future directions. *Brain, Behavior, & Immunity, 10*(2), 77–91.

Brenner, I. K., Shek, P. N., & Shephard, R. J. (1994). Infection in athletes. *Sports Medicine, 17*(2), 86–107.

Bruunsgaard, H., Hartkopp, A., Mohr, T., Konradsen, H., Heron, I., Mordhorst, C. H., & Pedersen, B. K. (1997). In vivo cell-mediated immunity and vaccination response following prolonged, intense exercise. *Medicine & Science in Sports & Exercise, 29*(9), 1176–1181.

Burns, V. E., Carroll, D., Ring, C., & Drayson, M. (2003). Antibody response to vaccination and psychosocial stress in humans: Relationships and mechanisms. *Vaccine, 21*(19–20), 2523–2534.

Campbell, J. P., Edwards, K. M., Ring, C., Drayson, M. T., Bosch, J. A., Inskip, A., . . . Burns, V. E. (2010). The effects of vaccine timing on the efficacy of an acute eccentric exercise intervention on the immune response to an influenza vaccine in young adults. *Brain, Behavior, & Immunity, 24*(4), 623–630. doi:S0889-1591(09)00465-6

Cohen, S., Miller, G. E., & Rabin, B. S. (2001). Psychological stress and antibody response to immunization: A critical review of the human literature. *Psychosomatic Medicine, 63*(1), 7–18.

Davidson, R. J., Kabat-Zinn, J., Schumacher, J., Rosenkranz, M., Muller, D., Santorelli, S. F., . . . Sheridan, J. F. (2003). Alterations in brain and immune function produced by mindfulness meditation. *Psychosomatic Medicine, 65*(4), 564–70.

Dhabhar, F. S., & McEwen, B. S. (1997). Acute stress enhances while chronic stress suppresses cell-mediated immunity in vivo: A potential role for leukocyte trafficking. *Brain, Behavior, & Immunity, 11*(4), 286–306.

Dhabhar, F. S., & McEwen, B. S. (2001). Bi-directional effects of stress on immune function: Possible explanations for salubrious as well as harmful effects. In R. Ader, D. L. Felten, & N. Cohen (Eds.), *Psychoneuroimmunology* (4th ed.). New York: Academic Press.

Edwards, K. M., Burns, V. E., Adkins, A. E., Carroll, D., Drayson, M., & Ring, C. (2008). Meningococcal A vaccination response is enhanced by acute stress in men. *Psychosomatuic Medicine, 70*(2), 147–151. doi:PSY.0b013e318164232e

Edwards, K. M., Burns, V. E., Allen, L. M., McPhee, J. S., Bosch, J. A., Carroll, D., Drayson, M., & Ring, C. (2007). Eccentric exercise as an adjuvant to influenza vaccination in humans. *Brain, Behavior, & Immunity, 21*(2), 209–217.

Edwards, K. M., Burns, V. E., Reynolds, T., Carroll, D., Drayson, M., & Ring, C. (2006). Acute stress exposure prior to influenza vaccination enhances antibody response in women. *Brain, Behavior, & Immunity, 20*(2), 159–168.

Edwards, K. M., Campbell, J. P., Ring, C., Drayson, M. T., Bosch, J. A., Downes, C., . . . Burns, V. E. (2010). Exercise intensity does not influence the efficacy of eccentric exercise as a behavioural adjuvant to vaccination. *Brain, Behavior, & Immunity, 24*(4), 623–630. doi:S0889-1591(10)00010-3

Edwards, K. M., Pung, M. A., Tomfohr, L. M., Ziegler, M. G., Campbell, J. P., Drayson, M. T., & Mills, P. J. (2012). Acute exercise enhancement of pneumococcal vaccination response: A randomised controlled trial of weaker and stronger immune response. *Vaccine, 30*(45), 6389–6395. doi:10.1016/j.vaccine.2012.08.022

Eskola, J., Ruuskanan, Soppi, E., Viljanen, M. K., Jarvinen, M., & Toivonen, H. (1978). Effect of sport stress on lymphocyte transformation and antibody formation. *Clinical & Experimental Immunology, 32*, 339–345.

Fielding, R. A., Manfredi, T. J., Ding, W., Fiatarone, M. A., Evans, W. J., & Cannon, J. G. (1993). Acute phase response in exercise. III. Neutrophil and IL-1 beta accumulation in skeletal muscle. *American Journal of Physiology, 265*(1 Pt 2), R166–R172.

Glaser, R., Kiecolt-Glaser, J. K., Malarkey, W. B., & Sheridan, J. F. (1998). The influence of psychological stress on the immune response to vaccines. *Annals of the New York Academy of Sciences, 840*, 649–655.

Gleeson, M., Pyne, D. B., McDonald, W. A., Clancy, R. L., Cripps, A. W., Horn, P. L., & Fricker, P. A. (1996). Pneumococcal antibody responses in elite swimmers. *Clinical & Experimental Immunology, 105*(2), 238–244.

Goldsby, R. A., Kindt, T. J., & Osborne, B. A. (2000). *Kuby immunology*. New York: Freeman and Company.

Grant, R. W., Mariani, R. A., Vieira, V. J., Fleshner, M., Smith, T. P., Keylock, K. T., . . . Woods, J. A. (2008). Cardiovascular exercise intervention improves the primary antibody response to keyhole limpet hemocyanin (KLH) in previously sedentary older adults. *Brain, Behavior, & Immunity, 22*(6), 923–932. doi:S0889-1591(08)00028-7

Hannoun, C., Megas, F., & Piercy, J. (2004). Immunogenicity and protective efficacy of influenza vaccination. *Virus Research, 103*(1–2), 133–138.

Havas, E., Parviainen, T., Vuorela, J., Toivanen, J., Nikula, T., & Vihko, V. (1997). Lymph flow dynamics in exercising human skeletal muscle as detected by scintography. *Journal of Physiology, 504*(Pt 1), 233–239.

Heath, G. W., Macera, C. A., & Nieman, D. C. (1992). Exercise and upper respiratory tract infections. Is there a relationship? *Sports Medicine, 14*(6), 353–365.

Hirose, L., Nosaka, K., Newton, M., Laveder, A., Kano, M., Peake, J., & Suzuki, K. (2004). Changes in inflammatory mediators following eccentric exercise of the elbow flexors. *Exercise Immunology Reviews, 10*, 75–90.

Ho, C. S., Lopez, J. A., Vuckovic, S., Pyke, C. M., Hockey, R. L., & Hart, D. N. (2001). Surgical and physical stress increases circulating blood dendritic cell counts independently of monocyte counts. *Blood, 98*(1), 140–145.

Hong, S., & Mills, P. J. (2008). Effects of an exercise challenge on mobilization and surface marker expression of monocyte subsets in individuals with normal vs. elevated blood pressure. *Brain, Behavior, & Immunity, 22*(4), 590–599. doi:S0889-1591(07)00335-2

Irwin, M. R., Olmstead, R., & Oxman, M. N. (2007). Augmenting immune responses to varicella zoster virus in older adults: A randomized, controlled trial of Tai Chi. *Journal of the American Geriatrics Society, 55*(4), 511–517. doi:JGS1109

Jahnke, R., Larkey, L., Rogers, C., Etnier, J., & Lin, F. (2010). A comprehensive review of health benefits of qigong and tai chi. *American Journal of Health Promotion, 24*(6), e1–e25. doi:10.4278/ajhp.081013-LIT-248

Keylock, K. T., Lowder, T., Leifheit, K. A., Cook, M., Mariani, R. A., Ross, K., . . . Woods, J. A. (2007). Higher antibody, but not cell-mediated, responses to vaccination in high physically fit elderly. *Journal of Applied Physiology, 102*(3), 1090–1098. doi:00790.2006

Kohut, M. L., Arntson, B. A., Lee, W., Rozeboom, K., Yoon, K. J., Cunnick, J. E., & McElhaney, J. (2004). Moderate exercise improves antibody response to influenza immunization in older adults. *Vaccine, 22*(17–18), 2298–2306.

Kohut, M. L., Cooper, M. M., Nickolaus, M. S., Russell, D. R., & Cunnick, J. E. (2002). Exercise and psychosocial factors modulate immunity to influenza vaccine in elderly individuals. *Journals of Gerontology Series A: Biological Sciences, 57*(9), M557–M562.

Krakauer, T. (1995). Levels of interleukin 6 and tumor necrosis factor in serum from humans vaccinated with live, attenuated Francisella tularensis. *Clinical & Diagnostic Laboratory Immunology, 2*(4), 487–488.

Lee, S. W., Youn, J. W., Seong, B. L., & Sung, Y. C. (1999). IL-6 induces long-term protective immunity against a lethal challenge of influenza virus. *Vaccine, 17*(5), 490–496.

MacIntyre, D. L., Sorichter, S., Mair, J., Berg, A., & McKenzie, D. C. (2001). Markers of inflammation and myofibrillar proteins following eccentric exercise in humans. *European Journal of Applied Physiology, 84*(3), 180–186.

Matzinger, P. (2002). The danger model: A renewed sense of self. *Science, 296*(5566), 301–305.

Millan, S., Gonzalez-Quijano, M. I., Giordano, M., Soto, L., Martin, A. I., & Lopez-Calderon, A. (1996). Short and long restraint differentially affect humoral and cellular immune functions. *Life Science, 59*(17), 1431–1442.

Paulsen, G., Benestad, H. B., Strom-Gundersen, I., Morkrid, L., Lappegard, K. T., & Raastad, T. (2005). Delayed leukocytosis and cytokine response to high-force eccentric exercise. *Medicine & Science in Sports & Exercise, 37*(11), 1877–1883. doi:00005768-200511000-00008

Peake, J., Nosaka, K., & Suzuki, K. (2005). Characterization of inflammatory responses to eccentric exercise in humans. *Exercise Immunology Reviews, 11*, 64–85.

Peake, J. M., Suzuki, K., Wilson, G., Hordern, M., Nosaka, K., Mackinnon, L., & Coombes, J. S. (2005). Exercise-induced muscle damage, plasma cytokines, and markers of neutrophil activation. *Medicine & Science in Sports & Exercise, 37*(5), 737–745. doi:00005768-200505000-00006

Pedersen, A. F., Zachariae, R., & Bovbjerg, D. H. (2009). Psychological stress and antibody response to influenza vaccination: A meta-analysis. *Brain, Behavior, and Immunity, 23*(4), 427–433. doi:S0889-1591(09)00007-5

Persoons, J. H., Berkenbosch, F., Schornagel, K., Thepen, T., & Kraal, G. (1995). Increased specific IgE production in lungs after the induction of acute stress in rats. *Journal of Allergy and Clinical Immunology, 95*(3), 765–770.

Powell, N. D., Allen, R. G., Hufnagle, A. R., Sheridan, J. F., & Bailey, M. T. (2011). Stressor-induced alterations of adaptive immunity to vaccination and viral pathogens. *Immunology and Allergy Clinics of North America, 31*(1), 69–79. doi:S0889-8561(10)00073-1

Schuerman, L., Prymula, R., Henckaerts, I., & Poolman, J. (2007). ELISA IgG concentrations and opsonophagocytic activity following pneumococcal protein D conjugate vaccination and relationship to efficacy against acute otitis media. *Vaccine, 25*(11), 1962–1968. doi:S0264-410X(06)01327-2

Silberman, D. M., Wald, M. R., & Genaro, A. M. (2003). Acute and chronic stress exert opposing effects on antibody responses associated with changes in stress hormone regulation of T-lymphocyte reactivity. *Journal of Neuroimmunology, 144*(1–2), 53–60.

Smith, T. P., Kennedy, S. L., & Fleshner, M. (2004). Influence of age and physical activity on the primary in vivo antibody and T cell-mediated responses in men. *Journal of Applied Physiology, 97*(2), 491–498.

Sorichter, S., Martin, M., Julius, P., Schwirtz, A., Huonker, M., Luttmann, W., . . . Berg, A. (2006). Effects of unaccustomed and accustomed exercise on the immune response in runners. *Medicine & Science in Sports & Exercise, 38*(10), 1739–1745. doi:10.1249/01.mss.0000230213.62743.fb

Sorichter, S., Puschendorf, B., & Mair, J. (1999). Skeletal muscle injury induced by eccentric muscle action: Muscle proteins as markers of muscle fiber injury. *Exercise Immunology Reviews, 5*, 5–21.

Tomiya, A., Aizawa, T., Nagatomi, R., Sensui, H., & Kokubun, S. (2004). Myofibers express IL-6 after eccentric exercise. *American Journal of Sports Medicine, 32*(2), 503–508.

Vedhara, K., Bennett, P. D., Clark, S., Lightman, S. L., Shaw, S., Perks, P., . . . Shanks, N. M. (2003). Enhancement of antibody responses to influenza vaccination in the elderly following a cognitive-behavioural stress management intervention. *Psychotherapy and Psychosomatics, 72*(5), 245–252. doi:10.1159/00007189571895

Viswanathan, K., & Dhabhar, F. S. (2005). Stress-induced enhancement of leukocyte trafficking into sites of surgery or immune activation. *Proceedings of the National Acadamy of Science USA, 102*(16), 5808–5813.

Woods, J. A., Keylock, K. T., Lowder, T., Vieira, V. J., Zelkovich, W., Dumich, S., . . . McAuley, E. (2009). Cardiovascular exercise training extends influenza vaccine seroprotection in sedentary older adults: The immune function intervention trial. *Journal of the American Geriatrics Society, 57*(12), 2183–2191. doi:JGS2563

Yang, Y., Verkuilen, J., Rosengren, K. S., Mariani, R. A., Reed, M., Grubisich, S. A., & Woods, J. A. (2007). Effects of a Taiji and Qigong intervention on the antibody response to influenza vaccine in older adults. *American Journal of Chinese Medicine, 35*(4), 597–607. doi:S0192415X07005090

PART 7

Pain

Edited by
Dane B. Cook

24

THE INTERACTION OF MUSCULOSKELETAL PAIN AND PHYSICAL ACTIVITY

Human studies

Thomas Graven-Nielsen, Henrik B. Madsen, and Lars Arendt-Nielsen

This chapter is intended to provide an overview of the research regarding exercise and muscle pain in humans, focusing on both the potential for exercise to reduce pain sensitivity and for pain to interfere with muscle function. In order to accomplish this, the chapter is divided into two sections. The first will describe the acute effects of exercise on pain in both healthy individuals and those with chronic pain conditions. The second will discuss the effects of pain on motor control systems with an emphasis on understanding how acute pain may translate into chronic pain conditions.

Effects of exercise on pain: exercise-induced hypoalgesia

Anecdotes about athletes who did not report pain following severe injuries during sports competition have contributed to the notion that exercise may alter pain perception. Over the past 30 years a number of studies have examined whether analgesia occurs during or following exercise. This area of research has produced evidence that one potential benefit for healthy individuals performing acute exercise is a reduction in pain sensitivity.

Exercise-induced hypoalgesia in healthy subjects

Several studies on healthy subjects have reported that pain intensity and unpleasantness are decreased (Koltyn, Garvin, Gardiner, & Nelson, 1996; Koltyn, 2000; Umeda, Newcomb, Ellingson, & Koltyn, 2010; Droste, 1991; Hoffman et al., 2004) and that pain thresholds as well as pain tolerance increased during and after aerobic, isometric and resistance exercise. Early research in this area was limited by significant methodological flaws (e.g., no control group), leading some to conclude that reduced pain sensitivity following exercise was simply a phenomenon of pre-exposure to painful stimuli (Padawer & Levine, 1992). However, subsequent research has clearly demonstrated that reduced pain sensitivity occurs following acute exercise when compared to no-exercise control conditions (Gurevich, Kohn, & Davis, 1994; Koltyn et al., 1996). This phenomenon has been referred to as exercise-induced analgesia or more recently, exercise-induced hypoalgesia (EIH). Most research on EIH has been conducted using aerobic exercise (bicycling or running), although studies using isometric exercise are common. Only a few studies have investigated the effect of resistance exercise on pain perception. Several types of experimental pain modalities, including mechanical, thermal and electrical stimuli, have been used to assess pain sensitivity following exercise. Although evidence exists that exercise reduces sensitivity to all the pain modalities tested, EIH is most consistently observed for mechanical and electrical stimuli (Koltyn, 2000; Hoeger Bement, 2009). Changes in pain intensity and unpleasantness occur not only in the exercised body part or within a few segmental levels, but also at distant sites, indicating that the central nervous system could play an important role in modulating pain during and following exercise (Kosek & Lundberg, 2003).

Exercise intensity and duration: Aerobic exercise most consistently produces a hypoalgesic effect when performed at intensities equal to or higher than 200 Watts or at 60–75% of maximal oxygen uptake ($\dot{V}O_2$ max) (Koltyn, 2002; Droste, 1991; Hoffman et al., 2004). Duration of exercise is also important and there appears to be an interaction between intensity and duration. Hoffman et al. (2004) assessed the pain sensitivity in healthy subjects before and after treadmill running and found that pain sensitivity decreased after exercise at high intensity (75% of $\dot{V}O_2$max) and longer duration (30 minutes). Pain sensitivity was not affected by exercise at the same intensity for a shorter time (10 minutes) or at reduced exercise intensity (50% of $\dot{V}O_2$max) that was of longer duration (30 minutes). Similar results have been reported in an animal study, where animals that run more have higher pain thresholds than animals that run less (Shyu, Andersson, & Thoren, 1982). Interestingly, in healthy subjects passive cycling induced pressure hypoalgesia compared with a control condition (Figure 24.1) (Nielsen, Mortensen, Sorensen, Simonsen, & Graven-Nielsen, 2009), indicating the role of joint movement or proprioception in EIH.

In contrast to aerobic exercise, EIH is produced with isometric exercise at both low and high intensity. Hoeger Bement and colleagues reported that isometric contractions at longer duration

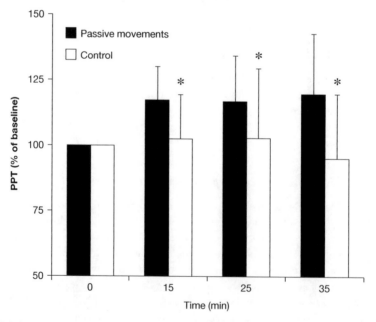

Figure 24.1 Average PPT (+ SD, N = 14, percentage of baseline) before and during passive physiological movements. Passive joint mobilization of the knee joint was implemented by an electrical bicycle (30 rpm) in blocks of 10–15 minutes in between assessment of the pressure pain thresholds. The pressure pain thresholds were increased at the lower leg compared with baseline and during control sessions (★: P < 0.05) (based on data from Nielsen, Mortensen, Sorensen, Simonsen, & Graven-Nielsen et al., 2009).

and lower intensity caused a greater decrease in pain sensitivity compared with contractions at low and high intensities of shorter duration (Hoeger Bement, Dicapo, Rasiarmos, & Hunter, 2008). However, Umeda and colleagues (Umeda, Newcomb, Ellingson, & Koltyn, 2010) failed to find a dose–response relationship for isometric handgrip performed at 25% of maximal voluntary contraction for 1, 3 and 5 minutes. Although blood pressure was found to increase in a dose–response manner, pain sensitivity did not differ among the three durations. Thus, it appears that isometric exercise can be performed at lower intensities to produce EIH and that the duration of exercise may be less important for isometric than aerobic exercise.

Compared to aerobic exercise, EIH to resistance exercise has been less studied. Koltyn and Arbogast (1998) assessed pain threshold and pain ratings in healthy subjects before and after 45 minutes of resistance exercise performed as four different exercises with three sets of ten repetitions at 75% of maximal voluntary contraction and found increased pain threshold and decreased pain ratings compared to quiet rest 5 minutes after exercise, but not 15 minutes after. Anshel and Russell (1994) studied the effect of 12 weeks of strength training compared to aerobic training and no training on pain tolerance and mood in unfit males and found that strength training had no positive influence on pain or mood, but, oddly, increased depressed mood.

Duration of exercise-induced analgesia: The hypoalgesic effect of exercise is larger during exercise compared with post-exercise measurements (Kosek, Ekholm, & Hansson, 1996), but the results on the duration of EIH are inconsistent. Hoffman et al. (2004) found a significant decrease in pain sensitivity 5 minutes after high-intensity aerobic exercise, which was not maintained after 10 minutes. However, Janal and colleagues (Janal, Colt, Clark, & Glusman, 1984) reported hypoalgesic effects 30 minutes after high-intensity aerobic exercise and Droste (1991) reported decreased pain sensitivity for up to 60 minutes post-exercise. In general, aerobic exercise appears to produce longer-lasting hypoalgesia than resistance exercise modalities (Koltyn & Arbogast, 1998).

Gender and exercise-induced analgesia: Most studies on EIH in healthy subjects have been conducted in males, but studies including both genders have shown comparable effects on pain sensitivity after exercise (Umeda et al., 2010; Hoffman et al., 2004; Kosek & Lundberg, 2003). Nonetheless, Sternberg, Bokat, Kass, Alboyadjian, and Gracely (2001) reported EIH in women but not men after treadmill running for 10 minutes at 85% of $\dot{V}O_2max$. Similarly, decreased pain sensitivity was found in women after submaximal isometric contractions, whereas male subjects did not present with decreased pain sensitivity. Phases of the menstrual cycle do not appear to influence the magnitude of EIH in women (Hoeger Bement et al., 2009). However, the complexity of the gender, pain and exercise relationship deserves more systematic study.

Exercise-induced hypoalgesia in chronic pain patients

Exercise is frequently used in pain management settings. Systematic reviews have concluded that exercise is beneficial for a variety of pain conditions, including neck pain, low back pain, pelvic girdle pain, osteoarthritis, knee osteoarthritis, fibromyalgia and rheumatoid arthritis (for a more detailed review refer to Chapter 27 in this volume). Decreased pain sensitivity to mechanical pressure at the index finger (Hoffman, Shepanski, Mackenzie, & Clifford, 2005), arm, leg and back (Meeus, Roussel, Truijen, & Nijs, 2010) has been reported after submaximal bicycling in chronic low back pain patients, and this decrease was similar to healthy controls (Meeus et al., 2010). In contrast to the EIH in chronic low back pain patients, exercise has been shown to induce pressure hyperalgesia post-exercise in patients with chronic fatigue syndrome (Meeus et al., 2010; Whiteside, Hansen, & Chaudhuri, 2004). To date, the influence of acute exercise on pain sensitivity and symptoms in patients with fibromyalgia has been equivocal. Several studies

(Kosek et al., 1996; Staud, Robinson, & Price, 2005; Vierck et al., 2001; Hoeger Bement et al., 2011; Lannersten & Kosek, 2010) have reported increased pain ratings and hyperalgesia during and after exercise while several others have reported decreases or no change (Newcomb, Koltyn, Morgan, & Cook, 2011; Kadetoff & Kosek, 2007; Staud, Robinson, Weyl, & Price, 2010). Newcomb and colleagues (Newcomb et al., 2011) recently reported that a low-intensity bout of cycle ergometry resulted in reduced sensitivity to pressure pain stimuli and improved symptoms up to 4 days following the acute exercise bout. In patients with chronic trapezius myalgia, multi-segmental increases in pressure pain thresholds were found post-exercise when performed by a body part distant from the painful muscles (Lannersten & Kosek, 2010), but not when exercise was performed in the area of the painful muscles (Lannersten & Kosek, 2010). Together, these data suggest that intensity, duration and exercise modality can influence EIH and symptom responses to acute exercise in chronic pain patients.

Effects of pain on motor control systems

There are dense synaptic connections from nociceptive fibres to both motoneurons and sensory neurons involved in motor control (tendon organs and muscle spindles) located in the ventral horn of the spinal cord (Schomburg, Steffens, & Kniffki, 1999). Moreover, fibres with nociceptive properties have a prominent influence on reflex control (Schomburg & Steffens, 2002). Because exercise involves increases in several physiological systems, including skeletal muscle activity, there are several mechanisms through which exercise may be communicating with the pain system. Based on this, there are several models that have been discussed with respect to the bilateral effects of pain on motor control systems.

An early explanatory model described the cause of muscle pain as based on muscle hyperactivity, which was maintained by a vicious cycle due to muscle ischemia (Travell, Rinzler, & Herman, 1942). In line with this, hyperactivity was also suggested to be important in the stress-causality and reflex-spasm models (deVries, 1966; Cohen, 1978). The model suggesting that muscle pain induces ongoing muscle hyperactivity was not systematically assessed in humans until the late 1990s. However, animal data indicate that muscle nociception results in muscle hyperactivity due to facilitation of γ-motoneurons (Schmidt, Kniffki, & Schomburg, 1981; Johansson & Sojka, 1991). The implication of such facilitation was discussed as a reflex-mediated spread of muscle stiffness and potentially the launch of a vicious cycle of hyperactivity. However, recent animal studies did not corroborate facilitation of the muscle spindle activity during muscle nociception (Ro & Capra, 2001; Masri, Ro, & Capra, 2005), but instead demonstrated that a modified spindle sensitivity was responsible for the change in proprioceptive function.

The pain-adaptation model links activity in nociceptive afferents, a central pattern generator, motor function and muscle coordination (Lund, Stohler, & Widmer, 1993). This model predicts that during muscle pain, muscle activity in antagonistic phases is facilitated and muscle activity in agonistic phases is inhibited, which may produce a decrease in movement amplitude and velocity. The pain-adaptation model is organized as inhibition and facilitation of motoneurons depending on the functional phases (agonist or antagonist) of the painful muscle. Recently this model was revised based on human experimental and clinical data, incorporating a more functional adaptation described by redistribution of activity between and within muscles to protect the painful structure (i.e., joint or muscle) instead of the specific agonist inhibition and increased antagonist activity originally proposed (Hodges, 2011).

The influence of muscle pain on the resting muscle

Increased resting muscle activity after experimental facial muscle pain compared with baseline recordings has been reported (Ashton-Miller, McGlashen, Herzenberg, & Stohler, 1990), but not compared with a sham pain condition where subjects recalled a painful condition without having the actual pain stimulation (Stohler, Zhang, & Lund, 1996). This indicates that the increased muscle activity is not related to the pain per se but rather is due to activities related to facial expressions. In a later study, a transient increase in the resting EMG activity was recorded during i.m. injection of hypertonic saline, which was not found after injection of the non-painful isotonic saline (Svensson, Graven-Nielsen, Matre, & Arendt-Nielsen, 1998). The transient increased muscle activity was not maintained during the ongoing muscle pain. Likewise, the resting EMG activity between repeated maximal voluntary contractions was not increased during experimental muscle pain (Graven-Nielsen, Svensson, & Arendt-Nielsen, 1997).

Musculoskeletal pain patients present both with increased and unchanged resting EMG activities. In fibromyalgia patients an increased resting EMG activity between contractions has been reported (Elert, Dahlqvist, Henriksson-Larsén, & Gerdle, 1989) in contrast to other studies where no changes in the resting muscle EMG activity was found in fibromyalgia (Zidar, Bäckman, Bengtsson, & Henriksson, 1990), low back pain (Collins, Cohen, Nailboff, & Schandler, 1982; Ahern, Follick, Council, Laser-Wolston, & Litchman, 1988), temporomandibular pain (Bodéré, Tea, Giroux-Metges, & Woda, 2005) and chronic neck pain due to trapezius myalgia (Larsson, Öberg, & Larsson, 1999). Spontaneous muscle activity (deVries, 1966) and unchanged (Howell, Chila, Ford, David, & Gates, 1985; Bobbert, Hollander, & Huijing, 1986) resting muscle activity were detected at the time for maximal soreness induced by eccentric exercise (delayed onset muscle soreness).

The influence of muscle pain on contractions without movement

In experimental muscle pain models, the maximal voluntary contraction (MVC) is attenuated as illustrated in Figure 24.2 (Graven-Nielsen, Lund, Arendt-Nielsen, Danneskiold-Samsøe, & Bliddal, 2002; Graven-Nielsen et al., 1997; Wang, Arima, Arendt-Nielsen, & Svensson, 2000).

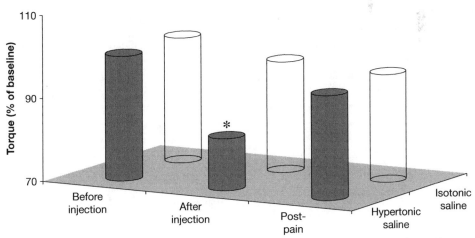

Figure 24.2 Mean maximal voluntary knee extension torque recorded before and after infusion (during, 10 minutes and 30 minutes post-infusion) of isotonic and hypertonic saline into m. rectus femoris. Significantly decreased torque compared with both pre-pain and post-pain recordings and compared with the recording immediately after infusion of isotonic saline is indicated (★) (based on data from Graven-Nielsen, Lund, Arendt-Nielsen, Danneskiold-Samsøe, & Biddell, 2002).

This decrease in MVC is not associated with modified contractile properties of muscle fibres and is likely better explained by a central inhibitory effect (Graven-Nielsen et al., 2002; Farina, Arendt-Nielsen, & Graven-Nielsen, 2005a). In fibromyalgia patients supramaximal stimulation of the ulnar nerve shows no difference in the strength of the adductor pollicis muscle between patients and control subjects, suggesting a deficient central activation of motor units in these patients explaining the reduced strength (Bäckman, Bengtsson, Bengtsson, Lennmarken, & Henriksson, 1988). Also, in localized pain conditions, attenuated MVC has been reported, e.g., in lateral epicondylalgia patients reduced strength is recorded in their sore arm compared to asymptomatic arms in controls (Slater, Arendt-Nielsen, Wright, & Graven-Nielsen, 2005). Interestingly, in trapezius myalgia patients, increased muscle activity during static contractions has been reported (Larsson et al., 1999).

Submaximal static contractions (e.g., 80% of the MVC before pain) are possible to maintain during experimental muscle pain, although with a significant reduction in endurance time (Ciubotariu, Arendt-Nielsen, & Graven-Nielsen, 2004). The different findings between the maximal contraction force, which is reduced by muscle pain, and submaximal contraction force, where the required force can be obtained during pain, is probably due to changes in descending neural drive to motoneurons. During MVC the descending neural drive cannot be voluntarily increased, and a pain-related inhibitory mechanism controlling the motoneurons may therefore explain the decreased MVC. In contrast, during submaximal contractions the voluntary neural drive can be increased and thus compensate for pain-related inhibitory mechanisms. Experimental muscle pain can also delay the recovery phase after fatiguing contractions (Ciubotariu, Arendt-Nielsen, & Graven-Nielsen, 2007), illustrating that the combination of pain and fatigue has a detrimental effect relevant in occupational conditions.

A decreased endurance time is reported in muscle pain patients performing a submaximal contraction compared with sex- and age-matched controls (Clark, Beemsterboer, & Jacobson, 1984; Elert, Dahlqvist, Almay, & Eisemann, 1993; Bengtsson, Bäckman, Lindblom, & Skogh, 1994; Gay, Maton, Rendell, & Majourau, 1994). When submaximal painful contractions are completed, at the cost of increased voluntary neural drive, then a more pronounced central fatigue may explain the decreased endurance time (James, Sacco, & Jones, 1995). Various physiological factors (e.g., microcirculation in the muscle) can influence endurance time in patients, which is not likely to occur in healthy volunteers exposed to experimental muscle pain. These results suggest that chronic pain can interfere with muscle activity/physical activity and that unique mechanisms may be involved.

Reduced muscle activity during pain has been recorded by surface EMG for contraction levels above 25% MVC (Falla, Farina, Dahl, & Graven-Nielsen, 2007) and impaired firing of single motor units during low contraction levels has been reported (Sohn, Graven-Nielsen, Arendt-Nielsen, & Svensson, 2000; Farina, Arendt-Nielsen, Merletti, & Graven-Nielsen, 2004; Tucker, Butler, Graven-Nielsen, Riek, & Hodges, 2009). The reduction in firing rate of motor units has been shown to be correlated with experimental muscle pain intensity (Farina et al., 2004). In fatiguing but non-painful contractions, reduced motor unit firing over time has also been found. During experimental muscle pain, the initial firing rate is reduced to the same level as at the end of fatiguing non-painful contractions (Farina, Arendt-Nielsen, & Graven-Nielsen, 2005b). This suggests that the nociceptive system in muscles is potentially linked with the mechanism causing reduced motor unit firing during fatigue.

The effect of muscle pain during static contractions not only decreases muscle activity of the painful muscle, but importantly also attenuates the synergistic muscles (Ciubotariu et al., 2004; Falla et al., 2007). Within muscles the spatial distribution of activity can be recorded by surface matrix EMG electrodes. With this method trapezius muscle activity was found to be fully reorganized and decreased by experimental muscle pain (Madeleine, Leclerc, Arendt-Nielsen, Ravier, & Farina, 2006). Generating the required contraction force and compensating for the muscle inhibition requires a new muscle coordination that eventually results in overload of otherwise non-painful muscles. This may also explain the larger movement variability seen in acute pain, whereas chronic or prolonged pain seems to reduce the movement variability (Madeleine, 2010). The contraction force is, among other factors, determined by the motor unit firing rate, and it is unclear how constant force can be maintained during muscle pain despite the decrease in motor unit firing rate. Motor unit twitch properties can change, which has been suggested as a compensatory mechanism for the decreased motor unit firing during pain. Accordingly, during experimental muscle pain, increased twitch force of low-threshold motor units has been reported (Sohn, Graven-Nielsen, Arendt-Nielsen, & Svensson, 2004; Farina, Arendt-Nielsen, Roatta, & Graven-Nielsen, 2008). On the contrary, muscle membrane properties seem to be unaffected by experimental muscle pain as both the M-wave (Farina et al., 2005a) and motor unit conduction velocity (Farina et al., 2005b) are unchanged. In post-pain conditions, when the motor unit firing rate returns to normal, the peak twitch force remains elevated (Farina et al., 2008), which strongly suggests that the facilitated twitch force is not the main mechanism compensating for the decline in motor unit firing rate. The maintenance of force may also be achieved if the nervous system increases the activity of muscles with a synergistic role to compensate for the decreased force produced by the painful muscle. Nevertheless, motor units in synergistic muscles neighbouring a painful muscle also demonstrate reduced firings (Figure 24.3) (Hodges, Ervilha, & Graven-Nielsen, 2008), and do not account for maintenance of force

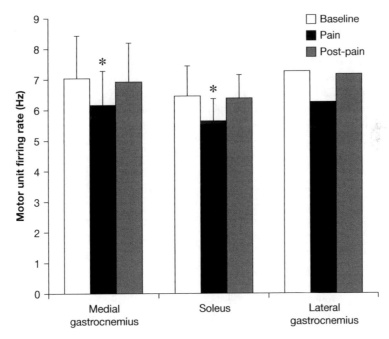

Figure 24.3 Mean discharge rate of single motor units during plantar-flexion at low-level contractions. Experimental pain was induced by injection of hypertonic saline in the lateral gastrocnemius muscle. The single motor units were identified and recorded before (open bars), during (solid bars) and post-pain (grey bars) in synergistic muscles (soleus, medial gastrocnemious). During pain the instantaneous firing rate is significantly reduced in synergistic motor units (★: P < 0.05). In one session a single motor unit was recorded in the lateral gastrocnemious (based on data from Hodges, Ervilha, & Graven-Nielsen, 2008).

during painful contractions without movements. Recruitment of additional motor units (e.g., high threshold units) during pain is an attractive mechanism to explain the maintained force with reduced motor unit firing. Recent data demonstrate such recruitment in combination with decreased motor unit firing in painful muscles (Tucker et al., 2009).

The experimental pain model, based on injections of hypertonic saline, does not affect the contractile apparatus (Graven-Nielsen et al., 2002). On the contrary, delayed onset muscle soreness (DOMS) is probably related to ultra-structural damage, which may affect the contractile properties resulting in loss of force. Reported loss of force within the first 24 hours of DOMS may be explained by inhibition of motor cortex and/or spinal motoneurons (Prasartwuth, Taylor, & Gandevia, 2005). Another study showed that eccentric contractions caused reduced EMG amplitude during sustained contractions, which was not found before DOMS, suggesting a modification of contractile properties (Hedayatpour, Falla, Arendt-Nielsen, & Farina, 2008). Increased (Kroon & Naeije, 1991), decreased (Nie, Arendt-Nielsen, Kawczynski, & Madeleine, 2007) and no differences in (Bajaj, Madeleine, Sjogaard, & Arendt-Nielsen, 2002) EMG activity during DOMS with constant contractions have also been reported. Therefore, when conditions include changes of the contractile properties in addition to modulation of motor control parameters by nociception, the results should be interpreted with caution.

The influence of muscle pain on contractions with movement

In conditions with experimental and clinical low back pain it was found that the low back muscle activity was increased in phases where the EMG activity normally is silent, and not affected or decreased in phases with strong EMG activity in control subjects (Arendt-Nielsen, Graven-Nielsen, Svarrer, & Svensson, 1996). Similarly, gait muscle pain often causes decreased EMG in the agonistic phase and increased EMG in the antagonistic phase of leg muscle activity (Graven-Nielsen et al., 1997). A similar finding is reported during trunk flexion-extension movements, where the antagonist phase showed increased activity in low back pain patients, which is normally silent in pain-free controls (Sihvonen, Partanen, Hänninen, & Soimakallio, 1991). The functional outcome of this reorganized motor control is reduced movement amplitudes in experimental and clinical musculoskeletal pain conditions (Graven-Nielsen & Arendt-Nielsen, 2008), which may protect the painful muscle by reducing the load on the painful structure. Individual combinations of increased, decreased and co-contraction activity of trunk flexors and extensors may be another strategy adopted to maintain spine stability in conditions of experimental low back pain (Hodges, Cholewicki, Coppieters, & MacDonald, 2006).

During muscle pain another strategy is characterized by decreased activity in both the agonistic and antagonistic muscles without significantly impairing the movement amplitude or acceleration (Ervilha, Arendt-Nielsen, Duarte, & Graven-Nielsen, 2004). Interestingly, the initial (100 ms) agonistic EMG burst activity was decreased during muscle pain suggesting a reorganized motor strategy. Reduced feed-forward responses of the abdominal muscles were found in conditions of experimental low back muscle pain and this change in motor planning may compromise spine stability (Hodges, Moseley, Gabrielsson, & Gandevia, 2003). Another example is gait initiation, which also depends on specific motor control strategies and is perturbed by experimental muscle pain (Madeleine, Voigt, & Arendt-Nielsen, 1999). In occupational settings abnormal motor planning results in compensatory action from other muscles to achieve the required movement, and this may possibly contribute to the development of musculoskeletal pain problems. During pointing movements increased trapezius activity was found with experimental pain induced in the biceps brachii muscle and this could constitute a compensatory response (Ervilha et al., 2004). Reorganized trapezius muscle activity during repetitive shoulder flexion has been characterized as reduced activity of the upper trapezius (with experimental pain) accompanied by increased muscle activity of the lower trapezius as compensation (Falla, Farina, & Graven-Nielsen, 2007).

The reorganized muscle coordination caused by muscle pain has strong biomechanical impact on the other skeletal structures. During experimental pain induced in the vastus medialis muscle, the functional significance of knee joint control during gait was assessed by three-dimensional gait analyses (Henriksen et al., 2007). The quadriceps muscle activity was reduced by muscle pain causing an impaired knee joint control and joint instability during walking. Similar changes have been observed in patients with osteoarthritic knee pain and experimental knee pain (Henriksen, Graven-Nielsen, Aaboe, Andriacchi, & Bliddal, 2010). The impaired joint control may place the knee joint prone to injury and as such participate in the chronicity of musculoskeletal problems. In recent studies, Hirata et al. (Hirata, Arendt-Nielsen, & Graven-Nielsen, 2010; Hirata, Ervilha, Arendt-Nielsen, & Graven-Nielsen, 2011) reported that pain induced in knee muscles challenged postural control, which may increase the risk of falls. Such biomechanical effects have important clinical implications for training and rehabilitation of patients with knee pain.

Summary and future directions

Aerobic, isometric and resistance exercises produce hypoalgesic effects in healthy subjects. Exercise-induced hypoalgesia following aerobic exercise is more likely to occur with higher intensity and longer duration, whereas EIH occurs after isometric contractions at both low and high intensity and may be independent of duration. Future studies are needed to examine chronic pain patients developing post-exercise pain in contrast to EIH, since hyperalgesia may block the mental health benefits of exercise.

A fundamental aspect of musculoskeletal pain conditions is motor control reorganization, which is most likely one crucial mechanism in understanding how acute pain may translate into a chronic pain condition. The interaction between musculoskeletal pain and motor control depends on the specific motor task. During dynamic exercise muscle pain causes a change in the coordination and changes in the co-contraction pattern. The functional adaptation to muscle pain may also involve increased muscle activity reflecting reorganized muscle coordination and strategy. In general, these findings do not support the 'vicious cycle' theory but rather an adaptive model predicting how muscle activity is reorganized in order to protect painful structures. Future pain models should address the variability and redundancy/reorganization in the motor control system, how this is affected by deep-tissue pain, and how this will interfere with motor performance and physical activity behaviours. Unfortunately the impaired functional effects caused by pain will counteract a potential positive effect of training on mental health.

References

Ahern, D. K., Follick, M. J., Council, J. R., Laser-Wolston, N., & Litchman, H. (1988). Comparison of lumbar paravertebral EMG patterns in chronic low back pain patients and non-patient controls. *Pain, 34*, 153–160.

Anshel, M. H., & Russell, K. G. (1994). Effect of aerobic and strength training on pain tolerance, pain appraisal and mood of unfit males as a function of pain location. *Journal of Sports Science, 12*, 535–547.

Arendt-Nielsen, L., Graven-Nielsen, T., Svarrer, H., & Svensson, P. (1996). The influence of low back pain on muscle activity and coordination during gait: A clinical and experimental study. *Pain, 64*, 231–240.

Ashton-Miller, J. A., McGlashen, K. M., Herzenberg, J. E., & Stohler, C. S. (1990). Cervical muscle myoelectric response to acute experimental sternocleidomastoid pain. *Spine, 15*, 1006–1012.

Bäckman, E., Bengtsson, A., Bengtsson, M., Lennmarken, C., & Henriksson, K. G. (1988). Skeletal muscle function in primary fibromyalgia. Effect of regional sympathetic blockade with guanethidine. *Acta Neurologica Scandinavica, 77*, 187–191.

Bajaj, P., Madeleine, P., Sjogaard, G., & Arendt-Nielsen, L. (2002). Assessment of postexercise muscle soreness by electromyography and mechanomyography. *Journal of Pain, 3,* 126–136.

Bengtsson, A., Bäckman, E., Lindblom, B., & Skogh, T. (1994). Long term follow-up of fibromyalgia patients: Clinical symptoms, muscular function, laboratory test – an eight year comparison study. *Journal of Musculoskeletal Pain, 2,* 67–80.

Bobbert, M. F., Hollander, A. P., & Huijing, P. A. (1986). Factors in delayed onset muscular soreness of man. *Medicine and Science in Sports and Exercise, 18,* 75–81.

Bodéré, C., Tea, S. H., Giroux-Metges, M. A., & Woda, A. (2005). Activity of masticatory muscles in subjects with different orofacial pain conditions. *Pain, 116,* 33–41.

Ciubotariu, A., Arendt-Nielsen, L., & Graven-Nielsen, T. (2004). The influence of muscle pain and fatigue on the activity of synergistic muscles of the leg. *European Journal of Applied Physiology, 91,* 604–614.

Ciubotariu, A., Arendt-Nielsen, L., & Graven-Nielsen, T. (2007). Localized muscle pain causes prolonged recovery after fatiguing isometric contractions. *Experimental Brain Research, 181,* 147–158.

Clark, G. T., Beemsterboer, P. L., & Jacobson, R. (1984). The effect of sustained submaximal clenching on maximum bite force in myofascial pain dysfunction patients. *Journal of Oral Rehabilitation, 11,* 387–391.

Cohen, M. J. (1978). Psychophysiological studies of headache: Is there similarity between migraine and muscle contraction headaches? *Headache, 18,* 189–196.

Collins, G. A., Cohen, M. J., Nailboff, B. D., & Schandler, S. L. (1982). Comparative analysis of paraspinal and frontalis EMG, heart rate and skin conductance in chronic low back pain patients and normals to various postures and stress. *Scandinavian Journal of Rehabilitation Medicine, 14,* 39–46.

deVries, H. A. (1966). Quantitative electromyographic investigation of the spasm theory of muscle pain. *American Journal of Physical Medicine, 45,* 119–134.

Droste, C. (1991). Physical exercise, endogenous opiates and pain regulation. *Schmerz, 5,* 138–147.

Elert, J. E., Dahlqvist, S. R., Almay, B., & Eisemann, M. (1993). Muscle endurance, muscle tension and personality traits in patients with muscle or joint pain – A pilot study. *Journal of Rheumatology, 20,* 1550–1556.

Elert, J. E., Dahlqvist, S. B. R., Henriksson-Larsén, K., & Gerdle, B. (1989). Increased EMG activity during short pauses in patients with primary fibromyalgia. *Scandinavian Journal of Rheumatology, 18,* 321–323.

Ervilha, U. F., Arendt-Nielsen, L., Duarte, M., & Graven-Nielsen, T. (2004). Effect of load level and muscle pain intensity on the motor control of elbow-flexion movements. *European Journal of Applied Physiology, 92,* 168–175.

Falla, D., Farina, D., Dahl, M. K., & Graven-Nielsen, T. (2007). Muscle pain induces task-dependent changes in cervical agonist/antagonist activity. *Journal of Applied Physiology, 102,* 601–609.

Falla, D., Farina, D., & Graven-Nielsen, T. (2007). Experimental muscle pain results in reorganization of coordination among trapezius muscle subdivisions during repetitive shoulder flexion. *Experimental Brain Research, 178,* 385–393.

Farina, D., Arendt-Nielsen, L., & Graven-Nielsen, T. (2005a). Experimental muscle pain decreases voluntary EMG activity but does not affect the muscle potential evoked by transcutaneous electrical stimulation. *Clinical Neurophysiology, 116,* 1558–1565.

Farina, D., Arendt-Nielsen, L., & Graven-Nielsen, T. (2005b). Experimental muscle pain reduces initial motor unit discharge rates during sustained submaximal contractions. *Journal of Applied Physiology, 98,* 999–1005.

Farina, D., Arendt-Nielsen, L., Merletti, R., & Graven-Nielsen, T. (2004). Effect of experimental muscle pain on motor unit firing rate and conduction velocity. *Journal of Neurophysiology, 91,* 1250–1259.

Farina, D., Arendt-Nielsen, L., Roatta, S., & Graven-Nielsen, T. (2008). The pain-induced decrease in low-threshold motor unit discharge rate is not associated with the amount of increase in spike-triggered average torque. *Clinical Neurophysiology, 119,* 43–51.

Gay, T., Maton, B., Rendell, J., & Majourau, A. (1994). Characteristics of muscle fatigue in patients with myofascial pain-dysfunction syndrome. *Archives of Oral Biology, 39,* 847–852.

Graven-Nielsen, T., & Arendt-Nielsen, L. (2008). Impact of clinical and experimental pain on muscle strength and activity. *Current Rheumatology Reports, 10,* 475–481.

Graven-Nielsen, T., Lund, H., Arendt-Nielsen, L., Danneskiold-Samsøe, B., & Bliddal, H. (2002). Inhibition of maximal voluntary contraction force by experimental muscle pain: A centrally mediated mechanism. *Muscle & Nerve, 26,* 708–712.

Graven-Nielsen, T., Svensson, P., & Arendt-Nielsen, L. (1997). Effects of experimental muscle pain on muscle activity and co-ordination during static and dynamic motor function. *Electroencephalography and Clinical Neurophysiology, 105,* 156–164.

Gurevich, M., Kohn, P. M., & Davis, C. (1994). Exercise-induced analgesia and the role of reactivity in pain sensitivity. *Journal of Sports Science, 12*, 549–559.

Hedayatpour, N., Falla, D., Arendt-Nielsen, L., & Farina, D. (2008). Sensory and electromyographic mapping during delayed-onset muscle soreness. *Medicine and Science in Sports and Exercise, 40*, 326–334.

Henriksen, M., Alkjaer, T., Lund, H., Simonsen, E. B., Graven-Nielsen, T., Danneskiold-Samsoe, B. et al. (2007). Experimental quadriceps muscle pain impairs knee joint control during walking. *Journal of Applied Physiology, 103*, 132–139.

Henriksen, M., Graven-Nielsen, T., Aaboe, J., Andriacchi, T. P., & Bliddal, H. (2010). Gait changes in patients with knee osteoarthritis are replicated by experimental knee pain. *Arthritis Care Research (Hoboken), 62*, 501–509.

Hirata, R. P., Arendt-Nielsen, L., & Graven-Nielsen, T. (2010). Experimental calf muscle pain attenuates the postural stability during quiet stance and perturbation. *Clinical Biomechanics (Bristol, Avon), 25*, 931–937.

Hirata, R. P., Ervilha, U. F., Arendt-Nielsen, L., & Graven-Nielsen, T. (2011). Experimental muscle pain challenges the postural stability during quiet stance and unexpected posture perturbation. *Journal of Pain, 12*, 911–919.

Hodges, P., Cholewicki, J., Coppieters, M., & MacDonald, D. (2006). *Trunk muscle activity is increased during experimental back pain, but the pattern varies between individuals.* In Proceedings of International Society for Electrophysiologyand Kinesiology, Turin.

Hodges, P. W. (2011). Pain and motor control: From the laboratory to rehabilitation. *Journal of Electromyography and Kinesiology, 21*, 220–228.

Hodges, P. W., Ervilha, U. F., & Graven-Nielsen, T. (2008). Changes in motor unit firing rate in synergist muscles cannot explain the maintenance of force during constant force painful contractions. *Journal of Pain, 9*, 1169–1174.

Hodges, P. W., Moseley, G. L., Gabrielsson, A., & Gandevia, S. C. (2003). Experimental muscle pain changes feedforward postural responses of the trunk muscles. *Experimental Brain Research, 151*, 262–271.

Hoeger Bement, M. K. (2009). Exercise-induced hypoalgesia: An evidence-based review. In K. A. Sluka (Ed.), *Mechanisms and management of pain for the physical therapist* (pp. 143–166). Seattle: IASP.

Hoeger Bement, M. K., Dicapo, J., Rasiarmos, R., & Hunter, S. K. (2008). Dose response of isometric contractions on pain perception in healthy adults. *Medicine and Science in Sports and Exercise, 40*, 1880–1889.

Hoeger Bement, M. K., Rasiarmos, R. L., DiCapo, J. M., Lewis, A., Keller, M. L., Harkins, A. L. et al. (2009). The role of the menstrual cycle phase in pain perception before and after an isometric fatiguing contraction. *European Journal of Applied Physiology, 106*, 105–112.

Hoeger Bement, M. K., Weyer, A., Hartley, S., Drewek, B., Harkins, A. L., & Hunter, S. K. (2011). Pain perception after isometric exercise in women with fibromyalgia. *Archives of Physical Medicine and Rehabilitation, 92*, 89–95.

Hoffman, M. D., Shepanski, M. A., Mackenzie, S. P., & Clifford, P. S. (2005). Experimentally induced pain perception is acutely reduced by aerobic exercise in people with chronic low back pain. *Journal of Rehabilitation Research and Development, 42*, 183–190.

Hoffman, M. D., Shepanski, M. A., Ruble, S. B., Valic, Z., Buckwalter, J. B., & Clifford, P. S. (2004). Intensity and duration threshold for aerobic exercise-induced analgesia to pressure pain. *Archives of Physical Medicine and Rehabilitation, 85*, 1183–1187.

Howell, J. N., Chila, A. G., Ford, G., David, D., & Gates, T. (1985). An electromyographic study of elbow motion during postexercise muscle soreness. *Journal of Applied Physiology, 58*, 1713–1718.

James, C., Sacco, P., & Jones, D. A. (1995). Loss of power during fatigue of human leg muscles. *Journal of Physiology (Lond.), 484*, 237–246.

Janal, M. N., Colt, E. W., Clark, W. C., & Glusman, M. (1984). Pain sensitivity, mood and plasma endocrine levels in man following long-distance running: Effects of naloxone. *Pain, 19*, 13–25.

Johansson, H., & Sojka, P. (1991). Pathophysiological mechanisms involved in genesis and spread of muscular tension in occupational muscle pain and in chronic musculoskeletal pain syndromes: A hypothesis. *Medical Hypotheses, 35*, 196–203.

Kadetoff, D., & Kosek, E. (2007). The effects of static muscular contraction on blood pressure, heart rate, pain ratings and pressure pain thresholds in healthy individuals and patients with fibromyalgia. *European Journal of Pain, 11*, 39–47.

Koltyn, K. F. (2000). Analgesia following exercise: A review. *Sports Medicine, 29*, 85–98.

Koltyn, K. F. (2002). Exercise-induced hypoalgesia and intensity of exercise. *Sports Medicine, 32*, 477–487.

Koltyn, K. F., & Arbogast, R. W. (1998). Perception of pain after resistance exercise. *British Journal of Sports Medicine, 32,* 20–24.

Koltyn, K. F., Garvin, A. W., Gardiner, R. L., & Nelson, T. F. (1996). Perception of pain following aerobic exercise. *Medicine and Science in Sports and Exercise, 28,* 1418–1421.

Kosek, E., Ekholm, J., & Hansson, P. (1996). Modulation of pressure pain thresholds during and following isometric contraction in patients with fibromyalgia and in healthy controls. *Pain, 64,* 415–423.

Kosek, E., & Lundberg, L. (2003). Segmental and plurisegmental modulation of pressure pain thresholds during static muscle contractions in healthy individuals. *European Journal of Pain, 7,* 251–258.

Kroon, G. W., & Naeije, M. (1991). Recovery of the human biceps electromyogram after heavy eccentric, concentric or isometric exercise. *European Journal of Applied Physiology and Occupational Physiology, 63,* 444–448.

Lannersten, L., & Kosek, E. (2010). Dysfunction of endogenous pain inhibition during exercise with painful muscles in patients with shoulder myalgia and fibromyalgia. *Pain, 151,* 77–86.

Larsson, R., Öberg, P. Å., & Larsson, S.-E. (1999). Changes of trapezius muscle blood flow and electromyography in chronic neck pain due to trapezius myalgia. *Pain, 79,* 45–50.

Lund, J. P., Stohler, C. S., & Widmer, C. G. (1993). The relationship between pain and muscle activity in fibromyalgia and similar conditions. In H. Værøy & H. Merskey (Eds.), *Progress in fibromyalgia and myofascial pain* (pp. 311–327). Amsterdam: Elsevier.

Madeleine, P. (2010). On functional motor adaptations: From the quantification of motor strategies to the prevention of musculoskeletal disorders in the neck-shoulder region. *Acta Physiologica (Oxf). 199 Suppl 679,* 1–46.

Madeleine, P., Leclerc, F., Arendt-Nielsen, L., Ravier, P., & Farina, D. (2006). Experimental muscle pain changes the spatial distribution of upper trapezius muscle activity during sustained contraction. *Clinical Neurophysiology, 117,* 2436–2445.

Madeleine, P., Voigt, M., & Arendt-Nielsen, L. (1999). Reorganisation of human step initiation during acute experimental muscle pain. *Gait and Posture, 10,* 240–247.

Masri, R., Ro, J. Y., & Capra, N. (2005). The effect of experimental muscle pain on the amplitude and velocity sensitivity of jaw closing muscle spindle afferents. *Brain Research, 1050,* 138–147.

Meeus, M., Roussel, N. A., Truijen, S., & Nijs, J. (2010). Reduced pressure pain thresholds in response to exercise in chronic fatigue syndrome but not in chronic low back pain: An experimental study. *Journal of Rehabilitation Medicine, 42,* 884–890.

Newcomb, L. W., Koltyn, K. F., Morgan, W. P., & Cook, D. B. (2011). Influence of preferred versus prescribed exercise on pain in fibromyalgia. *Medicine and Science in Sports and Exercise, 43,* 1106–1113.

Nie, H., Arendt-Nielsen, L., Kawczynski, A., & Madeleine, P. (2007). Gender effects on trapezius surface EMG during delayed onset muscle soreness due to eccentric shoulder exercise. *Journal of Electromyography and Kinesiology, 17,* 401–409.

Nielsen, M. M., Mortensen, A., Sorensen, J. K., Simonsen, O., & Graven-Nielsen, T. (2009). Reduction of experimental muscle pain by passive physiological movements. *Manual Therapy, 14,* 101–109.

Padawer, W. J., & Levine, F. M. (1992). Exercise-induced analgesia: Fact or artifact? *Pain, 48,* 131–135.

Prasartwuth, O., Taylor, J. L., & Gandevia, S. C. (2005). Maximal force, voluntary activation and muscle soreness after eccentric damage to human elbow flexor muscles. *Journal of Physiology, 567,* 337–348.

Ro, J. Y., & Capra, N. F. (2001). Modulation of jaw muscle spindle afferent activity following intramuscular injections with hypertonic saline. *Pain, 92,* 117–127.

Schmidt, R. F., Kniffki, K.-D., & Schomburg, E. D. (1981). Der Einfluss kleinkalibriger Muskelafferenzen auf den Muskeltonus. In H. Bauer, W. P. Koella, & H. Struppler (Eds.), *Therapie der spastic* (pp. 71–86). München: Verlag for angewandte Wissenschaft.

Schomburg, E. D., & Steffens, H. (2002). Only minor spinal motor reflex effects from feline group IV muscle nociceptors. *Neuroscience Research, 44,* 213–223.

Schomburg, E. D., Steffens, H., & Kniffki, K. D. (1999). Contribution of group III and IV muscle afferents to multisensorial spinal motor control in cats. *Neuroscience Research, 33,* 195–206.

Shyu, B. C., Andersson, S. A., & Thoren, P. (1982). Endorphin mediated increase in pain threshold induced by long-lasting exercise in rats. *Life Sciences, 30,* 833–840.

Sihvonen, T., Partanen, J., Hänninen, O., & Soimakallio, S. (1991). Electric behavior of low back muscles during lumbar pelvic rhythm in low back pain patients and healthy controls. *Archives of Physical Medicine and Rehabilitation, 72,* 1080–1087.

Slater, H., Arendt-Nielsen, L., Wright, A., & Graven-Nielsen, T. (2005). Sensory and motor effects of experimental muscle pain in patients with lateral epicondylalgia and controls with delayed onset muscle soreness. *Pain, 114,* 118–130.

Sohn, M. K., Graven-Nielsen, T., Arendt-Nielsen, L., & Svensson, P. (2000). Inhibition of motor unit firing during experimental muscle pain in humans. *Muscle & Nerve, 23*, 1219–1226.

Sohn, M. K., Graven-Nielsen, T., Arendt-Nielsen, L., & Svensson, P. (2004). Effects of experimental muscle pain on mechanical properties of single motor units in human masseter. *Clinical Neurophysiology, 115*, 76–84.

Staud, R., Robinson, M. E., & Price, D. D. (2005). Isometric exercise has opposite effects on central pain mechanisms in fibromyalgia patients compared to normal controls. *Pain, 118*, 176–184.

Staud, R., Robinson, M. E., Weyl, E. E., & Price, D. D. (2010). Pain variability in fibromyalgia is related to activity and rest: Role of peripheral tissue impulse input. *Journal of Pain, 11*, 1376–1383.

Sternberg, W. F., Bokat, C., Kass, L., Alboyadjian, A., & Gracely, R. H. (2001). Sex-dependent components of the analgesia produced by athletic competition. *Journal of Pain, 2*, 65–74.

Stohler, C. S., Zhang, X., & Lund, J. P. (1996). The effect of experimental jaw muscle pain on postural muscle activity. *Pain, 66*, 215–221.

Svensson, P., Graven-Nielsen, T., Matre, D., & Arendt-Nielsen, L. (1998). Experimental muscle pain does not cause long-lasting increases in resting electromyographic activity. *Muscle & Nerve, 21*, 1382–1389.

Travell, J. G., Rinzler, S., & Herman, M. (1942). Pain and disability of the shoulder and arm. *Journal of the American Medical Association, 120*, 417–422.

Tucker, K., Butler, J., Graven-Nielsen, T., Riek, S., & Hodges, P. (2009). Motor unit recruitment strategies are altered during deep-tissue pain. *Journal of Neuroscience, 29*, 10820–10826.

Umeda, M., Newcomb, L. W., Ellingson, L. D., & Koltyn, K. F. (2010). Examination of the dose-response relationship between pain perception and blood pressure elevations induced by isometric exercise in men and women. *Biological Psychology, 85*, 90–96.

Vierck, C. J., Jr., Staud, R., Price, D. D., Cannon, R. L., Mauderli, A. P., & Martin, A. D. (2001). The effect of maximal exercise on temporal summation of second pain (windup) in patients with fibromyalgia syndrome. *Journal of Pain, 2*, 334–344.

Wang, K., Arima, T., Arendt-Nielsen, L., & Svensson, P. (2000). EMG-force relationships are influenced by experimental jaw-muscle pain. *Journal of Oral Rehabilitation, 27*, 394–402.

Whiteside, A., Hansen, S., & Chaudhuri, A. (2004). Exercise lowers pain threshold in chronic fatigue syndrome. *Pain, 109*, 497–499.

Zidar, J., Bäckman, E., Bengtsson, A., & Henriksson, K. G. (1990). Quantitative EMG and muscle tension in painful muscles in fibromyalgia. *Pain, 40*, 249–254.

25

EFFECTS OF PHYSICAL ACTIVITY ON LABORATORY PAIN

Studies on animals

Kathleen A. Sluka

Pain is defined as a sensory and emotional experience associated with actual or potential tissue damage, or described in terms as such (www.iasp-pain.org). Chronic pain is a significant health problem affecting between 20% and 50% of the population; musculoskeletal pain is the most common. Chronic pain interferes with everyday activities including work, recreational activities, and activities of daily living. Acute pain, directly related to a tissue injury, also significantly impacts daily activities. Further, adequate treatment of acute pain is thought to prevent development of chronic pain. Interestingly, only 25% of respondents with pain participate in exercise: 45% of those with chronic pain and 14% of those with acute (for a review, see Sluka, 2009b). One effective treatment common for nearly all types of chronic pain, including those with musculoskeletal pain, is regular exercise (for a review, see Bement, 2009). Regular exercise also produces analgesia in uninjured animals and reduces pain behaviors after inflammatory, non-inflammatory, and neuropathic injury (Bement & Sluka, 2005; Blustein, McLaughlin, & Hoffman, 2006; Konarzewski, Sadowski, & Jozwik, 1997; Kuphal, Fibuch, & Taylor, 2007; Mathes & Kanarek, 2006; Shankarappa, Piedras-Renteria, & Stubbs, Jr., 2011; Stagg et al., 2011). In contrast to regular exercise, a single bout of exercise can enhance pain in both humans and animals (Lannersten & Kosek, 2010; Sluka & Rasmussen, 2010; Staud, Robinson, & Price, 2005; Vierck et al., 2001; Yokoyama, Lisi, Moore, & Sluka, 2007). Understanding the mechanisms that underlie these diverse effects of exercise will assist in the development of exercise protocols for patient populations.

As pain is a subjective experience in humans, measurement of pain in animals is inferred from the response of the animal to noxious stimuli. Several common tests are done that apply noxious heat or mechanical stimuli to a peripheral site (tail, paw, muscle, joint) and measure the withdrawal of the animal to the stimuli as latency (heat) or force (mechanical). Thus, a longer latency or greater force to withdrawal is indicative of analgesia and a shorter latency or lower force to withdrawal is indicative of pain and termed hypersensitivity (i.e., hyperalgesia). In addition, spontaneous pain behaviors – flinching or licking – are also measured in response to an acute injection of noxious chemical stimuli – formalin or acetic acid. To model pain conditions, several animal models have been developed. Neuropathic pain is induced by ligating a peripheral nerve and results in mechanical and heat hypersensitivity that lasts for months. Inflammatory pain is induced by injection of formalin, carrageenan, or complete Freund's adjuvant into paw, muscle, or joints. An initial acute inflammatory response is followed by a chronic inflammatory response and results in decreased weight bearing, limb guarding, heat hypersensitivity, and mechanical hypersensitivity. Non-inflammatory chronic muscle pain is induced by two intramuscular acidic saline injections (2–5 days apart) and results in mechanical hypersensitivity without tissue damage. Spontaneous acute pain is induced by intraperitoneal acetic acid injections or intraplantar formalin injections and results in flinching and licking behaviors for 10–60 minutes.

Nociceptors respond to noxious stimuli and transmit information to the central nervous system for perception of pain; a schematic diagram of this pathway is shown in Figure 25.1A. Briefly, the nociceptors innervating peripheral tissue are activated by tissue injury, or noxious stimuli, and subsequently transmit this information to nociceptive neurons in the spinal cord dorsal horn. These neurons, termed spinothalamic (STT) cells, then send information to the thalamus and to the cortex for the perception of pain. The somatosensory cortices (SI and SII) are primarily involved in the sensation of pain in terms of quality, location, duration, and intensity, while the anterior cingulate and insular cortices (IC and CC) mediate the emotional component of pain (Hofbauer, Rainville, Duncan, & Bushnell, 2001; Rainville, Duncan, Price, Carrier, & Bushnell, 1997). Figure 25.1B shows a schematic diagram of descending inhibitory pathways thought to be involved in exercise-induced analgesia. In particular, the periaqueductal gray (PAG) in the midbrain sends input through the rostral ventromedial medulla (RVM) in the brainstem, which subsequently projects to the spinal cord. Activation of this pathway inhibits activity of nociceptive dorsal horn neurons as well as activity of nociceptors entering the dorsal horn. Understanding of the activation of different pathways and receptors by exercise, as well as how exercise may interact with these pathways, is important to a better understanding of the effects of exercise on pain. This could lead to improved exercise prescription for individuals with pain.

As exercise can both reduce pain and increase pain, it is important to understand the different contexts and mechanisms underlying both phenomena to better manage people with painful conditions. To understand these mechanisms, animal models have been developed for both exercise-induced analgesia and exercise-induced pain. Recently several studies have begun to study these phenomena in more detail, and this chapter will review the underlying mechanisms for exercise-induced analgesia and exercise-induced pain focusing on animal models.

Exercise-induced analgesia

Effects of exercise on pain behaviors

There are a number of different types of exercises that have been used in animals to produce analgesia. These include (1) increased physical activity by allowing animals free access to running wheels in their cages generally for several weeks, (2) strengthening exercises where rats do resisted exercise training, and (3) aerobic conditioning exercises using either treadmill running or swimming. In general, these tasks have been done repetitively over days or weeks. More specifically, allowing rats free access to running wheels for 3 weeks increases withdrawal responses to noxious heat stimuli applied to the tail (tail flick) (Kanarek, Gerstein, Wildman, Mathes, & D'Anci, 1998; Mathes & Kanarek, 2006). Similarly, in mice bred for high running wheel activity, withdrawal thresholds to noxious heat (tail flick) are higher than control mice (Li, Rhodes, Girard, Gammie, & Garland, 2004). A single swimming exercise task at either a low intensity or high intensity also increases withdrawal responses to noxious heat (tail flick) (Blustein et al., 2006). A resistance strengthening exercise program for 12 weeks in rats increases the paw withdrawal latency to noxious mechanical stimulation; this analgesic effect lasts for 15 minutes after ending

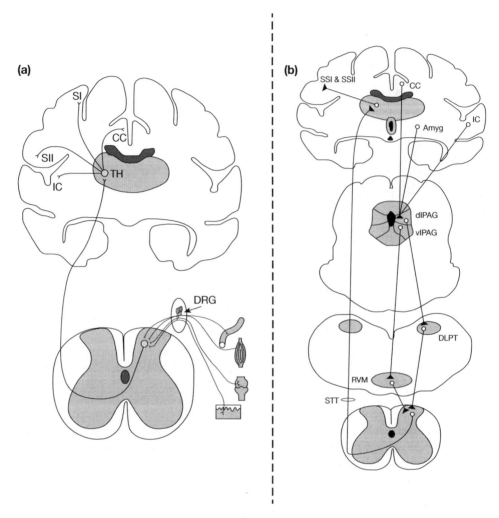

Figure 25.1 Schematic diagrams showing ascending nociceptive pathways (a) and inhibitory pathways (b). Nociceptors (first-order neuron) innervating joints send input to the spinal cord dorsal horn and synapse on spinothalamic tract cells (STT) (second-order neuron). STT cells then project supraspinally to the thalamus to synapse on a thalamic neuron (third-order neuron), which then projects to cortical sites, somatosensory cortex (SI, SII), insular cortex (IC), and anterior cingulate cortex (CC), resulting in perception of pain. B. Descending inhibitory pathways include the periaqueductual gray matter (vlPAG and dlPAG), which projects to the rostroventomedial medulla (RVM) and the dorsolateral pons (DLPT). The RVM and the DLPT then project to the spinal cord and inhibit activity in nociceptive neurons.

the task (Mazzardo-Martins et al., 2010). Thus, in uninjured rats, studies show that wheel running, swimming, and resistance training result in analgesia.

Repeated physical activity or exercise training prevents the development of acute pain behaviors to noxious stimuli, and reverses pain behaviors in animal models of muscle and nerve pain. For example, 5–9 days of swimming activity at moderate intensity prevents spontaneous pain-like behaviors induced by intraperitoneal acetic acid injection (Mazzardo-Martins et al., 2010) and by intraplantar formalin injection (Kuphal et al., 2007). In animals, repeated aerobic exercise tasks like swimming and treadmill running reduce neuropathic pain induced by nerve injury or diabetes, and chronic muscle pain induced by repeated acid injections (Bement & Sluka, 2005; Korb et al., 2010; Kuphal et al., 2007; Shankarappa et al., 2011; Sharma, Ryals, Gajewski, & Wright, 2010; Stagg et al., 2011). For example, after development of non-inflammatory muscle pain induced by repeated acid injections, 15–30 minutes of treadmill running for 4 days (6m/min; low intensity) reverses the existing mechanical hypersensitivity when compared to sedentary rats; this effect occurs after the first 15-minute task and continues throughout 4 days of exercise (Bement & Sluka, 2005). In the same model of non-inflammatory muscle pain, moderate-intensity treadmill running for 30–45 minutes (13–16m/min) attenuated development of mechanical hypersensitivity when compared to sedentary mice (Sharma et al., 2010). In this study, it is unknown if moderate intensity had an immediate effect since changes were not measured until after 1 week of exercise training. In animals with diabetic neuropathy induced by streptozotocin, treadmill running for 60 minutes/day, 5 days per week (18m/min; high intensity), started at the time of induction of diabetes, delays the onset of hypersensitivity to noxious heat without changing blood sugar concentration (Shankarappa et al., 2011). Similarly, in animals with neuropathic pain induced by sciatic nerve injury, treadmill running (16m/min, 8% grade, high intensity), started at the time of injury or 3 weeks later, decreased the duration of mechanical and heat hypersensitivity with significant reductions starting 3 weeks after exercise (Figure 25.2A) (Stagg et al., 2011). The analgesic effects were similar if the animals exercised 3 days per week or 5 days per week, but did not occur at a lower intensity (10m/min). In animals with neuropathic pain (sciatic nerve injury), a 2-week training session of 90 minutes/day forced swimming was performed prior to injury. Rats continued to swim for 90 minutes per day after the nerve injury. By the third week rats showed reduced hypersensitivity to noxious cold and heat stimuli when compared to sedentary animals (Kuphal et al., 2007). These studies show that regular exercise can prevent or reduce the duration of hypersensitivity in animal models of pain. It should be noted that forced exercise tasks such as treadmill running or swimming may produce analgesia through a stress response, and it is well known that stress can produce analgesia without the exercise task (Blustein et al., 2006; Hopkins, Spinella, Pavlovic, & Bodnar, 1998; King, Devine, Vierck, Rodgers, & Yezierski, 2003; Konarzewski et al., 1997). Exercise also produces a variety of effects that may influence pain including affecting the sympathetic, cardiovascular, and motor systems (Danion, Latash, Li, & Zatsiorsky, 2001; Morimoto, Tan, Nishiyasu, Sone, & Murakami, 2000; Roveda et al., 2003; Sacco, Hope, Thickbroom, Byrnes, & Mastaglia, 1999; Spierer et al., 2007). In summary, a variety of exercise programs in animals produce analgesia in uninjured animals, prevent the development of pain behaviors to acute noxious stimuli, and reduce pain behaviors in animals with chronic pain conditions.

Mechanisms underlying exercise-induced analgesia

Opioid mechanisms

It is generally thought that exercise produces analgesia by activating endogenous opioid mechanisms. Centrally, this classical opioid analgesic pathway involves activation of the PAG in the midbrain, which projects through the RVM and subsequently to the spinal cord to inhibit nociceptive information (for a review, see Sluka, 2009a) (Figure 25.1B). Endogenous opioid peptides include β-endorphin, endomorphins, enkephalins, and dynorphins. These peptides are located in the PAG, RVM, and spinal cord and bind to opioid receptors (μ, δ, or κ) located on central neurons and nociceptors. When the endogenous opioids bind their receptors they inhibit activity of the target neuron and reduce pain in humans and animals.

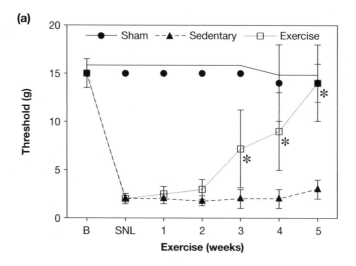

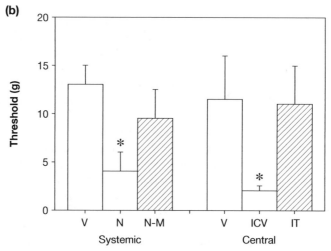

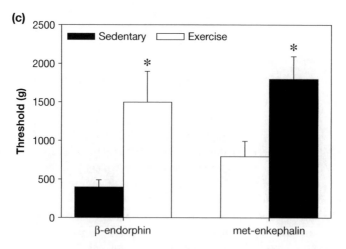

Figure 25.2 Treadmill running 5 days per week reverses the reduced mechanical withdrawal threshold induced by nerve injury when compared to sedentary rats with nerve injury. Normal withdrawal thresholds of the paw were 15 g; withdrawal thresholds decreased to between 2 and 3 g after nerve injury. B. Systemic naloxone (N) reversed the analgesic effects of exercise when compared to vehicle injection (V). Injection of naloxone methiodide (N-M) systemically, to block peripheral opioid receptors only, had no effect on the analgesia. C. Naloxone methiodide delivered supraspinally (i.c.v.) but not spinally (i.t.) reversed the analgesia produced by exercise in animals with neuropathic pain when compared to vehicle (V). D. Exercise increased the expression of β-endorphin in the PAG and met-enkephalin in the RVM when compared to sedentary rats. Data are mean ± S.E.M. ★, P<0.05 (redrawn from data presented in Stagg et al., 2011.)

In uninjured animals, β-endorphins are produced in a wide range of tissue types, including the PAG, RVM, spinal cord, and muscle (Denning et al., 2008; Sluka, 2009a). In human subjects, serum levels of β-endorphin increase in response to aerobic exercise; there is a minimum threshold of exercise duration and intensity for this release (Colt, Wardlaw, & Frantz, 1981; Rahkila, Hakala, Alen, Salminen, & Laatikainen, 1988; Rahkila, Hakala, Salminen, & Laatikainen, 1987). Blockade of opioid receptors systemically, reduces analgesia produced by chronic running wheel activity and by strength training in animals without tissue injury (Li et al., 2004; Mazzardo-Martins et al., 2010). In rats, 3 weeks of running wheel activity reduces the effectiveness of μ- and κ-opioid agonists given systemically or into the PAG in the midbrain (D'Anci, Gerstein, & Kanarek, 2000; Kanarek et al., 1998; Mathes & Kanarek, 2001, 2006; Smith & Yancey, 2003). Together these data support a role for opioid receptors in the analgesia produced by exercise.

In animal models of pain, several studies show that opioid receptors are also involved in the analgesia produced by regular exercise. There is release of β-endorphin in the PAG and enkephalin in the RVM after treadmill running in animals with neuropathic pain (Stagg et al., 2011) (Figure 25.2D). Systemic blockade of opioid receptors reverses the analgesia produced by regular aerobic exercise in neuropathic pain, chronic muscle pain, and acetic acid–induced pain (Bement & Sluka, 2005; Mazzardo-Martins et al., 2010; Shankarappa et al., 2011; Stagg et al., 2011) (Figure 25.2B). Blockade of opioid receptors centrally, giving naloxone intracerebroventricularly (i.c.v.) to block brainstem receptors, also reduces the analgesia produced by exercise in animals with neuropathic pain (Stagg et al., 2011) (Figure 25.2C). On the other hand, blockade of peripheral opioid receptors (naloxone methiodide) has no effect on the analgesia produced by treadmill running in animals with neuropathic pain (Stagg et al., 2011). In animals with chronic muscle pain, the analgesia produced on the first day of treadmill exercise is reduced by systemic naloxone and repeated exercise is reversed by daily naloxone injections, suggesting an acute release of endogenous opioid peptides (Bement & Sluka, 2005). In animals with diabetic neuropathy, analgesia produced by 2 weeks of treadmill running is reversed by a single injection of naloxone to block opioid receptors (Shankarappa et al., 2011), again supporting that opioids are continuously released in response to repeated exercise training. Together these data suggest that regular exercise reduces pain by activation of opioid receptors in descending inhibitory pathways in the central nervous system. However, recent studies show peripheral expression of opioid peptides in muscle (Denning et al., 2008), suggesting that exercise may also produce its effects by activation of peripheral opioid receptors.

Hippocampal changes
Interestingly, running wheel exercise increases c-fos expression (Lee et al., 2003; Oladehin & Waters, 2001), increases cell proliferation (Boehme et al., 2011; Ra et al., 2002; Sahay et al., 2011; Shors, Anderson, Curlik, & Nokia, 2012), and increases opioid receptor expression in the

hippocampus (de Oliveira et al., 2010), a brain structure involved in learning and memory. In fact regular running wheel activity increases learning and memory and neurogenesis (Boehme et al., 2011; Shors et al., 2012). In contrast, blockade of μ-opioid receptors reduces cell proliferation or neurogenesis induced by running wheel activity (Persson et al., 2004). Together these data suggest that regular exercise activates hippocampal neurons and may alter learning and memory through activation of opioid receptors. Voluntary exercise also reduces depressive behaviors in mice with concomitant changes in brain-derived neurotrophic factor (BDNF) in the hippocampus (Duman, Schlesinger, Russell, & Duman, 2008). Cognitive dysfunction and depression are co-morbid symptoms found in people with chronic pain conditions (Glass, 2009; Van, Kempke, & Luyten, 2010), and thus benefits of regular exercise in people with chronic pain could be to improve learning and reduce depression.

Serotonin

Serotonin is a major neurotransmitter found in descending inhibitory pathways and has been implicated in exercise-induced analgesia. Swimming-induced prevention of acetic-acid-induced spontaneous behavior is prevented by prior depletion of serotonin with p-chlorophenylalanine (PCPA) (Mazzardo-Martins et al., 2010). In contrast, nerve injury increases serotonin in the dorsal raphe nucleus of the midbrain, and this increase is prevented by regular treadmill exercise (Korb et al., 2010). Serotonin produces its effects through multiple different receptors, and is found in several different brain sites as well as the spinal cord and the periphery (Sluka, 2009a, 2009c). Future studies should investigate the role of serotonin receptors and different brain sites to more fully characterize the role of serotonin in exercise-induced analgesia and exercise-induced pain.

Ion channels

It is also possible that exercise has effects peripherally, reducing nociceptor activity. Enhanced activity of calcium channels would result in increased nociceptor excitability, which would be manifested as hypersensitivity to noxious stimuli. A recent study recorded calcium currents in dorsal root ganglia neurons (DRG) in animals with diabetic neuropathy, as a measure of excitability of nociceptive afferents (Shankarappa et al., 2011). Diabetic mice show enhanced calcium current density for both low- (T-; LVA) and high-voltage calcium currents (N-, P/Q, L-; HVA), indicative of increased calcium channel availability and activation. Treadmill running reduces the enhanced current densities of HVA and LVA calcium channels, suggesting reductions in nociceptor activity. Since prior studies show that genetic and pharmacological reduction of LVA or HVA calcium channels reduces pain behaviors in a variety of animal models (Chaplan, Pogrel, & Yaksh, 1995; Malmberg & Yaksh, 1994; Sluka, 1997, 1998; Todorovic & Jevtovic-Todorovic, 2011; Wang, Pettus, Gao, Phillips, & Bowersox, 2000), it is possible that regular exercise reduces pain hypersensitivity by normalization of enhanced ion channel activity of nociceptors.

Neurotrophic factors

Pain is influenced by neurotrophic factors, particularly members of the nerve-growth factor (NGF) family of neurotrophins, which include brain-derived neurotrophic factor (BDNF), neurotrophin-3 (NT-3), and neurotrophin-4 (NT-4). Increases in NT-3 are thought to be analgesic. After 3 weeks of exercise in mice with non-inflammatory muscle pain, there is increased expression of NT-3 mRNA and protein in the muscle tissue (Sharma et al., 2010), the same time period when significant reductions in pain behaviors are observed. Increased intramuscular expression of NT-3 (transgenic mice) or intramuscular injection of NT-3 reduces mechanical hypersensitivity induced by intramuscular acid injections (Gandhi, Ryals, & Wright, 2004). Together, these data suggest that increases in NT-3 could be one mechanism by which regular exercise produces analgesia.

Future directions

While research has begun to address the role of physical activity or exercise in animal models of pain there is limited data on mechanisms underlying the analgesic effects. Both central factors and peripheral factors need to be investigated in more detail in animal models of pain. For example, the data examining opioid receptor involvement in the analgesic effect of pain is primarily based on systemic delivery of naloxone, although one recent study showed an effect when given supraspinally. It is unclear which opioid receptors mediate the exercise-induced analgesia (μ, δ, or κ), or the location of opioid receptors (i.e., PAG, RVM, spinal cord, nociceptor) in the analgesic effect. Further comparisons between forced (swimming and treadmill) and voluntary exercise (running wheels) is critical to gain a better understanding of underlying mechanisms. In addition, peripheral effects of exercise on reducing injury-induced changes in nociceptor excitability are intriguing and suggest that exercise may have long-term effects. Could exercise change expression of factors at the peripheral level that can then inhibit nociceptor activity, such as NT-3, endogenous opioid peptides, or opioid receptors? While it is recognized that exercise has effects on a variety of systems including sympathetic, cardiovascular, and motor, in addition to the nociceptive system, it is unclear if these effects are directly related to the analgesia. Lastly, could regular physical activity prevent the development of chronic pain, or the conversion of acute pain to chronic pain? Understanding the molecular and cellular mechanisms underlying exercise-induced analgesia will help identify potential patient populations for treatment, and identify protocols that could be effective in treatment of painful conditions.

Exercise-induced pain

Eccentric exercise-induced pain

Exercise-induced pain in animals has been induced by eccentric exercise and running wheel activity. Eccentric exercise, lengthening contractions, produces pain and muscle soreness to pressure for several days in humans and has been termed delayed onset muscle soreness (DOMS) (Frey Law et al., 2008; Slater, Arendt-Nielsen, Wright, & Graven-Nielsen, 2005). Animal models have been developed to study the underlying mechanisms of eccentric exercise-induced pain (Alvarez, Levine, & Green, 2010; Dessem et al., 2010; Fujii et al., 2008). Eccentric exercise in animals is generally produced by electrically stimulating a muscle and having the joint movement occur in an eccentric manner. Eccentric exercise results in increased sensitivity to mechanical stimulation of the muscle measured behaviorally in awake animals (Dessem et al., 2010; Taguchi, Matsuda, & Mizumura, 2007; Taguchi, Sato, & Mizumura, 2005). In parallel, electrophysiological recordings from muscle nociceptors show increased sensitivity to mechanical stimulation of the muscle after eccentric exercise (Taguchi et al., 2005). Eccentric exercise results in muscle damage, increased pro-inflammatory cytokine release in muscle, and infiltration of inflammatory cells to muscle (Alvarez et al., 2010; Dessem et al., 2010; Fujii et al., 2008). Muscle nociceptors also show increased expression of the neuropeptide calcitonin gene-related peptide (CGRP) and of the ATP-receptor P2X3 (Dessem et al., 2010). Release of pro-inflammatory cytokines, neuropeptides, or ATP in response to eccentric exercise can directly activate and alter excitability of muscle nociceptors to result in mechanical hypersensitivity. In particular, the following potential mediators could be directly related to the observed behavioral increases in hypersensitivity – heat, decreases in pH, lactic acid, or ATP. Each of these mediators can bind specific receptors to produce their effects – transient receptor potential vanilloid receptor (TRPV1), acid sensing ion channels (ASICs), or purinergic receptors (P2X). Pharmacological blockade of TRPV1 channels (heat-effect) or ASICs (decreased pH/lactic acid-effect) prevents the eccentric exercise-induced mechanical hypersensitivity (Fujii et al., 2008). However, recording from nociceptive afferents after eccentric exercise shows no changes in response to decreases in pH or lactic acid, ATP, or heat (Taguchi et al., 2005). This would suggest that while these substances may be released and activate nociceptors their responses are not sensitized. Together the data suggest that eccentric exercise results in release of inflammatory mediators that subsequently activate nociceptors to result in enhanced sensitivity to mechanical stimuli and pain.

Exercise-enhanced pain

Interestingly, Levine and colleagues show that a prior eccentric exercise task enhances the response to a subsequent injection of the inflammatory mediator prostaglandin E-2 (PGE-2) (Alvarez et al., 2010), sometimes termed a priming effect. Specifically, after the hyperalgesia to eccentric exercise resolves, intramuscular injection of PGE-2 results in a long-lasting hyperalgesia (days) when compared to injection of PGE-2 without eccentric exercise (hours) (Alvarez et al., 2010). Reduction of the intracellular messenger protein kinase Cε (PKCε) or the inflammatory cytokine receptor to interleukin-6 in nociceptors (with oligonucleotide antisense injected intrathecally) prevents the enhanced effect of eccentric exercise-induced hyperalgesia to PGE2. This suggests that eccentric exercise results in a sensitization of nociceptors that involves IL-6 receptors and activation of PKCε so that a subsequent noxious stimulus results in an enhanced pain response.

Similarly, a non-damaging exercise stimulus in combination with a subthreshold muscle insult produces mechanical hypersensitivity. In this model the non-damaging exercise task was 2 hours of running wheel activity where animals were encouraged to continuously run (Sluka, Danielson, Rasmussen, & Dasilva, 2012; Sluka & Rasmussen, 2010; Yokoyama et al., 2007). This task alone did not produce mechanical hypersensitivity (Sluka & Rasmussen, 2010). However, when combined with a subthreshold muscle insult that does not produce hypersensitivity on its own, mechanical hypersensitivity develops 24 hours later (Sluka et al., 2012; Sluka & Rasmussen, 2010; Yokoyama et al., 2007) (Figure 25.3A). The muscle insult used in these studies was either two intramuscular pH 5.0 acid injections or intramuscular 0.03% carrageenan. These studies subsequently showed that the exercise task could be given up to 2 hours before or up to 2 hours after the muscle insult, and a 30-minute exercise task could produce the same enhanced hypersensitivity (Sluka et al., 2012; Sluka & Rasmussen, 2010). Further, while the effect occurs in both male and female mice, when 0.03% carrageenan is combined with the 2-hour fatigue task, female mice show greater hypersensitivity (Sluka & Rasmussen, 2010); ovariectomy prevents the enhanced hypersensitivity observed in females so that now the hyperalgesia is similar to that observed in males (Sluka & Rasmussen, 2010). Interestingly, there is no observable muscle damage, and no change in pH, lactic acid, creatinine kinase, phosphate, or oxygen in the muscle immediately after the exercise task. Although a 10% fatigue occurs with the 2-hour exercise task, no fatigue occurs with the 30-minute exercise task. Together these data suggest that non-damaging exercise can enhance pain to a subthreshold muscle insult and that peripheral metabolic factors related to fatiguing exercise do not mediate this enhanced hyperalgesia.

Using this model of exercise-induced pain, changes indicative of enhanced neuron excitability are observed in the central nervous system. Specifically, the 2-hour exercise task increases

(a)

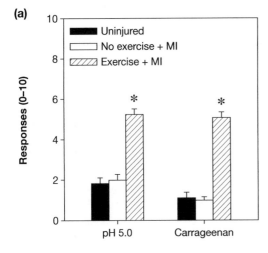

(b)

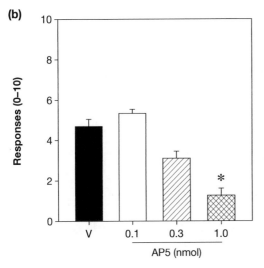

(c)

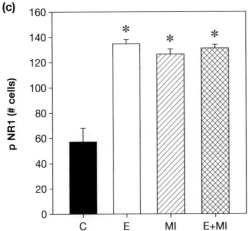

Figure 25.3 (a) Number of withdrawals to repeated mechanical stimuli (0.4 mN) applied to the paw of mice in uninjured animals, in animals that received a subthreshold muscle insult of either two injections of pH 5.0 into the gastrocnemius muscle or 0.03% carrageenan, or animals that received a 2-hour exercise task prior to the subthreshold muscle insult. Increased mechanical sensitivity occurred in the group that received muscle insult in combination with exercise (*, $p < 0.05$). (b) Microinjection of an NMDA receptor antagonist (AP5) into the caudal raphe nuclei (nucleus raphe pallidus and obscurus) during the exercise task prevents the development of mechanical sensitivity to the combination of exercise with a subthreshold muscle insult (0.03% carrageenan). *, $p < 0.05$. (c) The number of cells in the caudal raphe (NRM, NRO, and NRP) labeled for p-NR1 (NMDA receptor phosphorylation) are significantly increased after the exercise task (E), after the subthreshold muscle insult (MI; 0.03% carrageenan), and after the exercise task in combination with the subthreshold muscle insult (E+MI). Data are mean ± S.E.M. *, $p < 0.05$ (figures modified from data presented in Sluka, Danielson, Rasmussen, & daSilva, 2012; Sluka & Rasmussen, 2010).

activation of cells in the caudal raphe nuclei of the medulla–nucleus raphe magnus (NRM), nucleus raphe pallidus (NRO), and nucleus raphe obscurus (NRO) – as measured by c-fos expression (Sluka & Rasmussen, 2010). In addition to inhibiting pain, the caudal raphe nuclei are also involved in enhancement of pain (Porreca, Ossipov, & Gebhart, 2002; Tillu, Gebhart, & Sluka, 2008) (Figure 25.3B) and thus may underlie the exercise-induced pain in this model. The NRM is classically thought to modulate pain while the NRO and NRP are classically thought to modulate motor activity. However, the NRM can modulate motor responses and the NRO/NRP can respond to noxious stimuli. Thus, these nuclei may be ideal for an interaction between exercise and pain.

Glutamate is a major excitatory neurotransmitter within the nervous system and the NMDA glutamate receptor plays a critical role in pain modulation within the caudal raphe. In the caudal raphe, overexpression of NMDA glutamate receptors (NR1-subunit) enhances mechanical hypersensitivity in uninjured animals (da Silva, Walder, Davidson, Wilson, & Sluka, 2010) and blockade of NMDA glutamate receptors in the caudal raphe during the 2-hour exercise task prevents the development of exercise-induced muscle pain (Sluka et al., 2012). Phosphorylation of the NMDA receptor (p-NR1; increasing cAMP production) in nociceptive neurons enhances NMDA currents, enhances channel conductance, and increases trafficking of the NMDA receptor complex to the cell membrane (Chen & Roche, 2007; Ehlers, Tingley, & Huganir, 1995; Lin, Wu, & Willis, 2002) – thus phosphorylation of NR1 enhances neuron excitability. In response to the exercise task, there is enhanced p-NR1 in the caudal raphe nuclei, which occurs immediately after the 2-hour exercise task, 2 hours after the 2-hour exercise task, or immediately after the 30-minute exercise task (Sluka et al., 2012) (Figure 25.3C). Together these data suggest increased activation and sensitization of NMDA receptors on excitatory neurons in the caudal raphe are necessary for development of exercise-induced pain.

Future directions

Future research examining exercise-induced pain should focus on potential brain sites where exercise could enhance neuron hyperexcitability (as shown in the RVM) and the underlying neurotransmitters and receptors involved in this process. Exercise-induced pain could also involve changes peripherally and could enhance pain through fatigue-related factors, or through factors released from exercising muscle, either locally or systemically (as shown with IL-6). The role of the sympathetic system in modulating pain behaviors is well known, as is the role of the sympathetic system in exercise effects. Thus, future experiments should determine if changes in the sympathetic system underlie the effects of exercise-induced pain, as well as exercise-induced analgesia.

Summary

Animal models have begun to decipher the underlying mechanisms of exercise-induced analgesia and exercise-induced pain. Evidence suggests that exercise-induced analgesia involves activation of central opioid receptors, utilizes serotonin, and may normalize nociceptor hypersensitivity by modulating ion channels and growth factors. Regular exercise also produces neurogenesis in the hippocampus, which may underlie the improvements in learning and depressive symptoms. Eccentric exercise results in pain and enhances the nociceptive response to subsequent stimuli. Evidence suggests that changes associated with muscle damage and inflammation likely mediate the pain response – this includes increases in pro-inflammatory cytokines, ATP, and neuro-peptides after eccentric exercise. Further, a subthreshold muscle insult combined with a non-damaging exercise task results in enhanced mechanical hypersensitivity that involves neuron excitability in the central nervous system. Thus, exercise has multiple effects and can modulate pain by either preventing or reversing pain, or by enhancing pain. Understanding the underlying mechanisms of exercise-induced analgesia and exercise-induced pain can assist with management of individuals with chronic pain.

References

Alvarez, P., Levine, J. D., & Green, P. G. (2010). Eccentric exercise induces chronic alterations in musculoskeletal nociception in the rat. *European Journal of Neuroscience, 32*(5), 819–825.

Bement, M. K. (2009). Exercise-induced hypoalgesia: An evidence-based review. In K. A. Sluka (Ed.), *Mechanisms and Management of Pain for the Physical Therapist* (pp. 143–166). Seattle: IASP Press.

Bement, M. K., & Sluka, K. A. (2005). Low-intensity exercise reverses chronic muscle pain in the rat in a naloxone-dependent manner. *Archives of Physical Medicine and Rehabilitation, 86*(9), 1736–1740.

Blustein, J. E., McLaughlin, M., & Hoffman, J. R. (2006). Exercise effects stress-induced analgesia and spatial learning in rats. *Physiology and Behavior, 89*(4), 582–586.

Boehme, F., Gil-Mohapel, J., Cox, A., Patten, A., Giles, E., Brocardo, P. S., et al. (2011). Voluntary exercise induces adult hippocampal neurogenesis and BDNF expression in a rodent model of fetal alcohol spectrum disorders. *European Journal of Neuroscience, 33*(10), 1799–1811.

Chaplan, S. R., Pogrel, J. W., & Yaksh, T. L. (1995). Role of voltage-dependent calcium channel subtypes in experimental tactile allodynia. *Journal of Pharmacology and Experimental Therapeutics, 269*, 1117–1123.

Chen, B. S., & Roche, K. W. (2007). Regulation of NMDA receptors by phosphorylation. *Neuropharmacology, 53*(3), 362–368.

Colt, E. W., Wardlaw, S. L., & Frantz, A. G. (1981). The effect of running on plasma beta-endorphin. *Life Sciences, 28*(14), 1637–1640.

D'Anci, K. E., Gerstein, A. V., & Kanarek, R. B. (2000). Long-term voluntary access to running wheels decreases kappa-opioid antinociception. *Pharmacology Biochemistry and Behavior, 66*(2), 343–346.

da Silva, L. F. S., Walder, R. Y., Davidson, B. L., Wilson, S. P., & Sluka, K. A. (2010). Changes in expression of NMDA-NR1 receptor subunits in the rostral ventromedial medulla modulates pain behaviors. *Pain, 151*, 155–161.

Danion, F., Latash, M. L., Li, Z. M., & Zatsiorsky, V. M. (2001). The effect of a fatiguing exercise by the index finger on single- and multi-finger force production tasks. *Experimental Brain Research, 138*(3), 322–329.

de Oliveira, M. S., da Silva Fernandes, M. J., Scorza, F. A., Persike, D. S., Scorza, C. A., da Ponte, J. B., et al. (2010). Acute and chronic exercise modulates the expression of MOR opioid receptors in the hippocampal formation of rats. *Brain Research Bulletin, 83*, 278–283.

Denning, G. M., Ackermann, L. W., Barna, T. J., Armstrong, J. G., Stoll, L. L., Weintraub, N. L., et al. (2008). Proenkephalin expression and enkephalin release are widely observed in non-neuronal tissues. *Peptides, 29*(1), 83–92.

Dessem, D., Ambalavanar, R., Evancho, M., Moutanni, A., Yallampalli, C., & Bai, G. (2010). Eccentric muscle contraction and stretching evoke mechanical hyperalgesia and modulate CGRP and P2X(3) expression in a functionally relevant manner. *Pain, 149*(2), 284–295.

Duman, C. H., Schlesinger, L., Russell, D. S., & Duman, R. S. (2008). Voluntary exercise produces antidepressant and anxiolytic behavioral effects in mice. *Brain Research, 1199*, 148–158.

Ehlers, M. D., Tingley, W. G., & Huganir, R. L. (1995). Regulated subcellular distribution of the NR1 subunit of the NMDA receptor. *Science, 269*(5231), 1734–1737.

Frey Law, L. A., Evans, S., Knudtson, J., Nus, S., Scholl, K., & Sluka, K. A. (2008). Massage reduces pain perception and hyperalgesia in experimental muscle pain: A randomized, controlled trial. *Journal of Pain, 9*(8), 714–721.

Fujii, Y., Ozaki, N., Taguchi, T., Mizumura, K., Furukawa, K., & Sugiura, Y. (2008). TRP channels and ASICs mediate mechanical hyperalgesia in models of inflammatory muscle pain and delayed onset muscle soreness. *Pain, 140*(2), 292–304.

Gandhi, R., Ryals, J. M., & Wright, D. E. (2004). Neurotrophin-3 reverses chronic mechanical hyperalgesia induced by intramuscular acid injection. *Journal of Neuroscience, 24*(42), 9405–9413.

Glass, J. M. (2009). Review of cognitive dysfunction in fibromyalgia: A convergence on working memory and attentional control impairments. *Rheumatic Disease Clinics of North America, 35*(2), 299–311.

Hofbauer, R. K., Rainville, P., Duncan, G. H., & Bushnell, M. C. (2001). Cortical representation of the sensory dimension of pain. *Journal of Neurophysiology, 86*(1), 402–411.

Hopkins, E., Spinella, M., Pavlovic, Z. W., & Bodnar, R. J. (1998). Alterations in swim stress-induced analgesia and hypothermia following serotonergic or NMDA antagonists in the rostral ventromedial medulla of rats. *Physiology and Behavior, 64*(3), 219–225.

Kanarek, R. B., Gerstein, A. V., Wildman, R. P., Mathes, W. F., & D'Anci, K. E. (1998). Chronic running-wheel activity decreases sensitivity to morphine-induced analgesia in male and female rats. *Pharmacology Biochemistry and Behavior, 61*(1), 19–27.

King, C. D., Devine, D. P., Vierck, C. J., Rodgers, J., & Yezierski, R. P. (2003). Differential effects of stress on escape and reflex responses to nociceptive thermal stimuli in the rat. *Brain Research, 987*(2), 214–222.

Konarzewski, M., Sadowski, B., & Jozwik, I. (1997). Metabolic correlates of selection for swim stress-induced analgesia in laboratory mice. *American Journal of Physiology, 273*(1 Pt 2), R337–R343.

Korb, A., Bonetti, L. V., Da Silva, S. A., Marcuzzo, S., Ilha, J., Bertagnolli, M., et al. (2010). Effect of treadmill exercise on serotonin immunoreactivity in medullary raphe nuclei and spinal cord following sciatic nerve transection in rats. *Neurochemical Research, 35*(3), 380–389.

Kuphal, K. E., Fibuch, E. E., & Taylor, B. K. (2007). Extended swimming exercise reduces inflammatory and peripheral neuropathic pain in rodents. *Journal of Pain, 8*(12), 989–997.

Lannersten, L., & Kosek, E. (2010). Dysfunction of endogenous pain inhibition during exercise with painful muscles in patients with shoulder myalgia and fibromyalgia. *Pain, 151*(1), 77–86.

Lee, M. H., Kim, H., Lim, B. V., Chang, H. K., Lee, T. H., Jang, M. H., et al. (2003). Naloxone potentiates treadmill running-induced increase in c-Fos expression in rat hippocampus. *Life Sciences, 73*(24), 3139–3147.

Li, G., Rhodes, J. S., Girard, I., Gammie, S. C., & Garland, T., Jr. (2004). Opioid-mediated pain sensitivity in mice bred for high voluntary wheel running. *Physiology and Behavior, 83*(3), 515–524.

Lin, Q., Wu, J., & Willis, W. D. (2002). Effects of protein kinase a activation on the responses of primate spinothalamic tract neurons to mechanical stimuli. *Journal of Neurophysiology, 88*, 214–221.

Malmberg, A. B., & Yaksh, T. L. (1994). Voltage-sensitive calcium channels in spinal nociceptive processing: Blockade of N-and P-type channels inhibits formalin-induced nociception. *Journal of Neuroscience, 14*, 4882–4890.

Mathes, W. F., & Kanarek, R. B. (2001). Wheel running attenuates the antinociceptive properties of morphine and its metabolite, morphine-6-glucuronide, in rats. *Physiology and Behavior, 74*(1–2), 245–251.

Mathes, W. F., & Kanarek, R. B. (2006). Chronic running wheel activity attenuates the antinociceptive actions of morphine and morphine-6-glucouronide administration into the periaqueductal gray in rats. *Pharmacology Biochemistry and Behavior, 83*(4), 578–584.

Mazzardo-Martins, L., Martins, D. F., Marcon, R., Dos Santos, U. D., Speckhann, B., Gadotti, V. M., et al. (2010). High-intensity extended swimming exercise reduces pain-related behavior in mice: Involvement of endogenous opioids and the serotonergic system. *Journal of Pain, 11*(1384), 1393.

Morimoto, K., Tan, N., Nishiyasu, T., Sone, R., & Murakami, N. (2000). Spontaneous wheel running attenuates cardiovascular responses to stress in rats. *Pflugers Archiv, 440*(2), 216–222.

Oladehin, A., & Waters, R. S. (2001). Location and distribution of Fos protein expression in rat hippocampus following acute moderate aerobic exercise. *Experimental Brain Research, 137*(1), 26–35.

Persson, A. I., Naylor, A. S., Jonsdottir, I. H., Nyberg, F., Eriksson, P. S., & Thorlin, T. (2004). Differential regulation of hippocampal progenitor proliferation by opioid receptor antagonists in running and non-running spontaneously hypertensive rats. *European Journal of Neuroscience, 19*(7), 1847–1855.

Porreca, F., Ossipov, M. H., & Gebhart, G. F. (2002). Chronic pain and medullary descending facilitation. *Trends in Neurosciences, 25*(6), 319–325.

Ra, S. M., Kim, H., Jang, M. H., Shin, M. C., Lee, T. H., Lim, B. V., et al. (2002). Treadmill running and swimming increase cell proliferation in the hippocampal dentate gyrus of rats. *Neuroscience Letters, 333*(2), 123–126.

Rahkila, P., Hakala, E., Alen, M., Salminen, K., & Laatikainen, T. (1988). Beta-endorphin and corticotropin release is dependent on a threshold intensity of running exercise in male endurance athletes. *Life Sciences, 43*(6), 551–558.

Rahkila, P., Hakala, E., Salminen, K., & Laatikainen, T. (1987). Response of plasma endorphins to running exercises in male and female endurance athletes. *Medicine and Science in Sports and Exercise, 19*(5), 451–455.

Rainville, P., Duncan, G. H., Price, D. D., Carrier, B., & Bushnell, M. C. (1997). Pain affect encoded in human anterior cingulate but not somatosensory cortex. *Science, 277*(5328), 968–971.

Roveda, F., Middlekauff, H. R., Rondon, M. U., Reis, S. F., Souza, M., Nastari, L., et al. (2003). The effects of exercise training on sympathetic neural activation in advanced heart failure: A randomized controlled trial. *Journal of the American College of Cardiology, 42*(5), 854–860.

Sacco, P., Hope, P. A., Thickbroom, G. W., Byrnes, M. L., & Mastaglia, F. L. (1999). Corticomotor excitability and perception of effort during sustained exercise in the chronic fatigue syndrome. *Clinical Neurophysiology, 110*(11), 1883–1891.

Sahay, A., Scobie, K. N., Hill, A. S., O'Carroll, C. M., Kheirbek, M. A., Burghardt, N. S., et al. (2011). Increasing adult hippocampal neurogenesis is sufficient to improve pattern separation. *Nature, 472*(7344), 466–470.

Shankarappa, S. A., Piedras-Renteria, E. S., & Stubbs, E. B., Jr. (2011). Forced-exercise delays neuropathic pain in experimental diabetes: Effects on voltage-activated calcium channels. *Journal of Neurochemistry, 118*(2), 224–236.

Sharma, N. K., Ryals, J. M., Gajewski, B. J., & Wright, D. E. (2010). Aerobic exercise alters analgesia and neurotrophin-3 synthesis in an animal model of chronic widespread pain. *Physical Therapy, 90*(5), 714–725.

Shors, T. J., Anderson, M. L., Curlik, D. M., & Nokia, M. S. (2012). Use it or lose it: How neurogenesis keeps the brain fit for learning. *Behavioural Brain Research, 227*(450), 458.

Slater, H., Arendt-Nielsen, L., Wright, A., & Graven-Nielsen, T. (2005). Sensory and motor effects of experimental muscle pain in patients with lateral epicondylalgia and controls with delayed onset muscle soreness. *Pain, 114*(1–2), 118–130.

Sluka, K. A. (1997). Blockade of calcium channels can prevent the onset of secondary hyperalgesia and allodynia induced by intradermal injection of capsaicin in rats. *Pain, 71*(2), 157–164.

Sluka, K. A. (1998). Blockade of N- and P/Q-type calcium channels reduces the secondary heat hyperalgesia induced by acute inflammation. *Journal of Pharmacology and Experimental Therapeutics, 287*(1), 232–237.

Sluka, K. A. (2009a). Central mechanisms involved in pain processing. In K. A. Sluka (Ed.), *Mechanisms and Management of Pain for the Physical Therapist* (pp. 41–72). Seattle: IASP Press.

Sluka, K. A. (2009b). Definitions, concepts and models of pain. In K. A. Sluka (Ed.), *Mechanisms and Management of Pain for the Physical Therapist* (pp. 3–18). Seattle: IASP Press.

Sluka, K. A. (2009c). Peripheral mechanisms involved in pain processing. In K. A. Sluka (Ed.), *Mechanisms and Management of Pain for the Physical Therapist* (pp. 19–40). Seattle: IASP Press.

Sluka, K. A., Danielson, J., Rasmussen, L., & Dasilva, L. F. (2012). Exercise-induced pain requires NMDA receptor activation in the medullary raphe nuclei. *Medicine and Science in Sports and Exercise, 44*, 420–427.

Sluka, K. A., & Rasmussen, L. A. (2010). Fatiguing exercise enhances hyperalgesia to muscle inflammation. *Pain, 148*, 188–197.

Smith, M. A., & Yancey, D. L. (2003). Sensitivity to the effects of opioids in rats with free access to exercise wheels: Mu-opioid tolerance and physical dependence. *Psychopharmacology (Berl), 168*(4), 426–434.

Spierer, D. K., DeMeersman, R. E., Kleinfeld, J., McPherson, E., Fullilove, R. E., Alba, A., et al. (2007). Exercise training improves cardiovascular and autonomic profiles in HIV. *Clinical Autonomic Research, 17*(6), 341–348.

Stagg, N. J., Mata, H. P., Ibrahim, M. M., Henriksen, E. J., Porreca, F., Vanderah, T. W., et al. (2011). Regular exercise reverses sensory hypersensitivity in a rat neuropathic pain model: Role of endogenous opioids. *Anesthesiology, 114*(4), 940–948.

Staud, R., Robinson, M. E., & Price, D. D. (2005). Isometric exercise has opposite effects on central pain mechanisms in fibromyalgia patients compared to normal controls. *Pain, 118*(1–2), 176–184.

Taguchi, T., Matsuda, T., & Mizumura, K. (2007). Change with age in muscular mechanical hyperalgesia after lengthening contraction in rats. *Neuroscience Research, 57*(3), 331–338.

Taguchi, T., Sato, J., & Mizumura, K. (2005). Augmented mechanical response of muscle thin-fiber sensory receptors recorded from rat muscle-nerve preparations in vitro after eccentric contraction. *Journal of Neurophysiology, 94*(4), 2822–2831.

Tillu, D. V., Gebhart, G. F., & Sluka, K. A. (2008). Descending facilitatory pathways from the RVM initiate and maintain bilateral hyperalgesia after muscle insult. *Pain, 136*(3), 331–339.

Todorovic, S. M., & Jevtovic-Todorovic, V. (2011). T-type voltage-gated calcium channels as targets for the development of novel pain therapies. *British Journal of Pharmacology, 163*(3), 484–495.

Van, H. B., Kempke, S., & Luyten, P. (2010). Psychiatric aspects of chronic fatigue syndrome and fibromyalgia. *Current Psychiatry Reports, 12*(3), 208–214.

Vierck, C. J., Jr., Staud, R., Price, D. D., Cannon, R. L., Mauderli, A. P., & Martin, A. D. (2001). The effect of maximal exercise on temporal summation of second pain (windup) in patients with fibromyalgia syndrome. *Journal of Pain, 2*(6), 334–344. Retrieved from PM:14622813.

Wang, Y.-X., Pettus, M., Gao, D., Phillips, C., & Bowersox, S. S. (2000). Effects of intrathecal administration of ziconotide, a selective neruonal N-type calcium channel blocker, on mechanical allodynia and heat hyperalgesia in a rat model of postoperative pain. *Pain, 84*, 151–158.

Yokoyama, T., Lisi, T. L., Moore, S. A., & Sluka, K. A. (2007). Muscle fatigue increases the probability of developing hyperalgesia in mice. *Journal of Pain, 8*, 692–699.

26

EFFECTS OF ACUTE AND CHRONIC PHYSICAL ACTIVITY ON CHRONIC PAIN CONDITIONS

Aaron J. Stegner, Morgan R. Shields, Jacob D. Meyer, and Dane B. Cook

Patients with chronic pain are more likely to be sedentary and less likely to engage in regular physical activity or exercise than their healthy peers. Although individuals with chronic pain report many of the same obstacles to physical activity as healthy people, they also often attribute their lack of activity to disability or pain as a result of their condition and a fear of exacerbating symptoms. This perspective could be particularly detrimental for these individuals as their low levels of activity and large amounts of sedentary time put them at a greater risk for worsening their disability (McCracken & Samuel, 2007), as well as other medical conditions such as heart disease, cancer, and stroke. This process has been characterized by some as a vicious cycle; these patients are inactive, at least in part, as a result of their pain condition, which leads to greater disability, which in turn decreases the likelihood of them being physically active (Leeuw et al., 2007). The relatively low level of activity in these patients is especially troubling when considering the large and growing body of evidence demonstrating that exercise and increased levels of daily physical activity can provide benefits to individuals with chronic pain beyond enhanced physical fitness. The benefits of regular exercise for these patients may include improvements in pain symptoms, physical and functional capacity, fatigue, anxiety, depressed mood, and quality of life. For low to moderate intensity prescriptions, the consensus appears to be that chronic pain patients can engage in exercise safely and without fear of exacerbating symptoms. Clinicians, for the most part, no longer subscribe to the view that rest and activity avoidance are the best methods of managing chronic pain symptoms. In fact, following decades of research, a recommendation for exercise or increased physical activity has become a standard element of multicomponent therapies for all manner of chronic pain conditions (Iversen, 2012).

This chapter reviews the evidence for the influence of exercise and physical activity on symptoms associated with a number of chronic pain conditions including widespread musculo-skeletal pain (e.g., fibromyalgia), rheumatoid arthritis, osteoarthritis, low back pain, headache, and neck pain. When possible the immediate effects of acute exercise for pain patients as well as the long-term impact of more chronic changes in physical activity levels are discussed. Where they exist, published guidelines for exercise prescription for patients with particular conditions are also reviewed. The conditions covered were chosen due to their relatively high prevalence in the U.S. population and the extent of the body of research exploring the relationship between each condition and physical activity.

Chronic widespread musculoskeletal pain

Chronic widespread musculoskeletal pain (CMP) is defined as pain occurring axially, on both the right and left side of the body and in both the upper and lower body lasting for at least 3 months (Wolfe et al., 1990). In addition, the all-over body pain cannot be explained by other pathologically defined medical conditions (e.g., arthritis, lupus, etc.). Estimates for the prevalence of CMP indicate that approximately 4% of the population is affected (Hardt, Jacobsen, Goldberg, Nickel, & Buchwald, 2008; Lindell, Bergman, Petersson, Jacobsson, & Herrstrom, 2000). Although CMP is the hallmark of fibromyalgia (FM), it is also often reported by patients being treated for Gulf War illness, irritable bowel syndrome, chronic fatigue syndrome, or depression. Not incidentally, the conditions listed above often co-occur in the same patients (Clauw, 2009).

Exercise and chronic widespread musculoskeletal pain

The large majority of what we know about the relationship between physical activity and CMP comes from research with FM patients, but other populations have been studied (e.g., Gulf War veterans, patients with irritable bowel syndrome, etc.). In just the last 5 years (2007–2012), more than 30 randomized control trials and 12 systematic reviews have been published examining the efficacy of exercise as a therapeutic treatment for FM. The interaction of acute and chronic exercise and their impact on FM symptoms is complicated. Patients with CMP report exercise, even when relativized for the participant's fitness, to be more painful and effortful than their healthy peers (Cook, Stegner, & Ellingson, 2010; Cook et al., 2012; Kadetoff & Kosek, 2010; Mengshoel, Vøllestad, & Førre, 1995). Although common perception among FM patients and many clinicians is that acute exercise leads to a worsening of symptoms, research on this topic is equivocal. Similarly, findings from research exploring increased sensitivity in patients with CMP following exercise have also been inconsistent. Despite the apparent confusion over the responses to acute bouts of exercise in CMP patients, there is now a large body of evidence suggesting that regular physical activity can positively impact many of the complaints and concomitant issues related to CMP (Busch et al., 2011).

Although patients with FM tend to be more sedentary (McLoughlin, Colbert, Stegner, & Cook, 2011) and less aerobically fit compared to sex- and age-matched controls, changes in cardiovascular fitness as a result of regular exercise do not appear to differ from those observed in healthy, formerly sedentary exercisers (Valim et al., 2003). In other words, there is no evidence to suggest that aerobic training has a differential impact on the cardiovascular fitness of patients suffering from CMP compared to healthy sedentary controls. A wide range of outcomes have been examined in order to evaluate the benefits of aerobic exercise in CMP patients, with improvements in quality of life (Brosseau et al., 2008a), decreased interference of activities of daily living (Busch, Barber, Overend, Peloso, & Schachter, 2007), and greater physical function/capacity (Busch et al., 2007; Thomas & Blotman, 2010) being among the most consistent findings. Authors of more recent reviews, perhaps due to an increase in the quality of exercise studies in FM, are more confident in their conclusions that pain, fatigue, and depressive symptoms in CMP are also positively influenced by aerobic exercise (Busch et al., 2011; Häuser et al., 2010).

The success of aerobic exercise interventions with other patient groups frequently reporting CMP is less clear as these populations have been understudied in this context. The lone randomized controlled trial on the influence of an aerobic exercise program as a treatment for veterans suffering from Gulf War illness was conducted by Donta and colleagues (2003). The results of this large-scale (N=1092), 12-week training study suggested a small effect for exercise on fatigue, cognitive symptoms, and mental health with no improvement for pain. The conclusions of this study, however, should be interpreted with caution as the investigation suffered from poor adherence to the prescribed exercise. Likewise, a single aerobic exercise trial was conducted with patients diagnosed with irritable bowel syndrome (Daley et al., 2008). Although the patients completing this 12-week training study reported an improvement in feelings of constipation there was no significant change in symptom–related pain ratings.

In addition to muscle pain, CMP patients often report muscle fatigue and weakness. As such, resistance training may also be beneficial for patients. Similar to the changes in fitness resulting from aerobic interventions, it appears that the trainability of the neuromuscular system in patients with FM does not differ significantly from their healthy counterparts (Häkkinen, Häkkinen, Hannonen, & Alen, 2001; Valkeinen et al., 2004). Resistance training interventions with FM patients have demonstrated benefits for muscular strength and endurance without an acute increase in pain (Brossaeu et al., 2008b; Cazzola et al., 2010). Although research on this exercise modality lags in quantity behind aerobic exercise, there is evidence to suggest resistance training can be valuable for improving pain, mood, and quality of life in CMP patients (Brosseau et al., 2008b; Cazzola et al., 2010).

A number of health and wellness organizations (e.g., American College of Sports Medicine [ACSM], Centers for Disease Control, American Heart Association, American College of Rheumatology [ACR]) have made recommendations for physical activity by encouraging healthy individuals to incorporate both aerobic and strength training as part of their fitness routine. A head-to-head comparison of aerobic and strength training interventions in FM was undertaken by Bircan, Karasel, Akgun, El, and Alper (2008). The results from the study demonstrated similar improvements for both aerobic and strength training interventions in pain, sleep, fatigue, and depression. Rooks and colleagues (2007) evaluated the efficacy of three multifaceted exercise programs: (1) aerobic and flexibility training, (2) aerobic, flexibility, and strength training, and (3) aerobic, flexibility, and strength training in combination with an FM education program, in comparison to the education program alone. Improvements in physical function, FM impact, and pain were found for all exercise interventions, with no improvements for the patients receiving education alone.

In addition to traditional exercise programs, alternative therapies of which exercise is a component are also being explored. A number of studies have explored the potential for conducting exercise in warm-water pools, or aquatic exercise therapy, as a way to possibly combine the purported benefits of balneotherapy, or warm-water therapy, with exercise. Limited evidence shows aquatic exercise therapy to be at least as effective as land-based exercise in providing pain relief, but may be superior in regard to improved mood (Cazzola et al., 2010; Gowans & deHueck, 2007). Mind-body exercise approaches, such as tai chi, qigong, and yoga, are also gaining notoriety as potentially efficacious interventions for CMP and appear to offer similar benefits for pain symptoms, function, quality of life, and mood (Busch et al., 2011) as other, more traditional exercise regimens.

Guidelines for exercise in patients with chronic widespread pain

Despite the strong evidence supporting the use of exercise as a component of CMP therapy, the requisite information to create specific prescriptions for the optimal mode, frequency, duration, or intensity for treatment is currently lacking. In 2005, the American Pain Society published their aerobic exercise recommendation for patients with FM (Burckhardt et al., 2005), which advocated for moderately intense activity (60–75% of age-adjusted heart rate maximum), 2–3 times/week. This recommendation, however, was based on the false supposition that improved fitness was necessary to treat FM symptoms and has since been abandoned. Häuser et al. (2010)

published a meta-analytic review on aerobic exercise with a stated objective of identifying evidence-based recommendations for optimal intensity and volume. They concluded that land- or water-based exercise performed at a moderate intensity (>50% of age-adjusted heart rate maximum) 2–3 times/week, for at least 4 weeks should result in improved symptoms while minimizing the likelihood of exacerbation. It is our position that the evidence does not support such a specific recommendation. In point of fact, the authors relied on the effect sizes of interventions derived from their meta-analytical investigation to draw their conclusions and none of the studies included in their analysis directly compared interventions of varying intensity or volume.

Of course, precise recommendations in terms of mode, frequency, duration, and intensity for particular symptoms associated with CMP would be the ideal. Unfortunately, the accumulated knowledge on exercise as it affects CMP is insufficient to make those kinds of recommendations. However, numerous less specific, evidence-based guidelines have been put forward for consideration when using exercise or strategies to increase physical activity in patients with CMP. When initiating a new exercise regimen, CMP patients should start at a low intensity and progress slowly. Low-intensity exercise appears to be more conducive to adherence and less likely to provoke symptom exacerbation (Busch et al., 2008; Cazzola et al., 2010; Thomas & Blotman, 2010). While low-intensity exercise is less likely to positively impact fitness, it may be enough to improve symptoms (Busch et al., 2008). Interventions should be individualized, taking into account current fitness and symptoms of the patient (e.g., if muscular weakness and fatigue are particular problems then the program should include some strength training exercises (Busch et al., 2008; Cazzola et al., 2010; Thomas & Blotman, 2010)). Patient preferences for particular modes of exercise should shape the program, but various types of exercise should be incorporated (Cazzola et al., 2010). Patients should be counseled to expect some increases in pain when starting a new regimen. If symptoms are aggravated, patients should reduce their intensity while trying to maintain their frequency (Cazzola et al., 2010; Thomas & Blotman, 2010). Supervised exercise programs, especially for new exercisers, are recommended as a way to provide education and facilitate adherence (Busch et al., 2008; Thomas & Blotman, 2010).

Rheumatoid arthritis

Rheumatoid arthritis (RA) is diagnosed based on the ACR criteria (1987) and common symptoms include systemic inflammation of peripheral joints, pain, fatigue, stiffness, impaired range of motion, and difficulties in activities of daily living (Woolf & Pfleger, 2003; Bilberg, Ahlmen, & Mannerkorpi, 2005). Prevalence rates of RA have been reported to range from 0.45% to 1.16% of the female population and 0.19% to 0.44% of males, but rates appear to vary across geographic regions (Guillemin et al., 2005; Symmons et al., 2002). RA patients self-report significantly lower total energy expenditure and less moderate-intensity physical activity when compared to age- and gender-matched controls (Henchoz et al., 2012). Further, RA patients with higher amounts of sedentary behavior report significantly greater pain, fatigue, and disability compared to more physically active RA patients (Henchoz et al., 2012). Thus, exercise has been examined as an adjunct treatment in this population as a means to increase strength, aerobic capacity, and reduce the pain associated with RA.

Exercise in rheumatoid arthritis

Both aerobic exercise training and resistance training can be completed safely by patients with RA. Regular aerobic exercise results in significant reductions in pain and disability while increasing functional ability, aerobic capacity, and quality of life (Metsios et al., 2008; Baillet et al., 2010). Improvements are greater for patients with longer illness duration and for those who exercise more frequently (Baillet et al., 2010). Resistance training leads to significant improvements in strength and functional capacity, and decreases in swollen joint counts, but evidence for reductions in RA pain associated with resistance training is less consistent (Baillet, Vaillant, Guinot, Juvin, & Gaudin, 2012). Short- and long-term exercise interventions are both efficacious for lessening RA symptoms, but the specific exercise mode, duration, and intensity necessary to elicit these results is unknown (Hurkmans, van der Giesen, Vliet Vlieland, Schoones, & Van den Ende, 2009).

Guidelines for exercise in rheumatoid arthritis

Although there are a growing number of randomized controlled exercise trials that report significant reductions in pain in RA patients, the dose of exercise needed is unknown, which may explain why exercise is not explicitly present in most guidelines developed for the treatment for RA. The National Institute for Health and Clinical Excellence (NICE) in the United Kingdom recommends a multidisciplinary treatment of RA, including consultation with a specialized physiotherapist and increasing fitness and regular exercise for enhancing joint flexibility and strengthening (National Collaborating Centre for Chronic Conditions, 2009). Further, the ACR emphasizes the use of medications in their RA practice guidelines but also maintains a helpful web page dedicated to the beneficial aspects of engaging in physical activity for arthritis patients (Westby, 2012). On the other hand, the most recent Cochrane Review suggested that employing treatment strategies that will improve aerobic capacity and muscle strength should be routine practice for RA patients (Hurkmans et al., 2009). The Ottawa Panel, an expert commission of Canadian methodologists and researchers, published evidence-based guidelines recommending the use of exercise for specific joint and overall functional strengthening to manage RA symptoms but a detailed prescription is not provided (Brosseau et al., 2011).

Osteoarthritis

Osteoarthritis (OA) is a common chronic joint pain condition that has been reported to affect 12.8% of the population including approximately 15% of women and 10.5% of men (Grotle, Hagen, Natvig, Dahl, & Kvien, 2008). The symptoms associated with OA include joint pain, limitation of joint range of motion, impaired joint stability, inflammation, and tenderness (Woolf & Pfleger, 2003). Common joints that are affected by OA are the knee, hip, and hand. In addition to pain symptoms, this condition can impact activities of daily living and quality of life (van Es et al., 2011). Exercise is recommended with the goal of increasing the ability to complete activities of daily living, increasing muscle strength, improving overall physical function, and decreasing pain.

Exercise in osteoarthritis

Aerobic activity (weight-bearing and non-weight-bearing), strength training (dynamic and isometric), and combined (both aerobic and anaerobic) exercise interventions have been shown to be beneficial for pain reduction in OA (Focht, 2006; Iwamoto, Sato, Takeda, & Matsumoto, 2011). Further, walking and strengthening exercises are equally effective in reducing knee OA pain (Roddy, Zhang, & Doherty, 2005). There is clear evidence of symptom improvement immediately following exercise interventions, but the long-term follow-up effects on OA pain are less clear (Pisters et al., 2007).

Guidelines for exercise in osteoarthritis

Exercise as a treatment for OA appears more frequently in guidelines compared to RA. For example, recently the ACR published five nonpharmacologic recommendations for the management of knee and hip OA, which include participation in cardiovascular and/or resistance exercise (Hochberg et al., 2012). NICE suggests a holistic approach, which specifically emphasizes the role of general exercise and local strengthening as a core component of OA treatment (National Collaborating Centre for Chronic Conditions, 2008). The European League Against Rheumatism (EULAR) released 10 recommendations for hip OA treatment that involve non-pharmacological interventions including regular education, exercise, and weight reduction if overweight (Zhang et al., 2005). In normal-weight OA patients, the Ottawa Panel recommends strengthening exercises, general physical activity, and manual therapy combined with exercise for the management of pain and improvement in functional status (Loew et al., 2012). The Ottawa Panel also recommends knee OA patients participate in aerobic walking combined with stretching and strengthening exercises to clinically improve pain, functional status, and quality of life (Loew et al., 2012). The Ottawa Panel concluded that for overweight patients with OA, a combination of physical activity and diet would result in clinically relevant improvement in pain relief, strength, and functional status (Brosseau et al., 2011). Although the specific parameters for the most effective exercise interventions have not been defined, exercise in some form appears to be consistently recommended in the treatment of OA.

Low back pain

Low back pain (LBP) is usually defined by its etiology (specific vs. unspecific), and duration (acute, subacute, and chronic). Low back pain refers to pain that is localized near the lumbar vertebrae and can be accompanied by sciatic nerve pain. Specific back pain, or pain from a known cause (e.g., disc displacement, tumors, etc.), is rare, usually ~10% of LBP cases, and treatments in these cases are focused on the underlying condition and not the back pain itself. Thus, the majority of LBP cases are of unknown etiology and treatments are focused on symptoms. Acute back pain is generally defined as being present for less than 6 weeks, while subacute back pain is defined as being present for between 6 weeks and 3 months. Chronic LBP includes all incidents lasting longer than 3 months. The incidence of LBP in adults in the United States was estimated to be about 26% over a 3-month period (Deyo, Mirza, & Martin, 2006). In England, data suggests that 28% of adults report LBP in a 1-month period (Macfarlane et al., 2012). This is consistent with Andersson's 1999 report suggesting as many as 85% of people suffer from back pain at some point in their lives. Importantly, this report shows that 60–70% of patients recover from their LBP within 6 weeks and 80–90% of patients recover within 12 weeks. For those whose pain does become chronic LBP, recovery is uncertain and returning to work is rare and may take years.

Exercise and low back pain

With the push for evidence-based medicine, there have been a large number of studies conducted to determine the efficacy of different treatments for LBP. These interventions generally target chronic LBP symptoms, include some type of exercise (e.g., yoga, strengthening, aerobic exercise, etc.) and focus on changes in pain ratings as the primary outcome. A number of reviews detailing the effects of exercise on LBP exist (e.g., Bell & Burnett, 2009; van Middelkoop et al., 2011) and conclude that exercise is a generally efficacious treatment. Other studies have looked at exercise therapy compared to traditional treatments (e.g., Ferreira et al., 2007; Mannion, Muntener, Taimela, & Dvorak, 1999), finding that exercise is a favorable therapy compared to usual care and is the same as or better than motor control therapy or active physiotherapy. The negative side effects of exercise therapy for LBP appear to be nominal, as adverse events are rarely reported. Therefore, exercise has been shown to be a safe and effective treatment option for people suffering from chronic LBP. Macedo and colleagues (Macedo, Maher, Latimer, & McAuley, 2009) put together a critical review of studies using motor control therapy (an approach using motor learning principles to retrain the lower back muscles) in chronic LBP and found it to be a more effective treatment than usual care, but not any better than other exercise modes. The general consensus is that exercise decreases pain scores in patients with chronic LBP, although the most efficacious intensity, duration, and mode of exercise have not yet been identified. Regular exercise reduces the risk of LBP recurrences if continued following initial pain treatment (Choi, Verbeek, Tam, & Jiang, 2010).

Guidelines for exercise in lower back pain

A number of organizations have published guidelines for the effective management and treatment of LBP. Almost all guidelines include recommendations to increase physical activity through structured exercise, or at a minimum, focus on maintaining current levels of physical activity. The American College of Physicians and the American Pain Society jointly recommend both exercise and yoga as effective forms of treatment for acute and chronic LBP (Chou, Huffman, American Pain Society, & American College of Physicians, 2007). In 2001, the Philadelphia Panel for Evidence-Based Clinical Practice Guidelines (Philadelphia Panel, 2001a) recommended continued daily activities (no specific change in exercise, just maintenance) for acute LBP, with recommendations for both subacute and chronic back pain sufferers to use exercise as a frontline treatment for pain. However, the addition of aerobic exercise to conventional physiotherapy rather than in place of regular treatment is not always recommended and should be prescribed cautiously (Chan, Mok, & Yeung, 2011). Without evidence of specific exercise programs being superior, it seems practical to permit patients the option to select an activity they prefer and enjoy. Overall, most back pain treatment recommendations will include limited pharmaco-therapy in conjunction with exercise therapy with specific recommendations depending on the individual case.

Headache

Headaches can vary in type and their pain symptoms are often described in terms of intensity and duration. Lifetime prevalence for tension-type headaches (TTH) is reported to be 46%, migraine 14%, and chronic daily headache 2.9% (Stovner et al., 2007). In the United States, the general prevalence of migraines is estimated to be 18.2% for women and 6.5% for men, with the highest overall prevalence occurring between the ages of 30 and 39 years (Lipton, Stewart, Diamond, Diamond, & Reed, 2001).

Exercise in headache patients

Tension-type headaches have been suggested to involve muscular pathophysiology (Millea & Brodie, 2002) and as such various physical therapies have been explored. Biondi (2005) concluded that physical therapy is more effective than massage or acupuncture for TTH in individuals with migraine, although physical therapy in conjunction with other treatments is most effective.

Limited evidence suggests that stretching and posture exercises have modest positive effects for TTH and accompanying muscle pain, while the evidence for repetitive motion, resistance training, and conditioning exercises is inconclusive (Fricton, 2007).

Migraine headaches have been reported to be associated with severe impairment and reduction of daily activity and involve a disruption in neural vascular activity (Davies, 2011; Lipton et al., 2001). In general, exercise research for migraine has been of poor quality and recommendations for exercise have been cautiously supported (Busch & Gaul, 2008; Biondi, 2005). One study examined the effectiveness of 1 hour of supervised aerobic exercise 3 times/week over an 8-week treatment period compared to a control group taking medication (Narin, Pinar, Erbas, Ozturk, & Idiman, 2003). Both groups reported decreases in the frequency of pain and pain disability, but the exercise group reported significantly more pain relief compared to the control group, supporting a potentially therapeutic effect of aerobic exercise on migraine pain (Narin et al., 2003).

Guidelines for exercise in headache patients

Although there are several headache organizations (e.g., American Academy of Neurology) that advocate the use of exercise for headache treatment, they lack specific guidelines. One evidence-based guideline for the treatment of migraines focuses on the use of medication and recommends that behavioral and physical interventions be used primarily for prevention rather than acute alleviation (Silberstein, 2000). The British Association for the Study of Headaches (2010) suggests that relaxation therapy, stress reduction, and coping should be frontline therapies for migraine. The European Federation of Neurological Societies suggests that although physical therapy may be a viable therapy for TTH, the lack of scientific evidence prevents specific recommendations (Bendtsen et al., 2010).

Chronic neck pain

Chronic neck pain has been reported to affect nearly 10% of the general population and has been identified as an ailment associated with the changes in workplace environments over the past century (Cote et al., 2008). The 12-month prevalence rate is between 30% and 50%, and is accompanied by limited ability to work and engage in social activities (Hogg-Johnson et al., 2008). Because weak musculature surrounding the neck has been suggested to be a potential cause of neck pain, strengthening exercises have been proposed as an active treatment.

Exercise in chronic neck pain

Exercise interventions focused on the neck musculature have resulted in moderate to large improvements in neck pain when compared to mock treatment, advice therapy, or no-treatment controls, and small to moderate improvements when compared to general practitioner care (Miller et al., 2010). Though this body of literature generally supports strengthening of shoulder and neck muscles to treat chronic neck pain, the protocols used for strengthening have varied, have not been well defined, or have been used in combination with other therapies. Thus, the most effective intervention for chronic neck pain has yet to be determined.

Guidelines for exercise in chronic neck pain patients

The Philadelphia Panel concluded that there is scientific evidence to support and recommend the use of proprioceptive and therapeutic exercises for chronic neck pain, but not thermotherapy, therapeutic massage, EMG biofeedback, mechanical traction, therapeutic ultrasound, or electrical stimulation (Philadelphia Panel, 2001b). Further, the Oklahoma Physician Advisory Committee recommends that an exercise program used to treat neck pain should include strength, endurance, flexibility, and educational components (Physician Advisory Committee, 1997). Specifically, the guidelines suggest that a conservative exercise treatment should be adopted before progressing to regular aerobic exercise and supervised therapeutic exercises. The American Physical Therapy Association recommends cervical manipulation and mobilization along with coordinating, strengthening, and endurance exercises in the treatment of neck pain (Childs et al., 2008).

Conclusions

Summary and limitations of exercise research in chronic pain conditions

Overall, exercise appears to have consistent and positive benefits for a multitude of chronic pain conditions with few adverse outcomes. As is the case for healthy individuals, the most common side effects of exercise are positive and include improved cardiopulmonary and mental health. Although much is known about the effect of exercise on pain in a variety of conditions, conclusions need to be made in light of the limitations in study design and execution including (1) rare use of attention-control conditions, (2) frequent comparison of different exercise therapies in the absence of no-treatment control conditions, (3) poorly defined exercise protocols that limit replication, (4) failure to report extra-intervention treatments and compliance rates, and (5) failure to measure extra-intervention physical activity. Although blinding is difficult in exercise studies, it is almost never done, which detracts from internal validity. These weaknesses in study design minimize the impact of recommending exercise as a specific treatment, and need to be taken into account when planning future studies. Research that directly compares different modes, intensities, and durations of exercise are needed to provide evidence-based prescriptions about dose response and to determine whether reductions in pain are related to improved strength and/or aerobic capacity. In regard to exercise prescription, it would be a mistake to rely on previously generated guidelines designed for specific health and fitness outcomes using data collected from healthy individuals and assume they can be adapted to suit the needs of chronic pain patients. Health and fitness outcomes are important, but exercise prescription for chronic pain needs to be based on data from patients suffering from these conditions. There is a need for research aimed at determining for whom and why exercise is an efficacious treatment of chronic pain. Currently, there appears to be an absence of treatment trials designed to uncover the psychobiological mechanisms responsible for symptom improvement in chronic pain patients following exercise training.

References

Andersson, G. B. (1999). Epidemiological features of chronic low-back pain. *Lancet, 354*(9178), 581–585.

Baillet, A., Vaillant, M., Guinot, M., Juvin, R., & Gaudin, P. (2012). Efficacy of resistance exercises in rheumatoid arthritis: Meta-analysis of randomized controlled trials. *Rheumatology (Oxford, England), 51*(3), 519–527.

Baillet, A., Zeboulon, N., Gossec, L., Combescure, C., Bodin, L. A., Juvin, R., . . . Gaudin, P. (2010). Efficacy of cardiorespiratory aerobic exercise in rheumatoid arthritis: Meta-analysis of randomized controlled trials. *Arthritis Care & Research, 62*(7), 984–992.

Bell, J. A., & Burnett, A. (2009). Exercise for the primary, secondary and tertiary prevention of low back pain in the workplace: A systematic review. *Journal of Occupational Rehabilitation, 19*(1), 8–24.

Bendtsen, L., Evers, S., Linde, M., Mitsikostas, D. D., Sandrini, G., Schoenen, J., & EFNS. (2010). EFNS guideline on the treatment of tension-type headache – report of an EFNS task force. *European Journal of Neurology, 17*(11), 1318–1325.

Bilberg, A., Ahlmen, M., & Mannerkorpi, K. (2005). Moderately intensive exercise in a temperate pool for patients with rheumatoid arthritis: A randomized controlled study. *Rheumatology (Oxford, England), 44*(4), 502–508.

Biondi, D. M. (2005). Physical treatments for headache: A structured review. *Headache, 45*(6), 738–746.

Bircan, C., Karasel, S. A., Akgun, B., El, O., & Alper, S. (2008). Effects of muscle strengthening versus aerobic exercise program in fibromyalgia. *Rheumatology International, 28*, 527–532.

British Association for the Study of Headaches. (2010). 2010 BASH guidelines. Retrieved from http://www.bash.org.uk/

Brosseau, L., Wells, G. A., Tugwell, P., Egan, M., Wilson, K. G., Dubouloz, C. J., . . . Veilleux, L. (2008a). Ottawa Panel evidence-based clinical practice guidelines for aerobic fitness exercises in the management of fibromyalgia: Part 1. *Physical Therapy, 88*(7), 857–871.

Brosseau, L., Wells, G. A., Tugwell, P., Egan, M., Wilson, K. G., Dubouloz, C. J., . . . Veilleux, L. (2008b). Ottawa Panel evidence-based clinical practice guidelines for strengthening exercises in the management of fibromyalgia: Part 2. *Physical Therapy, 88*(7), 873–886.

Brosseau, L., Wells, G. A., Tugwell, P., Egan, M., Dubouloz, C. J., Casimiro, L., . . . Ottawa Panel. (2011). Ottawa Panel evidence-based clinical practice guidelines for the management of osteoarthritis in adults who are obese or overweight. *Physical Therapy, 91*(6), 843–861.

Burckhardt, C. S., Goldenberg, D., Crofford, L., Gerwin, R., Gowens, S., Jackson, K., . . . Turk, D. (2005). *Guideline for the management of fibromyalgia syndrome pain in adults and children (Clinical practice guideline No. 4)*. Glenview, IL: American Pain Society.

Busch, A. J., Barber, K. A. R., Overend, T. J., Peloso, P. M. J., & Schachter, C. L. (2007). Exercise for treating fibromyalgia syndrome. *Cochrane Database of Systematic Reviews, 2007* (4): CD003786. doi:10.1002/14651858.CD003786.pub2

Busch, V., & Gaul, C. (2008). Exercise in migraine therapy—is there any evidence for efficacy? A critical review. *Headache, 48*(6), 890–899.

Busch, A. J., Thille, P., Barber, K. A. R., Schachter, C. L., Biodonde, J., & Collacott, B. K. (2008). Best practice: E-model—prescribing physical activity and exercise for individuals with fibromyalgia. *Physiotherapy Theory and Practice, 24*(3), 151–166.

Busch, A. J., Webber, S. C., Brachniec, M., Bidonde, J., Dal Bello-Haas, V., Danyliw, A. D., . . . Schachter, C. L. (2011). Exercise therapy for fibromyalgia. *Current Pain and Headache Reports, 15*, 358–367.

Cazzola, M., Atzeni, F., Salaffi, F., Stisi, S., Cassisi, G., & Sarzi-Puttini, P. (2010). What kind of exercise is best in fibromyalgia therapeutic programmes? A practical review. *Experimental Rheumatology, 28*(Suppl. 63), S117–S124.

Chan, C. W., Mok, N. W., & Yeung, E. W. (2011). Aerobic exercise training in addition to conventional physiotherapy for chronic low back pain: A randomized controlled trial. *Archives of Physical Medicine and Rehabilitation, 92*(10), 1681–1685.

Childs, J. D., Cleland, J. A., Elliott, J. M., Teyhen, D. S., Wainner, R. S., Whitman, J. M., . . . American Physical Therapy Association. (2008). Neck pain: Clinical practice guidelines linked to the international classification of functioning, disability, and health from the orthopedic section of the American Physical Therapy Association. *Journal of Orthopaedic and Sports Physical Therapy, 38*(9), A1–A34.

Choi, B. K., Verbeek, J. H., Tam, W. W., & Jiang, J. Y. (2010). Exercises for prevention of recurrences of low-back pain. *Cochrane Database of Systematic Reviews (Online)* (1): CD006555.

Chou, R., Huffman, L. H., American Pain Society, & American College of Physicians. (2007). Nonpharmacologic therapies for acute and chronic low back pain: A review of the evidence for an American Pain Society/American College of Physicians clinical practice guideline. *Annals of Internal Medicine, 147*(7), 492–504.

Clauw, D. J. (2009). Fibromyalgia: An overview. *American Journal of Medicine, 122*(12, Supplement), S3–S13.

Cook, D. B., Stegner, A. J., & Ellingson, L. D. (2010). Exercise alters pain sensitivity in Gulf War veterans with chronic musculoskeletal pain. *Journal of Pain, 11*(8), 764–772.

Cook, D. B., Stegner, A. J., Nagelkirk, P. R., Meyer, J. D., Togo, F., & Natelson, B. H. (2012). Responses to exercise differ for chronic fatigue syndrome patients with fibromyalgia. *Medicine and Science in Sports and Exercise, 44*, 1186–1193.

Cote, P., van der Velde, G., Cassidy, J. D., Carroll, L. J., Hogg-Johnson, S., Holm, L. W., . . . Peloso, P. M. (2008). The burden and determinants of neck pain in workers result of the bone and joint decade 2000–2010 task force on neck pain and its associated disorders. *European Spine Journal, 17*(Supplement 1), S60–S74.

Daley, A. J., Grimmett, C., Roberts, L., Wilson, S., Fatek, M., Roalfe, A., & Singh, S. (2008). The effects of exercise upon symptoms and quality of life in patients diagnosed with irritable bowel syndrome: A randomised controlled trial. *International Journal of Sports Medicine, 29*(9), 778–782.

Davies, P. (2011). What has imaging taught us about migraine? *Maturitas, 70*(1), 34–36.

Deyo, R. A., Mirza, S. K., & Martin, B. I. (2006). Back pain prevalence and visit rates: Estimates from U.S. national surveys, 2002. *Spine, 31*(23), 2724–2727.

Donta, S. T., Clauw, D. J., Engel, C. C., Jr., Guarino, P., Peduzzi, P., Williams, D. A., . . . VA Cooperative Study #470 Study Group. (2003). Cognitive behavioral therapy and aerobic exercise for Gulf War veterans' illnesses: A randomized controlled trial. *Journal of the American Medical Association, 289*(11), 1396–1404.

Ferreira, M. L., Ferreira, P. H., Latimer, J., Herbert, R. D., Hodges, P. W., Jennings, M. D., . . . Refshauge, K. M. (2007). Comparison of general exercise, motor control exercise and spinal manipulative therapy for chronic low back pain: A randomized trial. *Pain, 131*(1–2), 31–37.

Focht, B. C. (2006). Effectiveness of exercise interventions in reducing pain symptoms among older adults with knee osteoarthritis: A review. *Journal of Aging and Physical Activity, 14*(2), 212–235.

Fricton, J. (2007). Myogenous temporomandibular disorders: Diagnostic and management considerations. *Dental Clinics of North America, 51*(1), 61–83, vi.

Gowans, S. E., & deHueck, A. (2007). Pool exercises for individuals with fibromyalgia. *Current Opinion in Rheumatology, 19*, 168–173.

Grotle, M., Hagen, K. B., Natvig, B., Dahl, F. A., & Kvien, T. K. (2008). Prevalence and burden of osteoarthritis: Results from a population survey in Norway. *Journal of Rheumatology, 35*(4), 677–684.

Guillemin, F., Saraux, A., Guggenbuhl, P., Roux, C. H., Fardellone, P., Le Bihan, E., . . . Coste, J. (2005). Prevalence of rheumatoid arthritis in France: 2001. *Annals of the Rheumatic Diseases, 64*(10), 1427–1430.

Häkkinen, A., Häkkinen, K., Hannonen, P., & Alen, M. (2001). Strength training induced adaptations in neuromuscular function of premenopausal women with fibromyalgia: Comparison with healthy women. *Annals of the Rheumatic Diseases, 60*(1), 21–26.

Hardt, J., Jacobsen, C., Goldberg, J., Nickel, R., & Buchwald, D. (2008). Prevalence of chronic pain in a representative sample in the United States. *Pain Medicine (Malden, Mass.), 9*(7), 803–812.

Häuser, W., Klose, P., Langhorst, J., Moradi, B., Steinbach, M., Schiltenwolf, M., & Busch, A. J. (2010). Efficacy of different types of aerobic exercise in fibromyalgia syndrome: A systematic review and meta-analysis of randomised controlled trials. *Arthritis Research & Therapy, 12*(3), R79.

Henchoz, Y., Bastardot, F., Guessous, I., Theler, J. M., Dudler, J., Vollenweider, P., & So, A. (2012). Physical activity and energy expenditure in rheumatoid arthritis patients and matched controls. *Rheumatology (Oxford, England), 51*(8):1500–1507.

Hochberg, M. C., Altman, R. D., April, K. T., Benkhalti, M., Guyatt, G., McGowan, J., . . . Tugwell, P. (2012). American College of Rheumatology 2012 recommendations for the use of nonpharmacologic and pharmacologic therapies in osteoarthritis of the hand, hip, and knee. *Arthritis Care & Research, 64*(4), 455–474.

Hogg-Johnson, S., van der Velde, G., Carroll, L. J., Holm, L. W., Cassidy, J. D., Guzman, J., . . . Bone and Joint Decade 2000–2010 Task Force on Neck Pain and Its Associated Disorders. (2008). The burden and determinants of neck pain in the general population: Results of the bone and joint decade 2000–2010 task force on neck pain and its associated disorders. *Spine, 33*(4 Suppl), S39–S51.

Hurkmans, E., van der Giesen, F. J., Vliet Vlieland, T. P., Schoones, J., & Van den Ende, E. C. (2009). Dynamic exercise programs (aerobic capacity and/or muscle strength training) in patients with rheumatoid arthritis. *Cochrane Database of Systematic Reviews (Online)* (4): CD006853.

Iversen, M. D. (2012). Rehabilitation interventions for pain and disability in osteoarthritis: A review of interventions including exercise, manual techniques, and assistive devices. *Orthopaedic Nursing, 31*, 103–108.

Iwamoto, J., Sato, Y., Takeda, T., & Matsumoto, H. (2011). Effectiveness of exercise for osteoarthritis of the knee: A review of the literature. *World Journal of Orthopedics, 2*(5), 37–42.

Kadetoff, D., & Kosek, E. (2010). Evidence of reduced sympatho-adrenal and hypothalamic pituitary activity during static muscular work in patients with fibromyalgia. *Journal of Rehabilitation Medicine, 42*, 765–772.

Leeuw, M., Goossens, M. E. J. B., Linton, S. J., Crombez, G., Boersma, K., & Vlaeyen, J. W. S. (2007). The fear-avoidance model of musculoskeletal pain: Current state of scientific evidence. *Journal of Behavioral Medicine, 30*, 77–94.

Lindell, L., Bergman, S., Petersson, I. F., Jacobsson, L. T., & Herrstrom, P. (2000). Prevalence of fibromyalgia and chronic widespread pain. *Scandinavian Journal of Primary Health Care, 18*(3), 149–153.

Lipton, R. B., Stewart, W. F., Diamond, S., Diamond, M. L., & Reed, M. (2001). Prevalence and burden of migraine in the United States: Data from the American Migraine Study II. *Headache, 41*(7), 646–657.

Loew, L., Brosseau, L., Wells, G. A., Tugwell, P., Kenny, G. P., Reid, R., . . . Longchamps, G. (2012). Ottawa Panel evidence-based clinical practice guidelines for aerobic walking programs in the management of osteoarthritis. *Archives of Physical Medicine and Rehabilitation.* Epub ahead of print.

Macedo, L. G., Maher, C. G., Latimer, J., & McAuley, J. H. (2009). Motor control exercise for persistent, nonspecific low back pain: A systematic review. *Physical Therapy, 89*(1), 9–25.

Macfarlane, G. J., Beasley, M., Jones, E. A., Prescott, G. J., Docking, R., Keeley, P., . . . MUSICIAN Study Team. (2012). The prevalence and management of low back pain across adulthood: Results from a population-based cross-sectional study (the MUSICIAN study). *Pain, 153*(1), 27–32.

Mannion, A. F., Muntener, M., Taimela, S., & Dvorak, J. (1999). A randomized clinical trial of three active therapies for chronic low back pain. *Spine, 24*(23), 2435–2448.

McCracken, L. M., & Samuel, V. M. (2007). The role of avoidance, pacing, and other activity patterns in chronic pain. *Pain, 130*, 119–125.

McLoughlin, M. J., Colbert, L. H., Stegner, A. J., & Cook, D. B. (2011). Are women with fibromyalgia less physically active than healthy women? *Medicine and Science in Sports and Exercise, 43*(5), 905–912.

Mengshoel, A. M., Vøllestad, N. K., & Førre, Ø. (1995). Pain and fatigue induced by exercise in fibromyalgia patients and sedentary healthy subjects. *Clinical and Experimental Rheumatology, 13*, 477–482.

Metsios, G. S., Stavropoulos-Kalinoglou, A., Veldhuijzen van Zanten, J. J., Treharne, G. J., Panoulas, V. F., Douglas, K. M., . . . Kitas, G. D. (2008). Rheumatoid arthritis, cardiovascular disease and physical exercise: A systematic review. *Rheumatology (Oxford, England), 47*(3), 239–248.

Millea, P. J., & Brodie, J. J. (2002). Tension-type headache. *American Family Physician, 66*(5), 797–804.

Miller, J., Gross, A., D'Sylva, J., Burnie, S. J., Goldsmith, C. H., Graham, N., . . . Hoving, J. L. (2010). Manual therapy and exercise for neck pain: A systematic review. *Manual Therapy, 15*, 334–354.

Narin, S. O., Pinar, L., Erbas, D., Ozturk, V., & Idiman, F. (2003). The effects of exercise and exercise-related changes in blood nitric oxide level on migraine headache. *Clinical Rehabilitation, 17*(6), 624–630.

National Collaborating Centre for Chronic Conditions (UK). (2008). *Osteoarthritis: The care and management of osteoarthritis in adults.* Available online at http://publications.nice.org.uk/osteoarthritis-cg59

National Collaborating Centre for Chronic Conditions (UK). (2009). *Rheumatoid arthritis: The management of rheumatoid arthritis in adults.* Available online at http://publications.nice.org.uk/osteoarthritis-cg79

Philadelphia Panel. (2001a). Philadelphia Panel evidence-based clinical practice guidelines on selected rehabilitation interventions for low back pain. *Physical Therapy, 81*(10), 1641–1674.

Philadelphia Panel. (2001b). Philadelphia Panel evidence-based clinical practice guidelines on selected rehabilitation interventions for neck pain. *Physical Therapy, 81*(10), 1701–1717.

Physician Advisory Committee. (1997). Neck pain treatment guidelines. Oklahoma City, OK: Oklahoma workers' compensation court.

Pisters, M. F., Veenhof, C., van Meeteren, N. L., Ostelo, R. W., de Bakker, D. H., Schellevis, F. G., & Dekker, J. (2007). Long-term effectiveness of exercise therapy in patients with osteoarthritis of the hip or knee: A systematic review. *Arthritis and Rheumatism, 57*(7), 1245–1253.

Roddy, E., Zhang, W., & Doherty, M. (2005). Aerobic walking or strengthening exercise for osteoarthritis of the knee? A systematic review. *Annals of the Rheumatic Diseases, 64*(4), 544–548.

Rooks, D. S., Gautman, S., Romeling, M., Cross, M. L., Stratigakis, D., Evans, B., Goldenberg, D. L., Iversen, M. D., & Katz, J. N. (2007). Group exercise, education, and combination self-management in women with fibromyalgia: A randomized trial. *Archives of Internal Medicine, 167*(20), 2192–2200.

Silberstein, S. D. (2000). Practice parameter: Evidence-based guidelines for migraine headache (an evidence-based review): Report of the quality standards subcommittee of the American Academy of Neurology. *Neurology, 55*(6), 754–762.

Stovner, L., Hagen, K., Jensen, R., Katsarava, Z., Lipton, R., Scher, A., . . . Zwart, J. A. (2007). The global burden of headache: A documentation of headache prevalence and disability worldwide. *Cephalalgia, 27*(3), 193–210.

Symmons, D., Turner, G., Webb, R., Asten, P., Barrett, E., Lunt, M., . . . Silman, A. (2002). The prevalence of rheumatoid arthritis in the United Kingdom: New estimates for a new century. *Rheumatology (Oxford, England), 41*(7), 793–800.

Thomas, E. N., & Blotman, F. (2010). Aerobic exercise in fibromyalgia: A practical review. *Rheumatology International, 30*, 1143–1150.

Valim, V., Oliveira, L., Suda, A., Silva, L., de Assis, M., Neto, T. B., . . . Natour, J. (2003). Aerobic fitness effects in fibromyalgia. *Journal of Rheumatology, 30*, 1060–1069.

Valkeinen, H., Alen, M., Hannonen, P., Häkkinen, A., Airaksinen, O., & Häkkinen, K. (2004). Changes in knee extension and flexion force, EMG and functional capacity during strength training in older females with fibromyalgia and healthy controls. *Rheumatology (Oxford, England)*, *43*(2), 225–228.

van Es, P. P., Luijsterburg, P. A., Dekker, J., Koopmanschap, M. A., Bohnen, A. M., Verhaar, J. A., . . . Bierma-Zeinstra, S. M. (2011). Cost-effectiveness of exercise therapy versus general practitioner care for osteoarthritis of the hip: Design of a randomised clinical trial. *BMC Musculoskeletal Disorders*, *12*, 232.

van Middelkoop, M., Rubinstein, S. M., Kuijpers, T., Verhagen, A. P., Ostelo, R., Koes, B. W., & van Tulder, M. W. (2011). A systematic review on the effectiveness of physical and rehabilitation interventions for chronic non-specific low back pain. *European Spine Journal*, *20*(1), 19–39.

Westby, M. (2012) Exercise and arthritis. Available online at http://www.rheumatology.org/practice/clinical/patients/diseases_and_conditions/exercise.asp

Wolfe, F., Smyth, H. A., Yunus, M. B., Bennett, R. M., Bombardier, C., Goldenberg, D. L., et al. (1990). The American College of Rheumatology 1990 criteria for the classification of fibromyalgia: Report of the multicenter criteria committee. *Arthritis & Rheumatism*, *3*(2), 160–172.

Woolf, A. D., & Pfleger, B. (2003). Burden of major musculoskeletal conditions. *Bulletin of the World Health Organization*, *81*(9), 646–656.

Zhang, W., Doherty, M., Arden, N., Bannwarth, B., Bijlsma, J., Gunther, K. P., . . . EULAR Standing Committee for International Clinical Studies Including Therapeutics (ESCISIT). (2005). EULAR evidence based recommendations for the management of hip osteoarthritis: Report of a task force of the EULAR standing committee for international clinical studies including therapeutics (ESCISIT). *Annals of the Rheumatic Diseases*, *64*(5), 669–681.

27

PHYSICAL ACTIVITY AND PAIN

Neurobiological mechanisms

Laura D. Ellingson and Dane B. Cook

This chapter is intended to introduce the reader to the neurobiological mechanisms that underlie pain perception and to discuss how exercise interacts with the central nervous system to both stimulate and decrease the experience of pain. The chapter is divided into four primary sections: the first provides a brief overview of the neurobiology of pain; the second and third discuss potential psychobiological mechanisms underlying the pain-inducing aspects of exercise; and the fourth addresses potential mechanisms, both opioid and non-opioid, that underlie the pain-relieving aspects of exercise and physical activity.

Neurobiology of pain

The processing of pain is complex and occurs throughout an integrated network of peripheral, spinal, and supraspinal pathways (for a more detailed overview of peripheral nociception please see Mense, 1993; Millan, 1999; and Schaible, Ebersberger & Natura, 2011). In most cases, the experience of pain results from nociception. However, pain perception is highly dependent upon interactions and modulations of afferent (bottom-up) and efferent (top-down) information at each level of processing. Further, psychological, cultural, and social factors can influence the central nervous system, ultimately shaping the pain experience.

Nociception begins in the periphery (skin, viscera, and muscles) with the stimulation of one or more nociceptors, free nerve endings with high thresholds for depolarization, designed to respond preferentially to a variety of noxious stimuli including mechanical, chemical, and thermal. Nociceptive fibers enter the spinal cord primarily through the dorsal horn delivering pain-relevant information to nociceptive-specific, wide-dynamic-range, and silent neurons before crossing to the contralateral ventral horn. Silent nociceptors are a unique class of neurons that become active following tissue damage and thus may play a role in the delayed onset muscle soreness that accompanies unaccustomed exercise. From the ventral horn, the nociceptive signal ascends in the spinal cord via second-order projection neurons primarily along the spinothalamic tract to the brainstem and diencephalon. Once there, it synapses in a variety of locations including the lateral and medial components of the thalamus, periaqueductal gray (PAG), parabrachial region, reticular formation, and hypothalamus. Third-order neurons then ascend to a number of brain regions associated with the sensory, affective, cognitive, and modulatory components of pain perception, thus highlighting the multidimensional nature of the pain experience. It is important to note that modulation of the nociceptive signal, both inhibition and facilitation, occurs at each level of processing from the periphery to the brain. This has relevance for a stimulus such as exercise, which has the capacity to both send nociceptive signals from the muscle and relieve pain through modulation via both peripheral and central mechanisms.

Although considerable research has accumulated regarding peripheral, spinal, and spinal-thalamic mechanisms underlying pain perception, less is known about the more integrated aspects of pain processing involving the brain. The most commonly reported brain regions responsible for processing pain include the thalamus, primary and secondary somatosensory cortices, anterior and posterior insular cortices, the anterior cingulate cortex, cerebellum, inferior parietal cortex, frontal cortex, especially dorsolateral and medial areas, and the lentiform nucleus. Less commonly reported areas include the PAG and hypothalamus, both thought to play an integral role in pain modulation. For several excellent reviews of pain processing in the brain please see Bingel & Tracey (2008) and Tracey (2007).

Exercise-induced muscle pain

Anecdotal and empirical evidence suggests that muscle pain is a natural consequence of exercise with pain threshold (the point at which pain in the exercising muscle becomes just noticeable) occurring at approximately 50% of maximum aerobic capacity (Cook, O'Connor, Eubanks, Smith, & Lee, 1997). The perception of muscle pain during exercise has been found to (a) increase as a positively accelerating function of exercise intensity (e.g., Watts and percent peak oxygen consumption), (b) be reproducible, (c) induce extremely intense pain at peak, and (d) to recover in two phases (fast initial and slower secondary).

Research in the area of muscle pain has often relied on unnatural stimuli such as hypertonic saline, electrical stimulation, and ischemia to induce pain. While these pain–induction methods have value (e.g., can be standardized and delivered under controlled conditions), one of the ideal qualities of a pain stimulus is that it mimics pain that individuals normally encounter in daily life. Muscle pain induced by exercise is one of the few natural pain-inducing stimuli enhancing its

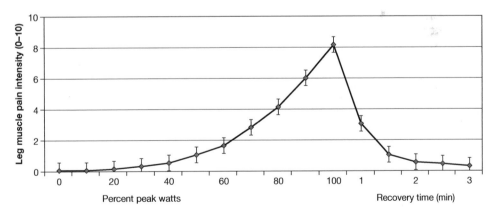

Figure 27.1 A typical muscle pain intensity response function that might occur during maximal cycle ergometry. Notable features include that (1) pain rarely occurs prior to 50% of peak exercise capacity for healthy individuals, (2) pain increases as a positively accelerating function of relative exercise intensity post pain threshold, and (3) pain during recovery is characterized by a fast initial decline in pain intensity (the first 30 seconds) and then a slower secondary decline over the next several minutes. Power functions, based on log10 transformation of pain ratings and exercise intensity (e.g., Watts), have been found to be greater than 2.0 prior to pain threshold and greater than 3.0 post pain threshold.

ecological validity. It can be delivered in a standardized fashion and it has proven to be a useful experimental pain stimulus in research settings (O'Connor & Cook, 1999).

As a naturally occurring pain stimulus, exercise-induced muscle pain (EIMP) may also have clinical relevance. EIMP is experienced as diffuse in nature and has been described as exhausting, intense, sharp, burning, tiring, cramping, pulling, and rasping (Cook et al., 1997). These words have also been used to characterize the experience of individuals suffering from chronic pain conditions such as fibromyalgia, arthritis, cancer pain, and chronic back pain (Cook, Lange, et al., 2004). Consequently, utilizing EIMP as an experimental pain stimulus may be more generalizable to chronic pain populations than other types of experimental pain stimuli.

Mechanisms

Although the mechanisms that underlie exercise-induced muscle pain have yet to be fully understood, there are a number of viable hypotheses. It is likely that elevated intramuscular pressure associated with high-intensity exercise leads to stimulation of mechanosensitive nociceptors. However, to date this has not been directly tested (O'Connor & Cook, 1999). This stimulation, in combination with the release of noxious biochemicals and deformation of tissue associated with muscular contraction, could be sufficient to stimulate nociceptive fibers (Cook et al., 1997; Mense, 1993). However, the exact combinations of pressure and biochemical accumulation that is both necessary and sufficient to result in the experience of muscle pain are currently unknown. Recent mouse studies have shown that exposing muscle nociceptors to a single biochemical that is normally released during exercise was insufficient to depolarize dorsal horn neurons, but that a combination of adenosine, hydrogen ions, and lactate was necessary for nociceptive transmission (Light et al. 2008). To date, research in humans has employed single agonist or antagonist drugs in an attempt to alter muscle pain during exercise. Of the biochemicals tested, prostaglandins, endogenous opioids, and adenosine have received the most attention. Other biochemicals that are candidates for involvement in exercise-induced muscle pain are bradykinin and hydrogen ions.

Prostaglandins

Prostaglandins are hormone-like lipid compounds that are found throughout a wide variety of tissues including muscle and are involved in pain processing. Research has demonstrated that prostaglandins are released within muscle during muscular contraction (Rotto & Kaufman, 1988). Prostaglandins facilitate pain perception primarily by sensitizing nociceptors (Diehl, Hoheisel, & Mense, 1993). However, it has been demonstrated that ingestion of aspirin, a prostaglandin antagonist, had no effect on perception of muscle pain during or following maximal cycling exercise (Cook et al., 1997). These results suggest that prostaglandins alone are not sufficient to induce muscle pain during exercise.

Opioids

The contribution of endogenous opioids to EIMP has also been explored. Opioid receptors are found peripherally in muscle as well as at spinal and supraspinal sites involved in pain processing (e.g., PAG, RVM). Endogenous opioids have a well-established role in pain modulation. Peripherally, concentrations of endogenous opioids have been consistently shown to increase during moderate and intense exercise (Boone, Sherraden, Pierzchala, Berger, & Van Loon, 1992; Schwartz & Kindermann, 1992). There is also limited evidence that central concentrations of endogenous opioids increase following long-duration aerobic exercise (Boecker et al., 2008). As such, endogenous opioids are a potential mechanism of muscle pain regulation. This regulation could occur through altering muscle sympathetic nerve activity (MSNA) responses to exercise, thus decreasing delivery of pain-related information to the spinal cord (Farrell, Ebert, & Kampine, 1991; Ray, Rea, Clary, & Mark, 1992). However, evidence in support of this is inconsistent. Research has shown that opioid antagonists (naloxone/naltrexone) can either increase (Farrell et al., 1991) or have no effect (Ray & Pawelczyk, 1994; Cook, O'Connor, & Ray, 2000; Ray & Carter, 2007) on MSNA during submaximal isometric handgrip exercise. Further, opioid agonists (morphine/codeine) have been shown to have no effect on MSNA during submaximal isometric handgrip exercise (Cook et al., 2000; Carter, Sauder, & Ray, 2002; Ray & Carter, 2007). Thus, the relationship between endogenous opioids, MSNA, and pain in response to exercise is currently equivocal.

Caffeine/adenosine

Caffeine is an adenosine antagonist and adenosine has been shown to have analgesic properties (Sawynok, 1998). Muscular contractions are associated with increased concentrations of adenosine in the exercising muscle (Costa et al., 2001; Langberg, Bjørn, Boushel, Hellsten, & Kjaer, 2002). Research has demonstrated that high doses of caffeine consistently attenuate muscle pain during both low-intensity and high-intensity aerobic exercise in both men and women and that this decrease occurs in a dose-response fashion (Motl, O'Connor, & Dishman, 2003; O'Connor, Motl, Broglio, & Ely, 2004; Motl, O'Connor, Tubandt, Puetz, & Ely, 2006).

Bradykinin

Bradykinin is a nonapeptide that has been shown to increase in a dose-response fashion during muscular contractions in humans (Blais, Adam, Massicotte, & Peronnet, 1999; Langberg et al., 2002). Bradykinin is also known to be potentiated under conditions of low pH and hypoxia, which both occur during exercise (Mense, 1993). Injection of bradykinin into muscle tissue induces pain (Babenko et al., 1999a, 1999b; Franz & Mense, 1975; Mørk, Ashina, Bendtsen, Olesen, & Jensen, 2003). Additionally, several studies have demonstrated that intramuscular concentrations of bradykinin increase during both isometric and low-intensity resistance exercise and that these increases are positively related to pain ratings taken during exercise (Boix, Roe, Rosenborg, & Knardahl, 2005; Gerdle et al., 2008). There is also some evidence that bradykinin may play a role in delayed onset muscle soreness (DOMS; Murase et al., 2010). Thus, bradykinin may be involved in muscle nociceptive signaling during exercise, as well as signaling from damaged muscle.

Hydrogen ions

Animal research shows that high extracellular concentrations of hydrogen ions induce both excitation and sensitization of the nociceptive fibers to mechanical stimuli applied to the skin (Steen, Reeh, Anton, & Handwerker, 1992). Research using rats has also shown that intramuscular injections of acidic phosphate buffer, which were designed to mimic extracellular hydrogen ion concentrations during exhaustive exercise, inflammation, or ischemia, led to excitation of chemosensitive nociceptive fibers within the muscle (Hoheisel, Reinohl, Unger, & Mense, 2004). Further, in humans, both cutaneous and intramuscular injections of acidic solutions elicit muscle pain (Birklin et al., 2000; Steen, Reeh, Geisslinger, & Steen, 2000).

Ischemic muscle contractions have been shown to lead to increases in muscle pain in humans, which are associated with decreases in extracellular pH on the surface of the contracting muscle (Graven-Nielsen et al., 2003; Issberner, Reeh, & Steen, 1996). However, to date no studies have been conducted that concurrently examine exercise-induced increases in hydrogen ions and changes in pain perception. Hydrogen ion accumulation during exercise may be involved in EIMP; however, it is not known whether this biochemical is sufficient to induce muscle pain under naturalistic conditions (i.e., daily physical activity).

Other psychobiological factors that could influence EIMP

Several potential modifiers and mediators of the relationship between pain and exercise have been examined including demographic factors (e.g,. sex), genetic factors (e.g., propensity for high blood pressure), and psychological factors (e.g., self-efficacy, personality). Both research and clinical evidence demonstrate that women are more sensitive to experimental pain stimuli and suffer from higher rates of chronic pain conditions than men (Berkley, 1997; Hurley & Adams, 2008; Riley, Robinson, Wise, Myers, & Fillingim, 1998). However, when EIMP was assessed relative to peak power output during cycling, women rated leg muscle pain as significantly less intense than men (Cook, O'Connor, Oliver, & Lee, 1998). Men and women have also been shown to have comparable exercise-induced hypoalgesic responses (see Chapter 26, this volume). These results highlight the implications of using an absolute as compared to a relative experimental pain stimulus. Delivery of an absolute stimulus (e.g., a 2000-gram pressure stimulus) may result in gender differences simply because the stimulus intensity represents a different relative stimulus.

Genetic factors and select psychological variables have also been investigated as possible moderators of EIMP. Cook, Jackson, O'Connor, and Dishman (2004) examined the influence of genetic susceptibility for hypertension (i.e., parental history) in normotensive African American women on leg muscle pain intensity during exercise. Results showed that participants with a family history of hypertension rated exercise as significantly less painful than those without a family history. These results support the potential influence of genetic factors on sensitivity for EIMP and are consistent with research demonstrating the involvement of genetics in pain perception as well as in risk for development of chronic pain conditions (Buskila, 2007; Kim et al., 2004; Mogil, 1999).

The influence of personality and self-efficacy on EIMP has also been explored. Based on Eysenck's personality theory and prior research regarding the relationship between personality and pain perception, Cook and colleagues (1998) examined whether personality characteristics (e.g., extraversion, neuroticism, psychoticism) were correlated with EIMP during cycling in college-aged men and women. Results showed that correlations between extraversion and pain perception were not significant for men or women and that only men demonstrated a moderate positive correlation between pain perception and neuroticism. Further, a moderate positive correlation was found between psychoticism and pain perception in women. These results suggest that personality variables such as neuroticism and psychoticism may influence pain perception. However, it is important to note that this sample consisted of healthy, college-aged men and women who all fell into the normal range for the personality variables assessed. Thus, further research using individuals whose scores fall outside the normal range is necessary to better understand how personality might affect pain perception. The influence of self-efficacy on EIMP tolerance was assessed in physically active, college-aged women before a maximal cycling test (Motl, Gliottoni, & Scott, 2007). Approximately 1 week later participants completed 30 minutes of cycling at 80% of maximum. Ratings of leg muscle pain intensity were assessed during both exercise bouts. Results showed that self-efficacy for tolerating pain was moderately and inversely correlated with ratings of muscle pain during both the maximal exercise test and the submaximal exercise, suggesting that self-efficacy may moderate the relationship between exercise and muscle pain.

Summary

Muscle pain is a natural consequence of exercise that has been relatively well characterized. From a muscle contractile perspective, it is likely that the elevated intramuscular pressure associated with high-intensity exercise and deformation of skeletal muscle tissue during contraction stimulates mechanosensitive nociceptors. Biochemical accumulation during intense exercise stimulates both mechano- and chemosensitive nociceptors, leading to naturally occurring muscle pain. This hypothesis has been tested with respect to several potential biochemicals including prostaglandins, endogenous opioids, adenosine, and bradykinin with only adenosine having a consistent hypoalgesic effect and bradykinin having a hyperalgesic effect. Several genetic and psychological factors have also been shown to influence EIMP. Although less rigorously tested than the biological factors, limited evidence suggests that a person's family history of hypertension, being female, being neurotic, and pain-specific self-efficacy can alter the EIMP relationship. The broad range of variables capable of influencing EIMP is an excellent example of pain perception as a complex psychobiological phenomenon.

Exercise-induced hypoalgesia

Despite its painful qualities, there is a growing body of evidence showing that a single bout of exercise results in a reduction in pain sensitivity to experimental pain stimuli. This reduction, termed exercise-induced hypoalgesia (EIH), is characterized by an increase in experimental pain thresholds and pain tolerances, and decreased intensity and unpleasantness ratings for a variety of painful stimuli delivered during and after exercise (Koltyn, 2000). These analgesic effects can last for up to an hour post exercise (Droste, Greenlee, Schreck, & Roskamm, 1991; Olausson et al., 1986). As discussed in Chapter 26, the effects of EIH have been examined most often following aerobic exercises such as running and cycling. However, it has been shown to occur after both resistance and isometric exercise. Research suggests that minimum thresholds exist for both the intensity and duration of exercise necessary to elicit a hypoalgesic effect (Hoffman et al., 2004). A qualitative review of exercise intensity and EIH found that intensities of approximately 70% of maximum aerobic capacity are more likely to elicit EIH than exercise at lower intensities (Koltyn, 2000).

Several theories have been developed in an attempt to explain the mechanism(s) responsible for EIH. These include release of stress mediators such as adrenocorticotrophic hormone and growth hormone, release of endogenous opioids, an interaction between the pain modulatory system and the cardiovascular system, activation of the endocannibinoid system, and activation of supraspinal pain inhibitory mechanisms via conditioned pain modulation. This phenomenon has been explored in both healthy populations and in clinical pain conditions (see Chapter 26).

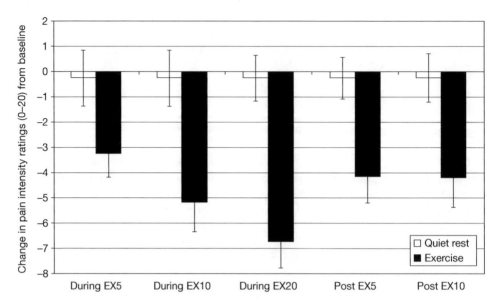

Figure 27.2 A representative hypoalgesic response (i.e., EIH) to 20 minutes of acute exercise and a 10-minute recovery period. Notable features include that (1) decreases in pain intensity are greater as exercise duration increases, (2) decreases in pain intensity are typically greater during exercise than at post-exercise time points, and (3) the hypoalgesic response lasts for upwards of 10 minutes following acute exercise. Data are expressed as a change from baseline using a 0–20 category-ratio type scale and are contrasted with a typical quiet rest response.

Mechanisms

Stress-induced analgesia

Various types of stressors (e.g., uncontrollable footshock in the rat; performance of cognitively challenging tasks in humans) have been shown to induce analgesia in both animal models and humans, warranting the term stress-induced analgesia (SIA) (Lewis, Cannon, & Liebeskind, 1980; Weiss et al., 1986; Fechir et al., 2009). Similar to other stressors, exercise affects stress mechanisms in a load-dependent manner (Galbo, 1982). Thus, exercise may induce hypoalgesia through stress-mediated mechanisms. Several early EIH studies reported an association between stress hormones such as adrenocorticotropin and growth hormone, cortisol, and prolactin and the EIH response (Pertovaara, Huopaniemi, Virtanen, & Johansson, 1984; Kemppainen, Pertovaara, Huopaniemi, Johansson, & Karonen, 1985). However, subsequent research blocking stress hormones has not consistently blocked the EIH response, making it unlikely that stress hormones are a primary mechanism of EIH (Kemppainen, Pertovaara, Huopaniemi, & Johansson, 1986; Kemppainen, Paalasmaa, Pertovaara, Alila, & Johansson, 1990).

Opioid mechanisms

Endorphins are peptides found throughout the body that are known to have pain-relieving properties similar to morphine. There are three major types including β-endorphins, enkephalins, and dynorphin, which bind to μ, δ, and κ receptors in order to reduce the intensity of pain in addition to other actions. Because endogenous opioids such as endorphins are activated by exercise and this activation is associated with decreases in pain sensitivity, it has been assumed that peripheral concentrations of opioids are a reflection of central opioidergic activity. Notwithstanding the flaws in this reasoning (Dishman and O'Connor, 2009), the powerful analgesic effects of opioids have made the "endorphin hypothesis" one of the more popular explanations for the pain-relieving effects of exercise.

In the central nervous system, β-endorphin may activate descending inhibitory pathways via its projections to the periaqueductal gray of the midbrain (for more detailed explanation see Chapter 25, this volume). However, less is known about central activation of the opioid system in response to exercise. One animal study reported elevated levels of β-endorphin in the amygdalae following prolonged treadmill running in rats, and a recent study in human male distance runners provided evidence of endogenous opioid release in the brain following 2 hours of running (Boecker et al., 2008). Overall, tests of opiodergic mechanisms in EIH have been inconsistent, with some research reporting blockage of EIH with the opioid antagonist naloxone (Haier, Quaid, & Mills, 1981; Janal, Colt, Clark, & Glusman, 1984; Droste, Meyer-Blankenburg, Greenlee, & Roskamm, 1988) and other research reporting no such effect (Black, Chesher, & Starmer, 1979; Janal et al., 1984; Olausson et al., 1986; Droste, Greenlee, Schreck, & Roskamm, 1991). Consequently, the involvement of endogenous opioids in EIH remains to be elucidated.

Non-opioid mechanisms

Exercise has a potent influence on the cardiopulmonary system including large changes in systolic blood pressure. Because resting blood pressure and parental history of hypertension have been negatively associated with pain sensitivity (Koltyn and Umeda, 2006), exercise-induced increases in blood pressure have been suggested as a mechanism of EIH. Specifically, it has been hypothesized that exercise could induce EIH through activation of arterial baroreceptors, sending afferent information along the nucleus tractus soltarius and stimulating several brainstem (periaqueductal gray, rostral ventromedial medulla), limbic (hypothalamus, amygdala), and cortical (insula, anterior cingulate) structures that are implicated in descending pain inhibition (Koltyn and Umeda, 2006; Ring, Edwards, & Kavussanu, 2008). However, there is no consistent dose-response relationship between changes in blood pressure and pain perception following exercise (Umeda, Newcomb, Ellingson, & Koltyn, 2010), and EIH research of cardiopulmonary mechanisms is necessarily confounded by other variables that change as a result of exercise intensity (e.g., biochemicals, respiration, blood flow).

Other, less tested hypotheses include EIH as a result of endocannabinoid release or EIH due to conditioned pain modulation (CPM) (Kosek & Lundberg, 2003). Neither of these hypotheses has been specifically tested in an EIH model. However, based on the literature showing stronger EIH effects with higher-intensity exercise, it is plausible that anandamide, an endogenous cannabionoid neurotransmitter, could be binding to receptors in the central nervous system. It is also possible that painful exercise stimulates descending inhibitory signals from the brain, a phenomenon termed CPM, and the descending inhibitory signal could partially account for reduced pain sensitivity post exercise. Overall the literature suggests an interaction between opioid and non-opioid mechanisms to explain EIH, but the exact mechanisms are not fully understood.

Conclusion

Exercise is a relatively unique behavior in that it has the capacity to both stimulate and relieve pain. There are a number of physiological mechanisms that interact to produce these effects and there is evidence that other psychobiological factors moderate both pain and hypoalgesia.

Understanding the relationships between exercise and pain and the associated mechanisms can contribute to a host of physical activity and mental health issues, including the role of pain in exercise adoption and adherence, the influence of pain on exercise performance, the interaction between EIH and mood during and following exercise, and the impact of exercise training on chronic muscle pain.

References

Babenko, V. V., Graven-Nielsen, T., Svensson, P., Drewes, A. M., Jensen, T. S., & Arendt-Nielsen, L. (1999a). Experimental human muscle pain induced by intramuscular injections of bradykinin, serotonin, and substance P. *European Journal of Pain*, *3*, 93–102.

Babenko, V. V., Graven-Nielsen, T., Svensson, P., Drewes, A. M., Jensen, T. S., & Arendt-Nielsen, L. (1999b). Experimental human muscle pain and muscular hyperalgesia induced by combinations of serotonin and bradykinin. *Pain*, *82*, 1–8.

Berkley, K. J. (1997). Sex differences in pain. *Behavioral and Brain Research*, *20*, 371–380.

Bingel, U., & Tracey, I. (2008). Imaging the CNS modulation of pain in humans. *Physiology*, *23*, 371–380.

Birklin, F., Weber, M., Ernst, M., Riedl, B., Neundorfer, B., & Handwerker, H. O. (2000). Experimental tissue acidosis leads to increased pain in complex regional pain syndrome (CRPS). *Pain*, *87*, 227–234.

Black, J., Chesher, G. B., & Starmer, G. A. (1979). The painlessness of the long distance runner. *Medical Journal of Australia*, *1*, 522–523.

Blais, C., Adam, A., Massicotte, D., & Peronnet, F. (1999). Increase in blood bradykinin concentration after eccentric weight-training exercise in men. *Journal of Applied Physiology*, *87*, 1197–1201.

Boecker, H., Sprenger, T., Spilker, M. E., Henriksen, G., Koppenhoefer, M., Wagner, K. J., Valet, M., Berthele, A., & Tolle, T. R. (2008). The runner's high: Opioidergic mechanisms in the human brain. *Cerebral Cortex*, *18*, 2523–2531.

Boix, F., Roe, C., Rosenborg, L., & Knardahl, S. (2005). Kinin peptides in human trapezius muscle during sustained isometric contraction and their relation to pain. *Journal of Applied Physiology*, *98*, 534–540.

Boone, J. B., Sherraden, T., Pierzchala, K., Berger, R., & Van Loon, G. R. (1992). Plasma met- enkephalin and catecholamine responses to intense exercise in humans. *Journal of Applied Physiology*, *72*, 388–392.

Buskila, D. (2007). Genetics of chronic pain states. *Best Practice and Research Clinical Rheumatology*, *21*, 535–547.

Carter, J. R., Sauder, C. L., & Ray, C. A. (2002). Effect of morphine on sympathetic nerve activity in humans. *Journal of Applied Physiology*, *93*, 1764–1769.

Cook, D. B., Jackson, E. M., O'Connor, P. J., & Dishman, R. K. (2004). Muscle pain during exercise in normotensive African American women: Effect of parental hypertension history. *Journal of Pain*, *5*, 111–118.

Cook, D. B., O'Connor, P. J., Eubanks, S. A., Smith, C. J., & Lee, M. (1997). Naturally occurring muscle pain during exercise: Assessment and experimental evidence. *Medicine and Science in Sports and Exercise*, *29*, 999–1012.

Cook, D. B., O'Connor, P. J., Oliver, S. E., & Lee, Y. (1998). Sex differences in naturally occurring muscle pain and exertion during maximal cycle ergometry. *International Journal of Neuroscience*, *95*, 183–202.

Cook, D. B., O'Connor, P. J., & Ray, C. A. (2000). Muscle pain perception and sympathetic nerve activity to exercise during opioid modulation. *American Journal of Physiology. Regulatory, Integrative and Comparative Physiology*, *279*, R1565–R1573.

Cook, D. B., Lange, G., Ciccone, D. S., Liu, W. C., Steffener, J., & Natelson, B. H. (2004). Functional imaging of pain in patients with primary fibromyalgia. *Journal of Rheumatology*, *31*, 364–378.

Costa, F., Diedrich, A., Johnson, B., Sulur, P., Farley, G., & Biaggioni, I. (2001). Adenosine, a metabolic trigger of the exercise pressor reflex in humans. *Hypertension*, *37*, 917–922.

Diehl, B., Hoheisel, U., & Mense, S. (1993). The influence of mechanical stimuli and of acetylsalicylic-acid on the discharges of slowly conducting afferent units from normal and inflamed muscle in the rat. *Experimental Brain Research*, *92*, 431–440.

Dishman, R. K., & O'Connor, P. J. (2009). Lessons in exercise neurobiology: The case of endorphins. *Mental Health and Physical Activity*, *2*, 4–9.

Droste, C., Greenlee, M. W., Schreck, M., & Roskamm, H. (1991). Experimental pain thresholds and plasma beta-endorphin levels during exercise. *Medicine and Science in Sports and Exercise*, *23*, 334–342.

Droste, C., Meyer-Blankenburg, H., Greenlee, M. W., & Roskamm, H. (1988). Effect of physical exercise on pain thresholds and plasma beta-endorphins in patients with silent and symptomatic myocardial ischemia. *European Heart Journal, 9,* 25–33.

Farrell, P. A., Ebert, T. J., & Kampine, J. P. (1991). Naloxone augments muscle sympathetic nerve activity during isometric exercise in humans. *American Journal of Physiology, 260,* E379–E388.

Fechir, M., Schlereth, T., Kritzmann, S., Balon, S., Pfeifer, N., Geber, C., et al. (2009). Stress and thermoregulation: Different sympathetic responses and different effects on experimental pain. *European Journal of Pain, 13,* 935–941.

Franz, M., & Mense, S. (1975). Muscle receptors with group IV afferent fibres responding to application of bradykinin. *Brain Research, 92,* 369–383.

Galbo, H. (1982). Endocrinology and metabolism in exercise. *Current Problem in Clinical Biochemistry, 11,* 26–44.

Gerdle, B., Hilgenfeldt, U., Larsson, B., Kristiansen, J., Sogaard, K., & Rosendal, L. (2008). Bradykinin and kallidin levels in the trapezius muscle in patients with work-related trapezius myalgia, in patients with whiplash associated pain, and in healthy controls – A microdialysis study of women. *Pain, 139,* 578–587.

Graven-Nielsen, T., Jansson, Y., Segerdahl, M., Kristensen, J. D., Mense, S., Arendt-Nielsen, L., et al. (2003). Experimental pain by ischaemic contractions compared with pain by intramuscular infusions of adenosine and hypertonic saline. *European Journal of Pain, 7,* 93–102.

Haier, R. J., Quaid, K., & Mills, J. S. C. (1981). Naloxone alters pain perception after jogging. *Psychiatry Research, 5,* 231–232.

Hoffman, M. D., Shepanski, M. A., Ruble, S. B., Valic, Z., Buckwalter, J. B., & Clifford, P. S. (2004). Intensity and duration threshold for aerobic exercise-induced analgesia to pressure pain. *Archives of Physical Medicine and Rehabilitation, 85,* 1183–1187.

Hoheisel, U., Reinohl, J., Unger, T., & Mense, S. (2004). Acidic pH and capsaicin activate mechanosensitive group IV muscle receptors in the rat. *Pain, 110,* 149–157.

Hurley, R. W., & Adams, M. C. (2008). Sex, gender, and pain: An overview of a complex field. *Anesthesia and Analgesia, 107,* 309–317.

Issberner, U., Reeh, P. W., & Steen, K. H. (1996). Pain due to tissue acidosis: A mechanism for inflammatory and ischemic myalgia? *Neuroscience Letters, 208,* 191–194.

Janal, M. N., Colt, E. W. D., Clark, W. C., & Glusman, M. (1984). Pain sensitivity, mood and plasma endocrine levels in man following long-distance running: Effects of naloxone. *Pain, 19,* 13–25.

Kemppainen, P., Paalasmaa, P., Pertovaara, A., Alila, A., & Johansson, G. (1990). Dexamethasone attenuates exercise-induced dental analgesia in man. *Brain Research, 519,* 329–332.

Kemppainen, P., Pertovaara, A., Huopaniemi, T., & Johansson, G. (1986). Elevation of dental pain threshold induced in man by physical exercise is not reversed by cyproheptadine-mediated suppression of growth hormone release. *Neuroscience Letters, 70,* 388–392.

Kemppainen, P., Pertovaara, A., Huopaniemi, T., Johansson, G., & Karonen, S. L. (1985). Modification of dental pain and cutaneous thermal sensitivity by physical exercise in man. *Brain Research, 360,* 33–40.

Kim, H., Neubert, J. K., San Miguel, A., Xu, K., Krishnaraju, R. K., Iadarola, M. J., et al. (2004). Genetic influence on variability in human acute experimental pain sensitivity associated with gender, ethnicity and psychological temperament. *Pain, 109,* 488–496.

Koltyn, K. F. (2000). Analgesia following exercise: A review. *Sports Medicine, 29,* 85–98.

Koltyn, K. F., & Umeda, M. (2006). Exercise, hypoalgesia and blood pressure. *Sports Medicine, 36,* 207–214.

Kosek, E., & Lundberg, L. (2003). Segmental and plurisegmental modulation of pressure pain thresholds during static muscle contractions in healthy individuals. *European Journal of Pain, 7,* 251–258.

Langberg, H., Bjørn, C., Boushel, R., Hellsten, Y., & Kjaer, M. (2002). Exercise-induced increase in interstitial bradykinin and adenosine concentrations in skeletal muscle and peritendinous tissue in humans. *Journal of Physiology, 542,* 977–983.

Lewis, J. W., Cannon, J. T., & Liebeskind, J. C. (1980). Opioid and nonopioid mechanisms of stress analgesia. *Science, 208,* 623–625.

Light, A. R., Hughen, R. W., Zhang, J., Rainier, J., Liu, Z., & Lee, J. (2008). Dorsal root ganglion neurons innervating skeletal muscle respond to physiological combinations of protons, ATP, and lactate mediated by ASIC, P2X and TRPV1. *Journal of Neurophysiology, 100,* 1184–1201.

Mense, S. (1993). Nociception from skeletal muscle in relation to clinical muscle pain. *Pain, 54,* 241–289.

Millan, M. J. (1999). The induction of pain: An integrative review. *Progress in Neurobiology, 57,* 1–164.

Mogil, J. S. (1999). The genetic mediation of individual differences in sensitivity to pain and its inhibition. *Proceedings of the National Academy of Sciences of the United States of America, 96,* 7744–7751.

Mørk, H., Ashina, M., Bendtsen, L., Olesen, J., & Jensen, R. (2003). Experimental muscle pain and tenderness following infusion of endogenous substances in humans. *European Journal of Pain, 7*, 145–153.

Motl, R. W., Glittoni, R. C., & Scott, J. A. (2007). Self-efficacy correlates with leg muscle pain during maximal and submaximal cycling exercise. *Journal of Pain, 8*, 583–587.

Motl, R. W., O'Connor, P. J., & Dishman, R. K. (2003). Effect of caffeine on perceptions of leg muscle pain during moderate intensity cycling exercise. *Journal of Pain, 4*, 316–321.

Motl, R. W., O'Connor, P. J., Tubandt, L., Puetz, T., & Ely, M. R. (2006). Effect of caffeine on leg muscle pain during cycling exercise among females. *Medicine and Science in Sports and Exercise, 38*, 598–604.

Murase, S., Terazawa, E., Queme, F., Ota, H., Matsuda, T., Hirate, K., . . . Mizumura, K. (2010). Bradykinin and nerve growth factor play pivotal roles in muscular mechanical hyperalgesia after exercise (delayed onset muscle soreness). *Journal of Neuroscience, 10*, 3751–3761.

O'Connor, P. J., & Cook, D. B. (1999). Exercise and pain: The neurobiology, measurement, and laboratory study of pain in relation to exercise in humans. *Exercise and Sport Sciences Reviews, 27*, 119–166.

O'Connor, P. J., Mod, R. W., Broglio, S. P., & Ely, M. R. (2004). Dose-dependent effect of caffeine on reducing leg muscle pain during cycling exercise is unrelated to systolic blood pressure. *Pain, 109*, 291–298.

Olausson, B., Eriksson, E., Ellmarker, L., Rydenhag, B., Shyu, B. C., & Anderson, S. A. (1986). Effects of naloxone on dental pain threshold following muscle exercise and low frequency transcutaneous nerve stimulation: A comparative study in man. *Acta Physiologica Scandinavica, 126*, 299–305.

Pertovaara, A., Huopaniemi, T., Virtanen, A., & Johansson, G. (1984). The influence of exercise on dental pain thresholds and the release of stress hormones. *Physiology and Behavior, 33*, 923–926.

Ray, C. A., & Carter, J. R. (2007). Central modulation of exercise-induced muscle pain in humans. *Journal of Physiology, 585*, 287–294.

Ray, C. A., & Pawelczyk, J. A. (1994). Naloxone does not affect the cardiovascular and sympathetic adjustments to static exercise in humans. *Journal of Applied Physiology, 77*, 231–235.

Ray, C. A., Rea, R. F., Clary, M. P., & Mark, A. L. (1992). Muscle sympathetic nerve responses to static leg exercise. *Journal of Applied Physiology, 73*, 1523–1529.

Riley, J. L., Robinson, M. E., Wise, E. A., Myers, C. D., & Fillingim, R. B. (1998). Sex differences in the perception of noxious experimental stimuli: A meta-analysis. *Pain, 74*, 181–187.

Ring, C., Edwards, L., & Kavussanu, M. (2008). Effects of isometric exercise on pain are mediated by blood pressure. *Biological Psychology, 78*, 123–128.

Rotto, D. M., & Kaufman, M. P. (1988). Effect of metabolic products of muscular contraction on discharge of group III and IV afferents. *Journal of Applied Physiology, 64*, 2306–2313.

Sawynok, J. (1998). Adenosine receptor activation and nociception. *European Journal of Pharmacology, 347*, 1–11.

Schaible, H. G., Ebersberger, A., & Natura, G. (2011). Update on peripheral mechanisms of pain: Beyond prostaglandins and cytokines. *Arthritis Research and Therapy, 13*, 210–218.

Schwarz, L., & Kindermann, W. (1992). Changes in beta-endorphin levels in response to aerobic and anaerobic exercise. *Sports Medicine, 13*, 25–36.

Steen, A. E., Reeh, P. W., Geisslinger, G., & Steen, K. H. (2000). Plasma levels after peroral and topical ibuprofen and effects upon low pH-induced cutaneous and muscle pain. *European Journal of Pain, 4*, 195–209.

Steen, K. H., Reeh, P. W., Anton, F., & Handwerker, H. O. (1992). Protons selectively induce lasting excitation and sensitization to mechanical stimulation of nociceptors in rat skin, in vitro. *Journal of Neuroscience, 12*, 86–95.

Tracey, I. (2007). Neuroimaging of pain mechanisms. *Current Opinion in Supportive and Palliative Care, 1*, 109–116.

Umeda, M., Newcomb, L. W., Ellingson, L. D., & Koltyn, K. F. (2010). Examination of the dose–response relationship between pain perception and blood pressure elevations induced by isometric exercise in men and women. *Biological Psychology, 85*, 90–96.

Weiss, J. M., Simson, P. G., Hoffman, L. J., Ambrose, M. J., Cooper, S., & Webster, A. (1986). Infusion of adrenergic receptor agonists and antagonists into the locus coeruleus and ventricular system of the brain. Effects on swim-motivated and spontaneous motor activity. *Neuropharmacology, 25*, 367–384.

PART 8

Energy and fatigue

Edited by
Justy Reed

28

EFFECT OF ACUTE AND REGULAR AEROBIC PHYSICAL ACTIVITY ON POSITIVE ACTIVATED AFFECT

Justy Reed

Physical activity promotes health and well-being (e.g., Warburton, Nicol, & Bredin, 2006). Positive activated affect (PAA) is a subjective mental state of energy and enthusiasm related to health and well-being. For example, PAA correlates favorably with longevity (Kubzansky, Sparrow, Vokonas, & Kawachi, 2001), immune function (Cohen, Doyle, Turner, Alper, & Skoner, 2003), stress response (Steptoe, Wardle, & Marmot, 2005), and marital satisfaction (Rogers & May, 2003). Given that physical activity is a healthy behavior and PAA is a positive mental state, the effect of physical activity on PAA offers a fertile area for health-related scientific inquiry. This chapter will review the quantitative effect of acute and regular physical activity on PAA, discuss a conceptual issue relative to PAA, and provide suggestions for future study. The chapter begins with definitions for the variables of interest: physical activity and PAA.

Definitions

Physical activity

Physical activity is aerobic or anaerobic movement produced by skeletal muscles that increases energy expenditure above resting (U.S. Department of Health and Human Services [USDHHS], 2008). Physical activity can range from very low in sedentary individuals to very high in well-conditioned athletes, and includes occupational, leisure time, household, and health-enhancing. Exercise is a form of physical activity. Exercise is planned and performed with the goal of improving health or fitness (USDHHS, 2008). Because physical activity is a broader concept than exercise, the term physical activity will be used in this chapter. Specifically, physical activity will refer to aerobic physical activity.

Positive activated affect (PAA)

Affect will be defined as the quality of a subjective mental state along the dimensions of valence and activation or what has been described as core affect (Russell, 2003). Valence describes affect along the positive versus negative quality of a mental state. Activation describes affect along the alertness versus sleepiness quality of a mental state. The core affect theory proposes that all affective states represent varying degrees of valence and arousal and therefore affect can be represented on

413

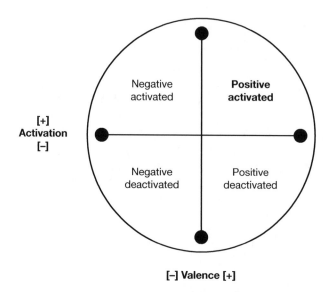

Figure 28.1 A circumplex model of self-reported affect. The activation dimension is the vertical axis and the valence dimension is the horizontal axis of the circumplex (adapted from Yik, Russell, and Feldman Barrett, 1999).

a two-dimensional circumplex (Posner, Russell, & Peterson, 2005). Several different names have been given to the upper right quadrant of the circumplex (see Yik, Russell, & Feldman Barrett, 1999). For this chapter, the upper right quadrant will be referred to as positive activated affect (PAA; Reed & Ones, 2006). See Figure 28.1 for a representation of the affect circumplex.

Affect-laden terms (e.g., gloomy or delighted) typically provide the link between a self-reported affective state and the circumplex. Similar affect-laden terms comprise the scales of common self-report affect instruments, for example, the Energy scale of the Activation-Deactivation Adjective Checklist (AD-ACL; Thayer, 1996) or the Positive Affect scale of the Positive and Negative Affect Schedule (PANAS; Watson, Clark, & Tellegen, 1988). Analyses conducted by Yik et al. (1999) revealed that affect terms and therefore affect scales having positive valence and moderately high levels of activation map to the upper right quadrant of the circumplex. This chapter examines the effect of acute and regular aerobic physical activity on the scale scores of self-report affect instruments that map to the PAA quadrant of the affect circumplex.

Effect of aerobic physical activity on PAA: meta-analytical evidence

Acute aerobic physical activity

This section discusses the review by Reed and Ones (2006). These authors conducted a meta-analysis on the effect of acute aerobic physical activity on post-activity self-reported PAA. The database consisted of 158 studies dated from 1979 to 2005. Studies examining affect in relation to aerobic exercise (e.g., aerobic dance, walking, jogging, running, swimming, and cycling) were identified using computer databases and manual searches of narrative reviews, quantitative reviews, and books. Reference lists of published articles, theses, and dissertations were checked for additional studies. The mean age of participants in the database was 24.50 years with a standard deviation (*SD*) of 11.64. Twenty-three percent of study samples were male, 35 percent female, and 40 percent mixed gender. Sixty-two percent of study samples were college students, 19 percent community participants, 8 percent athletes, 4 percent clinical participants, and 5 percent mixed samples of university faculty, staff, and students. Effect sizes (ESs) were obtained for physical activity groups and control groups. The majority of control samples were attention controls. ESs for each study were computed by subtracting the mean post-activity PAA from the mean pre-activity PAA and dividing the difference by the pooled *SD*, resulting in a *d*-value ES (Cohen, 1977). The random effects approach of Hunter and Schmidt (2004) was utilized to conduct the analysis and therefore *d*-values were corrected for measurement error and sampling error. Positive *d*-values reflected increased pre- to post-activity PAA.

The mean corrected ES ($\bar{d}_{corr}$) estimated the average population effect. The standard deviation of corrected *d* values (SD_{corr}) and 90 percent credibility interval (90 percent CrI) were used to detect the presence of moderators in the overall analysis and to verify whether the results of individual moderator analyses generalized across study settings. For the overall analysis, if SD_{corr} was large relative to $\bar{d}_{corr}$ or the 90 percent CrI included zero (Whitener, 1990), moderators were present. For moderator analyses, if the 90 percent CrI did not include zero, the $\bar{d}_{corr}$ effect generalized. That is, the moderator effect retains a positive or negative sign across study settings and situations (Ones, Viswesvaran, & Schmidt, 1993).

The overall activity $\bar{d}_{corr}$ of 0.47 indicated PAA increased by nearly one half of a *SD* on average from pre- to post-aerobic activity. The control $\bar{d}_{corr}$ of -0.17 indicated PAA decreased by roughly two-tenths of a *SD* from pre to post control. These results show that the effect of aerobic activity on PAA is nearly four times the magnitude of the effect in control conditions. The overall activity SD_{corr} of 0.37 and 90 percent CrI (lower limit, upper limit) of (-0.01, 0.94) signified the presence of moderators. Therefore, activity-related moderator analyses were conducted for pre-activity (baseline) PAA, activity intensity, duration, and dose, and post-activity PAA assessment times. Study-related moderator analyses included study quality (defined as the number of internal validity threats controlled) and source (published vs. unpublished). Moderator analyses were not conducted for control groups.

To examine whether pre-activity PAA moderated the effect of aerobic activity on post-activity PAA, pre-activity mean PAA scores were converted to standard scores (z scores). Studies were divided into three categories based on pre-activity z score: less than -0.5 z, -0.5 z to 0.5 z, and greater than 0.5 z. For studies in the less than -0.5 z category, $\bar{d}_{corr}$ = 0.63, twice the magnitude of the other two categories. The 90 percent CrI did not include zero (0.16, 1.10), indicating generalizable increases in PAA when baseline PAA is lower than average. Effects were not generalizable in the other two categories.

Intensity was coded using percent oxygen uptake reserve (percent $\dot{V}O_2R$). The data allowed formation of categories for low (15 to 39 percent $\dot{V}O_2R$), moderate (40 to 59 percent $\dot{V}O_2R$), and high (60 to 85 percent $\dot{V}O_2R$). The low-intensity $\bar{d}_{corr}$ of 0.57 (SD_{corr} = 0.33) indicated a generalizable effect nearly twice the magnitude of the other two categories. Moderate- and high-intensity effects were not generalizable.

Duration (session time) was coded in minutes per session, and studies were grouped into five time intervals. The $\bar{d}_{corr}$ (SD_{corr}) for the first three intervals were 7 to 15 minutes, 0.56 (0.38); 20 to 28 minutes, 0.46 (0.31); and 30 to 35 minutes, 0.57 (0.33). The 90 percent CrIs for these intervals did not include zero and all $\bar{d}_{corr}$ were within .10 *SD* indicating similar generalizable effects. Effects tapered in the 40- to 60-minute interval, 0.37 (0.31) and were markedly reduced in the fifth interval for studies having durations greater than 75 minutes, -0.72 (0.66).

Dose was quantified as the product of intensity and duration. Low doses (e.g., 20 minutes' brisk walking) increased post-activity PAA, $\bar{d}_{corr}$ = 0.45 (SD_{corr} = 0.30). Similar results were found for moderate doses (e.g., 30 minutes at 65 percent heart rate maximum), $\bar{d}_{corr} = 0.46$ ($SD_{corr} = 0.34$). High doses (e.g., 90 minutes at 70 percent heart rate maximum) produced null effects, $\bar{d}_{corr} = 0.09$ ($SD_{corr} = 0.27$). Very high doses (e.g., marathon) resulted in markedly reduced post-activity PAA, $\bar{d}_{corr} = -0.98$ ($SD_{corr} = 0.37$). The authors characterized the dose results in terms of "zones" of effect. Low and moderate doses are optimal because effects were positive and generalizable. High doses are unstable because the effect was null on average, but may increase or decrease depending on other moderators such as activity history (see Hallgren, Moss, & Gastin, 2010). Very high doses are unpleasant because they render considerable physiological and psychological fatigue and significantly lower post-activity PAA in virtually all situations.

PAA during recovery was examined using intervals of 0 to 2, 5 to 10, 15 to 30, and 40 to 1440 minutes post activity. The $\bar{d}_{corr}$ (SD_{corr}) ranged from a generalizable 0.61 (0.40) at 0 to 2 minutes to a non-generalizable 0.10 (0.31) at 40 to 1440 minutes' recovery. Effects for the other time intervals were not generalizable. Post-activity PAA is important because knowledge of response patterns may provide insight about conditions that maximize the effect.

Study quality was analyzed using categories of studies whose authors attempted to control 1 to 2, 3 to 4, 5 to 6, or 7 to 10 threats to internal validity. The results suggested a positive association between study quality and ES, indicating larger effects for studies with higher internal validity. However, the authors noted that this association should be interpreted cautiously due to the near complete overlap of the 90 percent CrIs for each of the categories. For study source, the effect in published studies, $\bar{d}_{corr} = 0.47$ ($SD_{corr} = 0.39$), was significantly greater than for unpublished studies, $\bar{d}_{corr} = 0.26$ ($SD_{corr} = 0.37$), pointing to a source bias.

Regular aerobic physical activity

This section summarizes the review by Reed and Buck (2009). These authors conducted a meta-analysis on the effect of aerobic activity programs on post-program self-reported PAA. The database consisted of 115 studies dated from 1980 to 2008. Whereas a single session provided the unit of inquiry in the acute activity meta-analysis (Reed & Ones, 2006), an activity program served as the unit of inquiry for this meta-analysis. Studies of affect in relation to aerobic exercise programs were identified using computer databases and manual searches of narrative reviews, quantitative reviews, and books. Reference lists of published articles, theses, and dissertations were checked for additional studies. The mean age of participants in the database was 42.41 years ($SD = 15.93$). Fourteen percent of study samples were male, 42 percent female, and 43 percent mixed gender. Fifty-eight percent of study samples were community participants, 22 percent clinical, 13 percent college students, 5 percent mixed samples of university faculty, staff, and students, and 2 percent athletes. ESs were obtained for physical activity groups and control groups. The majority of control samples were attention controls. Study ESs were computed by subtracting the mean post-program PAA from the mean pre-program PAA and dividing the difference by the pooled SD, resulting in a d-value ES (Cohen, 1977). Similar to Reed and Ones (2006), this review utilized a random effects model, ESs were corrected for measurement error and sampling error, and activity-related and study-related variables were coded as potential moderators.

The overall activity $\bar{d}_{corr}$ of 0.57 indicated PAA increased by six-tenths of a SD on average from pre to post program. The control $\bar{d}_{corr}$ of 0.03 ($SD_{corr} = 0.11$) indicated PAA remained unchanged on average from pre to post control. These results show that aerobic physical activity programs increase PAA and control conditions produce little change in PAA. The overall activity program SD_{corr} and 90 percent CrI (lower limit, upper limit) were 0.48 (-0.04, 1.18) signifying the presence of moderators. Therefore, activity-related moderator analyses were conducted for pre-program (baseline) PAA, activity frequency, intensity, and time, program duration, and activity dose. Study-related moderator analyses included study quality (defined as the number of internal validity threats controlled) and source (published vs. unpublished). Moderator analyses were not conducted for control groups.

The baseline analysis was conducted in a similar manner to that of Reed and Ones (2006). The effect for studies in the lower third of the z-score distribution (less than -0.5 z) was $\bar{d}_{corr}$ = 0.81 (SD_{corr} = 0.40), almost twice the magnitude of studies in the middle category (-0.5 z to 0.5 z) at $\bar{d}_{corr}$ = 0.45 (SD_{corr} = 0.34), and three times greater than studies in the upper category (greater than 0.5 z) with $\bar{d}_{corr}$ = 0.26 (SD_{corr} = 0.02). The results show a clear inverse relation between baseline PAA and the magnitude of improvement from aerobic exercise programs. Unlike Reed and Ones (2006), effects were generalizable for all baseline categories.

A moderating effect was found for frequency (days per week), with higher frequencies producing larger effects. The $\bar{d}_{corr}$ (SD_{corr}) for the three frequency categories were: less than 3 days per week, 0.57 (0.29); 3 days per week, 0.52 (0.37); and greater than 3 days per week, 0.79 (0.34). Activity intensity was coded as percent $\dot{V}O_2R$. The $\bar{d}_{corr}$ (SD_{corr}) for low- and high-intensity programs resulted in the largest PAA increases of 0.72 (0.00) and 0.68 (0.34), respectively. Moderate-intensity programs produced smaller, but respectable, effects of 0.50 (0.46). The effects for moderate-intensity programs did not generalize, however. The $\bar{d}_{corr}$ (SD_{corr}) for activity duration (session time) were 15 to 25 minutes, 0.55 (0.38); 30 to 35 minutes, 0.68 (0.43); and 40 to 60 minutes, 0.49 (0.37). Program duration was coded in weeks, and studies grouped into three categories. The $\bar{d}_{corr}$ (SD_{corr}) were 4 to 9 weeks, 0.51 (0.28); 10 to 12 weeks, 0.63 (0.42); and 13 to 32 weeks, 0.45 (0.28). The moderator analyses for session time and program duration showed a tendency toward smaller effects with longer session times and longer programs.

Dose was quantified as the product of activity intensity, time per session, frequency per week, and program duration, and coded into categories of low (e.g., 2 days per week, 20-minute sessions, moderate intensity, 8 to 10 weeks), moderate (e.g., 3 days per week, 30-minute sessions, moderate intensity, 10 to 12 weeks), and high (e.g., 4 days per week, 40-minute sessions, moderate intensity, 12 to 14 weeks). Dose effects ranged from $\bar{d}_{corr}$ = 0.56 (SD_{corr} = 0.40) for moderate to $\bar{d}_{corr}$ = 0.65 (SD_{corr} = 0.38) for high aerobic program doses. The maximum dose category ES difference was 0.09, signifying dose as a weak moderator. Importantly, however, with respect to the activity-related moderator analyses, 90 percent CrIs did not include zero for nearly all variable categories, suggesting that a variety of aerobic activity programs result in generalizable increases in PAA.

The authors analyzed study quality using categories of studies whose authors attempted to control 1 to 3, 4 to 5, 6 to 7, or 8 to 9 threats to internal validity. The results revealed a positive association between the number of threats controlled and ES. The $\bar{d}_{corr}$ (SD_{corr}) were 0.27 (0.00) for studies controlling 1 to 3 threats and 0.77 (0.00) in studies controlling 8 to 9 threats, indicating larger effects in studies with higher internal validity. There was no source bias: the effect in published studies of 0.56 (0.36) mirrored the result for unpublished studies of 0.54 (0.43).

Summary of meta-analytical findings

Considered together, the two meta-analyses show that acute and regular aerobic physical activity increase self-reported PAA by approximately one half a SD in experimental participants who perform aerobic activity compared to control participants who do not. Stated differently, the findings indicate that a randomly selected person who just completed aerobic activity would be about 65 to 70 percent more likely to report higher PAA than a randomly selected sedentary person (Ellis, 2010). Moderator analyses show effects are consistently positive under the following conditions: lower than average pre-activity or pre-program PAA, low-intensity activity, activity

417

sessions of 10 to 35 minutes, and low- to moderate-activity doses as quantified for single sessions or progams. Additionally, PAA for acute bouts is consistently positive during the first two minutes post activity (except after very high-intensity activity) and the analysis of regular aerobic activity shows that a variety of programs produce generalizable increases in PAA. Study-related moderator analyses revealed a weak study quality bias and a significant trend toward larger effects in published studies for the acute data and a strong study quality bias, but no source bias (published vs. unpublished) in the aerobic program data. Thus, in the acute literature, the data suggest a tendency for larger effects in published studies independent of study quality, but in the aerobic program literature, effect magnitude appears driven by study quality, not publication status. The number of studies was relatively small for some of the moderator analyses and these findings should therefore be considered preliminary (see Reed & Buck, 2009, and Reed & Ones, 2006, for more details). Finally, meta-analytical findings, in particular the results of moderator analyses, provide information only about the conditions under which ES magnitudes will differ, but not how or why the effects occur (Miller & Pollock, 1994).

A conceptual issue

Is PAA fundamentally core affect or natural kind?

A natural kind in science is a category from which researchers can form testable hypotheses and make valid and reliable generalizations from samples of the category to the whole category (Boyd, 1999). Some have argued core affect may be a natural kind (e.g., Barrett, 2006) and by deduction the dimensions of valence and arousal are natural kinds. Core affect theorists share the assumption that PAA is a blend of positive valence and moderately high activation. In other words, core affect theory implies that PAA occurs only because of the fundamental dimensions of arousal and valence. Others dispute these claims. Scarantino (2009) suggests the evidence supports only positive affect and negative affect separately as natural kinds. Martinez Bedard (2008) argues that the four quadrants of the affect circumplex are separate natural kinds because each of these categories, apart from the theory of core affect, share causally related properties and are therefore more scientifically homogeneous than core affect. PAA may therefore be a natural kind distinct from core affect per se. The important conceptual issue is whether PAA is fundamentally core affect or a natural kind and the point of this discussion is to remind readers that core affect and the associated circumplex model is not necessarily the only way to conceptualize the study of PAA or affect in general. See Watson (2000) for a similar, but alternative theory of affect.

Future research directions

Future research should help clarify why physical activity enhances PAA in some people and not in others. Cognitive and individual difference variables along with genetic factors are potentially productive avenues.

Cognitive variables associated with PAA before, during, and after physical activity such as attentional focus to pleasant or unpleasant stimuli (e.g., Tian & Smith, 2011) and cognitive appraisal differences related to gender, fitness, and activity status (e.g., Rose & Parfitt, 2010) are likely important for PAA change and physical activity adherence. Another viable area involves expectancies about the impact of physical activity on well-being (e.g., Anderson & Brice, 2011). Expectations are often mediated by changes in behavior and expectancy theory can account for any effect for which a person can develop an expectation, including the affective benefits of physical activity. Expectancies play a central part in placebo effects (Stewart-Williams, 2004) and investigators are encouraged to spend more effort understanding the role of placebo effects (if any) in the relationship between physical activity and PAA. Testing expectations, however, requires creative research designs to minimize experimenter bias.

Researchers should continue to explore individual differences. For example, "grit" defined as perseverance and passion for long-term goals (Duckworth, Peterson, Matthews, & Kelly, 2007) might correlate with PAA during and after physical activity and be related to intentions within the theory of planned behavior (Ajzen, 1991) or behavioral regulation constructs in self-determination theory (Deci & Ryan, 2000). Individual differences relative to an affective "home base" (Kuppens, Oravecz, & Tuerlinckx, 2010) could also shed light on activity-related PAA response variability.

Genetic factors likely influence voluntary physical activity and health outcomes and are perhaps a source of variation in affective responses to physical activity (de Geus & de Moor, 2008). Preliminary research suggests increased activity-related PAA might in part depend on variations in dopamine systems (Simonen et al., 2003) or brain-derived neurotrophic factor (BDNF), a gene possibly related to physical activity and activity-associated PAA (Bryan, Hutchison, Seals, & Allen, 2007). Understanding gene-by-physical activity interactions is undoubtedly an important future research topic.

Finally, researchers should replicate the important findings reviewed in this chapter to firmly establish the reliability of the results. As aptly noted by Hunter (2001), scientific progress in any field not only depends on new ideas but also requires a database of facts and replicated studies help establish scientific facts. A meta-analysis on the effect of aerobic activity on in-task PAA could now provide a constructive addition to the literature. There is also a need for more studies on the effect of weight training on PAA.

Conclusion

Positive activated affect (PAA) is a subjective mental state of positive energy and engagement. PAA is related to health and well-being. Aerobic physical activity increases self-reported PAA in aerobic activity groups compared to non-activity control groups (Reed & Buck, 2009; Reed & Ones, 2006). Several conditions result in consistent and generalizable increases in post-activity PAA including when pre-activity PAA is lower than average and with lower-intensity aerobic activity sessions of 10 to 35 minutes. A variety of aerobic physical activity programs appear to increase PAA. An important conceptual issue is whether PAA is fundamentally a function of valence and arousal or a scientific natural kind. Cognitive and individual difference variables along with genetic factors are suggested as productive research areas for further understanding the effect of aerobic physical activity on PAA.

References

Ajzen, I. (1991). The theory of planned behavior. *Organizational Behavior and Human Decision Processes, 50,* 179–211.

Anderson, R. J., & Brice, S. (2011). The mood enhancing benefits of exercise: Memory biases augment the effect. *Psychology of Sport and Exercise, 12,* 79–82.

Barrett, L. (2006). Are emotions natural kinds? *Perspectives on Psychological Science, 1*(1), 28–58.

Boyd, R. (1999). Kinds: Complexity and multiple realization. *Philosophical Studies, 95,* 67–98.

Bryan, A., Hutchison, K. E., Seals, D. R., & Allen, D. L. (2007). A transdisciplinary model integrating genetic, physiological, and psychological correlates of voluntary exercise. *Health Psychology, 26*(1), 30–39.

Cohen, J. (1977). *Statistical power analysis for the behavioral sciences* (Rev. ed.). New York: Academic Press.

Cohen, S., Doyle, W. J., Turner, R. B., Alper, C. M., & Skoner, D. P. (2003). Emotional style and susceptibility to the common cold. *Psychosomatic Medicine, 65,* 652–57.

Deci, E. L., & Ryan, R. M. (2000). The what and why of goal pursuits: Human needs and the self-determination of behavior. *Psychological Inquiry, 11*, 227–68.

de Geus, E. J. C., & de Moor, M. H. M. (2008). A genetic perspective on the association between exercise and mental health. *Mental Health and Physical Activity, 1*, 53–61.

Duckworth, A. L., Peterson, C., Matthews, M. D., & Kelly, D. R. (2007). Grit: Perseverance and passion for long-term goals. *Journal of Personality and Social Psychology, 92*(6), 1087–101.

Ellis, P. D. (2010). *The essential guide to effect sizes: Statistical power, meta-analysis, and the interpretation of research results.* New York: Cambridge University Press.

Hallgren, M. A., Moss, N. D., & Gastin, P. (2010). Regular exercise participation mediates the affective response to acute bouts of vigorous exercise. *Journal of Sports Science and Medicine, 9*, 629–37.

Hunter, J. E. (2001). The desperate need for replications. *Journal of Consumer Research, 28*(1), 149–58.

Hunter, J. E., & Schmidt, F. L. (2004). *Methods of meta-analysis: Correcting error and bias in research findings* (2nd ed.). Thousand Oaks, CA: Sage.

Kubzansky, L. D., Sparrow, D., Vokonas, P., & Kawachi, I. (2001). Is the glass empty or half full? A prospective study of optimism and pulmonary function in the Normative Aging Study. *Annals of Behavioral Medicine, 24*, 345–53.

Kuppens, P., Oravecz, Z., & Tuerlinckx, F. (2010). Feelings change: Accounting for individual differences in the temporal dynamics of affect. *Journal of Personality and Social Psychology, 99*(6), 1042–60.

Martinez Bedard, B. (2008). *Is core affect a natural kind?* (Unpublished Masters thesis). Georgia State University, Atlanta.

Miller, N., & Pollock, V. E. (1994). Meta-analytic synthesis for theory development. In H. Cooper & L. V. Hedges (Eds.), *The handbook of research synthesis* (pp. 457–83). New York: Russell Sage.

Ones, D. S., Viswesvaran, C., & Schmidt, F. L. (1993). Comprehensive meta-analysis of integrity test validities: Findings and implications for personnel selection and theories of job performance. *Journal of Applied Psychology, 78*(4), 679–703.

Posner, J., Russell, J. A., & Peterson, B. S. (2005). The circumplex model of affect: An integrative approach to affective neuroscience, cognitive development, and psychopathology. *Development and Psychopathology, 17*(3), 715–34.

Reed, J., & Buck, S. (2009). The effect of regular aerobic exercise on positive activated affect: A meta-analysis. *Psychology of Sport and Exercise, 10*, 581–94.

Reed, J., & Ones, D. (2006). The effect of acute aerobic exercise on positive activated affect: A meta-analysis. *Psychology of Sport and Exercise, 7*, 477–514.

Rogers, S. J., & May, D. C. (2003). Spillover between marital quality and job satisfaction: Long-term patterns and gender differences. *Journal of Marriage and the Family, 65*, 482–95.

Rose, E. A., & Parfitt, G. (2010). Pleasant for some and unpleasant for others: A protocol analysis of the cognitive factors that influence affective responses to exercise. *International Journal of Behavioral Nutrition and Physical Activity, 7*, 1–15.

Russell, J. A. (2003). Core affect and the psychological construction of emotion. *Psychological Review, 110*(1), 145–72.

Scarantino, A. (2009). Core affect and natural affective kinds. *Philosophy of Science, 76*, 940–57.

Simonen, R. L., Rankinen, T., Perusse, L., Leon, A. S., Skinner, J. S., Wilmore, J. H., . . . Bouchard, C. A. (2003). Dopamine D2 receptor gene polymorphism and physical activity in two family studies. *Physiology and Behavior, 78*, 751–57.

Steptoe, A., Wardle, J., & Marmot, M. (2005). Positive affect and health-related neuroendocrine, cardiovascular, and inflammatory processes. *Proceedings of the National Academy of Sciences of the United States of America, 102*(18), 6508–12.

Stewart-Williams, S. (2004). The placebo puzzle: Putting together the pieces. *Health Psychology, 23*(2), 198–206.

Thayer, R. E. (1996). *The origin of every day moods: Managing energy, tension, and stress.* New York: Oxford University Press.

Tian, Q., & Smith, J. C. (2011). Attentional bias to emotional stimuli is altered during moderate- but not high-intensity exercise. *Emotion, 11*(6), 1415–24.

United States Department of Health and Human Services. (2008). *Physical activity guidelines for Americans.* Atlanta: U.S. Department of Health and Human Services.

Warburton, D., Nicol, C., & Bredin, S. (2006). Health benefits of physical activity: The evidence. *Canadian Medical Association Journal, 174*(6), 801–9.

Watson, D. (2000). *Mood and temperament.* New York: Guilford Press.

Watson, D., Clark, L. A., & Tellegen, A. (1988). Development and validation of brief measures of positive and negative affect: The PANAS scales. *Journal of Personality and Social Psychology*, *54*(6), 1063–70.

Whitener, E. M. (1990). Confusion of confidence intervals and credibility intervals in meta-analysis. *Journal of Applied Psychology*, *75*(3), 315–21.

Yik, M., Russell, J., & Feldman Barrett, L. (1999). Structure of self-reported current affect: Integration and beyond. *Journal of Personality and Social Psychology*, *77*(5), 600–19.

29

PHYSICAL ACTIVITY AND FEELINGS OF FATIGUE

Timothy W. Puetz and Matthew P. Herring

Early investigators of fatigue despaired at the development of an acceptable definition and measure of fatigue and ultimately declared "that the term fatigue be absolutely banished from precise scientific discussion and consequently that attempts to obtain a fatigue test be abandoned" (Muscio, 1921, p. 45). In more recent years, fatigue has been acknowledged as a pervasive public health problem, well deserving of serious scientific query, in part because feelings of fatigue have a significant negative impact on quality of life and work productivity (Ricci, Chee, Lorandeau, & Berger, 2007). A better understanding of feelings of fatigue ultimately could contribute to enhancing quality of life as well as improving the diagnosis and treatment of a variety of fatigue-related health problems.

Physical activity is a healthful behavior that has promise for combating feelings of fatigue (O'Connor & Puetz, 2005; Puetz, 2006; Puetz, O'Connor, & Dishman, 2006a). However, there is surprisingly little empirical research on the relation of exercise to feelings of fatigue despite the routine anecdotal reports of reduced fatigue after periods of physical activity. This chapter provides a foundation for understanding the relationship between physical activity and feelings of fatigue by (a) discussing the prevalence and social impact of fatigue, (b) providing a brief history of physical activity and feelings of fatigue, (c) outlining the conceptualization, operationalization, and measurement of physical activity and fatigue, (d) examining the quality of the evidence investigating the impact of physical activity on feelings of fatigue, (e) addressing the impact of physical activity on feelings of fatigue in patient populations, and (f) examining future research needs in this area of study. This information will provide a background for understanding and rationale for examining the relationship between physical activity and feelings of fatigue.

Prevalence and social impact of fatigue

Approximately 20 percent of adults worldwide report persistent fatigue (Wessely, Hotopf, & Sharpe, 1998). This statistic is slightly higher in the United States where fatigue is reported by 24 percent of the population, with women having 1.5 times the risk of males for reporting fatigue (Chen, 1986; Kroenke & Price, 1993). The lifetime prevalence of unexplained fatigue lasting 2 weeks or more is estimated at about 14 percent (Addington, Gallo, Ford, & Eaton, 2001), and approximately 9 percent of adults at any point in time are experiencing fatigue of more than a 6-month duration (Darbishir, Ridsdale, & Seed, 2003). Among individuals experiencing unexplained fatigue during their lifetime, approximately 20 percent will likely have persistent fatigue over many years (Addington et al., 2001). Adolescents have similar trends in feelings of fatigue in that the 6-month incidence of fatigue is about 30 percent in 11- to 15-year-olds (Rimes et al., 2007).

Considering the prevalence of fatigue in the general population, it is not surprising that fatigue is a frequent complaint in primary (i.e., medical care provided by a physician who is the patient's first contact within the health care system) and secondary care (i.e., medical care provided by a specialist upon referral by a primary care physician), with prevalence rates ranging from 10 to 40 percent depending on the definition, duration, and setting (Wessely, Chalder, Hirsch, Wallace, & Wright, 1997). Each year fatigue is the primary reason for about 7 percent of all physician visits, resulting in approximately seven million visits annually (Ruffin & Cohen, 1994). However, only about 8 to16 percent of people who experience fatigue will actually consult their primary physician and only 32 percent of fatigued individuals in primary care will show improvement by 1 year (de Rijk, Schreurs, & Bensing, 2000; Joyce, Hotopt, & Wessely, 1997). This prognosis is worse in secondary care, where fewer than 10 percent return to pre-morbidity functioning (Joyce et al., 1997). Lost productivity in the United States workforce due to fatigue has amounted to a loss of approximately US$136 billion per year. This is an excess of US$101 billion in health-related lost productivity time when workers with fatigue are compared with workers without fatigue (Ricci et al., 2007).

A brief history of physical activity and feelings of fatigue

Based on a steadily growing body of literature during the past 10 to 15 years, the relationship between physical activity and feelings of fatigue has emerged as a serious area of research. The ideas underlying this area of research, however, have been around much longer. The physiology of fatigue, as opposed to the psychology of fatigue, was well studied during the nineteenth century. Italian physiologist Angelo Mosso (1846–1910) began to shift the focus of research from fatigue of the body to fatigue of the mind, which culminated in his book *La Fatica* (1891), the first text to recognize feelings of fatigue in a psychological context. Mosso, generally recognized as the father of fatigue research, acknowledged the multidimensional nature of the construct and integrated physiological, psychological, and psychosocial concepts into the study of fatigue (Di Giulio, Daniele, & Tipton, 2006). This biopsychosocial conceptualization would significantly impact multidisciplinary fatigue research on an international scale for years to come.

Early physicians recognized that fatigue could manifest as an acute or chronic generalized state. These feelings of fatigue were described as a reduced capacity to perform either mental or physical work and such disability was associated with the brain and nervous system (Poore, 1875). Influenced by the work of Mosso, clinicians began to make a sharp distinction between objective and subjective fatigue (Dearborn, 1902). The concept of subjective fatigue raised measurement issues related to the indirect measure of central nervous system activity. Despite these diagnostic limitations, treatment prescriptions for such feelings of fatigue became rest, proper diet, and light to moderate exercise (Cowles, 1893; MacDougall, 1899; Waterman, 1909).

By the mid-1940s, many physicians had adopted the holistic approach to fatigue in which both the physiological and psychological correlates of disease were considered. For example, Bartley and Chute (1947) recommended chronic fatigue research should examine the relative importance of multiple physical and psychological contributions to feelings of fatigue. These recommendations were supported by clinical reports in which fatigue was identified as being a chief complaint in most disease states such that physical and psychological disorders accounted for 20 and 80 percent of fatigue cases, respectively (Allen, 1944; Muncie, 1941). Such clinical observations in chronic disease populations blurred the line between physical and psychological etiologies, suggesting that several biopsychosocial factors contributed to feelings of fatigue. As the conceptualization of feelings of fatigue continued to evolve, the clinical management of fatigue remained a continuous dose of light to moderate exercise (Allen, 1945).

Today, feelings of fatigue remain a serious symptom that can severely impact quality of life in the general population and patient groups. Contemporary theories on physical activity and feelings of fatigue have changed little over the last century. Physical activity is still positively associated with decreased physical and mental fatigue and the mechanism for these psychological effects is likely an interaction among biopsychosocial variables (O'Connor & Puetz, 2005; Puetz, 2006; Puetz et al. 2006a). Unfortunately, the consistent recommendation of physical activity in the clinical treatment of fatigue has done little to move the research area of physical activity and feelings of fatigue forward. Against this historical background, scientific interest in the effects of physical activity on feelings of fatigue remains in its infancy.

Conceptualization, operationalization, and measurement of physical activity and fatigue

The relationship between physical activity and feelings of fatigue remains poorly understood partly because fatigue and physical activity are difficult to define. The following section outlines the conceptualization and operationalization of both physical activity and fatigue and then discusses measurement issues related to this area of research.

Definition: what is physical activity?

The field of exercise science has distinctly conceptualized physical activity. Physical activity refers to any skeletal muscle activation resulting in energy expenditure beyond that of a resting level (Caspersen, Powell, & Christenson, 1985). This is operationalized through kilocalories (kcal) per unit of time. The term exercise is often used synonymously with physical activity; however, exercise is a subcategory of physical activity. Exercise refers to planned, structured, repetitive bodily movements conducted for the purpose of improving or maintaining one or more components of health or physical fitness (Caspersen et al., 1985). Exercise can be acute or chronic. Acute exercise refers to a single, relatively short bout of exercise. Chronic exercise refers to cumulative, acute bouts of exercise carried out repeatedly over time. Chronic exercise is often quantified in terms of frequency, intensity, duration, and mode (Buckworth & Dishman, 2002).

Definition: what is fatigue?

Unlike physical activity, an accepted and sufficiently accurate definition of fatigue remains elusive. Feelings of fatigue have been described as an aversive, non-specific, subjective experience that cannot currently be measured by objective methods (Ream & Richardson, 1996). However, a number of conceptualizations of fatigue have developed along dualistic (i.e., bidirectional) lines, including acute and chronic fatigue, physiological and psychological fatigue, and central and peripheral fatigue. While dualistic approaches have proven to be popular, such definitions fail to capture the multidimensional aspects of fatigue (Shen, Barbera, & Shapiro, 2006). With no known biological markers and numerous proposed causes, the operationalization of fatigue through concrete indicators has failed to reflect the empirical reality of the construct.

Feelings of fatigue likely are multidimensional with emotional, behavioral, and cognitive components. However, for the purposes of this discussion, the focus is on fatigue conceptualized as a mood state. A mood is a transient feeling people report experiencing ranging in duration from minutes to weeks and ultimately has an influence on thoughts and behaviors (Buckworth & Dishman, 2002). The mood of fatigue specifically refers to feelings of having a reduced capacity to complete mental or physical activities (O'Connor, 2004). This reduced capacity to complete mental or physical activities is distinct from, but also often accompanies, other related moods, including depression, for example.

Some contend biological systems that regulate mood evolved through natural selection to facilitate the transfer of genes (Watson, 2000). Feelings of fatigue likely evolved to promote rest, thereby enhancing recovery from injury or illness. From this evolutionary perspective, fatigue mood states have been vital to the propagation and survival of the human species.

Measuring physical activity and feelings of fatigue

Measurement is a two-fold issue in research examining the relationship between physical activity and feelings of fatigue. There is no single standard for measuring physical activity (Montoye, Kemper, Saris, & Washburn, 1996; Paffenbarger, Blair, Lee, & Hyde, 1993) or feelings of fatigue (Aaronson et al., 1999; O'Connor, 2004). Thus, both the exposure and outcome variables must be assessed with imperfect measures. Establishing the validity of physical activity instruments has been a recognized, yet still unresolved, problem in exercise science research (LaPorte, Montoye, & Caspersen, 1985). However, the problem of establishing the validity of fatigue measures has only recently gained greater attention in the areas of medicine and mental health (Whitehead, 2009).

It is important to accurately measure physical activity because such measurement can help quantify the physiological responses that may directly or indirectly influence psychological variables (Buckworth & Dishman, 2002). There are at least 30 methods for measuring physical activity, including direct and indirect calorimetry, physiologic markers (e.g., doubly labeled water), monitors (e.g., accelerometers), surveys (e.g., exercise recall), and direct observation. The selection of methods depends on the target population and level of sensitivity and specificity necessary to answer the research question (Casperson, 1989). Thus, it is important to address the difficulty of comparing results across studies with non-uniform assessment methods when discussing physical activity.

Fatigue is a universal symptom not only associated with most acute and chronic illnesses, but also with normal, healthy function and everyday life. Over 30 fatigue scales have proliferated in the clinical and scientific community and no two scales have operationalized the construct of fatigue exactly the same (Dittner, Wessely, & Brown, 2004; O'Connor, 2004). While some measure phenomenology, fatigue severity, or impact, many assess a mixture of all of these. There is no consensus about whether fatigue is best conceptualized as a symptom, a mood, an aspect of quality of life, or in some other way (O'Connor, 2004; Ream & Richardson, 1996). The choice of scale ultimately depends on the conceptualization of fatigue, the clinical or research application, and the psychometric evidence to support interpretation of scores. Thus, fatigue research has been inundated with measures ranging widely in their ability to offer valid interpretation of the construct.

Eidelman (1979) stated, "The absence of an overall definition of fatigue preempts any scientific basis for measuring the condition, because logically that which cannot be defined cannot be measured, and is not understood" (p. 340). Although a rather bold statement, it is also quite honest. In an area of study in which exposure and outcome variables must be assessed with imperfect measures, one must be cognizant of the limitations of the research.

Research on physical activity and feelings of fatigue

The body of research on physical activity and feelings of fatigue is not as extensive as that addressing the relationship between physical activity and other psychological variables such as anxiety, depression, or quality of life. Although there are some limitations in the research related to study design and instrumentation, the overall evidence for the effects of physical activity on feelings of fatigue generally is both positive and consistent (Puetz, 2006; Puetz et al., 2006a). Epidemiological and experimental research that has addressed the relationship between physical activity and feelings of fatigue is described in the following sections.

Epidemiological evidence

Epidemiological evidence can help researchers examine the distribution and determinants of physical activity in the general population and how this health-related behavior is associated with fatigue outcomes. The application of such knowledge is vital in the prevention and control of disease and the promotion of health.

A meta-analysis was conducted to synthesize the available evidence of the effect of physical activity on feelings of energy and fatigue in the population. Twelve population-based studies examining the association between physical activity and feelings of fatigue, published between 1945 and 2005, were identified by searches of Current Contents, Google Scholar, PsycInfo, Web of Science, and PubMed databases using the following search terms: energy, fatigue, quality of life, SF-36, and vitality, combined with exercise, physical activity, epidemiology, population study, prevalence, or incidence (Puetz, 2006). Odds ratios (OR) and relative risks (RR) were calculated from studies such that scores were interpreted relative to a sedentary sample and increases in feelings of energy and decreases in feelings of fatigue resulted in positive effect sizes (ES).

Results showed that people who are physically active in their leisure time have about a 40 percent reduced risk of experiencing fatigue compared with sedentary individuals (Puetz, 2006). Figure 29.1 illustrates the ORs and 95 percent confidence intervals (lower limit, upper limit) for the seven cross-sectional studies, the RRs and 95 percent confidence intervals (lower limit, upper limit) for the five longitudinal studies, and the overall 40 percent lower risk of fatigue in physically active persons. All studies found a positive relationship between physical activity and reduced feelings of fatigue; however, these effects were moderated by the study design and fatigue measure. The magnitude of the effect was attenuated in the stronger design of longitudinal studies compared to cross-sectional studies and increased in studies that used the well-validated Medical Outcome Study Short Form 36 Vitality Scale (SF-36; Ware, 2000) compared to studies that used other less-accepted energy and fatigue measures. These results highlight the design and measurement issues that continue to limit physical activity and fatigue research.

Because epidemiological comparisons cannot establish direction of causality, such evidence should be interpreted with caution. However, the strength of epidemiological evidence can be evaluated with standard criteria (i.e., strength of association, temporal sequence, consistency, dose response, biological plausibility) in order to judge whether the observed association suggests causality in the absence of adequate experimental evidence (Hill, 1965). There was agreement among the aforementioned studies suggesting a strong, consistent, temporally appropriate, dose-response relationship between physical activity and feelings of fatigue. However, there was a lack of compelling evidence to confirm any plausible biological mechanisms to explain the apparent protective effect of physical activity against feelings of fatigue. This paucity of evidence regarding biological plausibility is another issue limiting physical activity and fatigue research.

Not all criteria must be met in order to establish direction of causality in epidemiological research. A longitudinal study by Lee and Russell (2003) of nearly 6,500 older women (aged

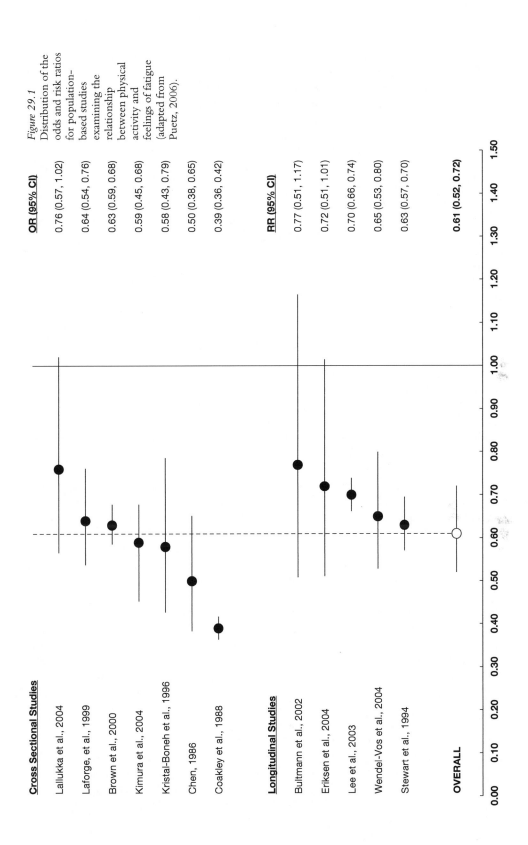

Cross Sectional Studies

	OR (95% CI)
Lallukka et al., 2004	0.76 (0.57, 1.02)
Laforge, et al., 1999	0.64 (0.54, 0.76)
Brown et al., 2000	0.63 (0.59, 0.68)
Kimura et al., 2004	0.59 (0.45, 0.68)
Kristal-Boneh et al., 1996	0.58 (0.43, 0.79)
Chen, 1986	0.50 (0.38, 0.65)
Coakley et al., 1988	0.39 (0.36, 0.42)

Longitudinal Studies

	RR (95% CI)
Bultmann et al., 2002	0.77 (0.51, 1.17)
Eriksen et al., 2004	0.72 (0.51, 1.01)
Lee et al., 2003	0.70 (0.66, 0.74)
Wendel-Vos et al., 2004	0.65 (0.53, 0.80)
Stewart et al., 1994	0.63 (0.57, 0.70)

OVERALL — **0.61 (0.52, 0.72)**

Figure 29.1
Distribution of the odds and risk ratios for population-based studies examining the relationship between physical activity and feelings of fatigue (adapted from Puetz, 2006).

70–75 years) particularly bolstered the argument for suggesting causality by examining the alterability of feelings of fatigue with the adoption or cessation of exercise. Women who reported exercise cessation during a 3-year observation period had greater decreases in SF-36 vitality scores than those who remained sedentary, those who remained physically active, or those who reported exercise adoption during that same period. The greatest increase in SF-36 vitality scores occurred among those who reported exercise adoption during the 3-year period. These changes were similar to those who remained physically active. These results not only provide evidence of temporal sequence, but also that these effects are alterable with increases or decreases in physical activity. Such epidemiological evidence is sufficiently strong to justify better-controlled prospective cohort studies and randomized controlled trials.

Experimental evidence

While experimental designs are often considered the most rigorous of all research designs, this is only the case if such a design is implemented well. Unfortunately, poor measurement and study design have limited experimental research in the area of physical activity and fatigue. This is often due to knowledge gaps as psychologists with limited background in exercise science, or physiologists with limited background in psychology, attempt to conduct physical activity and fatigue research (Buckworth & Dishman, 2002). Such issues regarding research design have been identified and discussed in a quantitative review (meta-analysis) of randomized controlled trials.

A meta-analysis of 70 randomized controlled trials examining the effects of chronic exercise on feelings of fatigue showed that exercise programs reduced fatigue in both healthy individuals and patient groups (Puetz et al., 2006a). Articles published from 1945 to November 2004 were located from searches of PsycInfo, PubMed, and Web of Science databases using the following keywords: energy, exercise, fatigue, mood, physical activity, Profile of Mood States (POMS), quality of life, resistance training, SF-36, and vitality. Articles included randomized allocation to either a chronic exercise condition or a non-exercise comparison condition and an energy or fatigue outcome measure assessed before and following the intervention. Effect sizes (ES) were computed by subtracting the mean change in fatigue for a non-exercise control group from the mean change in fatigue for an exercise group and dividing the difference by the pooled standard deviation of baseline scores (Hedges & Olkin, 1985).

The magnitude of the overall mean ES and 95 percent confidence interval (lower limit, upper limit) was moderate at 0.37 (0.29, 0.45), indicating that, on average, participants in exercise conditions reported approximately four-tenths of a standard deviation (*SD*) greater reduction in fatigue compared to participants in control conditions. The overall effect, however, was heterogeneous and moderated by a variety of study design issues. The effect varied according to the presence or absence of a usual care or placebo control (e.g., stretching or health education) and whether exercise training was completed alone or in combination with additional therapy. Investigations that used a placebo control and examined chronic exercise alone found no effect of chronic exercise on feelings of fatigue. This finding suggests that certain placebo controls may act as treatments in physical activity and fatigue studies, especially in populations of older adults and individuals with psychological distress. This could be attributed to the relative intensity of exercise in older adults who participate in stretching control interventions or placebo effects in individuals with psychological distress. Nonetheless, these results highlight the need for investigators to pursue more rigorous design methodology in physical activity and fatigue research.

Few exercise-training studies have been conducted with healthy adults characterized by feelings of fatigue (O'Connor & Puetz, 2005). Despite the lack of research specifically designed to examine changes in feelings of fatigue after exercise training in healthy, but fatigued individuals, available randomized controlled trials have shown reduced feelings of fatigue (Puetz, 2006). These experimental studies support the epidemiological evidence, suggesting a positive association between physical activity and reductions in fatigue. However, research design issues limit the strength of this evidence and preclude confirmation of the cause–effect nature of this relationship. These issues include confounded treatments in which exercise is combined with other treatments (e.g., behavior modification therapy), failure to match groups based on pre-treatment fatigue levels, inadequate description of the exercise stimulus, and failure to include no-treatment controls or placebo controls in the research design.

Such weaknesses in research design have made the effect of chronic exercise on feelings of fatigue difficult to interpret in terms of examining healthy, but fatigued, adult samples. Puetz, Flowers, and O'Connor (2008) addressed previous research limitations in a randomized controlled trial examining the effects of 6 weeks of exercise training on feelings of energy and fatigue in sedentary, healthy young adults reporting persistent fatigue. Thirty-six healthy young adults (mean age 23 years) who reported persistent feelings of fatigue were randomly assigned to a moderate-intensity, low-intensity, or no-treatment control group. Exercise conditions consisted of individually supervised cycling, 3 days per week for 30 minutes at the prescribed exercise intensity. The control condition consisted of sitting quietly on a cycle ergometer for the same frequency and duration as the exercise conditions. Results of the 6-week intervention showed significant benefits in energy and fatigue for both exercise conditions compared to the control condition. However, changes in feelings of fatigue were dependent on exercise intensity, whereas the effect on feelings of energy was similar for both the low-intensity and moderate-intensity conditions. More favorable outcomes for fatigue were seen in the low-intensity exercise group. It is noteworthy that changes in both energy and fatigue were unrelated to changes in aerobic fitness. Physical activity appears to be effective in healthy, sedentary populations. However, what is its efficacy in patient groups with chronic disease?

Physical activity and feelings of fatigue in patient populations

Physical activity may be especially beneficial in reducing feelings of fatigue in certain patient groups with chronic disease (Puetz, 2006). Three patient groups that have received significant examination of the effects of physical activity and feelings of fatigue in the scientific literature include fibromyalgia (Hauser, Bernardy, Arnold, Offenbächer, & Schiltenwolf, 2009a; Hauser et al., 2010), cardiovascular disease (Puetz, Beasman, & O'Connor, 2006b), and cancer patients (Brown et al., 2011; Cramp & Daniel, 2008; Velthuis, Agasi-Idenburg, Aufdemkampe, & Wittink, 2010). Research that has addressed the relationship between physical activity and feelings of fatigue is briefly described in the next section for each of these patient populations.

Fibromyalgia

Fibromyalgia is a disorder characterized by widespread musculoskeletal pain accompanied by fatigue, and sleep, memory, and mood dysfunction (Wolfe et al., 2010). While there is no cure for fibromyalgia, medications, cognitive behavior therapy, and exercise have consistently been recommended as a means to control symptoms (Clauw, 2009). A meta-analysis of 28 randomized controlled trials examining the effect of aerobic exercise treatment on feelings of fatigue in patients with fibromyalgia showed that aerobic exercise significantly reduced feelings of fatigue in this patient population (Hauser et al., 2010). The mean ES and 95 percent confidence interval (lower limit, upper limit) was −0.22 (−0.38, −0.05), supporting the positive effects of exercise on feelings of fatigue. The effect is slightly larger than the effect of cognitive behavior therapy (−0.09;

Bernardy, Fuber, Kollner, & Hauser, 2010) and antidepressants (−0.13; Hauser, Bernardy, Uceyler, & Sommer, 2009b) on feelings of the fatigue. This raises the question of whether a multidisciplinary therapy that combines exercise, cognitive behavioral therapy, and medical management is superior to exercise treatment alone.

The potential additive effect of a second treatment to an exercise intervention was addressed in another meta-analysis (Hauser et al., 2009a) that examined the magnitude of multicomponent treatments on feelings of fatigue in patients with fibromyalgia. Multicomponent treatments were defined as an intervention in which at least one educational or other psychological therapy was combined with exercise treatment. The mean effect for the nine randomized controlled trials included in the analysis was −0.85 (−1.50, −0.20), indicating an average of nearly nine-tenths of a *SD* greater reduction in fatigue among participants in exercise groups compared to participants in control groups. The cumulative meta-analytic evidence suggests that combination therapies incorporating exercise and behavioral therapies may provide an additive effect in the reduction of fatigue in patients with fibromyalgia. These results should be interpreted with caution because medication was not controlled in most studies. Therefore, there remains some uncertainty whether the effects reported are due only to the multicomponent treatment applied or to con-comitant medications.

Lera et al. (2009) directly addressed the additional efficacy of cognitive behavioral therapy in multicomponent treatments in a randomized controlled trial analyzing the effect of two multicomponent treatments on functional capability and symptom severity in patients with fibromyalgia. Eighty-three women (mean age 50 years) with fibromyalgia were randomly assigned to a 15-week multicomponent treatment or a multicomponent treatment combined with cognitive behavioral therapy. The multicomponent treatment included medical management, exercise training, and education classes. The exercise training consisted of 40 minutes of stretching and light aerobic exercise once a week for 10 of the 15 therapy sessions. The cognitive behavioral therapy focused on coping with stress, modifying lifestyles, and changing pain behaviors. After the 15-week program both multicomponent treatments exhibited similar improvements in functional capability and symptom severity. However, a sub-analysis of fibromyalgia patients with fatigue at baseline showed that the addition of cognitive behavioral therapy leads to a greater improvement in daily functioning and health status than is achieved through a multicomponent treatment alone. The significant improvements in functional capability and symptom severity were maintained at the 6-month follow-up.

Cardiovascular disease

Compared to the literature dealing with cardiac rehabilitation exercise programs in relation to other mental health areas such as anxiety, depression, and quality of life, there have been few reviews of research on exercise-based cardiac rehabilitation and feelings of fatigue. A meta-analysis of 36 cardiac rehabilitation studies showed that cardiac rehabilitation exercise programs were consistently associated with decreases in feelings of fatigue (Puetz et al., 2006b). The magnitude of the effect was 0.51 (0.42, 0.61) showing that participants in exercise programs reported on average one half a *SD* greater reduction in fatigue compared to control groups. However, features of the research design modified this effect. Non-controlled trials had a larger effect (ES = 0.58; 0.47, 0.68) than controlled trials (ES = 0.32; 0.14, 0.50). Nineteen cardiac rehabilitation studies concurrently measured anxiety, depression, and fatigue. Comparison of ESs in cardiac rehabilitation studies concurrently measuring anxiety, depression, and fatigue suggested that exercise-based cardiac rehabilitation programs have significantly larger effects on feelings of fatigue (ES = 0.59; 0.47, 0.71) compared with anxiety (ES = 0.40; 0.28, 0.52) and depression (ES =

0.35; 0.22, 0.48). These findings suggest that cardiac rehabilitation researchers and practitioners may benefit from examining, and perhaps even focusing on, feelings of fatigue as a salient outcome.

Stern, Gorman, and Kaslow (1983) have also provided convincing evidence to support the effect of cardiac rehabilitation exercise programs on reducing feelings of fatigue. One hundred and six post-myocardial infarction patients (mean age 54 years) meeting criteria for anxiety or depression were randomly assigned to a 12-week exercise therapy, group counseling, or usual care control. Exercise therapy consisted of supervised sessions of moderate aerobic exercise 3 days per week. Participants in the group counseling and usual care conditions were requested not to begin any formal exercise programs. Anxiety, depression, and fatigue were assessed before and after these treatments and during a 6-month and 12-month follow-up, during which time no formal exercise or group therapy occurred. Whereas exercise therapy initially reduced anxiety, depression, and fatigue, after the 12-week intervention, group counseling was only effective for depression and anxiety. Fatigue actually increased for those individuals in the counseling group. However, the most interesting result of this study was that fatigue actually increased in the exercise therapy condition at the 6-month and 12-month follow-up, while depression and anxiety reductions were maintained over the same time period. In addition, fatigue rates were reduced in the group counseling and usual care conditions at 6 and 12 months (Figure 29.2). Compliance rates following the intervention likely account for these trends in that 50 percent of exercise condition patients stopped exercising following the 12-week intervention whereas approximately 30 percent of group therapy and usual care patients began some form of exercise.

Cancer

Cancer-related fatigue is a persistent, subjective sense of tiredness related to cancer or cancer treatment that interferes with usual functioning and has been described as a nearly universal symptom among cancer patients (Mock et al., 2000). Exercise has been proposed as an effective intervention to improve feelings of fatigue in cancer patients both during and following treatment. Of four meta-analyses that have directly examined exercise effects on cancer-related fatigue, one examined cancer patients only during treatment (Velthuis et al., 2010) and another examined cancer patients only following treatment (Brown et al., 2011), precluding direct examination of differences between these two populations. The other two quantitative reviews allowed for comparisons of cancer patients both during and following treatment (Cramp & Daniel, 2008; Puetz & Herring, 2012).

Cramp and Daniel (2008) conducted a meta-analysis of 28 studies to examine differences in the magnitude of the effect of exercise on fatigue in cancer patients during and following treatment. There was a significant effect such that cancer patients following treatment (ES = −0.37; −0.55, −0.18) had a larger reduction in fatigue than cancer patients during treatment (ES = −0.18; −0.32, −0.05). The effect following treatment was similar to that of Brown et al. (2011), ES = 0.31, but the effect during treatment was significantly smaller than Velthuis et al. (2010), ES = 0.30 (note: positive ESs in Brown et al. and Velthuis et al. indicated greater fatigue reduction in cancer patients). The limitation of the Cramp and Daniel (2008) meta-analysis was that a moderator analysis was not conducted. This limited the understanding of how characteristics of study design, exercise interventions, and patient populations may influence exercise efficacy in cancer patients during and following treatment.

These limitations were addressed in a meta-analysis of 70 randomized controlled trials examining the differential effects of exercise treatment on cancer-related fatigue in cancer patients during and following treatment (Puetz & Herring, 2012). Compared with comparison conditions,

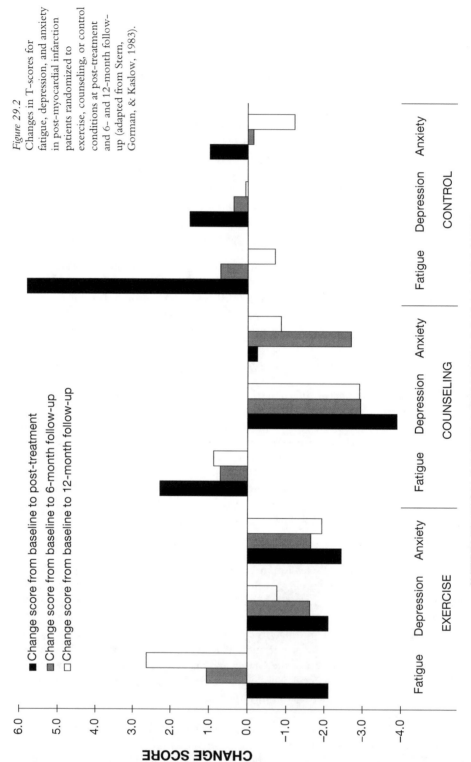

Figure 29.2
Changes in T-scores for fatigue, depression, and anxiety in post-myocardial infarction patients randomized to exercise, counseling, or control conditions at post-treatment and 6– and 12-month follow-up (adapted from Stern, Gorman, & Kaslow, 1983).

■ Change score from baseline to post-treatment
▨ Change score from baseline to 6-month follow-up
□ Change score from baseline to 12-month follow-up

CHANGE SCORE

6.0
5.0
4.0
3.0
2.0
1.0
0.0
-1.0
-2.0
-3.0
-4.0

Fatigue   Depression   Anxiety
EXERCISE

Fatigue   Depression   Anxiety
COUNSELING

Fatigue   Depression   Anxiety
CONTROL

INTERVENTION GROUP & PSYCHOLOGICAL MEASURE

exercise treatment significantly reduced fatigue for cancer patients during (ES = 0.32; 0.21, 0.43) and following (ES = 0.38; 0.21, 0.54) treatment. Improvements for cancer patients during treatment varied according to the patient's baseline fatigue scores and exercise adherence rates such that patients with lower baseline fatigue scores and higher intervention adherence rates realized the largest improvements. Among cancer patients following treatment, improvements were largest for those trials with longer durations between treatment completion and exercise initiation, trials with shorter exercise program lengths, and trials using waitlist comparisons. Perhaps the most interesting finding was related to the differential effects exercise treatment had on fatigue between exercise and control conditions in cancer patients during and following treatment. Fatigue symptoms were mitigated in cancer patients participating in an exercise intervention (4.2 percent decrease) compared to comparison interventions (29.1 percent increase) during treatment, while fatigue symptoms were reduced in cancer patients participating in exercise programs (20.5 percent decrease) compared to comparison interventions (1.3 percent decrease) following treatment. These findings suggest exercise has a palliative effect in patients during treatment and a recuperative effect in patients following treatment.

Evidence to support the positive effects of exercise on feelings of fatigue across the time course of cancer treatment and recovery were presented in a randomized controlled trial examining the effect of a self-administered exercise intervention before, during, and after allogeneic hematopoietic stem cell transplantation (Wiskermann et al., 2011). One hundred and five cancer patients were randomly assigned to a partly self-administered exercise or social contact control condition. The exercise intervention consisted of three 20- to 40-minute light aerobic sessions and two full-body resistance training (i.e., 8–20 repetitions, 2–3 sets) sessions per week. Participants in the exercise group started exercising on an outpatient basis 1 to 4 weeks before hospital admission, continued during the inpatient period, and sustained the program until 6 to 8 weeks after discharge from the hospital. The outpatient exercise period was self-directed at home, whereas the inpatient exercise period was supervised twice weekly. The control group wore pedometers during the outpatient period to measure physical activity and received the same frequency of social contact as the exercise intervention during the inpatient period. Over the entire time course of cancer treatment and recovery from the initial medical checkup to the 6- to 8-week follow-up, the exercise condition showed a 15 percent improvement in fatigue scores and the control condition showed 28 percent deterioration in fatigue during the same time period. Several important results from this study were (a) fatigue was reduced in the 1- to 4-week period following the medical checkup prior to hospital admission for the exercise condition compared to the control condition, (b) fatigue was significantly mitigated at discharge from the hospital following cancer treatment in the exercise group compared to the control group in which fatigue actually increased, and (c) fatigue was significantly reduced at the 6- to 8-week follow-up in the exercise group compared to the control group to the extent that the exercise condition participants had scores significantly lower than baseline (Figure 29.3). These results support the conclusion that exercise has a palliative effect in patients undergoing cancer treatment and a recuperative effect in patients following treatment, and that clinicians should consider prescribing exercise at cancer diagnosis.

Directions for future investigation

Although experimental evidence in patient and non-patient populations is largely supportive of the positive effects of physical activity on feelings of fatigue, the area of research is still in its formative years. One important next step in the evolution toward strong science-based practice is the need to better understand which biological, psychological, and psychosocial aspects of

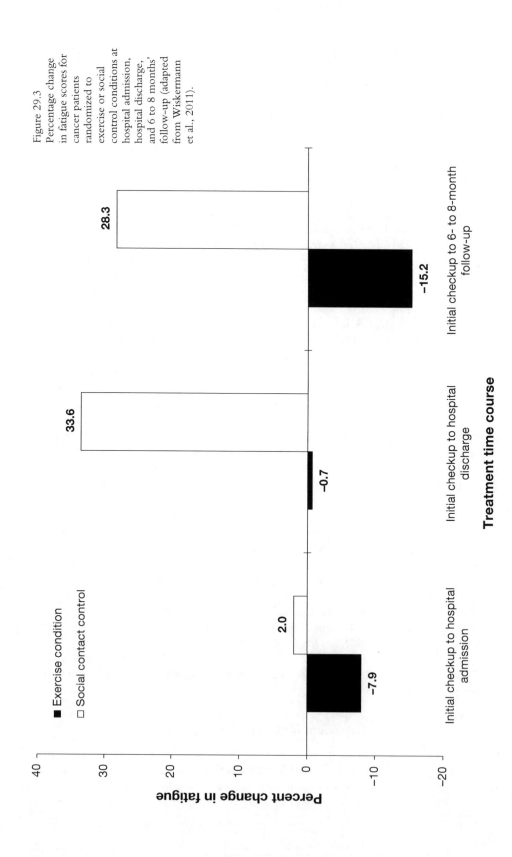

Figure 29.3
Percentage change
in fatigue scores for
cancer patients
randomized to
exercise or social
control conditions at
hospital admission,
hospital discharge,
and 6 to 8 months'
follow-up (adapted
from Wiskermann
et al., 2011).

physical activity contribute to improved feelings of fatigue. The following section will discuss two major directions for future investigations, namely identifying biological mechanisms behind the physical activity and fatigue relationship and recognizing the importance of interdisciplinary research in further developing this area of study.

Mechanisms

The brain has long been suspected as the primary driver of feelings of fatigue. It is now generally accepted that the brain controls mental, physiological, and behavioral processes. Although genes control brain functioning, social, developmental, and environmental factors can alter gene expression. These alterations in gene expression can induce changes in brain functioning and behavior (Dishman et al., 2006). It is unclear whether the origin of fatigue is in a particular brain structure, is the result of an integrative process involving a number of different brain regions, or is the result of electrophysiological synchronization of entire brain activity (St Clair Gibson et al., 2003). However, metabolic and neurochemical pathways within the central nervous system offer testable mechanisms that might help explain the effects of physical activity on feelings of fatigue.

The specific brain mechanisms that generate the moods of energy and fatigue are unknown, but monoamine-, histamine-, acetylcholine-, glutamate-, and gamma-aminobutyric acid (GABA)-mediated neurotransmission have been implicated (Demyttenaere, De Fruyt, & Stahl, 2005; Stahl, 2002; Stahl, Zhang, Damatarca, & Grady, 2003). There is evidence that physical activity can alter these neurotransmitters and neuromodulators (Dishman et al., 2006). Understanding the neurotransmitters and neuromodulators involved in generating feelings of fatigue is important, but perhaps more important is examining how these chemical messengers regulate potentially malfunctioning neurological circuits or brain areas associated with mental and physical fatigue. For example, brain cortical areas (e.g., dorsolateral prefrontal cortex) and central nervous system components regulating motor functioning (e.g., striatum, cerebellum, spinal cord) could be reasonable candidates in mediating moods of mental and physical fatigue, respectively (Demyttenaere et al., 2005; Stahl et al., 2003).

Unfortunately, there has been very little use of the traditions and methods of biology, psychology, and neuroscience in the study of physical activity and feelings of fatigue. Future research needs to incorporate the basics of neuroanatomy, neurophysiology, and psychopharmacology along with techniques of neuroscience to facilitate sound research on physical activity and fatigue. The best strategy to employ in this course of research development is effective trans-disciplinary collaboration.

Interdisciplinary research

Most research is conducted within the established boundaries of a given scientific discipline. Interdisciplinary research involves bringing together people and ideas from different disciplines to jointly frame a problem, agree on a methodological approach, and analyze data (Golde & Gallagher, 1999). As envisioned by Mosso over 120 years ago, this integration of traditional disciplines is vital in uncovering the multidimensional nature of fatigue (Mosso, 1891). The paucity of such research in the area of physical activity and fatigue is disheartening, but the few studies examining psychosocial pathways (e.g., McAuley, White, Rogers, Motl, & Courneya, 2010), immunological response (e.g., Kop, Weinstein, Deuster, Wittaker, & Tracy, 2008; Robson-Ansley et al., 2009), and neuroimaging (e.g., Dishman, Thom, Puetz, O'Connor, & Clementz, 2010) show the promise such interdisciplinary research can offer in advancing our understanding of the biopsychosocial aspects of fatigue. It is imperative that future investigators continue collaboration across scientific disciplines.

Although knowledge about physical activity and feelings of fatigue has significantly increased in the last decade, further investigation is important for the realization of increased public health and well-being. The following are some key critical objectives for future research:

- To more fully characterize the features of the physical activity or exercise stimulus (i.e., frequency, intensity, session duration, program length, and mode) on specific neurobiological and psychological outcome measures of feelings of fatigue.
- To examine the degree of overlap or independence of the effect of physical activity on feelings of fatigue with other mood states including anxiety and depression, and quality of life.
- To better understand the biological correlates and mechanisms for changes in feelings of fatigue that occur with regular exercise.
- To more closely examine the impact of physical activity on fatigue and various disease states and how sociodemographic factors such as age, sex, and socioeconomic status modify the effects of physical activity on feelings of fatigue.
- To investigate the similarities, interactions, and differences among different exercise training paradigms, psychosocial interventions, and pharmacological treatments employed to reduce feelings of fatigue.

Conclusions

Physical activity is a healthy behavior that has promise for combating feelings of fatigue (O'Connor & Puetz, 2005). Approximately 20 percent of adults worldwide report persistent fatigue (Wessely et al., 1998). Historically clinicians have recognized the physiological and psychological aspects of fatigue and have consistently recommended exercise as a treatment. The subjective nature of fatigue has made conceptualizing, operationalizing, and measuring the construct difficult. This, in conjunction with the imperfect measure of physical activity, has created some limitations in the area of physical activity and fatigue research. Despite such limitations, epidemiological evidence suggests that people who are physically active in their leisure time have about a 40 percent reduced risk of experiencing feelings of fatigue compared with sedentary comparison groups (Puetz, 2006). This population-based research has been substantiated with experimental evidence that shows physical activity does reduce feelings of fatigue across both healthy groups and patient populations. However, the quality of methodological rigor must continue to improve and evolve in a manner that integrates biological, psychological, and psychosocial factors into fatigue research. Future investigation can best meet these standards by incorporating interdisciplinary research into uncovering the biological mechanisms behind the effects of physical activity on feelings of fatigue.

References

Aaronson, L. S., Teel, C. S., Cassmeyer, V., Neuberger, G. B., Pallikkathayil, L., Pierce, J., . . . Wingate, A. (1999). Defining and measuring fatigue. *Journal of Nursing Scholarship, 31*, 45–50.

Addington, A. M., Gallo, J. J., Ford, D. E., & Eaton, W. W. (2001). Epidemiology of unexplained fatigue and major depression in the community: The Baltimore ECA Follow-up, 1981–1994. *Psychological Medicine, 31*, 1037–44.

Allen, F. N. (1944). The differential diagnosis of weakness and fatigue. *New England Journal of Medicine, 231*, 414–18.

Allen, F. N. (1945). The clinical management of weakness and fatigue. *Journal of the American Medical Association, 127*, 957–60.

Bartley, S. H., & Chute, E. (1947). *Fatigue and impairment in man.* New York: McGraw-Hill.

Bernardy, K., Fuber, N., Kollner, V., & Hauser, W. (2010). Efficacy of cognitive-behavioral therapies in fibromyalgia syndrome: A systematic review and meta-analysis of randomized controlled trials. *Journal of Rheumatology, 37,* 1991–2005.

Brown, J. C., Huedo-Medina, T. B., Pescatello, L. S., Pescatello, S. M., Ferrer, R. A., & Johnson, B. T. (2011). Efficacy of exercise interventions in modulating cancer-related fatigue among adult cancer survivors: A meta-analysis. *Cancer Epidemiology, Biomarkers, and Prevention, 20,* 123–33.

Buckworth, J., & Dishman, R. K. (2002). *Exercise psychology.* Champaign, IL: Human Kinetics.

Caspersen, C. J. (1989). Physical activity epidemiology: Concepts, methods and applications to exercise science. *Exercise and Sport Sciences Reviews, 17,* 423–73.

Caspersen, C. J., Powell, K. E., & Christenson, G. M. (1985). Physical activity, exercise, and physical fitness: Definitions and distinctions for health-related research. *Public Health Reports, 100,* 126–31.

Chen, M. K. (1986). The epidemiology of self-perceived fatigue among adults. *Preventive Medicine, 15,* 74–81.

Clauw, D. J. (2009). Fibromyalgia: An overview. *American Journal of Medicine, 122,* S3–S13.

Cowles, E. (1893). *The mental symptoms of fatigue.* New York: Fless & Ridge.

Cramp, F., & Daniel, J. (2008). Exercise for the management of cancer-related fatigue in adults. *Cochrane Database of Systematic Reviews, 2,* CD006145.

Darbishire, L., Ridsdale, L., & Seed, P. T. (2003). Distinguishing patients with chronic fatigue from those with chronic fatigue syndrome: A diagnostic study in UK primary care. *British Journal of General Practice, 53,* 441–5.

Dearborn, G. V. N. (1902). On the "fatigue" of nerve centers. *Psychological Review, 9,* 180–3.

Demyttenaere, K., De Fruyt, J., & Stahl, S. M. (2005). The many faces of fatigue in major depressive disorder. *International Journal of Neuropsychopharmacology, 8,* 93–105.

de Rijk, A. E., Schreurs, K. M. G., & Bensing, J. M. (2000). Patient factors related to the presentation of fatigue complaints: Results from a women's general health care practice. *Women and Health, 30,* 121–36.

Di Giulio, C., Daniele, F., & Tipton, C. M. (2006). Angelo Mosso and muscular fatigue: 116 years after the first congress of physiologists: IUPS commemoration. *Advances in Physiology Education, 30,* 51–7.

Dishman, R. K., Thom, N. J., Puetz, T. W., O'Connor, P. J., & Clementz, B. A. (2010). Effects of cycling exercise on vigor, fatigue, and electroenphalographic activity among young adults who report persistent fatigue. *Psychophysiology, 47,* 1066–74.

Dishman, R. K., Berthoud, H., Booth, F. W., Cotman, C. W., Edgerton, V. R., Fleshner, M. R., . . . Zigmond, M. J. (2006). The neurobiology of exercise. *Obesity, 14*(3), 345–56.

Dittner, A., Wessely, S., & Brown, R. (2004). The assessment of fatigue: A practical guide for clinicians and researchers. *Journal of Psychosomatic Research, 56,* 157–70.

Eidelman, D. (1979). "Fatigue on rest" and associated symptoms (headache, vertigo, blurred vision, nausea, tension, and irritability) due to locally asymptomatic, unerupted, impacted teeth. *Medical Hypotheses, 5,* 339–46.

Golde, C. M., & Gallagher, H. A. (1999). The challenges of conducting interdisciplinary research in traditional doctoral programs. *Ecosystems, 2,* 281–5.

Hauser, W., Bernardy, K., Arnold, B., Offenbächer, M., & Schiltenwolf, M. (2009a). Efficacy of multicomponent treatment in fibromyalgia syndrome: A meta-analysis of randomized controlled trials. *Arthritis and Rheumatism, 15,* 216–24.

Hauser, W., Bernardy, K., Uceyler, N., & Sommer, C. (2009b). Treatment of fibromyalgia syndrome with antidepressants: A meta-analysis. *Journal of the American Medical Association, 301,* 198–209.

Hauser, W., Klose, P., Langhorst, J., Moradi, B., Steinbach, M., Schiltenwolf, M., & Busch, A. (2010). Efficacy of different types of aerobic exercise in fibromyalgia syndrome: A systematic review and meta-analysis of randomized controlled trials. *Arthritis Research and Therapy, 12,* R79.

Hedges, L. V., & Olkin, I. (1985). *Statistical methods for meta-analysis.* New York: Academic Press.

Hill, A. B. (1965). The environment and disease: Association or causation. *Proceedings of the Royal Society of Medicine, 58,* 295–300.

Joyce, J., Hotopt, M., & Wessely, S. (1997). The prognosis of chronic fatigue and chronic fatigue syndrome: A systematic review. *Quarterly Journal of Medicine, 90,* 223–33.

Kop, W. J., Weinstein, A. A., Deuster, P. A., Wittaker, K. S., & Tracy, R. P. (2008). Inflammatory markers and negative mood symptoms following exercise withdrawal. *Brain, Behavior, and Immunity, 22,* 1190–96.

Kroenke, K., & Price, R. (1993). Symptoms in the community: Prevalence, classification, and psychiatric comorbidity. *Archives of Internal Medicine, 153,* 2474–80.

LaPorte, R. E., Montoye, H. L., & Caspersen, C. J. (1985). Assessment of physical activity in epidemiological research: Problems and prospects. *Public Health Reports, 100*, 131–46.

Lee, C., & Russell, A. (2003). Effects of physical activity on emotional well-being among older Australian women: Cross-sectional and longitudinal analyses. *Journal of Psychosomatic Research, 54*, 155–60.

Lera, S., Gelman, S. M., Lopez, M. J., Abenoza, M., Zorrilla, J. G., Castro-Fornieles, J., & Salamero, M. (2009). Multidisciplinary treatment of fibromyalgia: Does cognitive behavior therapy increase the response to treatment? *Journal of Psychosomatic Research, 67*, 433–41.

MacDougall, R. (1899). Fatigue. *Psychological Review, 6*, 203–8.

McAuley, E., White, S. M., Rogers, L. Q., Motl, R. W., & Courneya, K. S. (2010). Physical activity and fatigue in breast cancer and multiple sclerosis: Psychosocial mechanisms. *Psychosomatic Medicine, 72*, 88–96.

Mock, V., Atkinson, A., Barsevick, A., Cella, D., Cimprich, B., Cleeland, C., . . . Stahl, C. (2000). NCCN practice guidelines for cancer-related fatigue. *Oncology (Williston Park), 14*, 151–61.

Montoye, H. J., Kemper, H. C. G., Saris, W. H. M., & Washburn, R. A. (1996). *Measuring physical activity and energy expenditure.* Champaign, IL: Human Kinetics.

Mosso A. (1891). *La Fatica.* Milano, IT: Treves.

Muncie, W. (1941). Chronic fatigue. *Psychosomatic Medicine, 3*, 277–85.

Muscio, B. (1921). Is a fatigue test possible? *British Journal of Psychology, 12*, 31–46.

O'Connor, P. J. (2004). Evaluation of four highly cited energy and fatigue mood measures. *Journal of Psychosomatic Research, 57*, 435–41.

O'Connor, P. J. & Puetz, T. W. (2005). Chronic physical activity and feelings of energy and fatigue. *Medicine and Science in Sports and Exercise, 37*, 299–305.

Paffenbarger, R. S., Blair, S. N., Lee, I. M., & Hyde, R. T. (1993). Measurement of physical activity to assess health effects in free-living populations. *Medicine and Science in Sports and Exercise, 25*, 60–70.

Poore, G. V. (1875). On fatigue. *Lancet, 106*, 163–4.

Puetz, T. W. (2006). Physical activity and feelings of energy and fatigue: Epidemiological evidence. *Sports Medicine, 36*, 767–80.

Puetz, T. W., Beasman, K. M., & O'Connor, P. J. (2006b). The effect of cardiac rehabilitation exercise programs on feelings of energy and fatigue: A meta-analysis of research from 1945 to 2005. *European Journal of Cardiovascular Prevention and Rehabilitation, 13*, 886–93.

Puetz, T. W., Flowers, S. S., & O'Connor, P. J. (2008). A randomized controlled trial of the effect of aerobic exercise training on feelings of energy and fatigue in sedentary young adults with persistent fatigue. *Psychotherapy and Psychosomatics, 77*, 167–74.

Puetz, T. W., & Herring, M. P. (2012). Differential effects of exercise on cancer-related fatigue during and following treatment: A meta-analysis. *American Journal of Preventive Medicine, 43*, e1–e24.

Puetz, T. W., O'Connor, P. J., & Dishman, R. K. (2006a). Effects of chronic exercise on feelings of energy and fatigue: A quantitative synthesis. *Psychological Bulletin, 132*, 866–76.

Ream, E., & Richardson, A. (1996). Fatigue: A concept analysis. *International Journal of Nursing Studies, 33*, 519–29.

Ricci, J. A., Chee, E., Lorandeau, A. L., & Berger, J. (2007). Fatigue in the U.S. workforce: Prevalence and implications for lost productive work time. *Journal of Occupational and Environmental Medicine, 49*, 1–10.

Rimes, K. A., Goodman, R., Hotopf, M., Wessely, S., Meltzer, H., & Chalder, T. (2007). Incidence, prognosis, and risk factors for fatigue and chronic fatigue syndrome in adolescents: A prospective community study. *Pediatrics, 119*, 603–9.

Robson-Ansley, P., Barwood, M., Canavan, J., Hack, S., Eglin, C., Davey, S., . . . Ansley, L. (2009). The effect of repeated endurance exercise on IL-6 and sIL-6R and their relationship with sensations of fatigue at rest. *Cytokine, 45*, 111–16.

Ruffin, M., & Cohen, M. (1994). Evaluation and management of fatigue. *American Family Physician, 50*, 625–34.

Shen, J., Barbera, J., & Shapiro, C. M. (2006). Distinguishing sleepiness and fatigue: Focus on definition and measurement. *Sleep Medicine Review, 10*, 63–76.

Stahl, S. M. (2002). The psychopharmacology of energy and fatigue. *Journal of Clinical Psychiatry, 63*, 7–8.

Stahl, S. M., Zhang, L. S., Damatarca, C., & Grady, M. (2003). Brain-circuits determine destiny in depression: A novel approach to the psychopharmacology of wakefulness, fatigue, and executive dysfunction in major depressive disorder. *Journal of Clinical Psychiatry, 64*, 6–17.

St Clair Gibson, A., Baden, D. A., Lambert, M. I., Lambert, E. V., Harley, Y., & Hampson, D. (2003). The conscious perception of the sensation of fatigue. *Sports Medicine, 33*, 167–76.

Stern, M. J., Gorman, P. A., & Kaslow, L. (1983). The group counseling vs. exercise therapy study: A controlled intervention with subjects following myocardial infarction. *Archives of Internal Medicine, 143*, 1719–25.

Velthuis, M. J., Agasi-Idenburg, S. C., Aufdemkampe, G., & Wittink, H. M. (2010). The effect of physical exercise on cancer-related fatigue during cancer treatment: A meta-analysis of randomized controlled trials. *Clinical Oncology (Royal College of Radiologists), 22*, 208–21.

Ware, J. (2000). *SF-36 health survey manual and interpretation guide.* Lincoln, NE: Quality Metric.

Waterman, G. (1909). The treatment of fatigue states. *Journal of Abnormal Psychology, 4*, 128–39.

Watson, D. (2000). *Mood and temperament.* New York: Guilford Press.

Wessely, S., Chalder, T., Hirsch, S., Wallace, P., & Wright, D. (1997). The prevalence and morbidity of chronic fatigue and chronic fatigue syndrome: A prospective primary care study. *American Journal of Public Health, 87*, 1449–55.

Wessely, S., Hotopf, M., & Sharpe, M. (1998). *Chronic fatigue and its syndromes.* Oxford: Oxford University Press.

Whitehead, L. (2009). The measurement of fatigue in chronic illness: A systematic review of unidimensional and multidimensional fatigue measures. *Journal of Pain and Symptom Management, 37*, 107–28.

Wiskermann, J., Dreger, P., Schwerdtfeger, R., Bondong, A., Huber, G., Kleindienst, N., . . . Bohus, M. (2011). Effects of a partly self-administered exercise program before, during, and after allogeneic stem cell transplantation. *Blood, 117*(9), 2604–13.

Wolfe, F., Clauw, D. J., Fitzcharles, M. A., Goldenberg, D. L., Katz, R. S., Mease, P., . . . Yunus, M. B. (2010). The American College of Rheumatology preliminary diagnostic criteria for fibromyalgia and measurement of symptom severity. *Arthritis Care and Research, 62*, 600–10.

30

TIRED OF BEING SEDENTARY

Physical activity as a treatment goal in patients with chronic fatigue syndrome

Jo Nijs, Mira Meeus, Jessica Van Oosterwijck, Kelly Ickmans, Inge van Eupen, and Daphne Kos

Chronic fatigue syndrome (CFS) describes a disorder consisting of chronic debilitating fatigue that cannot be explained by any known chronic medical or psychological condition (Fukuda et al., 1994). While a variety of case definitions exist, often with varying nomenclatures (reviewed in Christley, Duffy, & Martin, 2011), the most widely accepted for research purposes remains the 1994 Centers for Disease Control and Prevention definition (Harvey, Wadsworth, Wessely, & Hotopf, 2008). The core feature of a CFS diagnosis is the exclusion of any active medical condition that may explain the presence of the symptoms (e.g., severe obesity, cancer hypo-thyroidism, primary sleep disorders, rheumatoid arthritis, multiple sclerosis, Hepatitis B or C, major depressive disorders with psychotic or melancholic features, bipolar affective disorders, schizophrenia, dementia, alcohol abuse; Fukuda et al., 1994). CFS is a disorder affecting approximately 0.5 percent of the population (Jason et al., 1999b).

A second requirement for CFS diagnosis entails the presence of a new onset, unexplained, and persistent fatigue, unrelated to exertion and not substantially relieved by rest. Importantly, the fatigue should be severely disabling, in a way that causes substantial reductions in physical activity levels. Finally, four or more of the following symptoms should be present for 6 months or longer: impaired memory or concentration; extreme, prolonged exhaustion and sickness as a result of physical or mental exertion (post-exertional malaise); unrefreshing sleep; muscle pain; pain in multiple joints; headaches of a new kind or greater severity; sore throat and tender lymph nodes (cervical or axillary).

Thus, CFS diagnostic criteria imply a substantial reduction in activity levels. In most cases, this implies a major decrease in physical activity level. Yet patients with CFS do not choose to be physically inactive. They are tired of being inactive. Without appropriate treatment, they are unable to increase their physical activity level without experiencing a relapse.

This chapter provides an overview of the current understanding of physical activity in patients with CFS. We discuss and summarize research data concerning CFS physical activity levels and patterns and explain that effective treatments are available to improve physical activity levels in patients with CFS. Finally, we address some methodological issues and directions for future research in this important area.

Physical activity level in patients with CFS

A large national birth cohort study revealed that continuing to be active despite increasing fatigue is likely a crucial step in the development of CFS (Harvey et al., 2008). Once CFS is established, the situation changes dramatically. Post-exertional malaise becomes a major characteristic of the illness. This implies that symptoms like fatigue and pain are typically made worse after modest amounts of exercise (Clapp et al., 1999), after increased daily physical activity (Black, O'Conner, & McCully, 2005), and after a submaximal exercise stress test (Bazelmans, Bleijenberg, Voeten, van der Meer, & Folgering, 2005; Lapp, 1997). Post-exertional malaise in CFS is accompanied by a delayed recovery from exercise (Paul, Wood, Behan, & Maclaren, 1999). Hence, rest and activity avoidance could be a way to cope with CFS-related post-exertional malaise (Vercoulen et al. 1996). These observations indirectly imply that patients with CFS perform less physical activity. In fact, it suggests that patients with CFS are too tired to be physically active. Is there research data to support this view?

Nijs et al. (2011) in a recent systematic literature review concluded that all published studies on physical activity in CFS found reduced habitual physical activity among patients with CFS compared to healthy controls (Bazelmans, Bleijenberg, van der Meer, & Folgering, 2001; Black, O'Conner, & McCully, 2005; Jason et al., 1999a; Sisto et al., 1998; Vercoulen et al., 1997). In total, 99 patients with CFS and 101 healthy control subjects were studied. Each of the studies used real-time continuous activity monitoring (accelerometers). Importantly, some studies used sedentary healthy participants for comparison. These findings provide research data to support the notion that patients with CFS, on average, are physically inactive and often perform less physical activity than sedentary control subjects (Nijs et al., 2011).

The question therefore arises, why are people with CFS physically inactive? Avoidance behavior toward physical activity is likely to influence physical activity level and exercise performance. CFS patients have been shown to perform less frequently specific activities expected to result in high fatigue levels and high fatigue expectations are related to low activity levels (Vercoulen et al., 1997). Kinesiophobia, a specific kind of fear-avoidance behavior, is defined as "an excessive, irrational, and debilitating fear of physical movement and activity resulting from a feeling of vulnerability to painful injury or reinjury" (Kori, Miller, & Todd, 1990). In patients with CFS, kinesiophobia represents a clinically important feature (i.e., related to disability), but does not appear to be a determinant of physiological exercise capacity (Nijs, De Meirleir, & Duquet, 2004; Nijs, Vanherberghen, Duquet, & De Meirleir, 2004; Silver et al., 2002). This observation is in line with a study showing stronger voluntary efforts (i.e., stronger brain signals recorded with electroencephalogram) during motor tasks in CFS patients compared to healthy controls (Siemionow, Fang, Calabrese, Sahgal, & Yue, 2004). This implies that during exercise capacity testing, patients with CFS do not avoid maximal exertion due to kinesiophobia; instead, their brain commands the muscles to exercise, but the body is incapable of performing.

On the other hand, overactivity or workaholism may be important predisposing and perpetuating factors for CFS. Patients with CFS are often perfectionists and frequently try very hard to meet their own and others' requirements (Van Houdenhove, Onghena, Neerinckx, & Hellin, 1995). Sustained physical or mental effort may, in susceptible individuals, eventually lead to neuro-endocrine and immunological dysfunctions (Van Houdenhove, Neerinckx, Onghena, Lysens, & Vertommen, 2001). This reasoning is in line with our current understanding of post-exertional malaise in people with CFS.

Several investigators have shown that overly vigorous exercise (De Becker, Roeykens, Reynders, McGregor, & De Meirleir, 2000; Lapp, 1997; Nijs, De Meirleir, Wolfs, & Duquet, 2004) or even merely a 30 percent increase in activity (Wong et al., 1992) frequently triggers a relapse, which may explain at least part of the physical inactivity seen in CFS patients. This post-exertional malaise has been linked to acute immune changes following physical activity that exceeds a CFS patient's physical capabilities (Jammes, Steinberg, Mambrini, Brégeon, & Delliaux, 2005; Nijs et al., 2010; Sorensen et al., 2003). Fatigue and other CFS characteristics like post-exertional malaise make it difficult, if not impossible, to be physically active. Anyone who has worked with CFS patients can confirm they do not choose to be physically inactive. On the contrary, patients with CFS are tired of living a sedentary life. Current rehabilitation approaches for CFS emphasize the importance of pacing daily activities and respect for the physical and mental limitations inherent to CFS (Nijs, Paul, & Wallman, 2008). This approach aims at preventing post-exertional malaise in patients with CFS (Nijs et al., 2008) and will be explained in more detail below.

Physical activity patterns in CFS patients

In addition to the reduced activity level compared to the premorbid level or to healthy controls, people with CFS display an abnormal activity pattern: their lifestyle appears to be characterized by activity peaks and longer bouts of rest after activity (Van der Werf, Prins, Vercoulen, van der Meer, & Bleijenberg, 2000). This was confirmed by a recent literature review, which concluded patients with CFS have lower and shorter average activity peaks, followed by longer rest periods (van Weering, Vollenbroek-Hutten, Kotte, & Hermens, 2007). Resting and activity avoidance could be a way to cope with the illness (Vercoulen et al., 1996).

Based on their behavior, patients with CFS can be categorized in two subgroups. One group comprises those who feel helpless and avoid activity, resulting in extremely passive behavior. The second group displays a highly variable activity pattern. At "good" moments they try to move mountains, leading to exhaustion and longer periods of recovery. Both types of physical behavior patterns appear to be maladaptive (Moss-Morris, Sharon, Tobin, & Baldi, 2005).

Given the nature of CFS it seems rational to assume patients with CFS present a more fluctuating activity pattern, with greater variations and a pronounced staggering of activities during the day. Concerning the staggering of activities during the day, we found higher ratios (peak activity/average activity) in patients with CFS (Meeus et al., 2011). Patients with CFS tended to concentrate their activities more in peaks (probably at their better moments), instead of dispersing them, although the difference in ratios (peak activity/average activity) between CFS and healthy controls was not statistically significant. Additionally, fluctuations in activity patterns during the complete assessment period were not significantly different between patients and controls. In summary, we found no evidence for important variations in the activity pattern of patients with CFS during the day, or day by day (Meeus et al., 2011).

In the same study (Meeus et al., 2011), we also asked the question: Is the physical activity pattern of patients with CFS related to symptom variations? Sedentary activities and staggering of physical activity were negatively correlated to symptom severity and variation on the same day and the following day (Meeus et al., 2011). This implies patients who concentrated their physical activity more in peaks did so on days they experienced fewer symptoms. Light, moderate, and vigorous activity, as well as average activity and the activity peak, were positively correlated with symptom severity and variation on the same day and the subsequent day, indicating patients experienced more symptoms when they were more active. In summary, the more patients with CFS are sedentary and the better activity is dispersed throughout the day, the fewer symptoms and variations they experience on the same and the following day (Meeus et al., 2011).

Finally, it is important to study biological factors in relation to physical activity in patients with CFS. Few studies have addressed this issue. We recently reported that activity-related symptom fluctuations in patients with CFS are not likely due to nitric oxide (NO) increases in response to normal physical activities (Meeus et al., 2010). NO was examined because it is known to increase the excitability of the central nervous system and regulate vascular tone in the tissues, including working muscles during exercise. When comparing CFS patients with healthy sedentary controls, no significant differences in serum NO amounts were observed. Variation in NO levels over the 1-week observation period was unrelated to daily activity levels in either group (Meeus et al., 2010). These findings corroborate our previous work, showing that neither post-exertional malaise nor impaired endogenous pain inhibition following exercise in patients with CFS is due to circulating NO levels (Meeus et al., 2010).

How to improve physical activity level and pattern during treatment

From what has been explained above, it seems plausible to include activity management in the comprehensive treatment of patients with CFS. Activity management is generally included in cognitive behavioral programs for CFS, and there is good evidence in support of the effectiveness of cognitive behavioral therapy for patients with CFS (Knoop, Bleijenberg, Gielissen, van der Meer, & White, 2007; Price, Mitchell, Tidy, & Hunot, 2008; Prins et al., 2001). Three weeks of pacing self-management is accompanied by a modest improvement in symptom severity and daily functioning (Nijs et al., 2009). The outcome of the latter study calls for a randomized controlled clinical trial to examine the effectiveness of pacing self-management for patients with CFS. Our group has completed such a trial and the results are in progress.

Self-management for people with CFS involves encouraging them to pace their activities and respect their physical and mental limitations (Pardaens, Haagdorens, Van Wambeke, Van den Broeck, & Van Houdenhove, 2006; Shephard, 2001). This strategy has been termed "pacing" and involves encouraging the patient to achieve an appropriate balance between activity and rest to avoid exacerbating symptoms. It requires the patient to set realistic activity goals on a daily basis (CFS/ME Working Group, 2001; Shephard, 2001) and to regularly monitor and manipulate activity in terms of intensity, duration, and rest periods to avoid possible over-exertion, which can result in worsening symptoms (CFS/ME Working Group, 2001; Shephard, 2001). Pacing takes into account the considerable fluctuations in symptom severity (Shephard, 2001) and delayed recovery from exercise that typically occurs in patients with CFS (Paul et al., 1999). This approach should not be confused with "adaptive pacing" (White et al., 2007), a strategy that advocates adapting to CFS. Such a strategy is based on the premise that people with CFS have a very low chance of recovery. In contrast, pacing activity self-management is an important aspect of the first phase of a comprehensive rehabilitation program for CFS, comprising a stabilization and subsequent grading phase (Nijs et al., 2008; Nijs, Van Oosterwijck, & Meeus, 2009). Graded activity and graded exercise therapy are typically used in the grading phase, and aim at increasing daily physical activity levels (e.g., Nijs et al., 2008). Graded activity implies the gradual increase of daily physical activity level, as well as the gradual increase in cognitive and social activities (Figure 30.1).

How should clinicians (physical therapists, occupational therapists, psychologists, etc.) provide activity self-management to their patients with CFS? The physical limits of the body should be respected in order to break out of the vicious circle of symptom exacerbations, avoidance, passivity, and further deconditioning. The pacing principle offers such a solution: limited periods (limits in proportion to the actual capabilities) of low-intensity activity, alternated with rest periods of the same duration.

Depending on the individual characteristics of the patient, activity self-management can be offered in a symptom- and time-contingent approach. Given mounting evidence supporting the

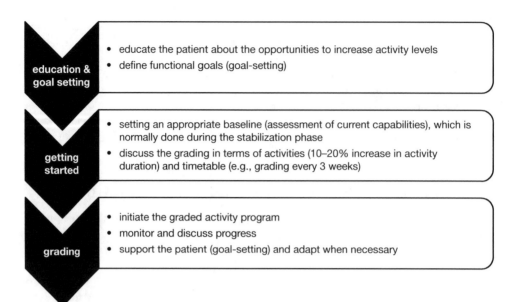

Figure 30.1 Grading phase: content of graded activity.

presence of central nervous system sensitization in CFS (Meeus, Nijs, Huybrechts, & Truijen, 2010; Meeus, Roussel, Truijen, & Nijs, 2010; Meeus, Nijs, Van de Wauwer, Toeback, & Truijen, 2008; Van Oosterwijck et al., 2010), small symptom variations should not be interpreted as signs of (new) tissue damage, but rather as "noise" produced by the hypersensitive central nervous system. Hence, a time-contingent approach seems rational even during the stabilization phase, and can prepare the patient for the graded activity approach during the grading phase. However, care must be taken not to over-exert the patient, because that may further increase the hypersensitivity of the central nervous system. The duration of daily activities should be adapted to the patient's capabilities, accounting for the physical and cognitive limitations inherent to the illness. Therefore, the duration of the activities should be carefully supervised by the clinician providing activity self-management. Pacing self-management techniques encourage a behavioral change and at the same time acknowledge the physical aspects of the illness.

Methodological issues in relation to physical activity research in CFS

The good thing about physical activity research in CFS is the fact that all findings point in the same direction (i.e., reduced physical activity in CFS). This is important for an illness with a long history of disagreement between scientists and conflicting data across studies. However, methodological issues should not be ignored. Physical activity monitoring in CFS research has been conducted with accelerometers worn at the wrist or the leg. Both of these anatomical locations might generate somewhat biased findings. However, accelerometers worn at the wrist are preferred. For example, many CFS patients experience ironing as a fatiguing task, but leg-worn activity monitors do not assess the motion associated with this activity.

Another issue is the fact that cognitive tasks are often experienced as fatiguing for patients with CFS. Physical activity monitors do not register such activities. Still, the fact that accelerometers now have omnidirectional sensors implies they permit valid real-time physical activity monitoring of movements in all directions. This represents an important methodological strength of physical activity research. Finally, patient employment status is an important concern because differences in activity level often appear between weekdays and weekend days. Further study in this area should consider possible bias due to work schedules and professional activities.

Future directions

Further work in this area should examine possible additional effects of physical activity interventions in patients with CFS. For example, to date, no data have been published on the extent that activity management contributes to the effectiveness of cognitive behavioral therapy in CFS patients. Cognitive behavioral therapy may be equally effective without inclusion of activity management. However, cognitive behavioral therapy might (in part) rely on activity management for its effectiveness. These are important questions, especially when we want to improve interventions targeting physical activity in patients with CFS.

Another future direction entails the study of the autonomic response of patients with CFS to daily physical activities like stair climbing or using a vacuum cleaner. Altered autonomic nervous system reactivity has been shown repeatedly in CFS patients (De Becker et al., 1998; Newton et al., 2009; Newton, Davidson, et al., 2007; Newton, Okonkwo, et al., 2007), but these studies used laboratory tests rather than real-life situations. It remains to be examined whether the stress response system of patients with CFS properly handles everyday physical stressors like stair climbing. This is important for rehabilitation purposes, as rehabilitation specialists should aim at increasing the physical capacity of CFS patients to cope with everyday stressors.

References

Bazelmans, E., Bleijenberg, G., van der Meer, J. W. M., & Folgering, H. (2001). Is physical deconditioning a perpetuating factor in chronic fatigue syndrome? A controlled study on maximal exercise performance and relations with fatigue, impairment and physical activity. *Psychological Medicine, 31*, 107–14.

Bazelmans, E., Bleijenberg, G., Voeten, M. J. M., van der Meer, J. W. M., & Folgering, H. (2005). Impact of a maximal exercise test on symptoms and activity in chronic fatigue syndrome. *Journal of Psychosomatic Research, 59*, 201–8.

Black, C. D., O'Conner, P. J., & McCully, K. K. (2005). Increased daily physical activity and fatigue symptoms in chronic fatigue syndrome. *Dynamic Medicine, 4*(1). doi:10.1186/1476-5918-4-3

CFS/ME Working Group. (2001). Report to the chief medical officer of an independent working group. London: Department of Health. Retrieved from: www.doh.gov.uk/cmo/cfsmereport/index.htm

Christley, Y., Duffy, T., & Martin, C. R. (2011). A review of the definitional criteria for chronic fatigue syndrome. *Journal of Evaluation Clinical Practice, 18* (1), 25–31. doi:10.1111/j.1365-2753.2010.01512.x

Clapp, L. L., Richardson, M. T., Smith, J. F., Wang, M., Clapp, A. J., & Pieroni, R. E. (1999). Acute effects of thirty minutes of light-intensity, intermittent exercise on patients with chronic fatigue syndrome. *Physical Therapy, 79*, 749–56.

De Becker, P., Dendale, P., De Meirleir, K., Campine, I., Vandenborne, I., & Hagers, Y. (1998). Autonomic testing in patients with chronic fatigue syndrome. *American Journal of Medicine, 105*, 22S–26S.

De Becker, P., Roeykens, J., Reynders, M., McGregor, N., & De Meirleir, K. (2000). Exercise capacity in chronic fatigue syndrome. *Archives of Internal Medicine, 160*, 3270–7.

Fukuda, K., Straus, S., Hickie, I., Sharpe, M., Dobbins, J., & Komaroff, A. (1994). The International Chronic Fatigue Syndrome Study Group. The chronic fatigue syndrome: A comprehensive approach to its definition and study. *Annals of Internal Medicine, 121*, 953–9.

Harvey, S. B., Wadsworth, M., Wessely, S., & Hotopf, M. (2008). Etiology of chronic fatigue syndrome: Testing popular hypotheses using a national birth study. *Psychosomatic Medicine, 70*, 488–95.

Jammes, Y., Steinberg, J. G., Mambrini, O., Brégeon, F., & Delliaux, S. (2005). Chronic fatigue syndrome: Assessment of increased oxidative stress and altered muscle excitability in response to incremental exercise. *Journal of Internal Medicine, 257*, 299–310.

Jason, L. A., King, C. P., Frankenberry, E. L., Jordan, K. M., Tryon, W. W., Rademaker, F., & Huang, C. F. (1999a). Chronic fatigue syndrome: Assessing symptoms and activity level. *British Journal of Clinical Psychology, 55*, 411–24.

Jason, L. A., Richman, J. A., Redmaker, A. W., Jordan, K. M., Plioplys, A. V., Taylor, R. R., . . . Plioplys, S. (1999b). A community-based study of chronic fatigue syndrome. *Archives of Internal Medicine, 159,* 2129–37.

Knoop, H., Bleijenberg, G., Gielissen, M. F., van der Meer, J. W., & White, P. D. (2007). Is full recovery possible after cognitive behavioural therapy for chronic fatigue syndrome? *Psychotherapy and Psychosomatics, 76,* 171–6.

Kori, S. H., Miller, R. P., & Todd, D. D. (1990). Kinesiophobia: A new view of chronic pain behavior. *Pain Management, 3,* 35–43.

Lapp, C. W. (1997). Exercise limits in chronic fatigue syndrome. *American Journal of Medicine, 103,* 83–4.

Meeus, M., Nijs, J., Huybrechts, S., & Truijen, S. (2010). Evidence for generalized hyperalgesia in chronic fatigue syndrome: A case control study. *Clinical Rheumatology, 29,* 393–8.

Meeus, M., Nijs, J., Van de Wauwer, N., Toeback, L., & Truijen, S. (2008). Diffuse noxious inhibitory control is delayed in chronic fatigue syndrome: An experimental study. *Pain, 139,* 439–48.

Meeus, M., Roussel, N., Truijen, S., & Nijs, J. (2010). Reduced pressure pain thresholds in response to exercise in chronic fatigue syndrome but not in chronic low back pain: An experimental study. *Journal of Rehabilitation Medicine, 42,* 884–90.

Meeus, M., van Eupen, I., Hondequin, J., Dehauwere, L., Kos, D., & Nijs, J. (2010). Nitric oxide concentrations are normal and unrelated to activity levels in chronic fatigue syndrome: A case-control study. *In Vivo, 24,* 865–9.

Meeus, M., van Eupen, I., Van Baarle, E., De Boeck, V., Luyckx, A., Kos, D., & Nijs, J. (2011) Symptom fluctuations and daily physical activity in patients with chronic fatigue syndrome: A case control study. *Archives of Physical Medicine and Rehabilitation, 92,* 1820–6.

Moss-Morris, R., Sharon, C., Tobin, R., & Baldi, J. C. (2005). A randomized controlled graded exercise trial for chronic fatigue syndrome: Outcomes and mechanisms of change. *Journal of Health Psychology, 10,* 245–59.

Newton, J. L., Davidson, A., Kerr, S., Bhala, N., Pairman, J., Burt, J., & Jones, D. E. (2007). Autonomic dysfunction in primary biliary cirrhosis correlates with fatigue severity. *European Journal of Gastroenterology and Hepatology, 19,* 125–32.

Newton, J. L., Okonkwo, O., Sutcliffe, K., Seth, A., Shin, J., & Jones, D. E. (2007). Symptoms of autonomic dysfunction in chronic fatigue syndrome. *Quarterly Journal of Medicine, 100,* 519–26.

Newton, J. L., Sheth, A., Shin, J., Parman, J., Wilton, K., Burt, J. A., & Jones, D. E. (2009). Low ambulatory blood pressure in chronic fatigue syndrome. *Psychosomatic Medicine, 71,* 361–5.

Nijs, J., Aelbrecht, S., Meeus, M., Van Oosterwijck, J., Zinzen, E., & Clarys, P. (2011). Tired of being inactive: A systematic literature review on physical activity, physiological exercise capacity, and muscle strength in patients with chronic fatigue syndrome. *Disability and Rehabilitation, 33,* 1493–500.

Nijs, J., De Meirleir, K., & Duquet, W. (2004). Kinesiophobia in chronic fatigue syndrome: Assessment and associations with disability. *Archives of Physical Medicine and Rehabilitation, 85,* 1586–92.

Nijs, J., De Meirleir, K., Wolfs, S., & Duquet, W. (2004). Disability evaluation in chronic fatigue syndrome: Associations between exercise capacity and activity limitations/participation restrictions. *Clinical Rehabilitation, 18,* 139–48.

Nijs, J., Paul, L., & Wallman, K. (2008). Chronic fatigue syndrome: An approach combining self-management with graded exercise to avoid exacerbations. *Journal of Rehabilitation Medicine, 40,* 241–47.

Nijs, J., van Eupen, I., Vandecauter, J., Augustinus, E., Bleyen, G., Moorkens, G., & Meeus, M. (2009). Can pacing self-management alter physical behaviour and symptom severity in chronic fatigue syndrome? A case series. *Journal of Rehabilitation Research and Development, 46,* 985–96.

Nijs, J., Vanherberghen, K., Duquet, W., & De Meirleir, K. (2004). Chronic fatigue syndrome: Lack of association between pain-related fear of movement and exercise capacity and disability. *Physical Therapy, 84,* 696–705.

Nijs, J., Van Oosterwijck, J., & Meeus, M. (2009). Myalgic encephalomyeltitis/chronic fatigue syndrome: Rehabilitation through activity management, stress management and exercise therapy. In J. H. Stone & M. Blouin (Eds.), *International Encyclopedia of Rehabilitation.* Retrieved from http://cirrie.buffalo.edu/encyclopedia/article.php?id=113&language=en

Nijs, J., Van Oosterwijck, J., Meeus, M., Lambrecht, L., Metzger, K., Frémont, M., & Paul, L. (2010). Unravelling the nature of post-exertional malaise in myalgic encephalomyeltitis/chronic fatigue syndrome: The role of elastase, complement C4a and interleukin 1beta. *Journal of Internal Medicine, 267,* 418–35.

Pardaens, K., Haagdorens, L., Van Wambeke, P., Van den Broeck, A., & Van Houdenhove, B. (2006). How relevant are exercise capacity measures for evaluating treatment effects in chronic fatigue syndrome? Results from a prospective, multidisciplinary outcome study. *Clinical Rehabilitation, 20,* 56–66.

Paul, L., Wood, L., Behan, W. M. H., & Maclaren, W. M. (1999). Demonstration of delayed recovery from fatiguing exercise in chronic fatigue syndrome. *European Journal of Neurology, 6,* 63–9.

Price, J. R., Mitchell, E., Tidy, E., & Hunot, V. (2008). Cognitive behaviour therapy for chronic fatigue syndrome in adults. *Cochrane Database of Systematic Reviews, 3:* CD001027. doi:10.1002/14651858.CD 001027.pub2

Prins, J. B., Bleijenberg, G., Bazelmans, E., Elving, L. D., de Boo, T. M., Severens, J. L. . . . van der Meer, J. W. (2001). Cognitive behaviour therapy for chronic fatigue syndrome: A multicentre randomised controlled trial. *Lancet, 357,* 841–7.

Shephard, C. (2001). Pacing and exercise in chronic fatigue syndrome. *Physiotherapy, 87,* 395–6.

Siemionow, V., Fang, Y., Calabrese, L., Sahgal, V., & Yue, G. H. (2004). Altered central nervous system signal during motor performance in chronic fatigue syndrome. *Clinical Neurophysiology, 115,* 2372–81.

Silver, A., Haeney, M., Vijayadurai, P., Wilks, D., Pattrick, M., & Main, C. J. (2002). The role of fear of physical movement and activity in chronic fatigue syndrome. *Journal of Psychosomatic Research, 52,* 485–93.

Sisto, S. A., Tapp, W. N., LaManca, J. J., Ling, W., Korn, L. R., Nelson, A.J., & Natelson, B. H. (1998). Physical activity before and after exercise in women with chronic fatigue syndrome. *Monthly Journal of the Association of Physicians, 91,* 465–73.

Sorensen, B., Streib, J. E., Strand, M., Make, B., Giclas, P. C., Fleshner, M., & Jones, J. F. (2003). Complement activation in a model of chronic fatigue syndrome. *Journal of Allergy and Clinical Immunology, 12,* 397–403.

Van der Werf, S., Prins, J., Vercoulen, J., van der Meer, J., & Bleijenberg, G. (2000). Identifying physical activity patterns in chronic fatigue syndrome using actigraph assessment. *Journal of Psychosomatic Research, 49,* 373–9.

Van Houdenhove, B., Neerinckx, E., Onghena, P., Lysens, R., & Vertommen, H. (2001). Premorbid "overactive" lifestyle in chronic fatigue syndrome and fibromyalgia: An etiological factor or proof of good citizenship? *Journal of Psychosomatic Research, 51,* 571–6.

Van Houdenhove, B., Onghena, P., Neerinckx, E., & Hellin, J. (1995). Does high "action-proneness" make people more vulnerable to chronic fatigue syndrome? A controlled psychometric study. *Journal of Psychosomatic Research, 39,* 633–40.

Van Oosterwijck, J., Nijs, J., Meeus, M., Lefever, I., Huybrechts, L., Lambrecht, L., & Paul, L. (2010). Pain inhibition and post-exertional malaise in myalgic encephalomyelitis/chronic fatigue syndrome: An experimental study. *Journal of Internal Medicine, 268,* 265–76.

van Weering, M., Vollenbroek-Hutten, M. M., Kotte, E .M., & Hermens, H. J. (2007). Daily physical activities of patients with chronic pain or fatigue versus asymptomatic controls. A systematic review. *Clinical Rehabilitation, 21,* 1007–23.

Vercoulen, J. H. M. M., Bazelmans, E., Swanick, C. M. A., Fennis, J. F. M., Galama, J. M. D., Jongen, P. J. H., . . . Bleijenberg, G. (1997). Physical activity in chronic fatigue syndrome: Assessment and its role in fatigue. *Journal of Psychiatric Research, 31,* 661–73.

Vercoulen, J. H., Hommes, O. R., Swanink, C. M., Jongen, P. J., Fennis, J. F., Galama, J. M., . . . Bleijenberg, G. (1996). The measurement of fatigue in patients with multiple sclerosis. A multidimensional comparison with patients with chronic fatigue syndrome and healthy subjects. *Archives of Neurology, 53*(7), 642–9.

White, P. D., Sharpe, M. C., Chalder, T., DeCesare, J. C., Walwyn, R., & PACE trial group. (2007). Protocol for the PACE trial: A randomised controlled trial of adaptive pacing, cognitive behaviour therapy, and graded exercise as supplements to standardised specialist medical care versus standardised specialist medical care alone for patients with the chronic fatigue syndrome/myalgic encephalomyelitis or encephalopthy. *BMC Neurology, 7*(6). doi:10.1186/1471-2377-7-6

Wong, R., Lopaschuk, G., Zhu, G., Walker, D., Catellier, D., Burton, D., . . . Montague, T. (1992). Skeletal muscle metabolism in the chronic fatigue syndrome: In vivo assessment by ^{31}P nuclear magnetic resonance spectroscopy. *Chest, 102*(6), 1716–22.

PART 9

Addictions

Edited by
Michael Ussher

31

PHYSICAL ACTIVITY AS AN AID IN SMOKING CESSATION

Adrian H. Taylor and Michael Ussher

Tobacco causes about five million deaths annually worldwide, and is the second leading cause of death (World Health Organization, 2011). Smoking cessation is a challenge due to the insidious nature of the addiction (American Psychiatric Association, 2000). Unaided quit attempts have a success rate (6–12 months abstinence) of around 3–5%, while aided quit attempts, particularly through a combination of behavioral counseling and nicotine replacement therapy (NRT), bupropion or varenicline, can improve success rates by around 7–9% (Cahill, Stead, & Lancaster, 2011; Hughes, Stead, & Lancaster, 2007; Stead, Perera, Bullen, Mant, & Lancaster, 2008). There is scope for new therapies. There is substantial research on why people relapse; notable reasons include cravings, low mood, and weight gain. Physical activity (PA) has the potential to influence all of these and has been recommended as an aid to smoking cessation by specialist smoking clinics (Everson-Hock, Taylor, & Ussher, 2010a; Everson-Hock, Taylor, Ussher, & Faulkner, 2010b), in self-help guides (Marcus, Hampl, & Fisher, 2004), and in national guidelines (US Department of Health & Human Services, 2008).

Many large-scale cross-sectional surveys have assessed associations between self-reported PA and smoking status. Kaczynski, Manske, Mannell, and Grewal (2008) identified 50 such studies, with almost 60% reporting a negative association, and the majority of the remaining studies had methodological issues. This evidence suggests that an increase in PA could help people to quit. It raises questions about how such an effect could occur and how PA interventions could be designed to maximize the effects on smoking.

Some randomized controlled trials, in a general primary care population, have shown increases in PA in a PA group relative to a control group but have shown no effect on smoking cessation (e.g., Taylor, Doust, & Webborn, 1998; Bull & Jamrozik, 1998). These studies are limited in that there is no information provided on whether smokers wish to quit. However, this research suggests that by simply increasing PA there is unlikely to be a spontaneous increase in smoking cessation. This raises the question of whether PA can aid smoking cessation when it is explicitly used for this purpose, and the remainder of the chapter will focus on this issue.

This chapter will provide an overview of research on:

- The chronic effects of PA on smoking cessation and dose-response issues.
- The acute effects of a single session of PA on smoking-related outcomes (e.g., cravings) and dose-response issues.

- Possible mechanisms underlying the effects of PA on smoking-related variables.
- Designing effective interventions that engage smokers.

The chronic effects of physical activity on smoking cessation

There have been a number of reviews of the chronic effects of exercise on smoking cessation (e.g., Nishi, Jenicek, & Tatara, 1998; Ussher, Taylor, West, & McEwen, 2000), but not all have clearly defined the research question, applied rigorous inclusion and exclusion criteria, or carefully considered the appropriateness of outcome measures (West, Hajek, Stead, & Stapleton, 2005). Ussher, Taylor, and Faulkner (2012) adopted a rigorous and conservative approach to understanding the effects of exercise. Their review identifies the excluded studies with a reason for their exclusion. The studies reviewed involved programs of supervised or unsupervised exercise alone or in addition to a smoking cessation intervention, compared with a smoking cessation program alone. Interventions involving exercise within a multiple component smoking cessation program were excluded because it would not be possible to attribute any effects solely to exercise. Studies involving interventions designed to target a number of health-related outcomes, including smoking, were excluded as, again, any effect could not be attributed to exercise. For example, a dietary intervention may hypothetically also enhance success at quitting by preventing weight gain, or it may reduce success at quitting due to elevated hunger during abstinence. Relapse in smoking cessation studies is notoriously high, so the review focused on trials with at least a 6-month follow-up (i.e., 6 months post quit or post treatment). Smoking cessation at the longest follow-up was reported as the main outcome.

The review identified 15 RCTs, seven of which had fewer than 25 people in each treatment arm, seven involved only females, and one, only males. The studies varied in the timing and intensity of the smoking cessation and exercise programs. In 13 studies a cognitive behavioral smoking cessation intervention was offered to both control and exercise groups, with six beginning before the quit date. In seven studies nicotine products were encouraged for all participants. Treatments lasted 5 to 15 weeks with the exception of one study with a single session, and another was undefined and involved an internet intervention. In terms of PA, nine, three, and two studies (with one not stating the timing) required participants to increase PA before, at the same time as, and after the quit date, respectively. Thus, in 12 studies the smokers set a quit date, and one study was unclear in its reporting.

Most studies involved a supervised group-based exercise program, with supplementary home-based exercises. A few studies also promoted free-living PA in addition to structured exercise, and one study exclusively focused on brief weekly counseling to increase PA (Ussher, West, McEwen, Taylor, & Steptoe, 2003, 2007). One study promoted resistance exercise (Ciccolo et al., 2011), but the others focused on cardiovascular-type exercise.

In terms of outcomes, three studies showed significantly higher abstinence rates in a physically active group versus a control group at end of treatment. One of these studies (Marcus et al., 1999) also showed a significant benefit for exercise versus control on abstinence at the 3-month follow-up (post-treatment) and a benefit for exercise of borderline significance ($p = 0.05$) at the 12-month follow-up (11.9% versus 5.4% abstinent). One study showed significantly higher abstinence rates for the exercise group versus a control group at the 3-month follow-up but not at the end of treatment or 12-month follow-up. The findings were reported using the most conservative outcomes for reporting smoking cessation. The other studies showed no significant effect for exercise on abstinence. The review concluded that only one study showed any long-term benefit of exercise on smoking cessation.

Most studies are efficacy studies with the recruitment of participants with an interest in exercise and generally high adherence to the exercise intervention, and thus may not represent what happens in real life. The study showing the greatest benefits of exercise (Marcus et al., 1999) involved 30–40 minutes of vigorous structured exercise classes three times a week for 12 weeks, which may not appeal to most smokers (see below).

Do trained smoking advisors routinely promote physical activity as an aid to quitting?

There are mixed views about whether smoking advisors should be encouraged to promote PA. McEwen, Hajek, McRobbie, and West (2006) suggest that behaviors such as PA should be initiated after a period of successful abstinence since the demands of planning, goal setting, and initiating two or more behavior changes simultaneously may be too much for some, and could result in smoking relapse. On the other hand, Marcus, Hampl, and Fisher (2004) advocate a need to prevent weight gain after smoking cessation through simultaneously changing multiple health behaviors that may reinforce each other.

In a survey of 170 smoking cessation advisors in England and Scotland, 56% claimed to promote PA, and the average time spent promoting PA was less than 5 minutes in a typical 45-minute counseling session (Everson, Taylor, & Ussher, 2010). Those holding more positive beliefs regarding pros and cons, self-efficacy, outcome efficacy, and importance of PA within smoking cessation were more likely to promote PA, and this was supported in interviews with the advisors (Everson-Hock, Taylor, Ussher, & Faulkner, 2010b). The advisors noted that PA was a valuable coping strategy for cravings and withdrawal symptoms, it redirected the focus toward something positive rather than stopping smoking, and could help with weight management and emotional eating (in the absence of a cigarette).

Are smokers interested in physical activity as an explicit aid for smoking cessation?

In a UK survey of 181 smokers attempting to quit, 22% reported currently using PA to control their smoking and 35% had used it during a previous quit attempt (Everson-Hock, Taylor, & Ussher, 2010a). Those in later stages of readiness for using PA as a cessation aid (i.e., action and maintenance) held more positive beliefs regarding self-efficacy to do PA and outcome efficacy (or the belief that PA would be useful). The survey focused on smokers' views on "physical activity" (e.g., short bouts of brisk walking) rather than vigorous "exercise" sessions, which may be more valuable on a daily basis and may minimize barriers to participation.

Acute effects of physical activity on smoking-related outcomes

Reviews have focused on the effects of a single session of PA on smoking-related outcomes (Taylor, Ussher, & Faulkner, 2007; Ussher et al., 2012), with studies involving either actual quitters or temporarily abstinent smokers.

Few studies have examined the acute effects from pre to post a single session of exercise among people receiving a smoking cessation intervention. Bock, Marcus, King, Borrelli, and Roberts (1999) reported significant reductions in cravings from pre to post exercise compared with a passive condition in weeks 5–10 of an 11-week trial, but the results reported for each session were not easy to disaggregate. Williams and colleagues (2010) reported that quitters who engaged in an 8-week smoking cessation program (i.e., counseling and NRT) plus three weekly 50-minute walks had no reduction in cravings compared with a passive control group. Finally,

Arbour-Nicitopoulos, Faulkner, Hsin, and Selby (2011) reported no acute effects on cravings among a sample of mental health patients receiving NRT to help with smoking cessation. Collectively, the results from these studies on the acute effects of exercise on cravings among those wishing to quit are unconvincing. This may be due to lower cravings at baseline, due to taking NRT, or because cravings tend to reduce over a few weeks after peaking within the first week of quitting.

Most acute studies have entailed a proof of concept approach in which cravings are initially exacerbated by a period of temporary nicotine abstinence (e.g., overnight) followed by either an exercise or control condition. Between- or within-subject crossover designs to compare pre to post exercise versus control changes in cravings and withdrawal symptoms have been used with smokers not receiving other smoking cessation aids.

Acute studies, following temporary abstinence, offer the opportunity to test the effects of a dose of exercise on smoking-related outcomes before promoting it within interventions. An example is the finding from an acute study that isometric exercises can reduce cravings (Ussher, West, Doshi, & Sampuran, 2006; Ussher, Cropley, Playle, Mohidin, & West, 2009), followed by the design of a study to test the feasibility and acceptability of offering isometric exercise within an NHS treatment (Al-Chalabi et al., 2008). Other research has looked at yoga in acute studies (Elibero, Janse van Rensburg, & Drobes, 2011) and as an intervention (Bock et al., 2010; Bock et al., 2012). Thus, acute studies allow us to examine what types of activity and what intensity and duration have the greatest effect on reducing cravings.

Two studies (Everson, Daley, & Ussher, 2008; Scerbo, Faulkner, Taylor, & Thomas, 2010) have shown that moderate and vigorous intensity exercise both reduce cravings, compared with a passive control group. Even short bouts (e.g., 5 minutes) of PA appear to temporarily reduce cravings, but the effects are more short-lived than for longer bouts. Together, these studies suggest that PA may be effective as a coping strategy for acutely reducing cravings and withdrawal symptoms.

Haasova and colleagues (2013) quantified the effects of a single bout of exercise on Strength of Desire to smoke (SoD; West, Hajek, & Belcher, 1989), which is a useful predictor of smoking cessation (Fidler, Shahab, & West, 2011). Using original individual patient data (IPD; Riley, Lambert, & Abo-Zaid, 2010) collated from 15 acute exercise studies, a linear regression was conducted with post-PA SoD as the main outcome and with various demographic and behavioral covariates added to the model, adjusting for study and baseline SoD. The pooled estimate for treatment effect (standardized mean difference) was -1.91 (95% CI -2.59; -1.22), with a high degree of between-study heterogeneity, as shown in Figure 31.1. In summary, these findings indicate a very strong acute effect of exercise on self-reported SoD.

Acute studies involving other measures of cravings and withdrawal symptoms (e.g., two-factor QSU-brief) have also shown reductions in cravings following exercise. Withdrawal symptoms include irritability, anger, poor concentration, depression, and hunger. Recent studies have begun to examine the acute effects of exercise on cue-elicited cravings. These studies are common in smoking cessation research and examine how a smoker responds to smoking triggers after exercise. Often such triggers elicit a craving, which may lead to smoking.

In terms of smoking topography, studies by Mikhail (1983), Reeser (1983), Thayer, Peters, Takahaski, and Birkhead-Flight (1993), Taylor and Katomeri (2007), and Faulkner, Arbour-Nicitopoulos, and Hsin (2010) have collectively shown that exercise acutely favorably influences time spent smoking and number of puffs smoking the next cigarette after exercise, and increases the time before smoking the next cigarette, compared with a passive control group.

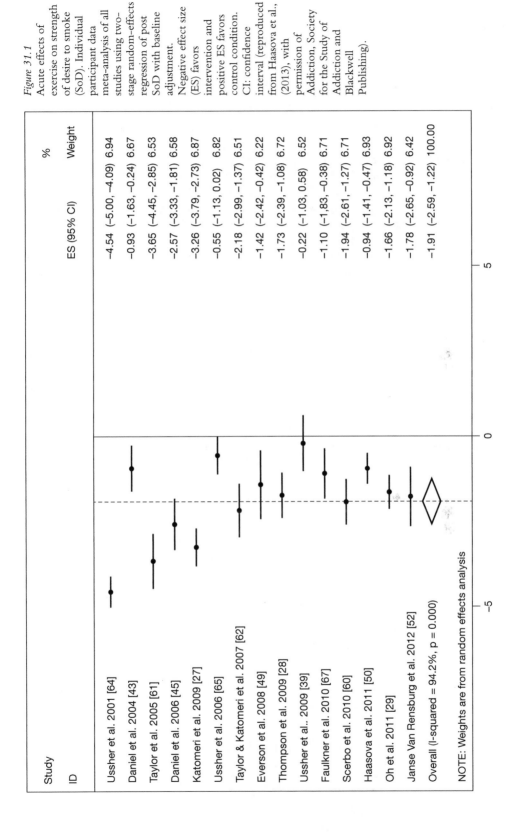

Figure 31.1
Acute effects of exercise on strength of desire to smoke (SoD). Individual participant data meta-analysis of all studies using two-stage random-effects regression of post SoD with baseline adjustment. Negative effect size (ES) favors intervention and positive ES favors control condition. CI: confidence interval (reproduced from Haasova et al., (2013), with permission of Addiction, Society for the Study of Addiction and Blackwell Publishing).

Mechanisms

There are a number of ways in which PA may help smokers to reduce or quit smoking, which are shown in Table 31.1. Some of these are discussed below.

Distraction: There is increasing interest in low-intensity "mindful" exercise (e.g., yoga, Tai Chi, isometrics, stretching) that may demand a greater cognitive focus (i.e., distraction from smoking) than walking, for example. Similarly, at a high intensity, above the ventilatory threshold, exercise may induce greater attentional demand or provide more introspective feedback associated with displeasure than at moderate intensities (Ekkekakis, Parfitt, & Petruzzello, 2011). In studies that have compared exercise with a distracting task (as a control condition) there was a greater reduction in cravings and withdrawal symptoms during and following moderate intensity exercise (e.g., Daniel, Cropley, & Fife-Schaw, 2006; Ussher, Nunziata, Cropley, & West, 2001), suggesting distraction is not the key mechanism. However, exercise appears to reduce attentional bias to smoking images (Janse van Rensburg, Taylor, & Hodgson, 2009; Oh & Taylor, in press), which may be an important indicator of addictive processes and inhibitory control (Field, Munafò, & Franken, 2009). Further research is needed to determine the role of exercise in building self-control and inhibitory strength as key elements of self-regulation (see Prime Theory by West, 2007; Baumeister & Vohs, 2011).

Affective changes: Another mechanism by which exercise may influence cigarette cravings is through changes in affect. Several studies have reported simultaneous changes in affective activation and feelings and cravings while exercising (e.g., Taylor, Katomeri, & Ussher, 2006). It may be that a single bout of moderate-intensity exercise provides a sense of pleasure or positively activated affective, and this replaces the hedonic expectancy from smoking a cigarette, thereby reducing the desire to smoke. Audrain-McGovern and colleagues (2011) suggested that the alternative reinforcement value from sport may prevent progression to smoking among adolescents.

Neuro-cognitive-affective effects: Two studies (Janse Van Rensburg, Taylor, Hodgson, & Benattayallah, 2009; Janse van Rensburg, 2010) have shown among abstinent smokers, using

Table 31.1 Possible mechanisms by which PA may help someone to reduce or quit smoking, and prevent relapse

---

- It may provide a useful distraction from smoking and reduce the frequency and intensity of tobacco cravings.
- Nicotine abstinence is associated with increased withdrawal symptoms such as anger, low mood, irritability, and hunger. PA may reduce these symptoms. The acute effects of exercise on mood and affect are widely recognized.
- Smokers experiencing depression have lower success in quitting. PA can have chronic positive effects on depression through a range of possible neurobiological and psychosocial mechanisms discussed elsewhere in this book.
- Doing some PA can remind a smoker just how breathless they have become, and this could prompt a desire to reduce or quit.
- Engaging in PA may displace certain behaviors and time spent in selected environments previously associated with smoking and could lead to a shift in identity away from that of a smoker.
- Weight gain and fear of weight gain can impact on whether a smoker quits and/or relapses. PA can help to prevent weight gain.
- PA may help to increase control capacity, and self-regulation of addiction to cigarettes has been described as a failure to self-regulate a habitual behavior in Prime Theory (West, 2007). Self-control involves overriding or inhibiting smoking, urges, or desire to smoke that would otherwise interfere with an attempt to cut down or quit smoking (Baumeister & Vohs, 2011).

---

functional magnetic resonance imagery (fMRI) while viewing smoking images, that after being passive, significant regional brain activations were identified in areas of the brain associated with visuospatial attention (e.g., parietal lobe, parahippocampal gyrus, and fusiform gyrus), drug use motivation (e.g., orbitofrontal cortex), and reward (e.g., caudate nucleus). Following a 10-minute bout of moderate-intensity exercise, none of these brain regions were activated. This suggests that exercise may implicitly regulate neuro-cognitive-affective processes that may lead from cues to developing an urge to smoke.

Weight gain prevention: A meta-analysis of 62 studies revealed that there was a mean increase of 4–5kg in body weight after 12 months of abstinence, with the greatest gain occurring within 3 months of quitting (Aubin, Farley, Lycett, Lahmek, & Aveyard, 2012). Untreated and pharmacologically treated quitters had similar weight gain but variation was large, with about 16% losing weight and 13% gaining more than 10kg.

Within 4–8 years, quitters gain about 9kg, compared with 2kg among continuing smokers, with 38% gaining over 10kg in weight (Lycett, Munafò, Johnstone, Murphy, & Aveyard, 2011). Weight gain concerns are often grounds for initiation of smoking behavior, reluctance to quit smoking, and smoking relapse (Klesges, Meyers, Klesges, & La Vasque, 1989), but not all studies support fear of weight gain as a reason for relapse (e.g., Xhou et al., 2009). In one study, just prior to quitting, 52% feared gaining weight, 84% were unwilling to accept a gain of more than 5kg in body weight, and 28% were not prepared to accept any weight gain (Tùnnesen et al., 1999). To account for this weight gain the basal metabolic rate reduces by the equivalent of 150–300kcals per day or about 10% of daily energy expenditure, partly explained by the fall in sympathetic drive. Also, some studies report an increased energy intake of about 250kcals/day at 3 months after smoking cessation, particularly among those prone to emotional or comfort eating (Perkins, 1993). Not surprisingly then, exercise has been recommended for preventing weight gain, both to address energy balance and also help self-regulate emotional eating (e.g., high-energy snacks) (Oh & Taylor, 2012; Taylor & Oliver, 2009; Thayer et al., 1993). In a laboratory study, temporarily abstinent smokers, who were also regular high-calorie snackers, showed reduced attentional bias to both smoking and snacking images, compared with neutral images, following 15 minutes of moderate-intensity exercise, relative to a passive control condition (Oh & Taylor, in press). Thus, short bouts of physical activity, compared with being sedentary, may reduce both cravings and salience of cues associated with reward.

The evidence for whether exercise prevents weight gain after quitting is mixed. When pooling the studies, Parsons and colleagues (2009) found no reduced gain at end of treatment, but did at 12 months' follow-up in a meta-analysis of three studies (Bize et al., 2010; Marcus et al., 1999; Ussher et al., 2003). In another meta-analysis of 10 studies (Spring et al., 2009) there was a significant reduction in weight gain from the exercise intervention in the short term (< 3 months), but not in the long term (> 6 months).

Practical and theoretical implications

Several pilot studies involving counseling, with detailed descriptions of behavioral change techniques, and novel exercise interventions (e.g., isometric exercise, yoga, resistance exercise; Al-Chalabi et al., 2008; Bock et al., 2010; Ciccolo et al., 2011) have been reported. Nevertheless, it is a challenge to determine how best to integrate exercise or PA into conventional pharmacological and behavioral support without overloading smokers (Jung, Fitzgeorge, Prapavessis, Faulkner, & Maddison, 2010; Maddison et al., 2010; Williams et al., 2010), and when to integrate any PA in relation to quitting. Most trials in the Cochrane review (Ussher et al., 2012) focused on increasing PA before quitting, but Taylor and colleagues (Taylor, Everson-Hock, & Ussher,

2010) described the development and piloting of a pragmatic "Walk to Quit" counseling intervention that incorporated a range of behavior change techniques, use of a pedometer, and a self-help guide at the same time as quitting. The focus was on building confidence to increase PA and also develop an expectation that PA would be a valuable cessation aid among smokers attempting to quit. In contrast, Prochaska and colleagues (2008) reported that a pedometer intervention helped to prevent relapse several months after quitting. Finally, it is important to note that our Cochrane review focused on trials in which smoking outcomes could clearly be attributed to PA. In contrast, more pragmatic trials have focused on more complex interventions to change multiple risk factors (e.g., McClure et al., 2011) with the focus on changing smoking, diet, and PA simultaneously.

There is little research on behavioral support to support smoking reduction among those who do not wish to quit immediately. In a pilot RCT with 99 disadvantaged smokers, an Exercise Assisted Reduction then Stop intervention, compared with a brief advice condition, resulted in 22% vs 6% making a quit attempt, 14% vs 4% with expired carbon monoxide confirmed 4–8 weeks' abstinence, and 10% vs 4% with CO confirmed abstinence at 16 weeks post baseline (Thompson et al., in press). A larger trial is needed to provide greater confidence in these findings, and further exploration of the value of physical activity as an aid for different smoking reduction strategies.

Exercise and smoking cessation for special populations

Adolescents, sport, and smoking

Research suggests there are complex relationships between type of sport, gender, and progression to smoking among adolescents (Larson, Story, Perry, Neumark-Sztainer, & Hannan, 2007; Audrain-McGovern, Rodriguez, & Moss, 2003), with competency beliefs and mood appearing to mediate an apparent protective effect of engaging in PA (Rodriguez, Duton, Tscherne, & Sass, 2008; Verkooijen, Nielsen, & Kremers, 2008). In contrast to adult research, only one study has looked at PA as an adolescent smoking cessation aid. Horn et al. (2011) conducted a cluster RCT to examine the effects of PA counseling in addition to a standard smoking cessation program. There was an increased likelihood of cessation at 6-month follow-up in the PA arm but mostly limited to male adolescents. Everson, Daley, and Ussher (2006) reported that, unlike research involving adult populations, 10 minutes of moderate-intensity cycle ergometry did not reduce desire to smoke in adolescents.

Mental illness, physical activity, and smoking

There is a much higher incidence of smoking among people with mental health problems (Williams & Ziedonis, 2004) and lower levels of PA (Janney et al., 2008). Depression is also associated with less success at smoking cessation (Berlin & Covey, 2006). As other chapters in this book will identify, it can be challenging to devise interventions that effectively increase PA among people with mental health problems. Faulkner and colleagues (2007) reported from survey data that 63% (n=109) of current or recently quit smokers receiving treatment for mental health disorders (e.g., schizophrenia or depression) were interested in becoming more physically active within the context of their smoking cessation efforts. PA was regarded as a useful behavioral strategy for coping with cravings and withdrawal symptoms. A pilot trial on the effects of exercise counseling among 44 female smokers with depression suggested the intervention was acceptable and feasible (Vickers et al., 2009). In the only acute study involving participants with severe mental illness, Arbour-Nicitopoulos and colleagues (2011) reported no effect of exercise on cravings and withdrawal symptoms. The use of NRT by all participants may have minimized baseline cravings, and hence created a floor effect.

Pregnancy, physical activity, and smoking

During pregnancy, smokers may be less inclined to use pharmaco-therapies, but appear interested in PA as an aid to quitting (Ussher, West, & Hibbs, 2004; Ussher, Ah-Yoon, West, & Straus, 2007). An ongoing trial is assessing the effects of an exercise intervention in this population (Ussher et al., 2008; Ussher et al., 2012).

Summary

This chapter has reviewed a wide range of literature that has considered the relationship between exercise, physical activity, and smoking, including cross-sectional studies, RCTs of exercise, or physical activity counseling interventions to aid smoking cessation, and acute studies to determine the temporary utility of physical activity for reducing cravings and withdrawal symptoms. In terms of the most rigorously conducted studies, there is some evidence that exercise may increase smoking cessation when used as an adjunctive treatment to usual care. Many previous studies have been too small-scale or had limitations that ongoing studies are currently addressing, so more definitive findings are expected in the coming years about the effectiveness of exercise as a smoking cessation aid.

In terms of acute exercise, there has been an exponential growth in the past decade in the number of studies designed to examine the effects on smoking-related outcomes. This research strongly suggests that, during temporary abstinence (when cravings and withdrawal symptoms are elevated), exercise reduces desire and strength of desire to smoke, withdrawal symptoms, attentional bias to smoking-related cues, and ad libitum smoking.

A variety of mechanisms for how exercise may have both acute and chronic effects have been considered and further research is required. Chronically, exercise may reduce weight gain following cessation and provide a useful behavioral coping strategy to manage cravings and withdrawal symptoms. Rather than just structured supervised exercise, a variety of approaches are being examined to help smokers to use physical activity as an aid to smoking reduction and cessation.

References

Al-Chalabi, L., Prasad, N., Steed, L., Stenner, S., Aveyard, P., Beach, J., & Ussher, M. (2008). A pilot randomised controlled trial of the feasibility of using body scan and isometric exercises for reducing urge to smoke in a smoking cessation clinic. *BMC Public Health, 8*, 349. doi:10.1186/1471-2458-8-349

American Psychiatric Association (APA), (2000). *Diagnostic and Statistical Manual of Mental Disorders* (4th Ed.). Washington, DC: American Psychiatric Association. doi:10.1176/appi.books.9780890423349

Arbour-Nicitopoulos, K., Faulkner, G. E., Hsin, A., & Selby, P. (2011). A pilot study examining the acute effects of exercise on craving reduction and affect among individuals with serious mental illness. *Mental Health & Physical Activity, 4*(2), 89–94. doi:10.1016/j.mhpa.2011.06.001

Aubin, H-J., Farley, A., Lycett, D., Lahmek, P., & Aveyard, P. (2012). How much weight do smokers gain after quitting cigarettes? A meta-analysis. *British Medical Journal, 345*, e4439–e4439. doi:10.1136/bmj.e4439

Audrain-McGovern, J., Rodriguez, D., & Moss, H. B. (2003).Smoking progression and physical activity. *Cancer Epidemiology, Biomarkers and Prevention, 12*(11), 1121–1129. Retrieved from http://cebp.aacr journals.org/content/12/11/1121.full

Audrain-McGovern, J., Rodriguez, D., Rodgers, K., & Cuevas, J. (2011). Declining alternative reinforcers link depression to young adult smoking. *Addiction, 106*(1), 178–187. doi:10.1111/j.1360-0443.2010.03113.x

Baumeister, R. F., & Vohs, K. D. (Eds.) (2011). *Handbook of Self-regulation: Research, Theory and Applications*. New York: Guilford Press.

Berlin, I., & Covey, L. S. (2006). Pre-cessation depressive mood predicts failure to quit smoking: The role of coping and personality traits. *Addiction, 101*(12), 1814–1821. doi:10.1111/j.1360-0443.2006.01616.x

Bize, R., Willi, C., Chiolero, A., Stoianov, R., Payot, S., Locatelli, I., & Cornuz, J. (2010). Participation in a population-based physical activity program as an aid for smoking cessation: A randomised trial. *Tobacco Control, 19*(6), 488–494. doi:10.1136/tc.2009.030288

Bock, B. C., Fava, J. L., Gaskins, R., Morrow, K. M., Williams, D. M., Jennings. E., . . . Marcus, B. H. (2012). Yoga as a complementary treatment for smoking cessation. *Journal of Women's Health, 21*(2), 240–248. doi:10.1089/jwh.2011.2963

Bock, B. C., Marcus, B. H., King, T. K., Borrelli, B., & Roberts, M. R. (1999). Exercise effects on withdrawal and mood among women attempting smoking cessation. *Addictive Behaviors, 24*(3), 399–410. doi:10.1016/S0306-4603(98)00088-4

Bock, B. C., Morrow, K. M., Becker, B. M., Williams, D. M., Tremont, G., Gaskins, R. B., . . . Marcus, B. H. (2010). Yoga as a complementary treatment for smoking cessation: Rationale, study design and participant characteristics of the Quitting-in-Balance study. *BMC Complementary and Alternative Medicine, 10*(1), 14. doi:10.1186/1472-6882-10-14

Bull, F. C., & Jamrozik, K. (1998). Advice on exercise from a family physician can help sedentary patients to become active. *American Journal of Preventive Medicine, 15*(2), 85–94. doi:10.1016/S0749-3797(98)00040-3

Cahill, K., Stead, L. F., & Lancaster, T. (2011). Nicotine receptor partial agonists for smoking cessation. *Cochrane Database of Systematic Reviews, 2*: CD006103. doi:10.1002/14651858.CD006103.pub3

Ciccolo, J. T., Dunsiger, S. I., Williams, D. M., Bartholomew, J. B., Jennings, E. G., Ussher, M. H., . . . Marcus, B. H. (2011). Resistance training as an aid to standard smoking cessation treatment: A pilot study. *Nicotine & Tobacco Research, 13*(8), 756–760. doi:10.1093/ntr/ntr068

Daniel, J. Z., Cropley, M., & Fife-Schaw, C. (2006). The effect of exercise in reducing desire to smoke and cigarette withdrawal symptoms is not caused by distraction. *Addiction, 101*(8), 1187–1192. doi:10.1111/j.1360-0443.2006.01457.x

Ekkekakis, P., Parfitt, G., & Petruzzello, S. J. (2011). The pleasure and displeasure people feel when they exercise at different intensities: Decennial update and progress towards a tripartite rationale for exercise intensity prescription. *Sports Medicine, 41*(8), 641–671. doi:10.2165/11590680-000000000-00000

Elibero, A., Janse Van Rensburg, K., & Drobes, D. (2011). Acute effects of aerobic exercise and hatha yoga on craving to smoke. *Nicotine & Tobacco Research, 13*(11), 1140–1148. doi:10.1093/ntr/ntr163

Everson, E. S., Daley, A. J., & Ussher, M. (2006). Does exercise have an acute effect on desire to smoke, mood and withdrawal symptoms in abstaining adolescent smokers? *Addictive Behaviors, 31*(9), 1547–1558. doi:10.1016/j.addbeh.2005.11.007

Everson, E. S., Daley, A. J., & Ussher, M. (2008). Moderate and vigorous intensity exercise acutely reduce cravings and withdrawal symptoms in abstaining young adult smokers. *Mental Health & Physical Activity, 1*(1), 26–31. doi:10.1016/j.mhpa.2008.06.001

Everson, E. S., Taylor, A. H., & Ussher, M. (2010). Determinants of physical activity promotion by smoking cessation advisors as an aid for quitting: Support for the Transtheoretical Model. *Patient Education & Counselling, 78*(1), 53–56. doi:10.1016/j.pec.2009.05.004

Everson-Hock, E. S., Taylor, A. H., & Ussher, M. (2010a). Readiness to use physical activity as a smoking cessation aid: A multiple behavior change application of the Transtheoretical Model among quitters attending Stop Smoking Clinics. *Patient Education & Counselling, 79*(2), 156–159. doi:10.1016/j.pec.2009.09.016

Everson-Hock, E. S., Taylor, A. H., Ussher, M., & Faulkner, G. (2010b). A qualitative perspective on multiple health behavior change: Views of smoking cessation advisors who promote physical activity. *Journal of Smoking Cessation, 5*(1), 7–14. doi:10.1375/jsc.5.1.7

Faulkner, G. E., Arbour-Nicitopoulos, K. P., & Hsin, A. (2010). Cutting down one puff at a time: The acute effects of exercise on smoking behavior. *Journal of Smoking Cessation, 5*(2), 130–135. doi:10.1375/jsc.5.2.130

Faulkner, G., Taylor, A. H., Munro, S., Selby, P., & Gee, C. (2007). Exploring the acceptability of physical activity programming within a smoking cessation service for individuals with severe mental illness. *Patient Education & Counseling, 66*(1), 123–126. doi:10.1016/j.pec.2006.11.003

Fidler, J. A., Shahab, L., & West, R. (2011). Strength of urges to smoke as a measure of severity of cigarette dependence: Comparison with the Fagerström Test for Nicotine Dependence and its components. *Addiction*, *106*(3), 631–638. doi:10.1111/j.1360-0443.2010.03226.x

Field, M., Munafò, M. R., & Franken, I. H. (2009). A meta-analytic investigation of the relationship between attentional bias and subjective craving in substance abuse. *Psychological Bulletin*, *135*(4), 589–607. doi:10.1037/a0015843

Filozof, C., Fernández Pinilla, M. C., & Fernández-Cruz, A. (2004). Smoking cessation and weight gain. *Obesity Reviews*, *5*(2), 95–103. doi:10.1111/j.1467-789X.2004.00131.x

Haasova, M., Warren, F. C., Ussher, M., Janse Van Rensburg, K., Faulkner, G., Cropley, M., ... Taylor, A. H. (2013). The acute effects of physical activity on cigarette cravings: Systematic review and meta-analysis with individual participant data (IPD). *Addiction*, *108*(1), 26–37. doi: 10.1111/j.1360-0443.2012.04034.x

Heatherton, T., Kozlowski, L., Frecker, J. R., & Fagerstrom, K. (1991). The Fagerstrom Test for Nicotine Dependence: A revision of the Fagerstrom Tolerance Questionnaire. *British Journal of Addiction*, *86*(9), 1119–1128. doi:10.1111/j.1360-0443.1991.tb01879.x

Horn, K., Dino, G., Branstetter, S., Zhang, J., Noerachmanto, N., Jarrett, T., & Taylor, M. (2011). The effects of physical activity on teen smoking cessation. *Pediatrics*, *128*(4), e801–e811. doi:10.1542/peds.2010-2599

Hughes, J. R., Stead, L. F., & Lancaster, T. (2007). Antidepressants for smoking cessation. *Cochrane Database of Systematic Reviews*, 1: CD000031. doi:10.1002/14651858.CD000031.pub3

Janney, C. A., Richardson, C. R., Holleman, R. G., Glasheen, C., Strath, S. J., Conroy, M. B., & Kriska, A. M. (2008). Gender, mental health service use and objectively measured physical activity: Data from the National Health and Nutrition Examination Survey (NHANES). *Mental Health & Physical Activity*, *1*(1), 9–16. doi:10.1016/j.mhpa.2008.05.001

Janse Van Rensburg, K. (2010). The effects of exercise on neuropsychological processes associated with a desire to smoke nicotine and cue-elicited cravings (PhD thesis). University of Exeter, UK. Retrieved from The Exeter Research and Institutional Content Archive (ERIC), http://hdl.handle.net/10036/106656

Janse Van Rensburg, K., Taylor A. H., & Hodgson, T. (2009). The effects of acute exercise on attentional biases to smoking-related stimuli during temporary abstinence from smoking. *Addiction*, *104*(11), 1910–1917. doi:10.1111/j.1360-0443.2009.02692.x

Janse Van Rensburg K., Taylor A. H., Hodgson, T., & Benattayallah, A. (2009). Acute exercise modulates cigarette cravings and brain activation in response to smoking-related images: An fMRI study. *Psychopharmacology*, *203*(3), 589–598. doi:10.1007/s00213-008-1405-3

Jung, M. E., Fitzgeorge, L., Prapavessis, H., Faulkner, G., & Maddison, R. (2010). The Getting Physical on Cigarettes trial: Rationale and methods. *Mental Health and Physical Activity*, *3*(10), 35–44. doi:10.1016/j.mhpa.2010.02.002

Kaczynski, A. T., Manske, S. R., Mannell, R. C., & Grewal, K. (2008). Smoking and physical activity: A systematic review. *American Journal of Health Behavior*, *32*(1), 93–110. doi:10.5555/ajhb.2008.32.1.93

Klesges, R. C., Meyers, A. W., Klesges, L. M., & La Vasque, M. E. (1989). Smoking, body weight, and their effects on smoking behavior: A comprehensive review of the literature. *Psychological Bulletin*, *106*(2), 204–230. doi:10.1037//0033-2909.106.2.204

Larson, N. I., Story, M., Perry, C. L., Neumark-Sztainer, D., & Hannan, P. J. (2007). Are diet and physical activity patterns related to cigarette smoking in adolescents? Findings from Project EAT. *Preventing Chronic Disease*, *4*(3), A51. Retrieved from http://www.ncbi.nlm.nih.gov/pmc/articles/PMC1955390/pdf/PCD43A51.pdf

Lycett, D., Munafò, M., Johnstone, E., Murphy, M., & Aveyard, P. (2011). Associations between weight change over 8 years and baseline body mass index in a cohort of continuing and quitting smokers. *Addiction*, *106*(1), 188–196. doi:10.1111/j.1360-0443.2010.03136.x

Maddison, R., Roberts, V., Bullen, C., McRobbie, H., Jiang, Y., Prapavessis, H., ... Brown, P. (2010). Design and conduct of a pragmatic randomized controlled trial to enhance smoking cessation outcomes with exercise: The Fit2Quit study. *Mental Health & Physical Activity*, *3*(2), 92–101. doi:10.1016/j.mhpa.2010.09.003

Marcus, B. H., Albrecht, A. E., King, T. K., Parisi, A. F., Pinto, B. M., Roberts, M., ... Abrams, D. B. (1999). The efficacy of exercise as an aid for smoking cessation in women: A randomised controlled trial. *Archives of Internal Medicine*, *159*(11), 1229–1234. Retrieved from http://archinte.ama-assn.org/cgi/content/full/159/11/1229

Marcus, B. H., Hampl, J. S., & Fisher, E. B. (2004). *How to Quit Smoking without Gaining Weight*. New York: Pocket Books.

McClure, J. B., Catz, S. L., Ludman, E. J., Richards, J., Riggs, K., & Grothaus, L. (2011). Feasibility and acceptability of a multiple risk factor intervention: The Step Up randomized pilot trial. *BMC Public Health, 11*(1), 167. doi:10.1186/1471-2458-11-167

McEwen, A., Hajek, P., McRobbie, H., & West, R. (2006). *Manual of Smoking Cessation: A Guide for Counsellors and Practitioners*. Oxford: Blackwell Publishing.

Mikhail, C. (1983). The acute effects of aerobic exercise on cigarette smoking (Master's thesis). University of Lethbridge, Canada. Retrieved from https://circle.ubc.ca/bitstream/handle/2429/25177/UBC_ 1984_A8%20M54.pdf?sequence=1

Nishi, N., Jenicek, M., & Tatara, K. (1998). A meta-analytic review of the effect of exercise on smoking cessation. *Journal of Epidemiology, 8*(2), 79–84. doi:10.2188/jea.8.79

Oh, H., & Taylor, A. H. (2012). Brisk walking reduces ad libitum chocolate snacking in breaks between both low and high demanding cognitive tasks. *Appetite, 58*(1), 387–392. doi:10.1016/j.appet.2011.11.006

Oh, H., & Taylor, A. H. (in press). Self-regulating smoking and snacking through physical activity. *Health Psychology*.

Parsons, A. C., Shraim, M., Inglis, J., Aveyard, P., & Hajek, P. (2009). Interventions for preventing weight gain after smoking cessation. *Cochrane Database of Systematic Reviews*, 1: CD006219. doi:10.1002/ 14651858.CD006219.pub2

Perkins, K. A. (1993). Weight gain following smoking cessation. *Journal of Consulting and Clinical Psychology, 61*(5), 768–777. doi:10.1037//0022-006X.61.5.768

Prochaska, J. J., Hall, S. M., Humfleet, G., Muñoz, R. F., Reus, V., Gorecki, J., & Hu, D. (2008). Physical activity as a strategy for maintaining tobacco abstinence: A randomized trial. *Preventive Medicine, 47*(2), 215–220. doi:10.1016/j.ypmed.2008.05.006

Reeser, K. A. (1983). The effects of repeated aerobic and non-aerobic exercise on cigarette smoking (Master's thesis). University of Alberta, Canada. Retrieved from cIRcle, University of British Columbia's digital repository, https://circle.ubc.ca/handle/2429/25203

Riley, R. D., Lambert, P. C., & Abo-Zaid, G. (2010). Meta-analysis of individual participant data: Rationale, conduct, and reporting. *British Medical Journal, 340*, c221.doi:10.1136/bmj.c221

Rodriguez, D., Duton, G. F., Tscherne, J., & Sass, J. (2008). Physical activity and adolescent smoking: A moderated mediator model. *Mental Health and Physical Activity, 1*(1), 17–25. doi:10.1016/j.mhpa. 2008.04.001

Scerbo, F., Faulkner, G., Taylor, A. H., & Thomas, S. (2010). Effects of exercise on cravings to smoke: The role of exercise intensity and cortisol. *Journal of Sports Sciences, 28*(1), 11–19. doi:10.1080/0264041 0903390089

Spring, B., Howe, D., Berendsen, M., McFadden, H. G., Hitchcock, K., Rademaker, A. W., & Hitsman, B. (2009). Behavioral intervention to promote smoking cessation and prevent weight gain: A systematic review and meta-analysis. *Addiction, 104*(9), 1472–1486. doi:10.1111/j.1360-0443.2009.02610.x

Stead, L. F., Perera, R., Bullen, C., Mant, D., & Lancaster, T. (2008).Nicotine replacement therapy for smoking cessation. *Cochrane Database of Systematic Reviews*, 1: CD000146. doi:10.1002/14651858. CD000146.pub3

Taylor, A. H., Doust, J., & Webborn, N. (1998). Randomised controlled trial to examine the effects of a GP exercise referral program in Hailsham, East Sussex, on modifiable coronary heart disease risk factors. *Journal of Epidemiology & Community Health, 52*(9), 595–601. doi:10.1136/jech.52.9.595

Taylor, A. H., Everson-Hock, E. S., & Ussher, M. (2010). Integrating the promotion of physical activity within a smoking cessation program: Findings from collaborative action research in UK Stop Smoking Services. *BMC Health Services Research, 10*(1), 317. doi:10.1186/1472-6963-10-317

Taylor, A. H., & Katomeri, M. (2007). Walking reduces cue-elicited cigarette cravings and withdrawal symptoms, and delays *ad libitum* smoking. *Nicotine & Tobacco Research, 9*(11), 1–8. doi:10.1080/146222007 01648896

Taylor, A. H., Katomeri, M., & Ussher, M. (2006). Effects of walking on cigarette cravings and affect in the context of Nesbitt's paradox and the circumplex model. *Journal of Sport & Exercise Psychology, 28*(1), 18–31.

Taylor, A. H., & Oliver, A. J. (2009). Acute effects of brisk walking on urges to eat chocolate, affect, and responses to a stressor and chocolate cue. An experimental study. *Appetite. 52*(1), 155–160. doi:10. 1016/j.appet.2008.09.004

Taylor, A. H., Ussher, M. H., & Faulkner, G. (2007). The acute effects of exercise on cigarette cravings, withdrawal symptoms, affect and smoking behavior: A systematic review. *Addiction, 102*(4), 534–543. doi:10.1111/j.1360-0443.2006.01739.x

Thayer, R., Peters, D., Takahaski, P., & Birkhead-Flight, A. (1993). Mood and behavior (smoking and sugar snacking) following moderate exercise: A partial test of self-regulation theory. *Personal and Individual Differences, 14*(1), 97–104. doi:10.1016/0191-8869(93)90178-6

Thompson, T. P., Aveyard, P., Greaves, C., Taylor, R., Warren, F., Green, C., . . . Taylor, A. H. (2013). An exploratory trial to evaluate the effects of a physical activity intervention as a smoking cessation induction and cessation aid among the "hard to reach": Exercise Assisted Reduction then Stop (EARS). Abstract in Proceedings of Society of Research on Nicotine and Tobacco Annual Conference, Boston, March.

Tùnnesen, P., Paoletti, P., Gustavsson, G., Russell, M. A., Saracci, R., Gulsvik, A., . . . Sawe, U., members of the Steering Committee of CEASE on behalf of the European Respiratory Society. (1999). Higher dosage nicotine patches increase one-year smoking cessation rates: Results from the European CEASE trial. *European Respiratory Journal, 13*(2), 238–246. doi:10.1034/j.1399-3003.1999.13b04.x

US Department of Health & Human Services. (2008). *Treating tobacco use and dependence: 2008 update. A report of the surgeon general.* Rockville, MD: Public Health Service. Retrieved from www.surgeongeneral. gov/tobacco/treating_tobacco_use08.pdf

Ussher, M., Ah-Yoon, M., West, R., & Straus, L. (2007). Factors associated with exercise participation and attitudes to exercise among pregnant smokers. *Journal of Smoking Cessation, 2*(1), 12–16. doi:10.1375/jsc.2.1.12

Ussher, M., Aveyard, P., Coleman, T., Straus, L., West, R., & Marcus, B. (2008). Physical activity as an aid to smoking cessation during pregnancy: Two feasibility studies. *BMC Public Health, 8*(1), 328. doi:10.1186/1471-2458-8-328

Ussher, M., Aveyard, P., Manyonda, I., Lewis, S., West, R., Lewis, B., . . . Coleman, T. (2012). Physical activity as an aid to smoking cessation during pregnancy: The LEAP randomised trial protocol. *Trials, 13*, 186. doi:10.1186/1745-6215-13-186

Ussher, M., Cropley, M., Playle, S., Mohidin, R., & West, R. (2009). Effect of isometric exercise and body scanning on cigarette cravings and withdrawal symptoms. *Addiction, 104*(7), 1251–1257. doi:10.1111/j.1360-0443.2009.02605.x

Ussher, M., Nunziata, P., Cropley, M., & West, R. (2001). Effect of a short bout of exercise on tobacco withdrawal symptoms and desire to smoke. *Psychopharmacology, 158*(1), 66–72. doi:10.1007/s002130100846

Ussher, M. H., Taylor, A., & Faulkner, G. (2012). Exercise interventions for smoking cessation. *Cochrane Database of Systematic Reviews, 1*.

Ussher, M. H., Taylor, A. H., West, R., & McEwen, A. (2000). Does exercise aid smoking cessation? A systematic review. *Addiction, 95*(2), 179–188. doi:10.1046/j.1360-0443.2000.9521996.x

Ussher, M., West, R., Doshi, R., & Sampuran, A. K. (2006). Acute effect of isometric exercise on desire to smoke and tobacco withdrawal symptoms. *Human Psychopharmacology: Clinical and Experimental, 21*(1), 39–46. doi:10.1002/hup.744

Ussher, M., West, R., & Hibbs, N. (2004). A survey of pregnant smokers' interest in different types of smoking cessation support. *Patient Education & Counseling, 54*(1), 67–72. doi:10.1016/S0738-3991(03)00197-6

Ussher, M., West, W., McEwen, A., Taylor, A. H., & Steptoe, A. (2003). Efficacy of exercise counselling as an aid for smoking cessation: A randomized controlled trial. *Addiction, 98*(4), 523–532. doi:10.1046/j.1360-0443.2003.00346.x

Ussher, M., West, W., McEwen, A., Taylor, A. H., & Steptoe, A. (2007). Randomized controlled trial of physical activity counseling as an aid to smoking cessation: A 12 month follow-up. *Addictive Behaviors, 32*(12), 3060–3064. doi:10.1016/j.addbeh.2007.04.009

Verkooijen, K. T., Nielsen, G. A., & Kremers, S. P. (2008). The association between leisure time physical activity and smoking in adolescence: An examination of potential mediating and moderating factors. *International Journal of Behavioral Medicine, 15*(2), 157–163. doi:10.1080/10705500801929833

Vickers, K. S., Patten, C. A., Lewis, B. A., Clark, M. M., Ussher, M., Ebbert, J. O., . . . Hurt, R. D. (2009). Feasibility of an exercise counseling intervention for depressed women smokers. *Nicotine and Tobacco Research, 11*(8), 985–995. doi:10.1093/ntr/ntp101

West, R. (2007). The PRIME Theory of motivation as a possible foundation for addiction treatment. In J. Henningfield, P. Santora, and W. Bickel (Eds.), *Drug Addiction Treatment in the 21st Century: Science and Policy Issues.* Baltimore, MD: Johns Hopkins University Press.

West, R., Hajek, P., & Belcher, M. (1989). Severity of withdrawal symptoms as a predictor of outcome of an attempt to quit smoking. *Psychological Medicine, 19*(4), 981–985. doi:10.1017/S0033291700005705

West, R., Hajek, P., Stead, L., & Stapleton, J. (2005). Outcome criteria in smoking cessation trials: Proposal for a common standard. *Addiction, 100*(3), 299–303. doi:10.1111/j.1360-0443.2004.00995.x

Williams, D. M., Whiteley, J. A., Dunsiger, S., Jennings, E. G., Albrecht, A. E., Ussher, M. H., . . . Marcus, B. H. (2010). Moderate intensity exercise as an adjunct to standard smoking cessation treatment for women: A pilot study. *Psychology of Addictive Behaviors, 24*(2), 349–354. doi:10.1037/a0018332

Williams, J. M., & Ziedonis, D. (2004). Addressing tobacco among individuals with a mental illness or an addiction. *Addictive Behaviors, 29*(6), 1067–1083. doi:10.1016/j.addbeh.2004.03.009

World Health Organization. (2011). *WHO Report on the Global Tobacco Epidemic.* Geneva: World Health Organization. Retrieved from http://www.who.int/tobacco/global_report/en/

Zhou, X., Nonnemaker, J., Sherrill, B., Gilsenan, A. W., Coste, F., & West, R. (2009). Attempts to quit smoking and relapse: Factors associated with success or failure from the ATTEMPT cohort study. *Addictive Behaviors, 34*(4), 365–373. doi:10.1016/j.addbeh.2008.11.013

32

PHYSICAL ACTIVITY AND ALCOHOL AND DRUG USE DISORDERS

Ana M. Abrantes, Stephen Matsko, Jessica Wolfe, and Richard A. Brown

Prevalence

Alcohol and drug use disorders are a major, global public health problem. Rates of use, abuse, and dependence are also high worldwide (Kessler et al., 2007). Approximately 8.9% of Americans aged 12 and older meet criteria for either substance abuse or dependence in the last year (Substance Abuse and Mental Health Services Administration, 2010). In Finland, 14.2% of young adults meet criteria for a lifetime substance use disorder (Latvala et al., 2009). In Japan, approximately 10.2% of the adult population has a lifetime alcohol use disorder (Orui, Kawakami, Iwata, Takeshima, & Fukao, 2011). Individuals with alcohol and drug use disorders experience significant mental health problems such as depression and anxiety as well as a number of negative health-related consequences, including health problems (Bloss, 2005), interpersonal violence (Stuart, 2005; Thompson & Kingree, 2006), risky sexual behavior (Justus, Finn, & Steinmetz, 2000), driving while under the influence (Cherpitel & Ye, 2008), and suicide (Wilcox, Conner, & Caine, 2004).

A number of treatment approaches for alcohol and drug use disorders have been shown to be effective, including cognitive behavioral therapies, 12-step programs, relapse prevention skills training, and pharmacotherapy (McGovern & Carroll, 2003). Despite the success of these approaches, relapse remains a major problem (Xie, McHugo, Fox, & Drake, 2005). Therefore, given the high prevalence of alcohol and drug use disorders as well as the associated economic impact, comorbidity, and mortality, it is crucial that accessible, affordable, and efficacious treatments to address drug and alcohol dependence continue to be developed.

The problem of relapse and the role of "lifestyle modification" in relapse prevention

In articulating their relapse model, Marlatt's (1985) primary focus was on the individual's ability to cope with situational factors that may precipitate relapse, and the need to deal with the negative cognitive-affective reactions following an initial lapse. An important aspect of this relapse model is the role of increasing lifestyle balance in preventing relapse (Marlatt & Witkiewitz, 2005). In the chapter on "Lifestyle Modification," Marlatt cites exercise as "a highly recommended lifestyle change activity" (Marlatt, 1985, p. 309) and discusses the advantages of physical activity as a relapse prevention strategy. Other writers have agreed that lifestyle-enhancing factors such as exercise and fitness may play an important role in the prevention and treatment of addictive disorders (Taylor, Sallis, & Needle, 1985; Tkachuk & Martin, 1999). For example, Larimer and colleagues (1999) describe the importance of helping the client develop "positive addictions" such as increased physical activity and meditation. Although lifestyle modification was one of the main components in Marlatt's relapse prevention model (Marlatt & Witkiewitz, 2005), the treatment outcome literature suggests that this component has received the least emphasis in relapse prevention programs for alcohol and drug dependence. Despite this lack of attention in the empirical literature, methods that attempt to foster healthy lifestyle changes may contribute to long-term maintenance of recovery, and interventions targeting physical activity, in particular, may be especially valuable as an adjunct to alcohol and drug use treatment.

Epidemiology of the relationship between physical activity and alcohol and drug use

There is a strong body of evidence pointing toward the significant deleterious effects of physical inactivity with respect to morbidity and mortality (USDHHS, 1996). The association between alcohol and drug use in relation to physical activity has been examined among adults and adolescents with large representative samples both cross-sectionally and longitudinally. Across a number of studies, alcohol use appears to be positively correlated with physical activity among adults (French, Popovici, & Maclean, 2009; Smothers & Bertolucci, 2001). However, at hazardous levels of drinking, physical activity decreases (Liangpunsakul, Crabb, & Qi, 2010). Similarly, while adolescents involved in competitive sports may have higher rates of alcohol consumption, physical activity outside competitive sports is related to decreased alcohol use (Peretti-Watel, Beck, & Legleye, 2002; Tur, Puig, Pons, & Benito, 2003). Interestingly, young adults in college demonstrate a somewhat different relationship, where binge drinking is associated with greater levels of physical activity (Vickers et al., 2004) and those who exercise regularly drink alcohol at significantly higher quantities than infrequent exercisers (Moore & Werch, 2008). With respect to illicit drug use, while the relationship between drug use and physical activity has yet to be examined in adults, youth engaging in regular physical activity use drugs at much lower levels than their sedentary counterparts (Duncan, Duncan, Strycker, & Chaumeton, 2002; Pate, Trost, Levin, & Dowda, 2000; Peretti-Watel et al., 2002).

Several studies have attempted to examine the directionality of the relationship between physical activity and substance use. For example, data collected from 11,741 high school seniors followed until 26 years of age showed that the extent of exercise participation in high school was associated with lower substance use frequency in high school and into early adulthood (Terry-McElrath & O'Malley, 2011). Similarly, in a sample of 4,240 twins in Finland, low levels of physical activity at ages 16–18 years were predictive of greater alcohol and illicit drug use at later timepoints (ages 22–27 years), even when controlling for familial factors (Korhonen, Kujala, Rose, & Kaprio, 2009). Further, in a 4-year prospective, longitudinal community study of 2,548 adolescents and young adults (ages 14–24), regular physical activity was significantly associated with decreased risk of substance use disorders (Strohle et al., 2007).

With respect to the extent that individuals with alcohol and drug use disorders engage in physical activity, information is limited. Data examined from the National Comorbidity Survey in the United States (n=5,877) showed that 63.5% of the alcohol-dependent respondents and 58.5% of the substance-dependent respondents reported regular physical activity (Goodwin, 2003), which did not significantly differ from the rates found among the general population without a mental disorder (60.3%). However, among substance abusing patients in addiction treatment, the rates of regular physical activity have been reported to be much lower (24% in Weinstock, Barry, & Petry, 2008, and 25% in Read & Brown, 2003).

In summary, alcohol (at problematic levels) and drug use are associated with lower levels of physical activity. Physical inactivity during adolescence has also been found to be predictive of higher levels of alcohol and drug use in adulthood. As such, alcohol- and drug-dependent patients in substance abuse treatment may benefit from increasing their levels of physical activity during and following treatment.

The role of exercise in addiction recovery: what has been done?

Alcohol use

There have been a small number of studies that have examined the effects of exercise in individuals with alcohol and drug use problems or disorders. In one of the first studies, Sinyor and colleagues (1982) engaged patients receiving inpatient alcohol rehabilitation treatment in 6 weeks of "tailored" exercise, consisting of progressively more rigorous physical exercise including stretching, calisthenics, and walking/running. Exercise participants demonstrated better abstinence outcomes post treatment than did non-exercising participants. Significant differences between exercisers and non-exercisers continued at 3-month and 18-month follow-up.

A later study by Murphy and colleagues (1986) randomly assigned heavy-drinking college students to running, meditation, or no treatment control. At post-intervention, participants assigned to either of the intervention conditions (running or meditation) demonstrated significant decreases in quantity of alcohol consumption compared with control participants. A number of exercise intervention studies have also been conducted with problem drinkers, and while drinking outcomes were not examined or reported, reductions in depression and anxiety as well as increases in fitness levels were observed (Donaghy, Ralston, & Mutrie, 1991; Ermalinski, Hanson, Lubin, Thornby, & Nahormek, 1997; Frankel & Murphy, 1974; Gary & Guthrie, 1972; Palmer, Vacc, & Epstein, 1988; Tsukue & Shohoji, 1981).

In our own work (R. A. Brown et al., 2009), we explored the efficacy of an aerobic exercise intervention as an adjunct to addiction treatment for alcohol-dependent patients. The 12-week exercise intervention involved attending our fitness facility once a week to participate in moderate-intensity aerobic exercise supervised by an exercise physiologist, with the expectation that participants exercise independently an additional two to three other times during the week. The results of this pilot study (n=19) suggest that, compared with the mean pretreatment percent days abstinent (PDA), significant increases in PDA were observed at the end of the 12-week exercise intervention and at the 3-month post-intervention follow-up. In addition, participants demonstrated good adherence to the intervention.

Other drug use

There are also few published studies examining the efficacy of exercise in adults with drug dependence. In an early study of softball team participation among homeless veteran substance abusers, compared with controls those in the exercise condition demonstrated higher abstinence rates 3 months post-discharge (Burling, Seidner, Robbins-Sisco, Krinsky, & Hanser, 1992). In one small uncontrolled pilot study of an exercise intervention conducted with substance-abusing offenders in outpatient treatment (Williams, 2000), a 12-week intervention consisting of once-weekly strength training groups plus recommendations for exercise during the rest of the week was examined. While substance abuse outcomes were not presented in the results, the authors reported that the 11 out of 20 participants who completed the intervention reported that exercise was helpful in maintaining abstinence. Other studies (Li, Chen, & Mo, 2002; Palmer, Palmer, Michiels, & Thigpen, 1995) have also demonstrated ancillary benefits related to improved anxiety and depression among substance abusers engaging in exercise. In addition, Li and colleagues (2002) found that, compared with pharmacotherapy, qigong therapy (a type of Chinese exercise involving slow, repetitive fluid movements) was associated with a more rapid detoxification of heroin.

In our own study (Brown et al., 2010) examining aerobic exercise as an adjunctive treatment for drug dependence, we found that following participation in a 12-week moderate-intensity aerobic exercise intervention, participants who attended at least 75% of the exercise sessions had significantly better substance use outcomes than those who did not. In terms of PDA for drug use, there was a significant increase and a trend towards increased PDA 3 months post-intervention. In addition, participants showed a significant increase in their cardiorespiratory fitness by the end of treatment.

A recent pilot study conducted in Denmark, in which participants took part in exercise groups three times a week for 2 to 6 months, found similar results (Roessler, 2010). Following the exercise intervention, which included both aerobic and group exercises (volleyball and badminton), participants reported a decrease in the urge to use substances from 65% to 47% as assessed by the Europe Addiction Severity Index. In addition, of the 20 participants who completed the intervention, when assessed "more than a year" following the exercise intervention, five reported no substance use and 10 reported reduced intake.

Another study examining cannabis use and aerobic exercise training reported decreases in daily cannabis use following the exercise intervention (Buchowski et al., 2011). In this pilot study, participants with cannabis dependence attended 10 exercise sessions over 2 weeks, during which they completed a 30-minute treadmill session. Significant changes in both cannabis craving and use were observed pre- to post-exercise.

Lastly, Weinstock and colleagues (2008) examined the extent to which exercise-related behaviors (e.g., buying a pair of sneakers) during a contingency management treatment for substance use disorders was related to abstinence outcomes in 187 outpatients. The results of the study revealed longer durations of abstinence for those who engaged in at least one exercise-related behavior during the 12-week contingency management intervention.

Adolescents

There exists scant research in the area of exercise interventions for adolescent populations with alcohol and drug use disorders. While Werch and colleagues (2003, 2005) have developed brief exercise interventions implemented in schools for the prevention of substance problems, much of the work in the area of introducing structured health promotion to adolescent substance abuse treatment has been conducted by Collingwood and colleagues (1991, 1994). Collingwood and colleagues (1991) conducted a study of a structured fitness program with adolescent substance abusers. The fitness program involved one to two meetings per week with an assignment to engage in two exercise sessions outside the meetings. Overall, participants showed improved physical fitness, reduced polysubstance use, and increased abstinence rates. In a larger-scale study, Collingwood, Sunderlin, and Kohl (1994) evaluated the effects of a fitness skills training program on substance use in a sample of approximately 1,500 "at-risk" adolescents. Although pre-post-data were available for only a subset of the sample, outcome data revealed general improvements in fitness and self-concept and in reduced substance use. Therefore, promising results have begun to emerge from these efforts to deliver exercise interventions to adolescent substance abusers.

Potential mechanisms

Exercise may benefit alcohol- and drug-dependent patients attempting recovery from substance problems through a number of different mechanisms of action. While none of the proposed mechanisms have been formally empirically tested, below is a description of some promising areas for further investigation. Possible neurobiological mechanisms are discussed in Chapter 33 by Smith and Lynch (this volume).

Reduced depressive symptoms

Although the relationship between substance use and depression is complex, studies in recent years have found an association between depressive symptomology and poor treatment outcome among patients with alcohol and drug use disorders (Brown et al., 1998; Nunes & Levin, 2004; Ouimette, Gima, Moos, & Finney, 1999; Poling, Kosten, & Sofuoglu, 2007). Physical activity has consistently been shown to have a positive impact on depressive symptoms across a broad array of populations (Dunn, Trivedi, & O'Neal, 2001; Doyne et al., 1987; Fremont & Craighead, 1987; Babyak et al., 2000).

Positive effects of exercise on psychological health have also been shown in individuals with alcohol and drug use disorders. For example, in studies where alcohol and drug use outcomes were not assessed, both aerobic and strength training exercise programs during the course of alcohol treatment have resulted in decreased depressive and anxiety symptoms (Frankel & Murphy, 1974; Palmer, Vacc, & Epstein, 1988; Palmer et al., 1995). Just as it has been found that improved drinking outcomes in alcohol-dependent patients receiving cognitive–behavioral treatment for depression were mediated by reduction of depressive symptoms (Brown, Evans, Miller, Burgess, & Mueller, 1997), so may exercise lead to improved drinking outcomes as a result of reductions in depressive and anxiety symptoms.

Positive mood states without use of alcohol or drugs

Through a pattern of escalating alcohol and drug use, dysregulation of brain reward pathways occurs (Froelich, 1997; Koob & Kreek, 2007; O'Malley et al., 1996). The brain attempts to compensate by producing less dopamine or reducing the number of dopamine receptors (e.g., Volkow et al., 2001). This, in turn, results in limited capacity of dependent individuals to experience pleasure in early recovery. Exercise has positive reinforcing properties that may be mediated by its effects on the endogenous opioid system and on dopaminergic reinforcement mechanisms (Meeusen, 2005). Further, more recent exercise intervention studies have shown that while decreases in negative affect are not always observed, significant increases in positive affect are consistently demonstrated (Brown, Liu-Ambrose, Tate, & Lord, 2009; Hoffman & Hoffman, 2008; Mutrie et al., 2007; Stroth, Hille, Spitzer, & Reinhardt, 2009). Therefore, alcohol- and drug-dependent patients in early recovery may find engaging in physical activity to be a viable means of experiencing pleasurable mood states and a positively reinforcing alternative to alcohol and drug use.

Decreased urges and coping-oriented motives

Urges to drink alcohol have been identified as an important relapse trigger for abstinent alcoholics (Monti, Rohsenow, & Hutchison, 2000). More recently it has been proposed that moderate-intensity exercise may provide short-term relief from urges to drink alcohol (Ussher, Sampuran,

Doshi, West, & Drummond, 2004). Therefore, decreases in urges to drink may mediate the effect of aerobic exercise on decreased likelihood for relapse.

In addition, recent studies have also examined the association between exercise and coping-oriented motives for alcohol and marijuana (Medina et al., 2011; Smits, Bonn-Miller, Tart, Irons, & Zvolensky, 2011). In one study, Medina and colleagues (2011) found that among trauma-exposed adults, vigorous-intensity exercise was inversely associated with their motivation toward using alcohol to cope. Similarly, Smits and colleagues (2011) found that, among young adult marijuana users, moderate-intensity exercise decreased anxiety sensitivity, which in turn decreased using marijuana as a coping strategy.

Improved cognitive functioning

Deficits in executive functioning, learning/memory, psychomotor speed, and visuospatial abilities (Ersche & Sahakian, 2007; Gruber, Silveri, & Yurgelun-Todd, 2007; Hildebrandt, Brokate, Eling, & Lanz, 2004; Jovanovski, Erb, & Zakzanis, 2005; Noel et al., 2007; Scott et al., 2007) are common neurocognitive consequences of chronic alcohol and drug use, and deficits in executive functioning may contribute to relapse in alcohol and drug use, especially given well-documented disinhibition and decision-making impairments that accompany early recovery (Baicy & London, 2007; Bowden-Jones, McPhillips, Rogers, Hutton, & Joyce, 2005). Regular physical activity is associated with both acute and sustained improvements in cognitive functioning (Stein, Collins, Daniels, Noakes, & Zigmond, 2007), particularly executive functioning (Coles & Tomporowski, 2008; Kramer & Erickson, 2007; Scisco, Leynes, & Kang, 2008; Sibley, Etnier, & LeMasurier, 2006). Therefore, increasing physical activity may result in critical improvements in regulation of attention, controlled information processing, and capacity for learning during early recovery for alcohol- and drug-dependent patients.

Improved sleep

Sleep disturbance is ubiquitous among those in early recovery (Brower, 2001; Stein et al., 2004). Indices of sleep disturbance have been found to be predictive of relapse to alcohol and drug use (Conroy et al., 2006; Liu, Xiaoping, Wei, & Zeng, 2000). Most often, sleep disturbances in early recovery are managed with pharmacotherapy. However, there has been reluctance among addiction experts to prescribe medication to patients in early recovery who are experiencing sleep disturbance (Friedmann et al., 2003). Exercise, on the other hand, has been considered an effective non-pharmacological treatment for sleep disturbance (Youngstedt, 2005) and it is feasible that it would have this benefit among those experiencing substance misuse.

Future directions

Relative to other areas of research, the role of exercise in alcohol and drug use recovery is still in its infancy. There is clearly much more research needed. Specifically, there is a critical need for well-designed, randomized controlled trials of clearly delineated exercise interventions, with objective measures of physical activity and biochemical verification of alcohol and drug use. In doing so, challenges related to recruitment and retention of patients in the exercise interventions (R. A. Brown et al., 2009, 2010; Roessler, 2010; Weinstock, 2010) must be addressed.

Weinstock (2010) identified factors that were associated with successfully initiating and maintaining an exercise program and these included social support, self-efficacy, motivation, having physical activity choices, goal setting and behavioral contracts, positive reinforcement, and feedback. Another important consideration in addressing recruitment and retention issues involves the "fit" of the exercise intervention to the patient population. For example, substance-dependent patients in early recovery may be in a sensitive period of transition that can include attending numerous outpatient treatment sessions as well as 12-step meetings, rebuilding strained familial and personal relationships, finding new jobs, and addressing physical health problems that may have resulted from prolonged periods of substance use. They may have specific preferences regarding the timing, type, and structure of an exercise intervention that would influence adoption and maintenance of regular physical activity (Abrantes et al., in press). As a result, focusing future research efforts on identifying exercise preferences among substance-abusing populations may contribute to the development of exercise interventions that are not only effective but also more feasible to administer.

In addition, considering barriers, particularly lack of motivation, in the development of exercise interventions will be important for adherence and retention issues. Alcohol- and drug-dependent patients may benefit from the use of tools to help bolster motivation. For example, pedometers have been used to improve self-monitoring, facilitate goal setting, and enhance motivation in numerous exercise intervention studies (Croteau, 2004; Merom et al., 2007; Murphy, Nevill, Murtagh, & Holder, 2007). In addition, monetary incentives have been utilized in previous exercise intervention studies as a means of increasing motivation and adherence (Jeffery, Wing, Thorson, & Burton, 1998; Robison et al., 1992). Given that contingency management approaches have been efficacious in substance-abusing populations (Higgins & Petry, 1999), utilizing a similar approach within exercise interventions for patients in substance abuse treatment may be an effective strategy for increasing motivation in this population.

Consideration may need to be given to gender differences when developing intervention programs for alcohol- and drug-dependent patients. Gender differences often emerge with regard to the type of exercise that appeals to women versus men, as well as the perceived benefits of engaging in an exercise-based intervention (Abrantes et al., in press). For example, women typically find walking and aerobics more appealing than men, whereas men endorse greater interest in sports, strength training, and running (Booth, Bauman, Owen, & Gore, 1997). These patterns may be important to consider given that interventions may be most successful if they are either tailored directly for women versus men, or if they are flexibly designed so that appealing options are available for both gender groups.

Conclusion

Relapse continues to pose a major problem to the substance abuse treatment field as a whole and to individuals attempting recovery from alcohol and drug use disorders. Studies evaluating strategies to enhance maintenance of treatment gains have devoted relatively little attention to lifestyle modification, and research in the area of exercise and recovery from alcohol and drug use disorders is still scant. Many patients in substance abuse programs express interest in incorporating exercise into their recovery (Read et al., 2001). In light of the promising findings from these studies, more research is clearly needed in this area.

A physical activity intervention with demonstrated generalizability and the potential for dissemination would have important clinical and public health implications for the treatment of alcohol and drug use disorders and would provide some definite advantages. Exercise offers the potential for improved health and wellness, as the physiological (e.g., USDHHS, 1996) and psychological (e.g., Tkachuk & Martin, 1999) health benefits of exercise have been well documented. Exercise also has the potential to be cost-effective, flexible, and accessible; many forms of exercise may be conducted independently, and associated costs are likely to be minimal.

Finally, exercise has minimal side effects compared with pharmacological treatment (Broocks et al., 1998), and carries with it far less risk of adverse events than does the use of psychotropic medication. Given each of these benefits, alcohol- and drug-dependent individuals may be afforded a valuable adjunct to traditional addiction treatment that could enhance alcohol and drug use outcomes, improve psychological well-being, and increase fitness and the overall health of patients.

References

Abrantes, A. M., Battle, C. L., Strong, D. R., Ing, E., Dubreuil, M. E., Gordon, A., & Brown, R. A. (in press). Exercise preferences of patients in substance abuse treatment. *Mental Health and Physical Activity.*

Babyak, M., Blumenthal, J. A., Herman, S., Khatri, P., Doraiswamy, M., Moore, K., . . . Krishnan, K. R. (2000). Exercise treatment for major depression: Maintenance of therapeutic benefit at 10 months. *Psychosomatic Medicine, 62,* 633–638. Retrieved from http://www.psychosomaticmedicine.org/

Baicy, K., & London, E. D. (2007). Corticolimbic dysregulation and chronic methamphetamine abuse. *Addiction, 102,* 5–15. doi:10.1111/j.1360-0443.2006.01777.x

Bloss, G. (2005). Measuring the health consequences of alcohol consumption: Current needs and methodological challenges. *Digestive Diseases, 23*(3–4), 162–169. doi:10.1159/000090162

Booth, M. L., Bauman, A., Owen, N., & Gore, C. J. (1997). Physical activity preferences, preferred sources of assistance, and perceived barriers to increased activity among physically inactive Australians. *Preventive Medicine, 26*(1), 131–137. doi:10.1006/pmed.1996.9982

Bowden-Jones, H., McPhillips, M., Rogers, R., Hutton, S., & Joyce, E. (2005). Risk-taking on tests sensitive to ventromedial prefrontal cortex dysfunction predicts early relapse in alcohol dependency: A pilot study. *Journal of Neuropsychiatry and Clinical Neuroscience, 17,* 417–420. doi:10.1176/appi.neuropsych.17.3.417

Broocks, A., Bandelow, B., Pekrun, G., George, A., Meyer, T., Bartmann, U., . . . Rüther, E. (1998). Comparison of aerobic exercise, clomipramine, and placebo in the treatment of panic disorder. *American Journal of Psychiatry, 155,* 603–609. Retrieved from http://ajp.psychiatryonline.org/

Brower, K. J. (2001). Alcohol's effects on sleep in alcoholics. *Alcohol Research and Health, 25,* 110–125. Retrieved from http://www.niaaa.nih.gov/Publications/AlcoholResearch/Pages/default.aspx

Brown, A. K., Liu-Ambrose, T., Tate, R., & Lord, S. R. (2009). The effect of group-based exercise on cognitive performance and mood in seniors residing in intermediate care and self-care retirement facilities: A randomised controlled trial. *British Journal of Sports Medicine, 43,* 608–614. doi:10.1136/bjsm.2008.049882

Brown, R. A., Abrantes, A. M., Read, J. P., Marcus, B. H., Jakicic, J., Strong, D. R., . . . Gordon, A. A. (2009). Aerobic exercise for alcohol recovery: Rationale, program description, and preliminary findings. *Behavior Modification, 33*(2), 220–249. doi:10.1007/s00213-011-2321-5

Brown, R. A., Abrantes, A. M., Read, J. P., Marcus, B. H., Jakicic, J., Strong, D. R., . . . Gordon, A. A. (2010). A pilot study of aerobic exercise as an adjunctive treatment for drug dependence. *Mental Health and Physical Activity, 3*(1), 27–34. doi:10.1016/j.mhpa.2010.03.001

Brown, R. A., Evans, D. M., Miller, I. W., Burgess, E. S., & Mueller, T. I. (1997). Cognitive-behavioral treatment for depression in alcoholism. *Journal of Consulting and Clinical Psychology, 65,* 715–726. doi:10.1037/0022-006X.65.5.715

Brown, R. A., Monti, P. M., Myers, M. G., Martin, R. A., Rivinus, T., Dubreuil, M. E., . . . Rohsenow, D. J. (1998). Depression among cocaine abusers in treatment: Relation to cocaine and alcohol use and treatment outcome. *American Journal of Psychiatry, 155,* 220–225. Retrieved from http://ajp.psychiatryonline.org/

Buchowski, M. S., Meade, N. N., Charboneau, E., Park, S., Dietrich, M. S., Cowan, R. L., & Martin, P. R. (2011). Aerobic exercise training reduces cannabis craving and use in non-treatment seeking cannabis-dependent adults. *PLoS One, 6,* e17465. doi:10.1371/journal.pone.0017465

Burling, T. A., Seidner, A. L., Robbins-Sisco, D., Krinsky, A., & Hanser, B. B. (1992). Batter up! Relapse prevention for homeless veteran substance abusers via softball team participation. *Journal of Substance Abuse, 4,* 407. doi:10.1016/0899-3289(92)90047-2

Cherpitel, C. J., & Ye, Y. (2008). Drug use and problem drinking associated with primary care and emergency room utilization in the US general population: Data from the 2005 National Alcohol Survey. *Drug and Alcohol Dependence, 97*(3), 226–230. doi:10.1016/j.drugalcdep.2008.03.033

Coles, K., & Tomporowski, P. D. (2008). Effects of acute exercise on executive processing, short-term and long-term memory. *Journal of Sports Science, 26*, 333–344. doi:10.1080/02640410701591417

Collingwood, T. R., Reynolds, R., Kohl, H. W., Smith, W., & Sloan, S. (1991). Physical fitness effects on substance abuse risk factors and use patterns. *Journal of Drug Education, 21*, 73–84. doi:10.2190/HV5J-4EYN-GPP7-Y3QG

Collingwood, T. R., Sunderlin, J., & Kohl, H. W., 3rd. (1994). The use of a staff training model for implementing fitness programming to prevent substance abuse with at-risk youth. *American Journal of Health Promotion, 9*, 20–23. Retrieved from http://ajhpcontents.org/loi/hepr

Conroy, D. A., Todd Arnedt, J., Brower, K. J., Strobbe, S., Consens, F., Hoffmann, R., . . . Armitage, R. (2006). Perception of sleep in recovering alcohol-dependent patients with insomnia: Relationship with future drinking. *Alcoholism: Clinical and Experimental Research, 30*, 1992–1999. doi:10.1111/j.1530-0277.2006.00245.x

Croteau, K. A. (2004). Strategies used to increase lifestyle physical activity in a pedometer-based intervention. *Journal of Allied Health, 33*, 278–281. Retrieved from http://www.asahp.org/journal_ah.htm

Donaghy, M., Ralston, G., & Mutrie, N. (1991). Exercise as a therapeutic adjunct for problem drinkers. *Journal of Sports Sciences, 9*, 440. doi:10.1080/02640419108729899

Doyne, E. J., Ossip-Klein, D. J., Bowman, E. D., Osborn, K. M., McDougall-Wilson, I. B., & Neimeyer, R. A. (1987). Running versus weight lifting in the treatment of depression. *Journal of Consulting and Clinical Psychology, 55*, 748–754. doi:10.1037/0022-006X.55.5.748

Duncan, S. C., Duncan, T. E., Strycker, L. A., & Chaumeton, N. R. (2002). Relations between youth antisocial and prosocial activities. *Journal of Behavioral Medicine, 25*, 425–438. doi:10.1023/A:1020466906928

Dunn, A. L., Trivedi, M. H., & O'Neal, H. A. (2001). Physical activity dose-response effects on outcomes of depression and anxiety. *Medicine and Science in Sports and Exercise, 33*, S587–597; discussion 609–510. doi:10.1097/00005768-200106001-00027

Ermalinski, R., Hanson, P. G., Lubin, B., Thornby, J. I., & Nahormek, P. A. (1997). Impact of a body-mind treatment component on alcohol inpatients. *Journal of Psychosocial Nursing, 35*, 39–45.

Ersche, K. D., & Sahakian, B. J. (2007). The neuropsychology of amphetamine and opiate dependence: Implications for treatment. *Neuropsychological Review, 17*, 317–336. doi:10.1007/s11065-007-9033-y

Frankel, A., & Murphy, J. (1974). Physical fitness and personality in alcoholism. Canonical analysis of measures before and after treatment. *Quarterly Journal on the Studies of Alcohol, 35*, 1272–1278.

Fremont, J., & Craighead, W. E. (1987). Aerobic exercise and cognitive therapy in the treatment of dysphoric moods. *Cognitive Therapy Research, 11*, 241–251. doi:10.1007/BF01183268

French, M. T., Popovici, I., & Maclean, J. C. (2009). Do alcohol consumers exercise more? Findings from a national survey. *American Journal of Health Promotion, 24*, 2–10. doi:10.4278/ajhp.0801104

Friedmann, P. D., Herman, D. S., Freedman, S., Lemon, S. C., Ramsey, S., & Stein, M. D. (2003). Treatment of sleep disturbance in alcohol recovery: A national survey of addiction medicine physicians. *Journal of Addictive Diseases, 22*, 91–103. doi:10.1300/J069v22n02_08

Froelich, J. C. (1997). Opioid peptides. *Alcohol Health and Research World, 21*, 132–135. Retrieved from http://www.niaaa.nih.gov/Publications/AlcoholResearch/Pages/default.aspx

Gary, V., & Guthrie, D. (1972). The effect of jogging on physical fitness and self concept on hospitalized alcoholics. *Quarterly Journal of Studies in Alcohol, 33*, 1073–1078.

Goodwin, R. D. (2003). Association between physical activity and mental disorders among adults in the United States. *Preventive Medicine, 36*(6), 698–703. doi:10.1016/S0091-7435(03)00042-2

Gruber, S. A., Silveri, M. M., & Yurgelun-Todd, D. A. (2007). Neuropsychological consequences of opiate use. *Neuropsychological Review, 17*, 299–315. doi:10.1007/s11065-007-9041-y

Higgins, S. T., & Petry, N. M. (1999). Contingency management. Incentives for sobriety. *Alcohol Research & Health, 23*, 122–127. Retrieved from http://www.niaaa.nih.gov/Publications/AlcoholResearch/Pages/default.aspx

Hildebrandt, H., Brokate, B., Eling, P., & Lanz, M. (2004). Response shifting and inhibition, but not working memory, are impaired after long-term heavy alcohol consumption. *Neuropsychology, 18*, 203–211. doi:10.1037/0894-4105.18.2.203

Hoffman, M. D., & Hoffman, D. R. (2008). Exercisers achieve greater acute exercise-induced mood enhancement than nonexercisers. *Archives of Physical Medicine and Rehabilitation, 89*, 358–363. doi:10.1016/j.apmr.2007.09.026

Jeffery, R. W., Wing, R. R., Thorson, C., & Burton, L. R. (1998). Use of personal trainers and financial incentives to increase exercise in a behavioral weight-loss program. *Journal of Consulting and Clinical Psychology, 66*, 777–783. doi:10.1037/0022-006X.66.5.777

Jovanovski, D., Erb, S., & Zakzanis, K. K. (2005). Neurocognitive deficits in cocaine users: A quantitative review of the evidence. *Journal of Clinical and Experimental Neuropsychology, 27,* 189–204. doi: 10.1080/13803390490515694

Justus, A. N., Finn, P. R., & Steinmetz, J. E. (2000). The influence of traits of disinhibition on the association between alcohol use and risky sexual behavior. *Alcoholism: Clinical and Experimental Research, 24,* 1028–1035. doi:10.1111/j.1530-0277.2000.tb04646.x

Kessler, R. C., Angermeyer, M., Anthony, J. C., Graaf R. D. E., Demyttenaere, K., Gasquet, I., . . . Ustun, T. B. (2007). Lifetime prevalence and age-of-onset distributions of mental disorders in the World Health Organization's World Mental Health Survey Initiative. *World Psychiatry, 6,* 168–176. Retrieved from http://www.wpanet.org/detail.php?section_id=10&content_id=421

Koob, G., & Kreek, M. J. (2007). Stress, dysregulation of drug reward pathways, and the transition to drug dependence. *American Journal of Psychiatry, 164,* 1149–1159. doi:10.1176/appi.ajp.2007.05030503

Korhonen, T., Kujala, U. M., Rose, R. J., & Kaprio, J. (2009). Physical activity in adolescence as a predictor of alcohol and illicit drug use in early adulthood: A longitudinal population-based twin study. *Twin Research and Human Genetics, 12,* 261–268. doi:10.1375/twin.12.3.261

Kramer, A. F., & Erickson, K. I. (2007). Capitalizing on cortical plasticity: Influence of physical activity on cognition and brain function. *Trends in Cognitive Science, 11,* 342–348. doi:10.1016/j.tics.2007.06.009

Larimer, M. E., Palmer, R. S., & Marlatt, G. A. (1999). Relapse prevention. An overview of Marlatt's cognitive-behavioral model. *Alcohol Research & Health, 23,* 151–160. Retrieved from http://www.niaaa.nih.gov/Publications/AlcoholResearch/Pages/default.aspx

Latvala, A., Tuulio-Henriksson, A., Perala, J., Saarni, S. I., Aalto-Setala, T., Aro, H., . . . Suvisaari, J. (2009). Prevalence and correlates of alcohol and other substance use disorders in young adulthood: A population-based study. *BMC Psychiatry, 9,* 73. doi:10.1186/1471-244X-9-73

Liangpunsakul, S., Crabb, D. W., & Qi, R. (2010). Relationship among alcohol intake, body fat, and physical activity: A population-based study. *Annals of Epidemiology, 20,* 670–675. doi:10.1016/j.annepidem.2010.05.014

Li, M., Chen, K., and Mo, Z. (2002). Use of qigong therapy in the detoxification of heroin addicts. *Alternative Therapies in Health and Medicine, 8,* 50–59. Retrieved from http://www.alternative-therapies.com/

Liu, T., Xiaoping, W., Wei, H., & Zeng, W. (2000). Frequency of withdrawal symptoms of natural detoxification in heroin addicts. *Chinese Mental Health Journal, 14*(2), 114–116. doi:CNKI:SUN: ZXWS.0.2000-02-017

Marlatt, G. A. (1985). Lifestyle modification. In G. A. Marlatt & J. R. Gordon (Eds.) *Relapse prevention: Maintenance strategies in the treatment of addictive behaviors,* pp. 280–348. New York: Guilford Press.

Marlatt, G. A., & Witkiewitz, K. (2005). Relapse prevention for alcohol and drug problems. In G. A. Marlatt & K. Witkiewitz (Eds.) *Relapse prevention: Maintenance strategies in the treatment of addictive behaviors* (2nd ed.), pp. 1–44. New York: Guilford Press.

McGovern, M. P., & Carroll, K. M. (2003). Evidence-based practices for substance use disorders. *Psychiatric Clinics of North America, 26,* 991–1010. doi:10.1016/S0193-953X(03)00073-X

Medina, J. L., Vujanovic, A. A., Smits, J. A., Irons, J. G., Zvolensky, M. J., & Bonn-Miller, M. O. (2011). Exercise and coping-oriented alcohol use among a trauma-exposed sample. *Addictive Behaviors, 36,* 274–277. doi:10.1016/j.addbeh.2010.11.008

Meeusen, R. (2005). Exercise and the brain: Insight in new therapeutic modalities. *Annals of Transplant, 10,* 49–51. Retrieved from http://www.annalsoftransplantation.com/

Merom, D., Rissel, C., Phongsavan, P., Smith, B. J., Van Kemenade, C., Brown, W. J., . . . Bauman, A. E. (2007). Promoting walking with pedometers in the community: The step-by-step trial. *American Journal of Preventive Medicine, 32,* 290–297. doi:10.1016/j.amepre.2006.12.007

Monti, P. M., Rohsenow, D. J., & Hutchison, K. E. (2000). Toward bridging the gap between biological, psychobiological and psychosocial models of alcohol craving. *Addiction, 95 Suppl 2,* S229–S236. doi:10.1046/j.1360-0443.95.8s2.11.x

Moore, M. J., & Werch, C. (2008). Relationship between vigorous exercise frequency and substance use among first-year drinking college students. *Journal of American College Health, 56*(6), 686–690. doi:10.3200/JACH.56.6.686-690

Murphy, M. H., Nevill, A. M., Murtagh, E. M., & Holder, R. L. (2007). The effect of walking on fitness, fatness and resting blood pressure: A meta-analysis of randomised, controlled trials. *Preventive Medicine, 44*(5), 377–385. doi:10.1016/j.ypmed.2006.12.008

Murphy, T. J., Pagano, R. R., & Marlatt, G. A. (1986). Lifestyle modification with heavy alcohol drinkers: Effects of aerobic exercise and meditation. *Addictive Behaviors, 11*(2), 175–186. doi:10.1016/0306-4603(86)90043-2

Mutrie, N., Campbell, A. M., Whyte, F., McConnachie, A., Emslie, C., Lee, L., . . . Ritchie, D. (2007). Benefits of supervised group exercise programme for women being treated for early stage breast cancer: Pragmatic randomised controlled trial. *BMJ, 334*(7592), 517. doi:10.1136/bmj.39094.648553.AE

Noel, X., Van der Linden, M., d'Acremont, M., Bechara, A., Dan, B., Hanak, C., . . . Verbanck, P. (2007). Alcohol cues increase cognitive impulsivity in individuals with alcoholism. *Psychopharmacology (Berlin), 192*(2), 291–298. doi:10.1007/s00213-006-0695-6

Nunes, E. V., & Levin, F. R. (2004). Treatment of depression in patients with alcohol or other drug dependence: A meta-analysis. *JAMA, 291*(15), 1887–1896. doi:10.1001/jama.291.15.1887

O'Malley, S. S., Jaffe, A. J., Chang, G., Rode, S., Schottenfeld, R., Meyer, R. E., & Rounsaville, B. (1996). Six-month follow-up of naltrexone and psychotherapy for alcohol dependence. *Archives of General Psychiatry, 53*(3), 217–224. Retrieved from http://archpsyc.ama-assn.org/

Orui, M., Kawakami, N., Iwata, N., Takeshima, T., & Fukao, A. (2011). Lifetime prevalence of mental disorders and its relationship to suicidal ideation in a Japanese rural community with high suicide and alcohol consumption rates. *Environmental Health and Preventive Medicine.* doi:10.1007/s12199-011-0209-y

Ouimette, P. C., Gima, K., Moos, R. H., & Finney, J. W. (1999). A comparative evaluation of substance abuse treatment IV. The effect of comorbid psychiatric diagnoses on amount of treatment, continuing care, and 1-year outcomes. *Alcohol: Clinical and Experimental Research, 23*(3), 552–557. doi:10.1111/j.1530-0277.1999.tb04152.x

Palmer, J. A., Palmer, L. K., Michiels, K., & Thigpen, B. (1995). Effects of type of exercise on depression in recovering substance abusers. *Perceptual and Motor Skills, 80*(2), 523–530. doi:10.2466/pms.1995.80.2.523

Palmer, J., Vacc, N., & Epstein, J. (1988). Adult inpatient alcoholics: Physical exercise as a treatment intervention. *Journal of Studies on Alcohol, 49*(5), 418–421. Retrieved from http://www.jsad.com/

Pate, R. R., Trost, S. G., Levin, S., & Dowda, M. (2000). Sports participation and health-related behaviors among US youth. *Archives of Pediatriatric Adolescent Medicine, 154*(9), 904–911. Retrieved from http://archpedi.ama-assn.org

Peretti-Watel, P., Beck, F., & Legleye, S. (2002). Beyond the U-curve: The relationship between sport and alcohol, cigarette and cannabis use in adolescents. *Addiction, 97*(6), 707–716. doi:10.1046/j.1360-0443.2002.00116.x

Poling, J., Kosten, T. R., & Sofuoglu, M. (2007). Treatment outcome predictors for cocaine dependence. *American Journal of Drug and Alcohol Abuse, 33*(2), 191–206. doi:10.1080/00952990701199416

Read, J. P., & Brown, R. A. (2003). The role of physical exercise in alcoholism treatment and recovery. *Professional Psychology: Research and Practice, 34*, 49–56. doi:10.1037/0735-7028.34.1.49

Read, J. P., Brown, R. A., Marcus, B. H., Kahler, C. W., Ramsey, S. E., Dubreuil, M. E., . . . Francion, C. (2001). Exercise attitudes and behaviors among persons in treatment for alcohol use disorders. *Journal of Substance Abuse Treatment, 21*(4), 199–206. doi:10.1016/S0740-5472(01)00203-3

Robison, J. I., Rogers, M. A., Carlson, J. J., Mavis, B. E., Stachnik, T., Stoffelmayr, B., . . .Van Huss, W. D. (1992). Effects of a 6-month incentive-based exercise program on adherence and work capacity. *Medicine and Science in Sports and Exercise, 24*(1), 85–93. Retrieved from http://journals.lww.com/acsm-msse/pages/default.aspx

Roessler, K. K. (2010). Exercise treatment for drug abuse—a Danish pilot study. *Scandinavian Journal of Public Health, 38*(6), 664–669. doi:10.1177/1403494810371249

Scisco, J. L., Leynes, P. A., & Kang, J. (2008). Cardiovascular fitness and executive control during task-switching: An ERP study. *International Journal of Psychophysiology, 69*(1), 52–60. doi:10.1016/j.ijpsycho.2008.02.009

Scott, J. C., Woods, S. P., Matt, G. E., Meyer, R. A., Heaton, R. K., Atkinson, J. H., . . . Grant, I. (2007). Neurocognitive effects of methamphetamine: A critical review and meta-analysis. *Neuropsychology Review, 17*(3), 275–297. doi:10.1007/s11065-007-9031-0

Sibley, B. A., Etnier, J. L., & LeMasurier, G. C. (2006). Effects of an acute bout of exercise on cognitive aspects of stroop performance. *Journal of Sport and Exercise Psychology, 28*, 285–299. Retrieved from http://journals.humankinetics.com/jsep

Sinyor, D., Brown, T., Rostant, L., & Seraganian, P. (1982). The role of a physical fitness program in the treatment of alcoholism. *Journal of Studies on Alcohol, 43*(3), 380–386. Retrieved from http://www.jsad.com/

Smits, J. A., Bonn-Miller, M. O., Tart, C. D., Irons, J. G., & Zvolensky, M. J. (2011). Anxiety sensitivity as a mediator of the relationship between moderate-intensity exercise and coping-oriented marijuana use motives. *American Journal of Addictions, 20*, 113–119. doi:10.1111/j.1521-0391.2010.00115.x

Smothers, B., & Bertolucci, D. (2001). Alcohol consumption and health-promoting behavior in a U.S. household sample: Leisure-time physical activity. *Journal of Studies on Alcohol, 62*(4), 467–476. Retrieved from http://www.jsad.com/

Stein, D. J., Collins, M., Daniels, W., Noakes, T. D., & Zigmond, M. (2007). Mind and muscle: The cognitive-affective neuroscience of exercise. *CNS Spectrum, 12*(1), 19–22. Retrieved from http://www.cnsspectrums.com/default.aspx

Stein, M. D., Herman, D. S., Bishop, S., Lassor, J. A., Weinstock, M., Anthony, J., . . . Anderson, B. J. (2004). Sleep disturbances among methadone maintained patients. *Journal of Substance Abuse Treatment, 26*(3), 175–180. doi:10.1016/S0740-5472(03)00191-0

Strohle, A., Hofler, M., Pfister, H., Muller, A. G., Hoyer, J., Wittchen, H. U., . . . Lieb, R. (2007). Physical activity and prevalence and incidence of mental disorders in adolescents and young adults. *Psychological Medicine, 37*(11), 1657–1666. doi:10.1017/S003329170700089X

Stroth, S., Hille, K., Spitzer, M., & Reinhardt, R. (2009). Aerobic endurance exercise benefits memory and affect in young adults. *Neuropsychological Rehabilitation, 19*(2), 223–243. doi:10.1080/0960 2010802091183

Stuart, G. L. (2005). Improving violence intervention outcomes by integrating alcohol treatment. *Journal of Interpersonal Violence, 20*(4), 388–393. doi:10.1177/0886260504267881

Substance Abuse and Mental Health Services Administration. (2010). *Results from the 2009 National Survey on Drug Use and Health: Volume I. Summary of National Findings* (Office of Applied Studies, NSDUH Series H-38A, HHS Publication No. SMA 10-4586Findings). Rockville, MD.

Taylor, C. B., Sallis, J. F., & Needle, R. (1985). The relation of physical activity and exercise to mental health. *Public Health Reports, 100*(195–201). Retrieved from http://www.publichealthreports.org/

Terry-McElrath, Y. M., & O'Malley, P. M. (2011). Substance use and exercise participation among young adults: Parallel trajectories in a national cohort-sequential study. *Addiction, 106*(10), 1855–1865.

Thompson, M. P., & Kingree, J. B. (2006). The roles of victim and perpetrator alcohol use in intimate partner violence outcomes. *Journal of Interpersonal Violence, 21*(2), 163–177. doi:10.1177/0886260505 282283

Tkachuk, G. A., & Martin, G. L. (1999). Exercise therapy for patients with psychiatric disorders: Research and clinical implications. *Professional Psychology: Research and Practice, 30*(3), 275–282. Retrieved from http://www.apa.org/pubs/journals/pro/index.aspx

Tsukue, I., & Shohoji, T. (1981). Movement therapy for alcoholic patients. *Journal of Studies on Alcohol, 42*, 144–149. Retrieved from http://www.jsad.com/

Tur, J. A., Puig, M. S., Pons, A., & Benito, E. (2003). Alcohol consumption among school adolescents in Palma de Mallorca. *Alcohol Alcohol, 38*(3), 243–248. doi:10.1093/alcalc/agg061

USDHHS (1996). *Physical Activity and Health: A Report of the Surgeon General.* Atlanta, GA: Centers for Disease Control and Prevention, National Center for Chronic Disease Control and Prevention.

Ussher, M., Sampuran, A. K., Doshi, R., West, R., & Drummond, D. C. (2004). Acute effect of a brief bout of exercise on alcohol urges. *Addiction, 99*(12), 1542–1547. doi:10.1002/hup.744

Vickers, K. S., Patten, C. A., Bronars, C., Lane, K., Stevens, S. R., Croghan, I. T., . . . Clark, M. M. (2004). Binge drinking in female college students: The association of physical activity, weight concern, and depressive symptoms. *Journal of American College Health, 53*(3), 133–140. doi:10.3200/JACH.53.3.133-140

Volkow, N. D., Chang, L., Wang, G. J., Fowler, J. S., Franceschi, D., Sedler, M., . . . Logan, J. (2001). Loss of dopamine transporters in methamphetamine abusers recovers with protracted abstinence. *Journal of Neuroscience, 21*(23), 9414–9418. Retrieved from http://www.jneurosci.org/

Weinstock, J. (2010). A review of exercise as intervention for sedentary hazardous drinking college students: Rationale and issues. *Journal of American College Health, 58*(6), 539–544. doi:10.1080/07448481003 686034

Weinstock, J., Barry, D., & Petry, N. M. (2008). Exercise-related activities are associated with positive outcome in contingency management treatment for substance use disorders. *Addictive Behaviors, 33*(8), 1072–1075. doi:10.1016/j.addbeh.2008.03.011

Werch, C., Moore, M., DiClemente, C. C., Owen, D. M., Jobli, E., & Bledsoe, R. (2003). A sport-based intervention for preventing alcohol use and promoting physical activity among adolescents. *Journal of School Health, 73*(10), 380–388. doi:10.1111/j.1746-1561.2003.tb04181.x

Werch, C. C., Moore, M. J., DiClemente, C. C., Bledsoe, R., & Jobli, E. (2005). A multihealth behavior intervention integrating physical activity and substance use prevention for adolescents. *Prevention Science, 6*(3), 213–226. doi:10.1007/s11121-005-0012-3

Wilcox, H. C., Conner, K. R., & Caine, E. D. (2004). Association of alcohol and drug use disorders and completed suicide: An empirical review of cohort studies. *Drug and Alcohol Dependence, 76 Suppl,* S11–S19. doi:10.1016/j.drugalcdep.2004.08.003

Williams, D. J. (2000). Exercise and substance abuse treatment: Predicting program completion using logistic regression. *Corrections Compendium, 25*(2), 4–7.

Xie, H., McHugo, G. J., Fox, M. B., & Drake, R. E. (2005). Substance abuse relapse in a ten-year prospective follow-up of clients with mental and substance use disorders. *Psychiatric Services, 56*(10), 1282–1287. doi:10.1176/appi.ps.56.10.1282

Youngstedt, S. D. (2005). Effects of exercise on sleep. *Clinical Sports Medicine, 24*(2), 355–365, xi. doi:10.1016/j.csm.2004.12.003

33

THE NEUROBIOLOGY OF EXERCISE AND DRUG-SEEKING BEHAVIOR

Mark A. Smith and Wendy J. Lynch

Epidemiological studies consistently report that physical activity is inversely related to substance use and abuse. Similar to many abused substances, physical activity produces positive affective states in both humans and animals. These positive affective states can be measured objectively and quantitatively, and have been demonstrated under a variety of experimental conditions (Belke & Wagner, 2005; Greenwood et al., 2011; Janal, Colt, Clark, & Glusman, 1984; Lett, Grant, Byrne, & Koh, 2000; Lett, Grant, & Koh, 2001; Nabetani & Tokunaga, 2001). Exercise also functions as a positive reinforcer, in that both humans and animals will perform an operant response (e.g., drive to a gym, press a lever) in order to engage in physical activity (Belke, 1997, 2000; Belke & Dunbar, 2001; Iversen, 1993; Schebendach, Klein, Foltin, Devlin, & Walsh, 2007). Preclinical studies report that aerobic exercise decreases drug self-administration and other measures of drug-seeking behavior. For instance, in laboratory rats, access to a running wheel decreases the acquisition (Smith & Pitts, 2011), maintenance (Cosgrove, Hunter, & Carroll, 2002; Smith, Schmidt, Iordanou, & Mustroph, 2008), and escalation (Smith, Walker, Cole, & Lang, 2011) of cocaine self-administration, and decreases the reinstatement of cocaine-seeking behavior after a period of abstinence (Lynch, Piehl, Acosta, Peterson, & Hemby, 2010; Smith, Pennock, & Walker, 2011; Zlebnik, Anker, Gliddon, & Carroll, 2010). Similar effects have been reported with other drugs of abuse, including alcohol (Crews, Nixon, & Wilkie, 2004; Ehringer, Hoft, & Zunhammer, 2009, but see Werme, Lindholm, Thorén, Franck, & Brené, 2002; McMillan, McClure, & Hardwick, 1995; Ozburn, Harris, & Blednov, 2008), morphine (Hosseini, Alaei, Naderi, Sharifi, & Zahed, 2009), and methamphetamine (Miller et al., 2011). A number of behavioral/psychological mechanisms likely contribute to the beneficial effects of exercise on drug-seeking behavior. For instance, exercise decreases several comorbid psychological conditions that are associated with substance abuse and dependence. Specifically, exercise decreases measures of depression and anxiety (see reviews by Herring, O'Connor, & Dishman, 2010; Perraton, Kumar, & Machotka, 2010), both of which are risk factors for developing a substance use disorder (Castle, 2008; Swendsen & Merikangas, 2000). Exercise also reliably increases measures of well-being, self-esteem, and self-efficacy (Fillipas, Oldmeadow, Bailey, & Cherry, 2006; Hughes et al., 2010; Muller et al., 2008). These positive psychological states are negatively correlated with substance use (Ellickson & Hays, 1991; Griffin, Scheier, Botvin, & Diaz, 2001; Zamboanga, Schwartz, Jarvis, & Van Tyne, 2009), and may offer protection against developing a substance use disorder. In addition to these mechanisms, exercise also produces functional adaptations in the central nervous system that may leave an individual less susceptible to developing compulsive patterns of drug intake. Although research into this latter area is still in its infancy, a growing number of studies reveal that many signaling molecules that mediate drug-seeking behavior are modulated by physical activity.

Dopamine

The mesolimbic reward pathway, which includes dopaminergic (DAergic) projections from the ventral tegmental area (VTA) to the nucleus accumbens (NAc) and prefrontal cortex (PFC), is believed to play a critical role in addiction, with results from numerous studies showing that many drugs of abuse, including cocaine, amphetamine, nicotine, alcohol, and opioids, increase extracellular DA in the NAc (Leshner & Koob, 1999). Five dopamine receptors, D1–D5, have been identified and further classified into two receptor subtypes: the D1 class, which includes the D1 and the D5 receptor subtypes, and the D2 class, which includes the D2, D3, and D4 receptor subtypes. The D1 class of receptors couple with stimulatory G proteins, which activate 3'–5'-cyclic adenosine monophosphate (cAMP) and protein kinase A (PKA), whereas the D2 class of receptors couple with inhibitory G proteins and have the opposite effects on cAMP and PKA. Pharmacological manipulation of DA via either D1 or D2 receptor blockade in the NAc is known to modulate responding for drugs of abuse, including cocaine, alcohol, and heroin (Cornish, Lontos, Clemens, & McGregor, 2005; Hodge, Samson, & Chappelle, 1997; McGregor & Roberts, 1993; Robledo, Maldonado-Lopez, & Koob, 1992). Evidence also suggests that enhanced DA signaling is involved in drug-seeking behavior. The neurobiology is best described for reinstatement of cocaine-seeking behavior, and results show that both D1 and D2 receptors play a critical role. Systemic pretreatment with D2 receptor antagonists inhibits cocaine-seeking behavior (Schenk & Gittings, 2003), whereas systemic pretreatment with D2 receptor agonists reinstates responding and potentiates cocaine-primed reinstatement (Self, Barnhart, Lehman, & Nestler, 1996). Systemic pretreatment with D1 receptor antagonists blocks reinstatement, and systemic pretreatment with D1 receptor agonists produces similar effects (Self et al., 1996). Fewer studies have examined the role of D1 and D2 receptor signaling for other drugs, but the available results for heroin (Bossert, Poles, Wihbey, Koya, & Shaham 2007; Shaham & Stewart, 1996), nicotine (Liu et al., 2010), and alcohol (Chaudhri, Sahuque, & Janak, 2009; Liu & Weiss, 2002) are similar to the results obtained with cocaine, suggesting that DAergic signaling is critically involved in mediating drug seeking and relapse for many drugs of abuse.

Exercise impacts DAergic signaling under many experimental conditions. For example, exercise increases the transport of calcium into the brain where it activates the synthesis of DA (Sutoo & Akiyama, 1996). Exercise also increases mRNA levels of tyrosine hydroxylase, the rate-limiting enzyme in DA synthesis, in the VTA and other brain regions (Greenwood et al., 2011). Exercise increases DA concentrations in numerous brain regions (Dishman, 1997), with recent evidence showing that animals selectively bred for high rates of wheel running have higher basal and exercise-induced concentrations of DA and DA metabolites and lower DA turnover in the NAc and striatum as compared with controls (Mathes et al., 2010). Exercise also normalizes DAergic signaling in the striatum and NAc of animals that have abnormally low levels of dopamine (e.g., epileptic mice, spontaneously hypertensive rats) by facilitating calcium/calmodulin-dependent DA synthesis (Sutoo & Akiyama, 2003). At the receptor level, chronic exercise, like chronic exposure to drugs of abuse, downregulates DA D2 receptors, with recent evidence showing that DA D2 receptor mRNA is reduced in the NAc of rats following chronic voluntary exercise (Greenwood et al., 2011). Similarly, transcripts encoding for both the D1 and D2 receptor genes are downregulated in the striatum of mice bred for high levels of running as compared with controls (Mathes et al., 2010). Recent data also indicate that pre-exposure to aerobic exercise blocks methamphetamine-induced conditioned place preference (Chen et al., 2008), methamphetamine-induced increases in DA release in the NAc (Chen et al., 2008), and amphetamine-induced DA release in the striatum (Marques et al., 2008). Collectively, these data show that exercise affects DA levels, synthesis, and metabolism, as well as DA receptor-mediated signaling. These data also suggest that exercise may interact with the reward pathway by serving as a substitute for drug reward, and may protect against drug relapse by countering neuro-adaptations in DAergic signaling that develop following chronic drug exposure.

Glutamate

Glutamate is the main excitatory neurotransmitter in the NAc, and it activates two ionotropic receptors: the N-methyl-D-aspartate (NMDA) receptor and the alpha-amino-3-hydroxy-5-methyl-4-isoxazole-propionic acid (AMPA) receptor. Although acute exposure to drugs of abuse does not generally alter glutamate release in the NAc, repeated administration decreases basal levels of glutamate and increases glutamate in response to subsequent drug exposure, suggesting that its role in mediating the reinforcing effects of drugs may become greater with repeated exposure (Schmidt & Pierce, 2010). Numerous studies have shown that chronic drug exposure produces long-lasting adaptations in glutamate receptors, including NMDA and AMPA receptors in the NAc and PFC of humans, non-human primates, and rats (Acosta et al., 2010; Hemby et al., 2005; Tang, Wesley, Freeman, Liang, & Hemby, 2004), as well as long-term decreases in AMPA receptor signaling (Beurrier & Malenka, 2002). Based on such findings, it has been suggested that glutamatergic projections from the PFC to the NAc represent a final common pathway toward the generation of drug-seeking and relapse (Kalivas & Volkow, 2005). Evidence in support of this idea is supported by findings showing that glutamate is increased in the NAc in response to both drug primes and drug-associated cues (Kalivas & McFarland, 2003), and by results showing that glutamate receptor antagonism in the NAc, particularly via AMPA receptors, attenuates drug-seeking behavior (Bäckström & Hyytiä, 2007; Cornish, Duffy, & Kalivas, 1999). Together, these findings suggest that adaptations in glutamatergic signaling modulate drug use following chronic administration and subsequent drug-seeking behavior.

Although few studies have examined the effects of exercise on glutamatergic signaling in the reward pathway, results from numerous studies show that it can affect glutamate signaling in several different areas in the brain. Most of the results have been obtained from animal models of cerebral ischemia, which results from the excessive release of glutamate and overstimulation of glutamate receptors, with results showing that exercise can normalize glutamate levels and improve functioning. Within the striatum, exercise blocks the increase in glutamate caused by ischemic injury (Jia et al., 2009). This result is important because it suggests that exercise may protect against overstimulation of glutamatergic receptors, which also occurs following chronic drug exposure. In non-ischemic "normal" animals, chronic exercise increases extracellular glutamate concentrations (Chang, Yang, Wang, & Wang, 2009) and AMPA receptor density (Dietrich et al., 2005; Real, Ferreira, Hernandes, Britto, & Pires, 2010) in the striatum. Exercise also increases striatal fos expression (a marker of functional activity), and this effect can be blocked by concurrent activation of NMDA and D1 receptors (Liste, Guerra, Caruncho, & Labandeira-Garcia, 1997). These findings suggest that the effects of exercise on reinstatement may involve both DAergic and glutamatergic signaling.

Norepinephrine

Norepinephrine plays an important role in drug-seeking behavior, particularly in later transitional stages that involve relapse to drug use after a period of abstinence. Preclinical studies have reported that norepinephrine is important for both stress-induced and cocaine primed-reinstatement (Erb et al., 2000; Léri, Flores, Rodaros, & Stewart, 2002; Zhang & Kosten, 2005). Stress-induced reinstatement is mediated by activation of beta-adrenergic receptors in the amygdala and bed nucleus of the stria terminalis (Erb et al., 2000; Léri et al., 2002), whereas cocaine-primed reinstatement is mediated, in part, by activation of alpha1-adrenergic receptors (Zhang & Kosten, 2005). Exercise decreases norepinephrine release in the frontal cortex (Soares et al., 1999), which may serve to attenuate the effects of stress and cocaine in reinstatement procedures. The mechanism by which exercise influences noradrenergic activity is not fully known, but the peptide neurotransmitter galanin is believed to play a role. Galanin is co-localized with norepinephrine in locus coeruleus neurons, and there is extensive galaninergic innervation of limbic and forebrain areas (Holets, Hökfelt, Rökaeus, Terenius, & Goldstein, 1988; Melander, Staines, & Rökaeus, 1986; Xu, Shi, & Hökfelt, 1998). Activation of G protein-coupled galanin receptors inhibits the firing of locus coeruleus neurons (Ma et al., 2001; Pieribone et al., 1995) and potentiates the inhibitory effects of norepinephrine at presynaptic alpha-2 adrenergic autoreceptors (Ma et al., 2001). Importantly, physical activity increases galanin gene expression in locus coeruleus neurons (O'Neal, Van Hoomissen, Holmes, & Dishman, 2001; Van Hoomissen, Holmes, Zellner, Poudevigne, & Dishman, 2004), and exercise output is positively correlated with levels of prepro-galanin mRNA (Eisenstein & Holmes, 2007; Holmes, Yoo, & Dishman, 2006). Thus, galanin-mediated decreases in norepinephrine signaling may be one way in which exercise decreases drug-seeking behavior in reinstatement procedures.

Opioids

Exercise increases plasma concentrations of endogenous opioid peptides. Studies have consistently reported increases in the mu- and delta-receptor ligands, beta-endorphin, met-enkephalin, and leu-enkephalin (Art, Franchimont, & Lekeux, 1994; Chen, Zhao, Yue, & Wang, 2007; Debruille et al., 1999) and the kappa-receptor ligand, dynorphin (Aravich, Rieg, Lauterio, & Doerries, 1993; Fontana et al., 1994) following aerobic activity. The positive affective states produced by exercise are blocked by the opioid antagonist naloxone (Lett et al., 2001), indicating that these effects are mediated by opioid receptors. Long-term exercise produces alterations in opioid binding proteins (de Oliveira et al., 2010; Houghten, Pratt, Young, Brown, & Spann, 1986) and decreases sensitivity to exogenously administered opioid agonists (Kanarek, Gerstein, Wildman, Mathes, & D'Anci, 1998; Mathes and Kanarek, 2001; Smith & Lyle, 2006; Smith & Yancey, 2003). In drug self-administration studies, voluntary wheel running decreases heroin self-administration (Smith & Pitts, 2012) and forced exercise on a treadmill decreases morphine self-administration (Hosseini et al., 2009). Reductions in the positive reinforcing effects of heroin and other opioids are likely mediated by changes in central opioid receptor populations following chronic exercise. Changes in opioid receptor populations may also play a role in the ability of exercise to decrease the self-administration of other drugs. Studies have shown that the opioid receptor system plays an important modulatory role in the reinforcing effects of cocaine (Herz, 1998; Mello & Negus, 2000) and alcohol (Roberts et al., 2000, 2001; Walker, Zorrilla, & Koob, 2011), and the kappa opioid receptor system is critically involved in the escalation of cocaine intake under extended-access conditions (Wee & Koob, 2010). Release of endogenous opioid peptides may thus be one way exercise produces generalized protective effects on drug-seeking behavior across multiple pharmacological classes.

PKA

Chronic exercise and chronic exposure to drugs of abuse produce a number of changes in second-messenger signaling systems. For example, chronic cocaine upregulates D1-cyclic adenosine monophosphate (cAMP)-PKA signaling, and the reinforcing capacity of various D1 agonists is positively correlated with their ability to stimulate cAMP production (Weed, Paul, Dwoskin, Moore, & Woolverton, 1997). Direct activation of PKA increases the reinforcing effects of drugs of abuse such as cocaine (Lynch & Taylor, 2005, but see Self et al., 1998), whereas inhibition of PKA decreases both motivation for the drug and subsequent drug-seeking behavior (Lynch and Taylor, 2005; Sanchez, Quinn, Torregrossa, & Taylor, 2010). Upregulation of PKA has been reported following both chronic high-dose cocaine administration (Terwilliger, Beitner-Johnson, Sevarino, Crain, & Nestler, 1991) and extended-access cocaine self-administration (Lu, Grimm, Shaham, & Hope, 2003; Lynch, Kiraly, Caldarone, Picciotto, & Taylor, 2007), but not following less intense chronic cocaine-treatment protocols (e.g., Crawford, Choi, Kohutek, Yoshida, & McDougall, 2004). Exercise also influences DAergic signaling via second-messengers, with results showing that mice bred for high levels of running have lower levels of the transcripts encoding for several different adenylate cyclase subtypes and activating polypeptides in the striatum, as compared with controls (Mathes et al., 2010). Exercise also modulates intracellular signaling proteins associated with DA-mediated signaling, including dopamine- and cAMP-regulated neuronal phosphoprotein (DARPP-32) (Aguiar et al., 2010), a well-known target of PKA that is essential for drug reinforcement (Svenningsson, Nairn, & Greengard, 2005).

Extracellular signal-regulated kinase

Extracellular signal-regulated kinase (ERK) is a molecule that is a key mediator of synaptic plasticity and is modulated by both drugs of abuse and exercise. ERK, which requires coincident activation of DA D1 and glutamate NMDA receptors, is critically involved in drug craving and relapse (Thomas, Kalivas, & Shaham, 2008). Specifically, levels of ERK in the NAc and projection sites of the NAc, including the PFC and amygdala, are correlated with levels of drug seeking across several different drug classes, including cocaine (Edwards, Bachtell, Guzman, Whisler, & Self, 2011; Koya et al., 2009; Lu, Koya, Zhai, Hope, & Shaham, 2006; Lynch et al., 2010), alcohol (Schroeder et al., 2008), and morphine (Li et al., 2008). Furthermore, like levels of drug-seeking behavior, phosphorylated levels of ERK increase over an abstinence period (Edwards et al., 2011; Kim & Kim, 2008; Koya et al., 2009; Li et al., 2008; Lu et al., 2006). Although very little is known with regard to the effects of exercise on ERK signaling in the NAc or PFC, there is a large literature indicating regulation of ERK by exercise in other brain regions and in peripheral tissue (muscle, heart; e.g., Kojda & Hambrecht, 2005; Smith & Zigmond, 2003). ERK contributes to long-term potentiation and regulates various learning tasks such as conditioned place preference, and both exercise and exposure to cocaine-associated cues upregulate phosphorylated levels of ERK in the hippocampus (Muller et al., 2008). There is also evidence to suggest that ERK activation is critical for the beneficial effects of exercise on mood (Gourley et al., 2008), raising the possibility that exercise may counter dysphoric mood states associated with drug withdrawal. Finally, a recent study reported that exercise attenuates cocaine-seeking behavior and blocks the increase in phosphorylated levels of ERK associated with enhanced cocaine seeking (Lynch et al., 2010). These findings suggest that exercise may reduce relapse vulnerability by preventing the increase in cocaine craving and associated neuroadaptations in ERK signaling.

Brain-derived neurotrophic factor

Synaptic changes occurring via brain-derived neurotrophic factor (BDNF) have also been implicated in drug addiction and are modulated by exercise. BDNF is synthesized in VTA DA neurons and enhances both DAergic and glutamatergic signaling (Blöchl & Sirrenberg, 1996; Lessman, 1998). Levels of BDNF increase incrementally in the reward pathway (i.e., VTA, NAc, and amygdala) over an abstinence period and are associated with progressive increases in drug-seeking behavior (i.e., Grimm et al., 2003). Exercise elevates BDNF, and through epigenetic mechanisms can modulate the chromatin structure containing the BDNF gene (Gomez-Pinilla, Zhuang, Feng, Ying, & Fan, 2011). Given that long-term changes in synaptic plasticity involving BDNF are strongly implicated in drug addiction, it is possible that exercise may be able to normalize some of these synaptic changes and reduce subsequent relapse vulnerability.

Other molecules

Evidence supports the effects of exercise on other signaling pathways (e.g., gamma-aminobutyric acid (GABA), serotonin, endocannabinoid, cortisol), but fewer studies have examined such pathways in the context of both exercise and drug-seeking behavior. Research on these systems will continue to expand, and it is likely that this research will show that exercise influences these molecules in ways that impact drug self-administration. Importantly, receptor-specific ligands are already available in most instances, which should expedite research into their role in drug abuse, as well as their modulation by physical activity.

Conclusions

Recent research has revealed that many signaling molecules associated with compulsive patterns of drug intake are influenced by physical activity. These findings represent a significant advancement in our understanding of the neurobiological effects of exercise, and contribute greatly to our understanding of the neurobiology of substance abuse and dependence. Additional research is still needed to determine which of these various molecules are related causally to the protective effects of exercise on drug-seeking behavior. Studies that target individual proteins through site-specific antagonists, genetic knockouts/knockdowns, and antisense oligonucleotides should determine which neurotransmitters and intracellular signaling molecules are mediating this relationship. Future research in this area will aid in the development of behavioral and pharmacological interventions to prevent compulsive patterns of drug intake in at-risk populations, and to reduce or eliminate compulsive drug use in populations already diagnosed with a substance use disorder. Although research examining aerobic exercise and substance abuse is far from complete, a sufficient amount of preclinical data now exists to support the design and implementation of exercise-based interventions in substance-abusing populations.

Acknowledgments

This research was supported by grants from the National Institute on Drug Abuse (R01-DA024716-WJL; R01-DA024716-S1-WJL; R01-DA027485-MAS; R01DA031725-MAS) and the Virginia Youth Tobacco Projects Research Coalition (Darlene Brunzell, PI; WJL).

References

Acosta, G., Hasenkamp, W., Daunais, J.B., Friedman, D.P., Grant, K.A., & Hemby, S.E. (2010). Ethanol self-administration modulation of NMDA receptor subunit and related synaptic protein mRNA expression in prefrontal cortical fields in cynomolgus monkeys. *Brain Research, 1318*, 144–154. doi:10.1016/j.brainres.2009.12.050

Aguiar, A.S., Jr, Boemer, G., Rial, D., Cordova, F.M., Mancini, G., Walz, R., . . . Prediger, R.D. (2010). High-intensity physical exercise disrupts implicit memory in mice: Involvement of the striatal glutathione antioxidant system and intracellular signaling. *Neuroscience, 171*, 1216–1227. doi:10.1016/j.neuroscience.2010.09.053

Aravich, P.F., Rieg, T.S., Lauterio, T.J., & Doerries, L.E. (1993). Beta-endorphin and dynorphin abnormalities in rats subjected to exercise and restricted feeding: Relationship to anorexia nervosa. *Brain Research, 622*, 1–8. doi:10.1016/0006-8993(93)90794-N

Art, T., Franchimont, P., & Lekeux, P. (1994). Plasma beta-endorphin response of thoroughbred horses to maximal exercise. *Veterinary Record, 135*, 499–503.

Bäckström, P., & Hyytiä, P. (2007). Involvement of AMPA/kainate, NMDA, and mGlu5 receptors in the nucleus accumbens core in cue-induced reinstatement of cocaine seeking in rats. *Psychopharmacology 192*, 571–580. doi:10.1007/s00213-007-0753-8

Belke, T.W. (1997). Running and responding reinforced by the opportunity to run: Effect of reinforcer duration. *Journal of the Experimental Analysis of Behavior, 67*, 337–351. doi:10.1901/jeab.1997.67-337

Belke, T.W. (2000). Varying wheel-running reinforcer duration within a session: Effect on the revolution-postreinforcement pause relation. *Journal of the Experimental Analysis of Behavior, 73*, 225–239. doi:10.1901/jeab.2000.73-225

Belke, T.W., & Dunbar, M.J. (2001). Effects of cocaine on fixed-interval responding reinforced by the opportunity to run. *Journal of the Experimental Analysis of Behavior, 75*, 77–91. doi:10.1901/jeab.2001.75-77

Belke, T.W., & Wagner, J.P. (2005). The reinforcing property and the rewarding aftereffect of wheel running in rats: A combination of two paradigms. *Behavioral Processes, 68*, 165–172. doi:10.1016/j.beproc.2004.12.006

Beurrier, C., & Malenka, R.C. (2002). Enhanced inhibition of synaptic transmission by dopamine in the nucleus accumbens during behavioral sensitization to cocaine. *Journal of Neuroscience, 22*, 5817–5822.

Blöchl, A., & Sirrenberg, C. (1996). Neurotrophins stimulate the release of dopamine from rat mesencephalic neurons via Trk and p75(Lntr) receptors. *Journal of Biological Chemistry, 271*, 21100–21107.

Bossert, J.M., Poles, G.C., Wihbey, K.A., Koya, E., & Shaham, Y. (2007). Differential effects of blockade of dopamine D1-family receptors in nucleus accumbens core or shell on reinstatement of heroin seeking induced by contextual and discrete cues. *Journal of Neuroscience, 27*, 12655–12663. doi:10.1523/JNEUROSCI.3926-07.2007

Castle, D.J. (2008). Anxiety and substance use: Layers of complexity. *Expert Review of Neurotherapeutics, 8*, 493–501. doi:10.1586/14737175.8.3.493

Chang, H.C., Yang, Y.R., Wang, S.G., & Wang, R.Y. (2009). Effects of treadmill training on motor performance and extracellular glutamate level in striatum in rats with or without transient middle cerebral artery occlusion. *Behavioural Brain Research, 205*, 450–455. doi:10.1016/j.bbr.2009.07.033

Chaudhri, N., Sahuque, L.L., & Janak, P.H. (2009). Ethanol seeking triggered by environmental context is attenuated by blocking dopamine D1 receptors in the nucleus accumbens core and shell in rats. *Psychopharmacology, 207*, 303–314. doi:10.1007/s00213-009-1657-6

Chen, H.I., Kuo, Y.M., Liao, C.H., Jen, C.J., Huang, A.M., Cherng, C.G., . . . Yu, L. (2008). Long-term compulsive exercise reduces the rewarding efficacy of 3,4-methylenedioxymethamphetamine. *Behavioural Brain Research, 187*, 185–189. doi:10.1016/j.bbr.2007.09.014

Chen, J.X., Zhao, X., Yue, G.X., & Wang, Z.F. (2007). Influence of acute and chronic treadmill exercise on rat plasma lactate and brain NPY, L-ENK, DYN A1-13. *Cellular and Molecular Neurobiology, 27*, 1–10. doi:10.1007/s10571-006-9110-4

Cornish, J.L., Duffy, P., & Kalivas, P.W. (1999). A role for nucleus accumbens glutamate transmission in the relapse to cocaine-seeking behavior. *Neuroscience, 93*, 1359–1367. doi:10.1016/S0306-4522(99)00214-6

Cornish, J.L., Lontos, J.M., Clemens, K.J., & McGregor, I.S. (2005). Cocaine and heroin ("speedball") self-administration: The involvement of nucleus accumbens dopamine and mu-opiate, but not delta-opiate receptors. *Psychopharmacology, 180*, 21–32. doi:10.1007/s00213-004-2135-9

Cosgrove, K.P., Hunter, R.G., & Carroll, M.E. (2002). Wheel-running attenuates intravenous cocaine self-administration in rats: Sex differences. *Pharmacology Biochemistry and Behavior, 73*, 663–671. doi:10.1016/S0091-3057(02)00853-5

Crawford, C.A., Choi, F.Y., Kohutek, J.L., Yoshida, S.T., & McDougall, S.A. (2004). Changes in PKA activity and Gs alpha and Golf alpha levels after amphetamine- and cocaine-induced behavioral sensitization. *Synapse, 51*, 241–248. doi:10.1002/syn.10301

Crews, F.T., Nixon, K., & Wilkie, M.E. (2004). Exercise reverses ethanol inhibition of neural stem cell proliferation. *Alcohol, 33*, 63–71. doi:10.1016/S0741-8329(04)00081-3

de Oliveira, M.S., da Silva Fernandes, M.J., Scorza, F.A., Persike, D.S., Scorza, C.A., da Ponte, J.B., . . . Arida, R.M. (2010). Acute and chronic exercise modulates the expression of MOR opioid receptors in the hippocampal formation of rats. *Brain Research Bulletin, 83*, 278–283. doi:10.1016/j.brainresbull. 2010.07.009

Debruille, C., Luyckx, M., Ballester, L., Brunet, C., Odou, P., Dine, T., . . . Cazin, J.C. (1999). Serum opioid activity after physical exercise in rats. *Physiological Research, 48*, 129–133.

Dietrich, M.O., Mantese, C.E., Porciuncula, L.O., Ghisleni, G., Vinade, L., Souza, D.O., & Portela, L.V. (2005). Exercise affects glutamate receptors in postsynaptic densities from cortical mice brain. *Brain Research, 1065*, 20–25. doi:10.1016/j.brainres.2005.09.038

Dishman, R.K. (1997). Brain monoamines, exercise, and behavioral stress: Animal models. *Medicine and Science in Sports and Exercise, 29*, 63–74. doi:10.1097/00005768-199701000-00010

Edwards, S., Bachtell, R.K., Guzman, D., Whisler, K.N., & Self, D.W. (2011). Emergence of context-associated GluR(1) and ERK phosphorylation in the nucleus accumbens core during withdrawal from cocaine self-administration. *Addiction Biology, 16*, 450–455. doi:10.1111/j.1369-1600.2010.00291.x

Ehringer, M.A., Hoft, N.R., & Zunhammer, M. (2009). Reduced alcohol consumption in mice with access to a running wheel. *Alcohol, 43*, 443–452. doi:10.1016/j.alcohol.2009.06.003

Eisenstein, S.A., & Holmes, P.V. (2007). Chronic and voluntary exercise enhances learning of conditioned place preference to morphine in rats. *Pharmacology Biochemistry and Behavior, 86*, 607–615. doi:10.1016/ j.pbb.2007.02.002

Ellickson, P.L., & Hays, R.D. (1991). Beliefs about resistance self-efficacy and drug prevalence: Do they really affect drug use? *International Journal of the Addiction, 25*, 1353–1378.

Erb, S., Hitchcott, P.K., Rajabi, H., Mueller, D., Shaham, Y., & Stewart, J. (2000). Alpha-2 adrenergic receptor agonists block stress-induced reinstatement of cocaine seeking. *Neuropsychopharmacology, 23*, 138–150. doi:10.1016/S0893-133X(99)00158-X

Fillipas, S., Oldmeadow, L.B., Bailey, M.J., & Cherry, C.L. (2006). A six-month, supervised, aerobic and resistance exercise program improves self-efficacy in people with human immunodeficiency virus: A randomised controlled trial. *Australian Journal of Physiotherapy, 52*, 185–190.

Fontana, F., Bernardi, P., Merlo Pich, E., Boschi, S., De Iasio, R., Capelli, M., . . . Spampinato, S. (1994). Endogenous opioid system and atrial natriuretic factor in normotensive offspring of hypertensive parents at rest and during exercise test. *Journal of Hypertension, 12*, 1285–1290.

Gomez-Pinilla, F., Zhuang, Y., Feng, J., Ying, Z., & Fan, G. (2011). Exercise impacts brain-derived neurotrophic factor plasticity by engaging mechanisms of epigenetic regulation. *European Journal of Neuroscience, 33*, 383–390. doi:10.1111/j.1460-9568.2010.07508.x

Gourley, S.L., Wu, F.J., Kiraly, D.D., Ploski, J.E., Kedves, A.T., Duman, R.S., & Taylor, J.R. (2008). Regionally specific regulation of ERK MAP kinase in a model of antidepressant-sensitive chronic depression. *Biological Psychiatry, 63*, 353–359. doi:10.1016/j.biopsych.2007.07.016

Greenwood, B.N., Foley, T.E., Le, T.V., Strong, P.V., Loughridge, A.B., Day, H.E., & Fleshner, M. (2011). Long-term voluntary wheel running is rewarding and produces plasticity in the mesolimbic reward pathway. *Behavioural Brain Research, 217*, 354–362. doi:10.1016/j.bbr.2010.11.005

Griffin, K.W., Scheier, L.M., Botvin, G.J., & Diaz, T. (2001). Protective role of personal competence skills in adolescent substance use: Psychological well-being as a mediating factor. *Psychology of Addictive Behaviors, 15*, 194–203. doi:10.1037//0893-164X.15.3.194

Grimm, J.W., Lu, L., Hayashi, T., Hope, B.T., Su, T.P., & Shaham, Y. (2003). Time-dependent increases in brain-derived neurotrophic factor protein levels within the mesolimbic dopamine system after withdrawal from cocaine: Implications for incubation of cocaine craving. *Journal of Neuroscience, 23*, 742–747.

Hemby, S.E., Tang, W., Muly, E.C., Kuhar, M.J., Howell, L., & Mash, D.C. (2005). Cocaine-induced alterations in nucleus accumbens ionotropic glutamate receptor subunits in human and non-human primates. *Journal of Neurochemistry, 95*, 1785–1793. doi:10.1111/j.1471-4159.2005.03517.x

Herring, M.P., O'Connor, P.J., & Dishman, R.K. (2010). The effect of exercise training on anxiety symptoms among patients: A systematic review. *Archives of Internal Medicine, 170*, 321–331.

Herz, A. (1998). Opioid reward mechanisms: A key role in drug abuse? *Canadian Journal of Physiology and Pharmacology, 76*, 252–258. doi:10.1139/cjpp-76-3-252

Hodge, C.W., Samson, H.H., & Chappelle, A.M. (1997). Alcohol self-administration: Further examination of the role of dopamine receptors in the nucleus accumbens. *Alcoholism-Clinical and Experimental Research, 21*, 1083–1091. doi:10.1111/j.1530-0277.1997.tb04257.x

Holets, V.R., Hökfelt, T., Rökaeus, A., Terenius, L., & Goldstein, M. (1988). Locus coeruleus neurons in the rat containing neuropeptide Y, tyrosine hydroxylase or galanin and their efferent projections to the spinal cord, cerebral cortex and hypothalamus. *Neuroscience, 24*, 893–906. doi:10.1016/0306-4522(88)90076-0

Holmes, P.V., Yoo, H.S., & Dishman, R.K. (2006). Voluntary exercise and clomipramine treatment elevate prepro-galanin mRNA levels in the locus coeruleus in rats. *Neuroscience Letters, 408*, 1–4. doi:10.1016/j.neulet.2006.04.057

Hosseini, M., Alaei, H.A., Naderi, A., Sharifi, M.R., & Zahed, R. (2009). Treadmill exercise reduces self-administration of morphine in male rats. *Pathophysiology, 16*, 3–7. doi:10.1016/j.pathophys.2008.11.001

Houghten, R.A., Pratt, S.M., Young, E.A., Brown, H., & Spann, D.R. (1986). Effect of chronic exercise on beta-endorphin receptor levels in rats. *NIDA Research Monographs, 75*, 505–508.

Hughes, D., Baum, G., Jovanovic, J., Carmack, C., Greisinger, A., & Basen-Engquist, K. (2010). An acute exercise session increases self-efficacy in sedentary endometrial cancer survivors and controls. *Journal of Physical Activity and Health, 7*, 784–793.

Iversen, I.H. (1993). Techniques for establishing schedules with wheel running as reinforcement in rats. *Journal of the Experimental Analysis of Behavior, 60*, 219–238. doi:10.1901/jeab.1993.60-219

Janal, M.N., Colt, E.W., Clark, W.C., & Glusman, M. (1984). Pain sensitivity, mood and plasma endocrine levels in man following long-distance running: Effects of naloxone. *Pain, 19*, 13–25. doi:10.1016/0304-3959(84)90061-7

Jia, J., Hu, Y.S., Wu, Y., Liu, G., Yu, H.X., Zheng, Q.P., . . . Cao, Z.J. (2009). Pre-ischemic treadmill training affects glutamate and gamma aminobutyric acid levels in the striatal dialysate of a rat model of cerebral ischemia. *Life Sciences, 84*, 505–511. doi:10.1016/j.lfs.2009.01.015

Kalivas, P.W., & McFarland, K. (2003). Brain circuitry and the reinstatement of cocaine-seeking behavior. *Psychopharmacology, 168*, 44–56. doi:10.1007/s00213-003-1393-2

Kalivas, P.W., & Volkow, N.D. (2005). The neural basis of addiction: A pathology of motivation and choice. *American Journal of Psychiatry, 162*, 1403–1413. doi:10.1176/appi.ajp.162.8.1403

Kanarek, R.B., Gerstein, A.V., Wildman, R.P., Mathes, W.F., & D'Anci, K.E. (1998). Chronic running-wheel activity decreases sensitivity to morphine-induced analgesia in male and female rats. *Pharmacology Biochemistry and Behavior, 61*, 19–27. doi:10.1016/S0091-3057(98)00059-8

Kim, S., & Kim, J.H. (2008). Time-dependent change of ERK phosphorylation levels in the nucleus accumbens during withdrawals from repeated cocaine. *Neuroscience Letters, 436*, 107–110. doi:10.1016/j.neulet.2008.02.068

Kojda, G., & Hambrecht, R. (2005). Molecular mechanisms of vascular adaptations to exercise. Physical activity as an effective antioxidant therapy? *Cardiovascular Research, 67*, 187–197. doi:10.1016/j.cardiores.2005.04.032

Koya, E., Uejima, J.L., Wihbey, K.A., Bossert, J.M., Hope, B.T., & Shaham, Y. (2009). Role of ventral medial prefrontal cortex in incubation of cocaine craving. *Neuropharmacology, 56*, 177–185. doi:10.1016/j.neuropharm.2008.04.022

Leri, F., Flores, J., Rodaros, D., & Stewart, J. (2002). Blockade of stress-induced but not cocaine-induced reinstatement by infusion of noradrenergic antagonists into the bed nucleus of the stria terminalis or the central nucleus of the amygdala. *Journal of Neuroscience, 22*, 5713–5718.

Leshner, A.I., & Koob, G.F. (1999). Drugs of abuse and the brain. *Proceedings of the Association of American Physicians, 111*, 99–108. doi:10.1046/j.1525-1381.1999.09218.x

Lessmann, V. (1998). Neurotrophin-dependent modulation of glutamatergic synaptic transmission in the mammalian CNS. *General Pharmacology, 31*, 667–674.

Lett, B.T., Grant, V.L., Byrne, M.J., & Koh, M.T. (2000). Pairings of a distinctive chamber with the aftereffect of wheel running produce conditioned place preference. *Appetite, 34*, 87–94. doi:10.1006/appe.1999.0274

Lett, B.T., Grant, V.L., & Koh, M.T. (2001). Naloxone attenuates the conditioned place preference induced by wheel running in rats. *Physiology and Behavior, 72*, 355–358. doi:10.1016/S0031-9384(00)00427-3

Li, Y.Q., Li, F.Q., Wang, X.Y., Wu, P., Zhao, M., Xu, C.M., . . . Lu, L. (2008). Central amygdala extracellular signal-regulated kinase signaling pathway is critical to incubation of opiate craving. *Journal of Neuroscience, 28*, 13248–13257. doi:10.1523/JNEUROSCI.3027-08.2008

Liste, I., Guerra, M.J., Caruncho, H.J., & Labandeira-Garcia, J.L. (1997). Treadmill running induces striatal Fos expression via NMDA glutamate and dopamine receptors. *Experimental Brain Research, 115*, 458–468. doi:10.1007/PL00005715

Liu, X., Jernigen, C., Gharib, M., Booth, S., Caggiula, A.R., & Sved, A.F. (2010). Effects of dopamine antagonists on drug cue-induced reinstatement of nicotine-seeking behavior in rats. *Behavioural Pharmacology, 21*, 153–160. doi:10.1097/FBP.0b013e328337be95

Liu, X., & Weiss, F. (2002). Reversal of ethanol-seeking behavior by D1 and D2 antagonists in an animal model of relapse: Differences in antagonist potency in previously ethanol-dependent versus nondependent rats. *Journal of Pharmacology and Experimental Therapeutics, 300*, 882–889. doi:10.1124/jpet.300.3.882

Lu, L., Grimm, J.W., Shaham, Y., & Hope, B.T. (2003). Molecular neuroadaptations in the accumbens and ventral tegmental area during the first 90 days of forced abstinence from cocaine self-administration in rats. *Journal of Neurochemistry, 85*, 1604–1613. doi:10.1046/j.1471-4159.2003.01824.x

Lu, L., Koya, E., Zhai, H., Hope, B.T., & Shaham, Y. (2006). Role of ERK in cocaine addiction. *Trends in Neurosciences, 29*, 695–703. doi:10.1016/j.tins.2006.10.005

Lynch, W.J., Kiraly, D.D., Caldarone, B.J., Picciotto, M.R., & Taylor, J.R. (2007). Effect of cocaine self-administration on striatal PKA-regulated signaling in male and female rats. *Psychopharmacology, 191*, 263–271. doi:10.1007/s00213-006-0656-0

Lynch, W.J., Piehl, K.B., Acosta, G., Peterson, A.B., & Hemby, S.E. (2010). Aerobic exercise attenuates reinstatement of cocaine-seeking behavior and associated neuroadaptations in the prefrontal cortex. *Biological Psychiatry, 68*, 774–777. doi:10.1016/j.biopsych.2010.06.022

Lynch, W.J., & Taylor, J.R. (2005). Persistent changes in motivation to self-administer cocaine following modulation of cyclic AMP-dependent protein kinase A (PKA) activity in the nucleus accumbens. *European Journal of Neuroscience, 22*, 1214–1220. doi:10.1111/j.1460-9568.2005.04305.x

Ma, X., Tong, Y.G., Schmidt, R., Brown, W., Payza, K., Hodzic, L., . . . Xu, Z.Q. (2001). Effects of galanin receptor agonists on locus coeruleus neurons. *Brain Research, 919*, 169–174. doi:10.1016/S0006-8993(01)03033-5

Marques, E., Vasconcelos, F., Rolo, M.R., Pereira, F.C., Silva, A.P., Macedo, T.R., & Ribeiro, C.F. (2008). Influence of chronic exercise on the amphetamine-induced dopamine release and neurodegeneration in the striatum of the rat. *Annals of the New York Academy of Sciences, 1139*, 222–231. doi:10.1196/annals.1432.041

Mathes, W.F., & Kanarek, R.B. (2001). Wheel running attenuates the antinociceptive properties of morphine and its metabolite, morphine-6-glucuronide, in rats. *Physiology and Behavior, 74*, 245–251. doi:10.1016/S0031-9384(01)00577-7

Mathes, W.F., Nehrenberg, D.L., Gordon, R., Hua, K., Garland, T., Jr., & Pomp, D. (2010). Dopaminergic dysregulation in mice selectively bred for excessive exercise or obesity. *Behavioural Brain Research, 210*, 155–163. doi:10.1016/j.bbr.2010.02.016

McGregor, A., & Roberts, D.C. (1993). Dopaminergic antagonism within the nucleus accumbens or the amygdala produces differential effects on intravenous cocaine self-administration under fixed and progressive ratio schedules of reinforcement. *Brain Research, 624*, 245–252. doi:10.1016/0006-8993(93)90084-Z

McMillan, D.E., McClure, G.Y., & Hardwick, W.C. (1995). Effects of access to a running wheel on food, water and ethanol intake in rats bred to accept ethanol. *Drug and Alcohol Dependence, 40*, 1–7. doi:10.1016/0376-8716(95)01162-5

Melander, T., Staines, W.A., & Rökaeus, A. (1986). Galanin-like immunoreactivity in hippocampal afferents in the rat, with special reference to cholinergic and noradrenergic inputs. *Neuroscience, 19*, 223–240. doi:10.1016/0306-4522(86)90017-5

Mello, N.K., & Negus, S.S. (2000). Interactions between kappa opioid agonists and cocaine – Preclinical studies. *Annals of the New York Academy of Sciences, 909*, 104–132.

Miller, M.L., Vaillancourt, B.D., Wright, M.J., Jr, Aarde, S.M., Vandewater, S.A., Creehan, K.M., & Taffe, M.A. (2011). Reciprocal inhibitory effects of intravenous d-methamphetamine self-administration and wheel activity in rats. *Drug and Alcohol Dependence.* Advance Online Publication. doi:10.1016/j.drugalcdep.2011.08.013

Muller, A.P., Cammarota, M., Dietrich, M.O., Rotta, L.N., Portela, L.V., Souza, D.O., . . . Perry, M.L. (2008). Different effect of high fat diet and physical exercise in the hippocampal signaling. *Neurochemical Research, 33*, 880–885. doi:10.1007/s11064-007-9530-7

Nabetani, T., & Tokunaga, M. (2001). The effect of short-term (10- and 15-min) running at self-selected intensity on mood alteration. *Journal of Physiological Anthropology and Applied Human Science, 20*, 231–239. doi:10.2114/jpa.20.233

O'Neal, H.A., Van Hoomissen, J.D., Holmes, P.V., & Dishman, R.K. (2001). Prepro-galanin messenger RNA levels are increased in rat locus coeruleus after treadmill exercise training. *Neuroscience Letters, 299*, 69–72. doi:10.1016/S0304-3940(00)01780-8

Ozburn, A.R., Harris, R.A., & Blednov, Y.A. (2008). Wheel running, voluntary ethanol consumption, and hedonic substitution. *Alcohol, 42*, 417–424. doi:10.1016/j.alcohol.2008.04.006

Perraton, L.G., Kumar, S., & Machotka, Z. (2010). Exercise parameters in the treatment of clinical depression: A systematic review of randomized controlled trials. *Journal of Evaluation in Clinical Practice, 16*, 597–604. doi:10.1111/j.1365-2753.2009.01188.x

Pieribone, V.A., Xu, Z.Q., Zhang, X., Grillner, S., Bartfai, T., & Hökfelt, T. (1995). Galanin induces a hyperpolarization of norepinephrine-containing locus coeruleus neurons in the brainstem slice. *Neuroscience, 64*, 861–874. doi:10.1016/0306-4522(94)00450-J

Real, C.C., Ferreira, A.F., Hernandes, M.S., Britto, L.R., & Pires, R.S. (2010). Exercise-induced plasticity of AMPA-type glutamate receptor subunits in the rat brain. *Brain Research, 1363*, 63–71. doi:10.1016/j.brainres.2010.09.060

Roberts, A.J., Gold, L.H., Polis, I., McDonald, J.S., Filliol, D., Kieffer, B.L., & Koob, G.F. (2001). Increased ethanol self-administration in delta-opioid receptor knockout mice. *Alcoholism-Clinical and Experimental Research, 25*, 1249–1256. doi:10.1097/00000374-200109000-00002

Roberts, A.J., McDonald, J.S., Heyser, C.J., Kieffer, B.L., Matthes, H.W., Koob, G.F., & Gold, L.H. (2000). Mu-Opioid receptor knockout mice do not self-administer alcohol. *Journal of Pharmacology and Experimental Therapeutics, 293*, 1002–1008.

Robledo, P., Maldonado-Lopez, R., & Koob, G.F. (1992). Role of dopamine receptors in the nucleus accumbens in the rewarding properties of cocaine. *Annals of the New York Academy of Sciences, 654*, 509–512. doi:10.1111/j.1749-6632.1992.tb26015.x

Sanchez, H., Quinn, J.J., Torregrossa, M.M., & Taylor, J.R. (2010). Reconsolidation of a cocaine-associated stimulus requires amygdalar protein kinase A. *Journal of Neuroscience, 30*, 4401–4407. doi:10.1523/JNEUROSCI.3149-09.2010

Schebendach, J.E., Klein, D.A., Foltin, R.W., Devlin, M.J., & Walsh, B.T. (2007). Relative reinforcing value of exercise in inpatients with anorexia nervosa: Model development and pilot data. *International Journal of Eating Disorders, 40*, 446–453. doi:10.1002/eat.20392

Schenk, S., & Gittings, D. (2003). Effects of SCH 23390 and eticlopride on cocaine-seeking produced by cocaine and WIN 35,428 in rats. *Psychopharmacology, 168*, 118–123. doi:10.1007/s00213-002-1276-y

Schmidt, H.D., & Pierce, R.C. (2010). Cocaine-induced neuroadaptations in glutamate transmission: Potential therapeutic targets for craving and addiction. *Annals of the New York Academy of Sciences, 1187*, 35–75. doi:10.1111/j.1749-6632.2009.05144.x

Schroeder, J.P., Spanos, M., Stevenson, J.R., Besheer, J., Salling, M., & Hodge, C.W. (2008). Cue-induced reinstatement of alcohol-seeking behavior is associated with increased ERK1/2 phosphorylation in specific limbic brain regions: Blockade by the mGluR5 antagonist MPEP. *Neuropharmacology, 55*, 546–554. doi:10.1016/j.neuropharm.2008.06.057

Self, D.W., Barnhart, W.J., Lehman, D.A., & Nestler, E.J. (1996). Opposite modulation of cocaine-seeking behavior by D1- and D2-like dopamine receptor agonists. *Science, 271*, 1586–1589. doi:10.1126/science.271.5255.1586

Self, D.W., Genova, L.M., Hope, B.T., Barnhart, W.J., Spencer, J.J., & Nestler, E.J. (1998). Involvement of cAMP-dependent protein kinase in the nucleus accumbens in cocaine self-administration and relapse of cocaine-seeking behavior. *Journal of Neuroscience, 18*, 1848–1859.

Shaham, Y., & Stewart, J. (1996). Effects of opioid and dopamine receptor antagonists on relapse induced by stress and re-exposure to heroin in rats. *Psychopharmacology, 125*, 385–391. doi:10.1007/BF02246022

Smith, A.D., & Zigmond, M.J. (2003). Can the brain be protected through exercise? Lessons from an animal model of Parkinsonism. *Experimental Neurology, 184*, 31–39. doi:10.1016/j.expneurol.2003.08.017

Smith, M.A., & Lyle, M.A. (2006). Chronic exercise decreases sensitivity to mu opioids in female rats: Correlation with exercise output. *Pharmacology Biochemistry and Behavior, 85*, 12–22. doi:10.1016/j.pbb.2006.06.020

Smith, M.A., Pennock, M.M., & Walker, K.L. (2011). Access to a running wheel decreases cocaine-primed and cue-induced reinstatement in male and female rats. *Drug and Alcohol Dependence, 121*, 54–61. doi:10.1016/j.drugalcdep.2011.08.006

Smith, M.A. & Pitts, E.G. (2011). Access to a running wheel inhibits the acquisition of cocaine self-administration. *Pharmacology Biochemistry and Behavior, 100,* 237–243. doi:10.1016/j.pbb.2011.08.025

Smith, M.A. & Pitts, E.G. (2012). Wheel running decreases the positive reinforcing effects of heroin. *Pharmacological Reports, 64,* 960–964.

Smith, M.A., Schmidt, K.T., Iordanou, J.C., & Mustroph, M.L. (2008). Aerobic exercise decreases the positive-reinforcing effects of cocaine. *Drug and Alcohol Dependence, 98,* 129–135. doi:10.1016/j.drugalcdep.2008.05.006

Smith, M.A., Walker, K.L., Cole, K.T., & Lang, K.C. (2011). The effects of aerobic exercise on cocaine self-administration in male and female rats. *Psychopharmacology, 218,* 357–369. doi:10.1007/s00213-011-2321-5

Smith, M.A., & Yancey, D.L. (2003). Sensitivity to the effects of opioids in rats with free access to exercise wheels: Mu opioid tolerance and physical dependence. *Psychopharmacology, 167,* 426–434. doi:10.1007/s00213-003-1471-5

Soares, J., Holmes, P.V., Renner, K.J., Edwards, G.L., Bunnell, B.N., & Dishman, R.K. (1999). Brain noradrenergic responses to footshock after chronic activity-wheel running. *Behavioral Neuroscience, 113,* 558–566. doi:10.1037//0735-7044.113.3.558

Sutoo, D.E., & Akiyama, K. (1996). The mechanism by which exercise modifies brain function. *Physiology and Behavior, 60,* 177–181. doi:10.1016/0031-9384(96)00011-X

Sutoo, D., & Akiyama, K. (2003). Regulation of brain function by exercise. *Neurobiology of Disease, 13,* 1–14. doi:10.1016/S0969-9961(03)00030-5

Svenningsson, P., Nairn, A.C., & Greengard, P. (2005). DARPP-32 mediates the actions of multiple drugs of abuse. *AAPS Journal, 7,* E353–E360.

Swendsen, J.D., & Merikangas, K.R. (2000). The comorbidity of depression and substance use disorders. *Clinical Psychology Review, 20,* 173–189. doi:10.1016/S0272-7358(99)00026-4

Tang, W., Wesley, M., Freeman, W.M., Liang, B., & Hemby, S.E. (2004). Alterations in ionotropic glutamate receptor subunits during binge cocaine self-administration and withdrawal in rats. *J Neurochemistry, 89,* 1021–1033. doi:10.1111/j.1471-4159.2004.02392.x

Terwilliger, R.Z., Beitner-Johnson, D., Sevarino, K.A., Crain, S.M., & Nestler, E.J. (1991). A general role for adaptations in G-proteins and the cyclic AMP system in mediating the chronic actions of morphine and cocaine on neuronal function. *Brain Research, 548,* 100–110. doi:10.1016/0006-8993(91)91111-D

Thomas, M.J., Kalivas, P.W., & Shaham, Y. (2008). Neuroplasticity in the mesolimbic dopamine system and cocaine addiction. *British Journal of Pharmacology, 154,* 327–342. doi:10.1038/bjp.2008.77

Van Hoomissen, J.D., Holmes, P.V., Zellner, A.S., Poudevigne, A., & Dishman, R.K. (2004). Effects of beta-adrenoreceptor blockade during chronic exercise on contextual fear conditioning and mRNA for galanin and brain-derived neurotrophic factor. *Behavioral Neuroscience, 118,* 1378–1390. doi:10.1037/0735-7044.118.6.1378

Walker, B.M., Zorrilla, E.P., & Koob, G.F. (2011). Systemic κ-opioid receptor antagonism by nor-binaltorphimine reduces dependence-induced excessive alcohol self-administration in rats. *Addiction Biology, 16,* 116–119. doi:10.1111/j.1369-1600.2010.00226.x

Wee, S., & Koob, G.F. (2010). The role of the dynorphin-kappa opioid system in the reinforcing effects of drugs of abuse. *Psychopharmacology, 210,* 121–135. doi:10.1007/s00213-010-1825-8

Weed, M.R., Paul, I.A., Dwoskin, L.P., Moore, S.E., & Woolverton, W.L. (1997). The relationship between reinforcing effects and in vitro effects of D1 agonists in monkeys. *Journal of Pharmacology and Experimental Therapeutics, 283,* 29–38.

Werme, M., Lindholm, S., Thorén, P., Franck, J., & Brené, S. (2002). Running increases ethanol preference. *Behavioural Brain Research, 133,* 301–308. doi:10.1016/S0166-4328(02)00027-X

Xu, Z.Q., Shi, T.J., & Hökfelt, T. (1998). Galanin/GMAP- and NPY-like immunoreactivities in locus coeruleus and noradrenergic nerve terminals in the hippocampal formation and cortex with notes on the galanin-R1 and -R2 receptors. *Journal of Comparative Neurology, 392,* 227–251. doi:10.1002/(SICI)1096-9861(19980309)392:2<227::AID-CNE6>3.0.CO;2-4

Zamboanga, B.L., Schwartz, S.J., Jarvis, L.H., & Van Tyne, K. (2009). Acculturation and substance use among Hispanic early adolescents: Investigating the mediating roles of acculturative stress and self-esteem. *Journal of Primary Prevention, 30,* 315–333. doi:10.1007/s10935-009-0182-z

Zhang, X.Y., & Kosten, T.A. (2005). Prazosin, an alpha-1 adrenergic antagonist, reduces cocaine-induced reinstatement of drug-seeking. *Biological Psychiatry, 57,* 1202–1204. doi:10.1016/j.biopsych.2005.02.003

Zlebnik, N.E., Anker, J.J., Gliddon, L.A., & Carroll, M.E. (2010). Reduction of extinction and reinstatement of cocaine seeking by wheel running in female rats. *Psychopharmacology, 209,* 113–125. doi:10.1007/s00213-010-1776-0

PART 10

Quality of life in special populations

Edited by
S. Nicole Culos-Reed

34

ROLE OF PHYSICAL ACTIVITY IN OLDER ADULTS' QUALITY OF LIFE

Steriani Elavsky and Edward McAuley

At the forefront of gerontological science is the promotion of successful aging, the foundation of which is maintaining quality of life (QOL). Accordingly, extending the quality of years lived is an integral part of extending lifespan. The urgency of helping older adults maintain high QOL has become evident in light of the changing US demographics. The life expectancy has been increasing steadily over a number of decades and an average American is now expected to live to 78.3 years of age. Currently, there are 38.9 million adults 65 years of age and older in the United States, accounting for 13% of the total population, but this number is projected to grow to 88.5 million by the year 2050 when older adults are expected to comprise 20% of the total US population (U.S. Census Bureau, 2008, 2011).

This extended survival is often accompanied by increases in declining health status, functional limitations, and disability. These adverse outcomes are not an inevitable part of the aging process, however, and even when these occur they do not necessarily translate to poor QOL. Lifestyle plays a major role in determining how successfully individuals age and physical (in)activity in particular is a major determinant of health and functional decline with age. There is also a growing body of evidence supporting the role of physical activity in enhancing QOL in the older adult population. In this chapter, we review the current state of the literature regarding physical activity and QOL in older adults. After defining QOL, we proceed with the discussion of how physical activity modulates the impact of aging on QOL, and conclude by identifying fruitful areas for future research.

What is quality of life?

Dijkers (2003, 2005) identified three prevalent conceptualizations of QOL in the medical, rehabilitative, social, and psychological sciences: QOL as utility, QOL as achievements, and QOL as subjective well-being. Measures of QOL as utility, such as morbidity and mortality indices, life expectancy, quality- or disability-adjusted life years, have been used in physical activity studies when making conclusions regarding QOL. For example, in the Canadian Community Health Survey (Sawatzky, Liu-Ambrose, Miller, & Marra, 2007), a utility-based measure (Health Utility Index Mark 3 or HUI3; Furlong, Feeny, Torrance, & Barr, 2001) was used to show that physical activity mediated the association between chronic conditions and the HUI3 score, which was used as an index of overall QOL.

In the QOL as achievements tradition, the most predominant approach has been viewing QOL as health-related QOL. The focus on health as a QOL index is understandable in older adults who are impacted by age-related declines in health and functional status. Presumably, most older adults also value their health and therefore both actual and perceived quality of health should correlate highly with general QOL. Nevertheless, whereas good health and functional capacity facilitate good QOL in older adults, they do not ensure it, nor do poor health and functional limitations automatically translate to poor QOL (Thomas, 2001). For example, a recent longitudinal study of a large community-based sample of older adults showed that changes in mental well-being cannot be fully explained by physical health and functional status in older adults (Turvey, Schultz, Beglinger, & Klein, 2009). Although multidimensional conceptualizations of QOL have been proposed in the physical activity literature (e.g., Stewart & King, 1991), these models have not been extensively empirically tested, nor do they explicitly address the extent to which each of the assessed domains is valued by older individuals or whether older adults truly rely on representations from these domains when evaluating their life as a whole.

In the QOL as subjective well-being tradition, the most frequently used conceptualization is that of Ed Diener, positing that subjective well-being is the sum reflection of cognitive and emotional evaluations of one's life. QOL has thus been consistently represented by a cognitive judgment of satisfaction with one's life (Diener, 1984; Pavot & Diener, 1993). Assessing QOL as global life satisfaction is potentially useful because it (1) allows for comparative judgments (i.e., evaluation of current state in relation to own ideal/desired standard, without predefining what are presumably relevant/valued domains to the individual); (2) places importance on cognitive evaluation; (3) is well suited for theory testing; and (4) is easily accomplished given that most life satisfaction measures are brief and easy to administer (Rejeski & Mihalko, 2001).

The conceptualization of QOL as life satisfaction also fits well with recent advances in the area of positive psychology, which has expanded our understanding of what facilitates life satisfaction and happiness. Among the core tenets of positive psychology is improving the quality of people's lives by building strength as well as repairing damage/weakness (Seligman & Csikszentmihalyi, 2000). The ultimate goal of a positive psychologist is thus to enable individuals to "flourish" or lead a fulfilling life. Taking this perspective, to have a high level of life satisfaction and to achieve happiness, individuals need to have pleasant emotional experiences and perceive having strong engagement and meaning in their daily lives. Although positive emotions or affect have been routinely studied as key aspects of QOL, little effort has been made to determine whether physical activity may contribute to feelings of engagement and life purpose aspects of well-being. Seligman (2011) recently proposed the concept of PERMA representing key elements of well-being: positive emotion, engagement, relationships, meaning and purpose, and accomplishment. Each of these elements must be present to contribute to well-being and each must be measured independently of the other elements (Seligman, 2011). It is easy to see the relevance of each of these elements for well-being of older adults. Older adults value social relationships and often initiate physical activity to derive social benefits. The high level of volunteerism and philanthropy seen in older adults also suggests that older adults seek out not only pleasurable and engaging activities but also activities that give them a sense of purpose and meaning (Eakman, Carlson, & Clark, 2010). Mastery and accomplishments are also key sources of self-efficacy beliefs that have been shown to mediate effects of physical activity on well-being and QOL in older adults.

In summary, although there is no consensus regarding how to define and assess QOL, past research indicates that the construct of QOL can be characterized as (1) reflecting both subjective (perceived) as well as objective conditions; (2) being comparative (i.e., involving comparison of a current standard to an ideal/desired state); (3) multidimensional (cannot be represented only by one domain such as health); and (4) involving both hedonic (pleasant emotions) and cognitive (satisfaction, engagement, meaning) properties. Clearly, no single measure is likely to capture effectively all of these dimensions, nor should it. It is our contention that, in line with Diener (1984), viewing QOL as global life satisfaction remains a useful and practical approach, especially when QOL is studied as an outcome of physical activity. Life satisfaction judgments reflect both subjective and objective conditions of one's life, how these compare to desired states and expectations, as well as valuation across a range of different life domains that take on varying levels of importance to individuals. Individuals are also likely to be more satisfied with their lives if they perceive having high levels of engagement and meaning in their lives.

Effects of physical activity on quality of life

As noted earlier, the most commonly researched perspectives on QOL in older adults involve health-related QOL and QOL as psychological well-being. Evidence from observational (cross-sectional and longitudinal) as well as experimental studies regarding the former indicates fairly consistent and robust effects of physical activity on health-related QOL. One of the first reviews of this literature was conducted by Rejeski, Brawley, and Shumaker (1996) who evaluated 28 studies targeting various aspects of health-related QOL in both healthy and diseased older adults. Their review was followed by an updated review with a broader focus on both health-related and well-being-based QOL (Rejeski & Mihalko, 2001). Across both of these reviews, the conclusion regarding health-related QOL was that physical activity enhances most aspects of health-related QOL regardless of age, activity, and health status, and that the effects can be observed across different physical activity settings and modes. However, the degree to which individuals benefited from physical activity appeared to depend on initial status, with normally functioning individuals showing smaller improvement than those scoring functionally below the norm. This higher responsiveness by individuals with low and compromised levels of functioning has been confirmed by subsequent studies. For example, in a study of community-dwelling older adults, which compared the effects of a group-mediated cognitive behavioral physical activity intervention program (GMCB) to a traditional cardiac rehabilitation program (CRP), it was the individuals with low baseline values (men in both groups and women in the GMCB program) who exhibited largest improvements in health-related QOL (Focht, Brawley, Rejeski, & Ambrosius, 2004).

There is also evidence that physical activity levels at any given time can have implications for health-related QOL years later, as well as evidence of robust long-term associations between changes in physical activity and health-related QOL. For example, women from the Nurse's Health Study who increased their physical activity levels across a 10-year period had higher health-related QOL compared to those women whose activity levels remained stable over that time, with effects being largest for limitations due to physical problems (Wolin, Glynn, Colditz, Lee, & Kawachi, 2007). In another prospective cohort study, older adults who were more active and less sedentary at baseline had higher health-related QOL 6 years later (Balboa-Castillo, León-Muñoz, Graciani, Rodríguez-Artalejo, & Guallar-Castillón, 2011), indicating that both physical activity as well as inactivity may serve as independent predictors of health-related QOL. Another 2-year prospective study of older community-dwelling women suggested that the effects of increased physical activity on improved physical and mental health aspects of health-related QOL can be explained in part by increased levels of self-efficacy (McAuley et al., 2008).

Relative to QOL as well-being, the updated review by Rejeski and Mihalko (2001) found weaker support for the link between physical activity and QOL defined as life satisfaction. In general, cross-sectional studies showed a stronger association with life satisfaction as compared to the intervention findings, which were more inconsistent. Only three of the six reviewed randomized controlled trials had positive physical activity effects on life satisfaction. Exercise protocols as well as measurement of life satisfaction varied across the studies, possibly accounting for the discrepancies. Nonetheless, given the global nature of satisfaction with life as a QOL index, and the multitude of other influences that impact judgments of life satisfaction, it is not entirely unexpected to see associations of weak to moderate magnitude. That is, unless physical activity positively impacts areas of life that are viewed as particularly relevant and that are highly valued by older individuals (e.g., physical function in individuals with functional limitations), it is unlikely that engaging in physical activity will translate into marked improvements in global QOL.

For example, in a study of previously low active but otherwise healthy community-dwelling older adults, McAuley et al. (2000) showed that both walking and toning/stretching exercise had a similar positive but small to moderate effect on life satisfaction during a 6-month intervention and that sustained physical activity following the intervention slowed the decline in life satisfaction only somewhat at 12-month follow-up. In another study of European older adults from three countries (>70) participating in the Better Ageing Project (Fox, Stathi, McKenna, & Davis, 2007), there was a weak association between objectively measured physical activity and QOL ($r = 0.20–0.28$). In spite of a high adherence rate to the intervention (95%) and high compliance with recommended home-based exercise (83%), there were no statistically significant improvements in well-being measures (including satisfaction with life) following the 12-month program as compared to the control group. A meta-analytic review of 36 studies of physical activity and well-being outcomes in healthy older adults (Netz, Wu, Becker, & Tenenbaum, 2005) arrived at the same conclusion. Although physical activity had a positive significant impact on different psychological well-being indicators overall (weighted mean-change effect sizes for the treatment and control groups were 0.24 and 0.09, respectively), effects on life satisfaction were the smallest. This finding supports the idea of differential magnitude of effects on more proximal outcomes of physical activity (e.g., anxiety, self-efficacy, self-perceptions, physical symptoms) that may determine QOL assessed as life satisfaction. Similarly, in a 5-year follow-up investigation of older adults previously enrolled in a 6-month randomized controlled trial of walking versus stretching/toning, increases in physical activity over time were shown to positively impact changes in life satisfaction primarily as a function of enhancing affect (Elavsky et al., 2005).

The rather modest associations between physical activity and well-being-defined QOL can reflect numerous issues. As noted earlier, physical activity would only be expected to influence global QOL (i.e., life satisfaction) when positive effects occur on outcomes highly valued by older adults and outcomes that also serve to enhance other key elements of well-being (i.e., positive emotion, engagement, relationships, meaning and purpose, accomplishment, or PERMA). Measurement issues may be also partially implicated in why more robust associations are not being detected (McAuley & Elavsky, 2006). Yet another possibility is the issue of uncertainty about the proper dosage and mode of the physical activity stimulus needed to influence QOL. A number of studies attempted to answer whether a dose-response relationship exists between physical activity and QOL in older adults, although the majority did so indirectly, including two reviews. Spirduso and Cronin (2001) found little support for a dose-response relationship and speculated that inconsistencies in measurement may have contributed to this finding. Schechtman and Ory (2001) explored the issue of dose response by conducting a preplanned meta-analysis of effects on health-related QOL from four randomized controlled physical activity interventions targeting frail older adults. In terms of dose response, interventions were categorized into high-, medium-, or low-intensity categories based on the exertion level of the actual activity and kilocalories burned per week as indicated by frequency and duration of activity. Overall, there was no support for a dose-response relationship. The authors speculated that the failure to detect a dose-response effect could be due to low precision in their compliance data, the relatively crude categorization of the interventions based on intensity, or their measurement of QOL.

To date, only one randomized controlled trial (RCT) directly tested the dose-response relationship between physical activity and health-related QOL. In a 6-month RCT of 430 sedentary postmenopausal women (ages 45–75), Martin and colleagues (Martin, Church, Thompson, Earnest, & Blair, 2009) compared the effects of three doses of exercise on health-related QOL (assessed using SF-36). The doses corresponded to 50%, 100%, and 150% of the physical activity recommendations based on estimates of energy expenditure (corresponding to 4, 8, and 12 kilocalories per kilogram body weight per week, respectively). The intensity of prescribed exercise was consistent (50% of peak $\dot{V}O_2$) and completed across three to four sessions per week. As compared to the non-exercise control group, all three exercise groups significantly improved on the physical and mental functions scores of SF-36, and exercise dose was a significant predictor of changes in all aspects of health-related QOL except for bodily pain. The findings thus demonstrated a dose-response relationship between physical activity and health-related QOL, and indicate that performing even less than recommended levels of physical activity can result in significant improvements in some aspects of health-related QOL in postmenopausal, sedentary women. Importantly, the magnitude of QOL improvement was unrelated to changes in weight or fitness, indicating that changes in these physical parameters are not needed to experience QOL improvements. This conclusion is corroborated by other reviews (e.g., Rejeski et al., 1996; Rejeski & Mihalko, 2001).

Unfortunately, there are no RCTs that would similarly compare the dose-response effect of physical activity on QOL at the psychological construct level (either as life satisfaction or along the conceptualization of Seligman's well-being theory). Similarly, it is unknown whether the effects observed in the Martin et al. (2009) study would generalize to other populations of older adults. Arguably, the effects of physical activity on QOL would be expected to be stronger in populations with compromised functioning or low levels of well-being, such as older adults and individuals with disabilities and cancer patients. The risk of both disability and cancer increase with age, and coupled with age-related declines in health status, these conditions make older individuals particularly vulnerable to poor QOL. For example, older adults at risk for disability enrolled in the multi-site Lifestyle Interventions and Independence for Elders Pilot (LIFE-P) RCT were shown to have poorer scores on a health-related QOL measure that combines preference-weighted values for symptoms and functioning when compared to healthy older adults (Groessl et al., 2007). The risk factors for lower health-related QOL in this trial further included white ethnicity, more comorbid conditions, slower 400-m walk times, and lower performance on tests on the Short Physical Performance Battery (SPPB; Guralnik, Ferrucci, Simonsick, Salive, & Wallace, 1995), which focused on balance and lower extremity function (i.e., chair stand scores). Encouragingly, the 12-month LIFE-P intervention, which consisted of a structured walking-focused exercise program with group-mediated behavioral counseling, resulted in significantly improved SPPB scores, faster walking speed, and lower incidence of major mobility disability (defined as incapacity to complete a 400-meter walk) as compared to the comparison successful aging education group (LIFE Study Investigators, 2006). Higher adherence to the program (Fielding et al., 2007) and lower depressive symptoms (Matthews et al., 2011) were associated with larger improvements, and those assigned to the LIFE-P intervention group continued to engage in more moderate-intensity physical activity and tended to maintain better physical function scores (Rejeski et al., 2009). Whether these functional performance improvements translate to short-term or long-term improvements in health-related QOL or well-being-defined QOL remains to be determined. Nonetheless, the literature on the links between physical activity, QOL, and disability suggests that positive effects of physical activity on impairment and function may translate to observable improvements in health-related QOL in functionally compromised older adults at risk for disability (Motl & McAuley, 2010). Whereas the effect of physical activity on reducing or preventing disability and its impact on well-being-defined QOL is less clear, it may occur as a result of reducing functional limitations and enhancing social cognitive factors such as self-efficacy beliefs (Motl & McAuley, 2010).

Mechanisms of physical activity and QOL relationship

So far, we have considered available evidence supporting the role of physical activity on enhancing both heath-related QOL and QOL defined from the psychological perspective as life satisfaction. Although health-related QOL represents an important outcome variable in its own right, especially in patient or diseased populations, it cannot be substituted for global QOL. In fact, several studies have now demonstrated that although impairments in perceived health status may represent one potential influence on QOL, they do not translate to equivalent decrements in life satisfaction. For example, although perceived physical health was found as one of four predictors of life satisfaction in frail elderly at risk for nursing home placement, approximately 40% of these frail older adults still rated their life satisfaction as high (Abu-Bader, Rogers, & Barusch, 2002). In another study of older Jamaican men, happiness and life satisfaction were correlated with each other but neither was associated with health status. Instead, health status was determined by social factors such as age, income, education, and area of residence, but these were not determinants of happiness or life satisfaction (Bourne, Morris, & Eldemire-Shearer, 2010). These findings are consistent with our theorizing that health-related QOL should not be presumed equivalent to global QOL, but instead should be viewed as a potential determinant of global QOL.

McAuley and Morris (2007) proposed such a conceptual model for physical activity effects on QOL in older adults that can be further elaborated. In this model, physical activity is presumed to impact global QOL indirectly through its effects on functional outcomes (physical, self-related, cognitive), which influence health status. Physical and mental health status further determine global QOL. However, any effect of physical activity on function, health status, and QOL is suggested to be moderated by how much value or importance individuals place on each of the functional and health domains, although no empirical data exist testing this position. Of particular importance in this model are self-related functional outcomes such as self-efficacy, self-esteem, and affect, which have been consistently shown to mediate the effects of physical activity on psychologically defined QOL. In other words, physical activity is expected to exert positive effects on QOL primarily by influencing areas of function and life valued highly by individuals. For example, in a 2-year prospective study of community-dwelling older women, McAuley et al. (2008) showed that changes in physical activity were associated with changes in QOL (assessed as life satisfaction) indirectly through its effects on self-efficacy, which further influenced self-rated physical and mental health status. In this observational study, mental health status was the primary (and only) direct determinant of changes in QOL, highlighting the importance of perceived mental health on ratings of life satisfaction in older women with few physical limitations.

Clearly, the pathways from physical activity to QOL in older adults are complex and multi-faceted. The model proposed by McAuley and Morris (2007) is particularly useful for characterizing effects of physical activity on QOL in an intervention context. It is also a good starting point in understanding the different types of influences that physical activity has on evaluations of QOL in older adults, but it is not all-encompassing. Theoretically speaking, one could characterize influences on QOL into two general categories of top-down and bottom-up influences (Diener, 1984). Top-down influences represent influences that are time-invariant or slow-changing. Common top-down influences on QOL studied in older adults include individual difference characteristics such as demographics, personality factors, or measures of initial status (e.g., health, obesity, depression, or disability status). Bottom-up influences are represented by different contextual or process variables that change over time, many of which have been shown to be modifiable by physical activity. Such influences may for example include daily affective and stress experiences, behavioral changes, or interpersonal interactions. Many psychosomatic factors such as level of fatigue, severity of disease/somatic symptoms, or sleep quality may be particularly potent bottom-up influences on QOL in older adults, with some potentially modifiable by physical activity.

Importantly, physical activity can operate both as a top-down and bottom-up influence on QOL. Differences in QOL have been observed between active and inactive older adults (Acree et al., 2006), demonstrating that physical activity status impacts QOL ratings. At the same time, changes in physical activity over time have been linked to changes in QOL in older adults, albeit indirectly (Elavsky et al., 2005). Similarly, many of the factors proposed as mediators of the physical activity and QOL relationship by McAuley and Morris (2007) can operate on both levels. For example, in an observational study of 185 community-dwelling older adults with advanced chronic disease (Solomon, Kirwin, Van Ness, O'Leary, & Fried, 2010), initial functional status, a top-down influence, was a determinant of differences in overall QOL; however, substantial variability in QOL ratings was observed over time. Poorer QOL ratings over time were associated with more depressed mood and greater disability related to activities of daily living, whereas higher QOL ratings were associated with better self-rated health and feeling closer to one's religious community (Solomon et al., 2010). These results suggest that changing, time-variant functional outcomes (i.e., physical, social, self-related) also operate as bottom-up influences on QOL. In the context of physical activity, then, one would expect overall physical activity status as well as deviations from usual levels of physical activity to be reflected in QOL evaluations, albeit mostly through indirect pathways. Physical activity status was shown to correlate with other measures of health and functional status (Bodde, Seo, & Frey, 2009) that impact QOL. Simultaneously, one would expect fluctuations in physical activity (i.e., deviations from usual activity) to be reflected in changes in different physical, self-related, and cognitive functional outcomes that are likely to impact domain-specific or global QOL ratings. Once again, the effects would be strongest in areas of function most valued by individuals.

Although we emphasized indirect pathways from physical activity to QOL in older adults, we do not discard the possibility that physical activity may be directly related to QOL (as life satisfaction), especially when physical activity represents a personally valued domain with high relevance for QOL. It should also be noted that in addition to top-down and bottom-up influences co-determining QOL, over time effects of bottom-up influences can accumulate and change top-down factors. Consider, for example, how a newly initiated regimen of physical activity can impact daily functioning of a previously inactive older adult scoring highly on a measure of disability relative to activities of daily living. Over time, as physical activity increases, an individual may experience improvements in different areas of functioning resulting from improved muscle strength and lower daily fatigue levels, as well as higher self-efficacy. Improvements in these (bottom-up) processes may improve the ability to perform activities of daily living and improve areas of social functioning, ultimately translating to changes in disability status (a top-down factor). Physical activity would thus be expected to enhance QOL through both pathways, bottom-up processes and top-down status factors, as well as interactive influences of top-down factors and bottom-up processes on how physical activity impacts QOL. A schematic of such a conceptual view of the physical activity and QOL relationship is presented in Figure 34.1.

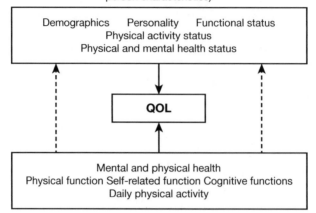

Top-down influences
(time invariant, individual difference or between-person characteristics)

Figure 34.1 A conceptual model representing the influence of different top-down and bottom-up factors on QOL of older adults. This figure is an adapted representation of relationships previously proposed by McAuley and Morris (2007) and Maher et al. (2012). Both top-down and bottom-up factors can influence QOL directly (solid lines). Fluctuations in bottom-up factors (e.g., daily behaviors or experiences) may also accumulate over time to influence top-down status factors (dashed lines). Although not depicted here, all influences should also be understood in the broader context of lifespan development.

Future directions for research

Our discussion has been focused on the role that physical activity plays in enhancing QOL in older adults. Data collected on samples of older adults also represent the majority of existing evidence for the link between physical activity and QOL. Little consideration of the physical activity and QOL relationship in other stages of the lifespan has inadvertently framed QOL as the "older adult problem," with other population segments being substantially less studied. However, just as individuals' physical activity behavior cannot be fully understood without knowledge of past physical activity habits, perceived QOL in older years cannot be separated from QOL experiences earlier in life. A better understanding of how both physical activity and QOL change across the lifespan would serve to further enlighten our understanding of how physical activity impacts QOL of older adults. Worth noting is the fact that it remains unclear exactly how well-being changes across the lifespan, and that although some level of consistency has been demonstrated both in lifespan trajectories of physical activity (e.g., Friedman et al., 2008; Malina, 2001) and well-being, there are notable individual differences in how older adults may adapt to age-related change. For example, some studies suggest that life satisfaction increases in a linear fashion with age (Prenda & Lachman, 2001), whereas other studies suggest a curvilinear change with life satisfaction peaking in midlife (Lang & Heckhausen, 2001) or between ages 65 and 70 (Mroczek & Spiro, 2005). There are also other studies that show little change in life satisfaction as a function of age alone (Fujita & Diener, 2005; Hamarat, Thompson, Steele, Matheny, & Simons, 2002; Hsu, 2010), indicating that other influences such as socioeconomic conditions, health status changes, or lifestyle factors may be more potent modulators of global

QOL than aging alone. More studies are needed to elaborate on the lifespan trajectories of both physical activity and QOL as well as the mechanisms of how one can influence the other at different stages of the lifespan.

The majority of studies focusing on physical activity and older adults have also investigated between-person differences in physical activity and QOL. Although such studies help identify potential risk factors or targets for interventions, they are not particularly revealing of the underlying mechanisms through which physical activity can impact QOL. More studies investigating within-person changes in physical activity and QOL are needed to better understand how both change over time, as well as what mechanisms may be at work when a change in QOL is observed are a function of change in physical activity. These mechanisms are likely to be dynamic, involving both slow-changing processes (e.g., disease or functional impairment) as well as short-term, more acute changes as a result of deviations from usual levels of physical activity from day to day, week to week, or across seasons. Life satisfaction ratings have been shown to be moderately stable over time (e.g., Fujita & Diener, 2005), but few studies have investigated to what extent short-term (daily or weekly) variability in life satisfaction may be driven by changes in physical activity within persons over time. Although there are no such studies in older adults, associations between life satisfaction ratings and deviations in daily physical activity have been reported in two daily diary studies of emerging adults (Maher et al., 2012). Further research is needed to determine whether deviations from usual physical activity impact life satisfaction at different timescales in older adults as well as the mechanisms through which such effects can occur. To this end, more longitudinal as well as intervention studies with QOL as the primary outcome variable are needed.

Any such studies must also include more representative samples of older adults. There are important qualitative changes occurring in the composition of American older adults. Just as other segments of the population, older adults are growing in diversity in terms of ethnic/racial, socioeconomic, as well as health status. For example, minorities now make up about 20% of the US older adult population but they are projected to represent about 43% of adults aged 65 and older in 2050 (U.S. Census Bureau, 2009). Nearly 10% of older adults currently live at or below the federal poverty level, and about a third (31.4%) are considered economically insecure (i.e., living at or below the poverty line) (National Council on Aging, 2010). These underserved groups remain underrepresented in physical activity and QOL research.

Summary

As individuals, we hope to live long while simultaneously enjoying our lives. As researchers, clinicians, and health care providers, our efforts are specifically aimed at maximizing people's QOL through maintenance of health, function, and well-being. Although aging is associated with reductions in one's functional capacity and health, older adults possess the same capacity to lead a happy life as young adults do. While the age-related changes in health and functional status bring about notable behavioral and psychological adaptations, there nonetheless remains much reserve and plasticity in terms of enhancing both function and health, while maintaining good QOL.

The good news is that a considerable proportion of the research on physical activity and QOL is based on samples of older adults, providing a solid evidence base for some of the key pathways through which physical activity can impact QOL in this population. Unfortunately, this predominant focus on aging (and patient) populations has led to an overemphasis of the health-related aspects of QOL. In biomedical circles, in particular, health status is often equated with QOL or the concept of health-related QOL is used as synonymous with general QOL. Although the evidence supports a positive effect of physical activity on health-related QOL, such effects cannot be viewed as synonymous with improvements in global QOL. Perceived health status should thus be more appropriately viewed as a determinant of global QOL, which is best viewed and assessed as life satisfaction. Other potent determinants of global QOL in older adults include social cognitive factors such self-efficacy and functional outcomes, although the exact mechanisms of the physical activity and QOL relationship remain to be determined.

Efforts to extend our understanding of how physical activity influences QOL in older adults must also be complemented by efforts to increase physical activity engagement in this population. Age-related decreases in physical activity levels have been demonstrated based on both objective and subjective measures of physical activity. In a large study with objective physical activity surveillance data, only about 17% of men and 12% of women aged 60–69 and 9% of men and 5% of women aged 70+ were found to spend the recommended daily time engaged in moderate and/or vigorous PA at 10+-minute sessions (Troiano et al., 2008). Another study estimated that older adults average about two-thirds of the estimated physical activity energy expenditure of young adults, engage in twice as many bouts of sedentary time as young adults, and perform half as many minutes of moderate PA as young adults, with older old ages and women faring worse than younger old ages and men (Davis & Fox, 2007). It is paramount to wage sustained efforts to increase physical activity in the older adult population so that they can harness the numerous benefits of physical activity, including improved QOL.

References

Abu-Bader, S. H., Rogers, A., & Barusch, A. S. (2002). Predictors of life satisfaction in frail elderly. *Journal of Gerontological Social Work, 38*(3), 3–17.

Acree, L. S., Longfors, J., Fjeldstad, A. S., Fjeldstad, C., Schank, B., Nickel, K. J., . . . Gardner, A. W. (2006). Physical activity is related to quality of life in older adults. *Health and Quality of Life Outcomes, 30*(4), 37.

Balboa-Castillo, T., León-Muñoz, L. M., Graciani, A., Rodríguez-Artalejo, F., & Guallar-Castillón, P. (2011). Longitudinal association of physical activity and sedentary behavior during leisure time with health-related quality of life in community-dwelling older adults. *Health and Quality of Life Outcomes, 9*, 47.

Bodde, A. E., Seo, D. C., & Frey, G. (2009). Correlation between physical activity and self-rated health status of non-elderly adults with disabilities. *Preventive Medicine, 49*(6), 511–514.

Bourne, P. A., Morris, C., & Eldemire-Shearer, E. (2010). Re-testing theories on the correlations of health status, life satisfaction and happiness. *North American Journal of Medical Sciences, 2*(7), 311–319.

Davis, M. G., & Fox, K. R. (2007). Physical activity patterns assessed by accelerometry in older people. *European Journal of Applied Physiology, 100*(5), 581–589.

Diener, E. (1984). Subjective well-being. *Psychological Bulletin, 95*(3), 542–575.

Dijkers, M. P. J. M. (2003). Individualization in quality of life measurement: Instruments and approaches. *Archives of Physical Medicine and Rehabilitation, 84*(4 Suppl 2), S3–S14.

Dijkers, M. P. J. M. (2005). Quality of life of individuals with spinal cord injury: A review of conceptualization, measurement, and research findings. *Journal of Rehabilitation Research and Development, 42*(3), 87–110.

Eakman, A. M., Carlson, M., & Clark, F. (2010). The meaningful activity participation assessment: A measure of engagement in personally valued activities. *International Journal of Aging and Human Development, 70*, 339–357.

Elavsky, S., McAuley, E., Motl, R. W., Konopack, J. F., Marquez, D. X., Hu, L., . . . Diener, E. (2005). Physical activity enhances long-term quality of life in older adults: Efficacy, esteem, and affective influences. *Annals of Behavioral Medicine, 30*(2), 138–145.

Fielding, R. A., Katula, J., Miller, M. E., Abbott-Pillola, K., Jordan, A., Glynn, N. W., . . . Life Study Investigators. (2007). Activity adherence and physical function in older adults with functional limitations. *Medicine & Science in Sports & Exercise, 39*(11), 1997–2004.

Focht, B. C., Brawley, L. R., Rejeski, W. J., & Ambrosius, W. T. (2004). Group-mediated activity counseling and traditional exercise therapy programs: Effects on health-related quality of life among older adults in cardiac rehabilitation. *Annals of Behavioral Medicine, 28*(1), 52–61.

Fox, K. R., Stathi, A., McKenna, J., & Davis, M. G. (2007). Physical activity and mental well-being in older people participating in the Better Ageing Project. *European Journal of Applied Physiology, 100*(5), 591–602.

Friedman, H. S., Martin, L. R., Tucker, J. S., Criqui, M. H., Kern, M. L., & Reynolds, C. A. (2008). Stability of physical activity across the lifespan. *Journal of Health Psychology, 13*(8), 1092–1104.

Fujita, F., & Diener, E. (2005). Life satisfaction set point: Stability and change. *Journal of Personality and Social Psychology, 88*(1), 158–164.

Furlong, W. J., Feeny, D. H., Torrance, G. W., & Barr, R. D. (2001). The health utilities index (HUI) system for assessing health-related quality of life in clinical studies. *Annals of Medicine, 33*(5), 375–384.

Groessl, E. J., Kaplan, R. M., Rejeski, W. J., Katula, J. A., King, A. C., Frierson, G., . . . Pahor, M. (2007). Health-related quality of life in older adults at risk for disability. *American Journal of Preventive Medicine, 33*(3), 214–218.

Guralnik, J. M., Ferrucci, L., Simonsick, E. M., Salive, M. E., & Wallace, R. B. (1995). Lower-extremity function in persons over the age of 70 years as a predictor of subsequent disability. *New England Journal of Medicine, 332*(9), 556–561.

Hamarat, E., Thompson, D., Steele, D., Matheny, K., & Simons, C. (2002). Age differences in coping resources and satisfaction with life among middle-aged, young-old, and oldest-old adults. *Journal of Genetic Psychology, 163*(3), 360–367.

Hsu, H. C. (2010). Trajectory of life satisfaction and its relationship with subjective economic status and successful aging. *Social Indicators Research, 99*(3), 455–468.

Lang, F. R., & Heckhausen, J. (2001). Perceived control over development and subjective well-being: Differential benefits across adulthood. *Journal of Personality and Social Psychology, 81*, 509–523.

LIFE Study Investigators. (2006). Effects of a physical activity intervention on measures of physical performance: Results of the Lifestyle Interventions and Independence for Elders Pilot (LIFE-P) study. *Journal of Gerontology: Medical Sciences, 61A*(11), 1157–1165.

Maher, J. P., Doerksen, S. E., Elavsky, S., Hyde, A. L., Pincus, A. L., Ram, N., & Conroy, D. E. (2012). A daily analysis of physical activity and life satisfaction in emerging adults. *Health Psychology*, October 22. [Epub ahead of print] PMID:23088171

Malina, R. M. (2001). *Tracking of physical activity across the lifespan*. Washington, DC: President's Council on Physical Fitness and Sports.

Martin, C. K., Church, T. S., Thompson, A. M., Earnest, C. P., & Blair, S. N. (2009). Exercise dose and quality of life: A randomized controlled trial. *Archives of Internal Medicine, 169*(3), 269–278.

Matthews, M. M., Hsu, F. C., Walkup, M. P., Barry, L. C., Patel, K. V., & Blair, S. N. (2011). Depressive symptoms and physical performance in the Lifestyle Interventions and Independence for Elders Pilot study. *Journal of the American Geriatrics Society, 59*(3), 495–500.

McAuley, E., Blissmer, B., Marquez, D. X., Jerome, G. J., Kramer, A. F., & Katula, J. (2000). Social relations, physical activity, and well-being in older adults. *Preventive Medicine, 31*(5), 608–617.

McAuley, E., Doerksen, S. E., Morris, K. S., Motl, R. W., Hu, L., Wójcicki, T. R., . . . Rosengren, K. R. (2008). Pathways from physical activity to quality of life in older women. *Annals of Behavioral Medicine, 36*(1), 13–20.

McAuley, E., & Elavsky, S. (2006). Physical activity, aging, and quality of life: Implications for measurement. In W. Zhu & W. Chodzko-Zajko (Eds.), *Measurement issues in aging and physical activity* (pp. 57–68). Champaign, IL: Human Kinetics.

McAuley, E., & Morris, K. (2007). Advances in physical activity and mental health: Quality of life. *American Journal of Lifestyle Medicine, 1*, 389–396.

Motl, R. W., & McAuley, E. (2010). Physical activity, disability, and quality of life in older adults. *Physical Medicine and Rehabilitation Clinics of North America, 21*(2), 299–308.

Mroczek, D. K., & Spiro, A. (2005). Change in life satisfaction during adulthood: Findings from the Veterans Affairs normative aging study. *Journal of Personality and Social Psychology, 88*(1), 189–202.

National Council on Aging. (2010). Current economic status of older adults in the United States: A demographic analysis, January 2010. Retrieved June 20, 2011 from http://www.ncoa.org/assets/files/pdf/Economic-Security-Trends-for-Older-Adults-65-and-Older_March-2010.pdf

Netz, Y., Wu, M. J., Becker, B. J., & Tenenbaum, G. (2005). Physical activity and psychological wellbeing in advanced age: A meta-analysis of intervention studies. *Psychological Aging, 20*, 272–284.

Pavot, W., & Diener, E. (1993). The affective and cognitive context of self-reported measures of subjective well-being. *Social Indicators Research, 28*(1), 1–20.

Prenda, K. M., & Lachman, M. E. (2001). Planning for the future: A life management strategy for increasing control and life satisfaction in adulthood. *Psychology and Aging, 16*, 206–216.

Rejeski, W. J., Brawley, L. R., & Shumaker, S. A. (1996). Physical activity and health-related quality of life. *Exercise and Sport Sciences Reviews, 24*, 71–108.

Rejeski, W. J., Marsh, A. P., Chmelo, E., Prescott, A. J., Dobrosielski, M., Walkup, M. P., . . . Kritchevsky, S. (2009). The Lifestyle Interventions and Independence for Elders Pilot (LIFE-P): 2-year follow-up. *Journal of Gerontology: Biological and Social Sciences, 64*(4), 462–467.

Rejeski, W. J., & Mihalko, S. L. (2001). Physical activity and quality of life in older adults. *Journals of Gerontology: Biological Sciences and Medical Sciences, 56A*(Special Issue No. 2), 23–35.

Sawatzky, R., Liu-Ambrose, T., Miller, W. C., & Marra, C. A. (2007). Physical activity as a mediator of the impact of chronic conditions on quality of life in older adults. *Health and Quality of Life Outcomes, 5*, 68.

Schechtman, K. B., & Ory, M. G. (2001). The effects of exercise on the quality of life of frail older adults: A preplanned meta-analysis of the FICSIT trials. *Annals of Behavioral Medicine, 23*(3), 186–197.

Seligman, M. E. P. (2011). *Flourish: A visionary new understanding of happiness and well-being.* Sydney: William Heinamann.

Seligman, M. E. P., & Csikszentmihalyi, M. (2000). Positive psychology: An introduction. *American Psychologist, 55*(1), 5–14.

Solomon, R., Kirwin, P., Van Ness, P. H., O'Leary, J., & Fried, T. R. (2010). Trajectories of quality of life in older persons with advanced illness. *Journal of the American Geriatrics Society, 58*(5), 837–843.

Spirduso, W. W., & Cronin, D. L. (2001). Exercise dose-response effects on quality of life and independent living in older adults. *Medicine & Science in Sports & Exercise, 33*(6 Suppl), S598–S608.

Stewart, A. L., & King, A. C. (1991). Evaluating the efficacy of physical activity for influencing quality-of-life outcomes in older adults. *Annals of Behavioral Medicine, 13*(3), 108–116.

Thomas, D. R. (2001). Critical link between health-related quality of life and age-related changes in physical activity and nutrition. *Journals of Gerontology: Medical Sciences, 56A*(10), M599–M602.

Troiano, R. P., Berrigan, D., Dodd, K. W., Mâsse, L. C., Tilert, T., & McDowell, M. (2008). Physical activity in the United States measured by accelerometer. *Medicine & Science in Sports & Exercise, 40*(1), 181–188.

Turvey, C. L., Schultz, S. K., Beglinger, L., & Klein, D. M. (2009). A longitudinal community-based study of chronic illness, cognitive and physical function, and depression. *American Journal of Geriatric Psychiatry, 17*(8), 632–641.

U.S. Census Bureau. (2008). *Annual estimates of the resident population by sex and selected age groups for the United States: April 1, 2000 to July 1, 2008 (NC-EST2008-02).* Retrieved June 20, 2011 from http://www.census.gov/popest/national/asrh/NC-EST2008-sa.html

U.S. Census Bureau. (2009). *U.S. population projections.* Retrieved June 20, 2011 from http://www.census.gov/population/www/projections/summarytables.html

U.S. Census Bureau. (2011). *Cumulative estimates of the components of resident population change by race and Hispanic origin for the United States: April 1, 2000 to July 1, 2009.* Retrieved June 20, 2011 from www.census.gov/popest/national/asrh/NC-EST2009-compchg.html

Wolin, K. Y., Glynn, R. J., Colditz, G. A., Lee, I. M., & Kawachi, I. (2007). Long-term physical activity patterns and health-related quality of life in U.S. women. *American Journal of Preventive Medicine, 32*(6), 490–499.

35

PHYSICAL ACTIVITY AND QUALITY OF LIFE IN CARDIOVASCULAR AND PULMONARY DISEASES

Charles F. Emery, Risa N. Long, and KayLoni L. Olson

"Physical activity" (PA) and "exercise" are often used interchangeably, but may refer to different concepts. PA typically refers to all types of activities in which body movement and muscle contraction are required, including most activities of daily living (ADLs) such as household chores and PA in the workplace. In contrast, exercise activity generally refers to planned and structured activities undertaken with the purpose of improving components of physical fitness such as muscular strength, flexibility, or physical endurance. The literature on PA and quality of life (QOL) in cardiovascular and pulmonary diseases includes studies of both daily PA as well as intervention studies evaluating the effects of exercise on QOL. Studies of both types of PA were included in this selective review with the goal of identifying the best data available for understanding the relationship between PA and QOL.

QOL is a multi-dimensional construct and various self-report measures have been utilized in the research literature to operationalize the multi-faceted components of QOL (e.g., self-rated health, social functioning, physical functioning, mood, and life satisfaction). The Medical Outcomes Study Short Form-36 (SF-36; Ware & Sherbourne, 1992) is the most commonly used QOL measure in health-related research and is considered a "generic" indicator because it can be used to evaluate QOL across a wide range of health conditions. The SF-36 provides eight subscale scores (physical functioning, physical role, bodily pain, general health, vitality, social functioning, emotional role, and mental health) as well as a mental component score and a physical component score. In addition to generic measures of QOL, research and clinical applications typically also assess QOL with illness-specific measures (e.g., Kansas City Cardiomyopathy Questionnaire (KCCQ); Quality of Life after Myocardial Infarction (QLMI) scale; St. George's Respiratory Questionnaire (SGRQ); Cystic Fibrosis Questionnaire – Revised). Most prior studies of QOL among cardiac patients have relied primarily on the SF-36.

Physical activity and quality of life in cardiovascular disease

Cardiovascular disease (CVD) refers broadly to disorders of the heart and vascular system. Thus, a number of distinct clinical disorders are encompassed including coronary heart disease (CHD), stroke, hypertension (HTN), and congestive heart failure (CHF). Although exercise was believed to be dangerous for patients with cardiac disease until the 1970s, during the past three decades it has been well documented that PA is both safe and beneficial for patients with CVD (Smart

Table 35.1 Quality of life outcomes of physical activity among patients with cardiovascular disease

Patient population	Physical activity and quality of life outcome	Caveats
Coronary heart disease	Exercise-based rehabilitation leads to increased QOL but changes generally do not exceed improvements due to treatment as usual.	– Benefits of exercise-based programs may only emerge during follow-up period. – Combined aerobic and resistance training may be more beneficial than aerobic alone in women. – Evidence of a dose-response relationship. – Age and sex may moderate the relationship between exercise and QOL.
Stroke	Exercise interventions lead to improvements in physical QOL but not necessarily mental QOL.	– Results are not maintained in follow-up (ranging from 12–24 months post-intervention). – Cardiorespiratory fitness may not be the mechanism through which exercise impacts QOL. Gait-speed may be alternative mechanism.
Hypertension	Exercise programs lead to improvements in QOL.	– Aerobic training may be more beneficial than resistance training. – Few studies of young adults.
Congestive heart failure	Lack of change in exercise capacity has been associated with lack of change in QOL.	– Inconsistent results limit reliability of conclusions.

QOL=quality of life

& Marwick, 2005). Table 35.1 provides a summary of QOL outcomes of exercise among patients with CVD.

Coronary heart disease

CHD (also referred to as coronary artery disease (CAD) or ischemic heart disease) is the most common form of heart disease, affecting 7.9% of Americans, and is the leading cause of death in the United States (Lloyd-Jones et al., 2010). CHD is characterized by an inadequate blood supply to the heart tissue resulting from narrowing of the coronary arteries. Reduced blood flow to the heart may result in symptoms of chest pain (angina), and blockage of blood flow may result in a myocardial infarction (MI or heart attack).

Cross-sectional studies generally reflect positive associations of PA with enhanced QOL across a wide range of patients with CVD, including older women (age $\geq$ 60 years; Janz et al., 2001). Among 262 cardiac patients entering a rehabilitation program, $\dot{V}O_2$max was associated with higher ratings on several SF-36 QOL dimensions (Jette & Downing, 1996). Conversely, in a large sample (n=1024) of patients diagnosed with CAD, low exercise capacity was associated with worse QOL and poorer overall health (Ruo et al., 2003).

In contrast to positive data from cross-sectional studies, longitudinal studies and exercise intervention studies indicate that PA may not be essential for improved QOL among patients with CVD. Emery and colleagues (2004) found that physical and mental QOL improved for men and women with CVD over a 12-month period following hospital admission, regardless of physical activity level. Likewise, improvements in QOL associated with exercise interventions often do not exceed improvements observed in control groups, as reflected in a review of randomized controlled trials (RCTs) by Taylor and colleagues (2004). However, several studies suggest that exercise treatment is associated with improvement in QOL at longer-term follow-ups of 6 months, 8 months, and 12 months (Belardinelli et al., 2001; Dugmore et al., 1999; Elley, Kerse, Arroll, & Robinson, 2003). In these studies, improved QOL is associated with increased functional capacity, as reflected by increases in peak $\dot{V}O_2$ and 6-minute walk distance, although not all studies included indicators of mental health. In addition, more intensive training has been associated with greater gains in QOL. Aerobic training combined with strength training resulted in more substantial improvements in QOL than aerobic exercise alone among women with CHD (Arthur et al., 2007; Hung et al., 2004). Similarly, Nieuwland and colleagues (2000) found that 6 weeks of high-intensity exercise led to significantly greater improvements in mental QOL (SF-36) than did low-intensity exercise.

Studies suggest possible age-related effects of exercise among patients with CVD. Marchionni and colleagues (2003) found that exercise was associated with improved physical QOL among post-MI participants over age 75, but individuals under age 75 reported improvements in physical QOL regardless of exercise status. Also, Seki and colleagues (2003) found improved mental QOL among older men (mean age = 70 years) with CHD following exercise training in the absence of increased functional capacity.

Stroke

Stroke occurs when there is disturbance of blood flow to one or more regions of the brain resulting from a clot in the bloodstream or a burst blood vessel. Consequences range from minimal damage to death, but many stroke survivors experience long-term impairment of functioning, including difficulty with ADLs and with cognitive tasks. Stroke is the fourth leading cause of death in the United States, and the leading cause of long-term disability. Additionally, one in eight stroke survivors experiences a subsequent stroke.

Cross-sectional data from 118 individuals 1 year after stroke indicate that degree of disability is associated with reductions in both PA and QOL (Carod-Artal, Egido, Gonzalez, & de Seijas, 2000). Among stroke survivors (2.4% of total sample of 51,193), self-report of regular exercise was associated with less impairment in health-related QOL (HRQOL) during the previous 30 days (Greenlund et al., 2002). However, recent data suggest that exercise may be associated with only select aspects of QOL. In a group of 40 stroke survivors, Rand and colleagues (Rand, Eng, Tang, Hung, & Jeng, 2010) found that PA measured both via accelerometer and via self-report was associated with physical QOL but not mental QOL (SF-36).

De Weerd and colleagues (De Weerd, Rutgers, Groenier, & van der Meer, 2011) conducted at-home longitudinal interviews of stroke patients (n = 57) immediately after hospital discharge and at 1-year follow-up. Patients who maintained or increased PA during the 1-year interval reported enhanced QOL, specifically better physical functioning and reduced physical role limitations.

Conflicting evidence emerged from a Cochrane review of exercise effects on QOL among stroke survivors (Saunders, Greig, Mead, & Young, 2009), but a recent review of RCTs reported positive effects of exercise on QOL (Chen & Rimmer, 2011). Across studies, exercise is associated with improved mental and physical QOL post intervention with a small to medium effect, but improvements in QOL are reduced at follow-up (ranging from 12–24 months post-intervention). Langhammer, Stanghelle, and Lindmark (2008) found that non-cardiorespiratory factors associated with self-initiated exercise may account for enhanced QOL outcomes, possibly reflecting increased self-efficacy or sense of responsibility among self-initiators.

Due to the nature of physical deficits associated with stroke, gait-specific exercise is often a focus of rehabilitation programs. Schmid and colleagues (2007) found that gait-speed increases during exercise rehabilitation were associated with improvements in physical QOL, but a recent review found no evidence that improvement in gait-speed affects QOL (Van de Port, Wood-Dauphinee, Lindeman, & Kwakkel, 2007). Combs and colleagues (2010) found improved QOL and physical fitness following treadmill-based exercise among 19 stroke patients, but changes in physical fitness were not correlated with changes in physical QOL at program completion or at 6-month follow-up, suggesting that cardiorespiratory fitness may not be the mechanism by which exercise influences physical QOL among post-stroke patients.

Hypertension

Essential, or primary, HTN is a condition marked by high blood pressure that is not secondary to another identifiable medical condition. HTN can lead to vascular weakness, scarring, increased risk of blood clots, and accumulation of plaque in the arteries. In turn, HTN places increased burden on the circulatory system and contributes to greater risk of future cardiac events as well as other medical conditions. HTN is one of the most common chronic health problems in the United States, affecting one out of three individuals.

In a cross-sectional study of 361 hypertensive patients, Fernandez and colleagues (Fernandez, Garcia, Alvarez, Giron, & Aguirre-Jaime, 2007) found that self-reported PA was positively associated with select domains of QOL in men and in those under age 65, but PA was more broadly associated with QOL among women and older participants (over age 65). Short-term, 24-hour PA measured with the actigraph among hypertensive patients has been positively associated with specific components of QOL such as emotional role functioning and physical functioning (SF-36; Okano et al., 2004).

Among hypertensive individuals, exercise programs typically lead to improvements in functional capacity and most aspects of QOL, including mental QOL, for middle-aged adults (Tsai et al., 2004) and older adults (Park et al., 2010), as well as women (Povoa et al., 2010). The latter study found that aerobic training was associated with greater QOL improvements than resistance training.

Congestive heart failure

CHF occurs when the heart cannot sufficiently pump blood throughout the body. It is a progressive disorder in which the heart continues to function but at a suboptimal level, leading to complications. Most often, individuals with CHF experience symptoms of fatigue, fluid accumulation in the lungs, and exercise intolerance.

Among CHF patients, the cross-sectional relationship between exercise capacity and QOL varies depending on the measure of activity. Better performance on the 6-minute walk test is associated with higher self-reported QOL (Santos & Brofman, 2008), while $\dot{V}O_2$max has been associated with some domains of QOL (physical function, role-physical, general health, vitality, mental health) but not other domains (bodily pain, social function, role-emotional; Juenger et al., 2002). In a recent study of 36 patients with CHF, PA measured via accelerometer was not associated with physical or mental QOL (van den Berg-Emmons, Bussmann, Balk, & Stam, 2005).

Results of intervention studies among individuals with CHF are equivocal (e.g., Pihl, Cider, Stromberg, Fridlund, & Martensson, 2011). Following a systematic review of the literature,

Lloyd-Williams and colleagues (Lloyd-Williams, Mair, & Leitner, 2002) found that method-ological concerns regarding the types of measures and the timing of assessments precluded firm conclusions. However, exercise programs of varying lengths (3 to 12 months) have been associated with improvements in QOL and increased functional capacity (Patwala et al., 2009; Bocalini, dos Santos, & Serra, 2008; Flynn et al., 2009), and failure to achieve increased $\dot{V}O_2$max or 6-minute walk distance has been associated with failure to experience changes in QOL (Brubaker, Moore, Stewart, Wesley, & Kitzman, 2009). However, studies do not consistently evaluate mental QOL. Data suggest that older individuals (<70 years) and very old individuals (≥70 years) with CHF experience exercise-associated increases in QOL (Miche et al., 2009), as do women with CHF (Gary et al., 2004).

Although some studies indicate that improvements in aerobic capacity may be the mechanism by which PA influences QOL (e.g., Mandic et al., 2008), other studies suggest that PA may not lead to improved QOL among patients with CHF (Van Tol, Huijsmans, Kroon, Schothorst, & Kwakkel, 2006). Additionally, a recent review of RCTs failed to find enhanced QOL among patients with CHF despite significant improvements in functional capacity (Chien, Lee, Wu, Chen, & Wu, 2006).

Methodological problems/concerns in this line of research

There is promising evidence of positive effects of exercise on QOL among patients with CVD, but there are a number of problems with this line of research, including methodological variability across studies in measures of QOL and PA/exercise capacity, type and length of exercise training programs, and absence of randomized controlled studies. Inconsistent findings may result from variability in measures of similar domains (e.g., 6-minute walk, $\dot{V}O_2$max, and actigraph are not consistently associated with QOL).

Although a generic QOL measure such as the SF-36 allows for comparison across patient groups and studies, generic measures may not be sensitive to illness-specific changes in QOL. In addition, prior studies have routinely addressed physical QOL but have not consistently assessed mental QOL.

Physical activity and quality of life in pulmonary disease

Pulmonary disease refers to disorders of the lungs and respiratory system. Thus, pulmonary disease incorporates a number of distinct conditions including chronic obstructive pulmonary disease (COPD), asthma, interstitial lung disease (ILD), cystic fibrosis (CF), and pulmonary hypertension, all of which have been associated with reduced QOL. Table 35.2 provides a summary of QOL outcomes of exercise among patients with pulmonary disease.

Chronic obstructive pulmonary disease

Chronic obstructive pulmonary disease (COPD) is the third leading cause of death in the United States and a major cause of disability. It is estimated that 12 million Americans have been diagnosed with COPD and another 12 million are living with COPD, but have not yet been diagnosed. COPD encompasses both emphysema and chronic bronchitis. Common symptoms include shortness of breath, cough with sputum production, fatigue, and insomnia. Risk factors include a history of smoking, genetics, and exposure to environmental toxins. Historically, COPD has affected more men than women, but the prevalence among women has increased in recent decades, primarily due to increased smoking rates among women (Mannino & Buist, 2007).

Table 35.2 Quality of life outcomes of physical activity among patients with pulmonary disease

Patient population	Physical activity and quality of life outcome	Caveats
Chronic obstructive pulmonary disease	Exercise-based rehabilitation leads to improvement in QOL immediately following intervention.	– Gains in QOL following exercise-based programs diminish during follow-up (12–24 months). – Maintenance programs plagued by poor compliance.
Asthma	– Greater physical activity associated with better QOL in children. – Exercise training improves QOL in adults.	– More randomized studies of QOL outcomes are needed, especially among children.
Interstitial lung disease – Pulmonary fibrosis – Sarcoidosis	Evidence for exercise-related increases in QOL.	– Randomized studies are needed to further explicate mechanisms of change.
Cystic fibrosis	Aerobic and anaerobic training may lead to improvements in physical domains of QOL among children and adolescents.	– Unclear whether supervised training is more effective than unsupervised training. – More studies examining QOL as a primary outcome are needed.
Pulmonary hypertension	Exercise-based rehabilitation may lead to improvements in QOL.	– Duration and intensity of exercise-based programs vary based on disease severity.

QOL=quality of life

Cross-sectional studies of patients with COPD generally indicate that lower PA is associated with poorer QOL (e.g., Belza et al., 2001). Greater PA, as measured by the 6-minute walk test, has been positively associated with physical QOL (Katsura, Yamada, Wakabayashi, & Kida, 2005).

Observational studies (e.g., Verril, Barton, Beasley, & Lippard, 2005) and randomized studies (e.g., Emery, Schein, Hauck, & MacIntyre, 1998) among patients with COPD indicate that exercise interventions (10–12 weeks) are associated with significant increases in HRQOL. Longitudinal studies of exercise training and maintenance indicate improvements in physical and mental QOL immediately following treatment, but improvements diminish during the year following treatment (Ringbaek, Brøndum, Martinez, Thøgersen, & Lange, 2010; Ries, Kaplan, Myers, & Prewitt, 2003). A recent meta-analysis of 31 RCTs of exercise rehabilitation found a positive effect of exercise on HRQOL, with effect sizes for physical and mental QOL exceeding a minimally important clinical difference (Lacasse, Goldstein, Lasserson, & Martin, 2006).

Asthma

Asthma is a common respiratory disease among all ages, but the disease originates primarily during childhood. Approximately 25 million people in the United States have asthma, and most cases are diagnosed among individuals aged 5–17 years. Asthma is characterized by airway inflammation, reversible airflow obstruction, and recurring symptoms including wheezing, dyspnea (i.e., shortness of breath), chest tightness, and coughing. The etiology is unknown, but asthma tends to be hereditary and is associated with repeated respiratory infections in childhood or exposure to specific allergens. More women than men are affected by asthma, but more boys than girls are diagnosed with asthma. Asthma is incurable, but can be managed with a variety of pharmacological treatments.

Cross-sectional data generally reveal a positive association between PA and QOL. In a population-based study of patients (n = 12,111) with asthma, lower PA was associated with poorer physical QOL (Ford, Mannino, Redd, Moriarty, & Mokdad, 2004). In a survey of PA among children with asthma, Cheng and colleagues (2010) found that individuals with higher levels of PA reported better physical and mental QOL than those with lower PA.

Outcomes of supervised exercise interventions among older patients with asthma have revealed improvements in asthma-related QOL (Mendes et al., 2010; Turner, Eastwood, Cook, & Jenkins, 2011), and self-administered exercise has been associated with maintaining gains in physical QOL during a 12-week follow-up (Dogra, Kuk, Baker, & Jamnik, 2011). Basaran and colleagues (2006) found that an 8-week basketball training program in children with asthma led to a significantly larger increase in physical and mental QOL than in a control group. Fanelli and colleagues (Fanelli, Cabral, Neder, Martins, & Carvalho, 2007) also found increases in physical and mental QOL following 16 weeks of aerobic training versus no training among children with moderate to severe asthma. Most exercise intervention studies in children with asthma have not included measures of QOL, limiting the ability to draw conclusions about the effects of PA on QOL.

Interstitial lung disease

Interstitial lung disease (ILD) refers to a large group of disorders classified by scarring of the lung tissue (interstitium). There are many causes of ILD, including autoimmune diseases, medication side effects, and occupational exposure. The most common type of ILD is idiopathic pulmonary fibrosis (IPF).

Idiopathic pulmonary fibrosis

Pulmonary fibrosis is a condition characterized by thickening and scarring (fibrosis) of the lung tissue over time. Symptoms of IPF include dyspnea, clubbing (rounding and/or widening of the finger tips and toes), chronic dry cough, fatigue, and unintentional weight loss. The etiology of IPF is unknown in most cases, but risk factors include history of tobacco use, viral infections, and medication use (e.g., cancer medications, antibiotics, and propanolol). It is estimated that 128,000 Americans have IPF, but this may be an underestimate due to the lack of standardized diagnostic criteria (Raghu, Weycker, Edelsburg, Bradford, & Oster, 2006).

Poorer exercise performance (measured by 6-minute walk distance) has been associated with lower QOL among patients with IPF in Japan (Tomioka, Imanaka, Hashimoto, & Iwaski, 2007). Nishiyama et al. (2008) found marked improvements in exercise capacity and physical QOL in patients with IPF following 10 weeks of exercise training compared to controls.

Sarcoidosis

Pulmonary sarcoidosis is another form of ILD characterized by inflammation and formation of tiny lumps of cells (granulomas) in the lungs. Symptoms of sarcoidosis include shortness of breath, coughing, and wheezing. During non-active phases of illness, inflammation decreases and granulomas may lessen in size, but symptoms can still occur. Sarcoidosis is known to affect African Americans more often than Caucasian Americans, but the cause of the disease remains unknown.

Poor exercise performance, as indexed by the 6-minute walk test, has been associated with decreased physical and mental QOL among patients with sarcoidosis (Baughman, Sparkman, & Lower, 2007; Bourbonnais & Samavati, 2010). Additionally, skeletal muscle weakness, as measured by quadriceps peak torque, was associated with poorer physical and mental QOL among 25 patients with sarcoidosis complaining of fatigue (Spruit et al., 2005).

Due to the broad categorization of ILDs, studies often comprise various diagnoses. Observational studies including mixed samples of patients with ILD (IPF and sarcoidosis) report positive associations of exercise capacity with physical and mental QOL (Chang, Curtis, Patrick, & Raghu, 1999), and increased general and disease-specific QOL following 6 weeks of exercise (Jastrzębski, Gumola, Gawlik, & Kozielski, 2006). Additionally, improvements in disease-specific QOL have been observed in a randomized study of 57 patients with ILD (34 IPF, 4 sarcoidosis) following 8 weeks of supervised exercise compared to controls (Holland, Hill, Conron, Munro, & McDonald, 2008), but there was a significant decrease in these gains 6 months following completion of the program.

Cystic fibrosis

Cystic fibrosis (CF) is a genetic disease characterized by excessive mucus buildup affecting the respiratory, endocrine, and digestive systems. The most prominent symptoms appear in the lungs, with mucus buildup contributing to shortness of breath and increased production of bacteria leading to infection and lung damage. There are approximately 30,000 Americans with CF, primarily individuals of northern European ancestry. The average lifespan for individuals with CF is currently 30 years, but advancements in treatment have contributed to a steady rise in the estimated life expectancy during the past 50 years.

Cross-sectional data indicate a positive relationship between activity level and QOL among children with CF. Children with the highest level of activity report better QOL than children with lower activity levels (Selvadurai, Blimkie, Cooper, Mellis, & Van Asperen, 2004).

Observational data evaluating effects of a 6-month home-cycling program among children with CF indicated improvements in QOL, as reflected by increases in perceived physical appearance and general self-worth (Gulmans et al., 1999). In addition, the short-term effects of anaerobic training have been associated with increased physical QOL among children with CF and this effect was sustained at 12-week follow-up (Klijn et al., 2004).

A randomized study of home-based, individualized exercise training among patients with CF led to improved health perception at follow-ups of 6, 18, and 24 months (Hebestreit et al., 2010). Inpatient aerobic training (but not strength training) contributed to improvements in physical QOL 1 month following discharge from the hospital among adolescents with CF (Selvadurai et al., 2002).

Pulmonary hypertension

Pulmonary hypertension (PH) is characterized by a progressive increase in blood pressure in the pulmonary arteries. The increase in pulmonary resistance results from narrowing of the blood vessels within the lungs, causing the right side of the heart to work harder to pump blood through the lungs. Over time the increased workload results in the enlargement of the right side of the heart, leading to right ventricular failure. PH can also develop secondary to primary pulmonary diseases such as COPD or ILD. Among patients with COPD, mild comorbid PH is common. Symptoms of PH include shortness of breath upon exertion, dizziness, chest pain, swelling of the legs and ankles, and fatigue.

Poorer exercise performance (measured by 6-minute walk distance) has been associated with lower QOL among patients with PH (Taichman et al., 2005), but increases in physical and mental QOL were observed among patients with PH who participated in 15 weeks of home-based exercise training following a 3-week in-hospital program (Mereles et al., 2006).

Methodological problems/concerns in this line of research

Limitations of the extant research include reliance on self-report measures of QOL, some of which have limited data on validity and reliability. Studies examining PA and QOL among patients with various pulmonary diseases generally use QOL measures that were validated for use in patients with COPD (e.g., SGRQ and SF-36), thereby limiting the validity of QOL assessment in some studies. Disease-specific measures of QOL have been developed for CF and asthma, but are not used regularly.

In addition, most studies rely on convenience samples of patients from clinical or hospital settings, thereby reducing the generalizability of results to community settings. Further limitations include small sample sizes, variability in measures of exercise capacity, and few longitudinal studies investigating change in HRQOL over time. Although mental QOL generally appears to be positively associated with PA, studies have not consistently assessed mental QOL.

Directions for future research

The gaps in the current literature suggest directions for further research. There remain relatively few studies addressing PA and QOL among patients with pulmonary disease, especially less common pulmonary diseases such as CF and IPF. Overall, there are relatively few RCTs evaluating the effects of exercise on QOL, although there are well-controlled studies among patients with CHD and COPD. Instead, most studies provide observational evidence of the relationship between PA and QOL. However, observational studies provide only preliminary evidence of the influence of PA levels on QOL. In the future, additional experimental studies would help to further explicate the relationship between PA and QOL, as well as help identify mechanisms by which PA may influence QOL in different patient groups.

Measurement problems also plague studies of PA and QOL. The gold standard for assessing PA is exercise stress testing. However, stress testing is impractical and cost-prohibitive in larger, community-based studies of PA. Therefore, studies in the field have typically used self-report measures of PA, but these measures are subject to responder bias. Studies also make use of PA measurement devices such as pedometers and accelerometers, but these devices also may introduce bias due to variability in adherence to measurement procedures, especially among patients with chronic cardiovascular and pulmonary illnesses.

QOL measurement is routinely conducted via self-report because the construct of QOL is typically reliant on participant perception. However, as with any self-report measure, responses may be biased due to desire for positive self-presentation. Utilization of both generic and illness-specific measures may help mitigate these biases. In addition, inclusion of objective QOL indicators and attention to components of QOL is critical to clarify effects in both physical and mental domains of functioning.

Conclusions

The preponderance of evidence from studies of both cardiovascular and pulmonary disease supports a positive relationship between PA and QOL (both physical and mental), although past studies have focused more on physical QOL than mental QOL. Differences across diagnostic groups have been observed. For example, PA may not be critical for short-term improvements in QOL among patients with CHD, but appears to be related to longer-term increases in QOL. In contrast, among stroke patients, PA is associated with short-term improvement in QOL, but not with longer-term QOL outcomes. Among patients with CHD and CHF, increased exercise capacity appears to be a mechanism of improved QOL, but not necessarily among stroke patients. Studies of patients with pulmonary disease do not reflect a consistent association between increased functional capacity and increased QOL. In general, the research literature in QOL outcomes of exercise among patients with pulmonary disease is less developed than the literature among patients with cardiovascular disease.

References

Arthur, H., Gunn, E., Thorpe, K., Martin Ginis, K., Mataseje, L., McCartney, N., & McKelvie, R.S. (2007). Effect of aerobic vs combined aerobic-strength training on 1-year, post-cardiac rehabilitation outcomes in women after a cardiac event. *Journal of Rehabilitation Medicine, 39*, 730–735.

Basaran, S., Guler-Uysal, F., Ergen, N., Seydaoglu, G., Bingol-Karakoç, G., & Altintas, D.U. (2006). Effects of physical exercise on quality of life, exercise capacity, and pulmonary function in children with asthma. *Journal of Rehabilitation Medicine, 38*, 130–135.

Baughman, R.P., Sparkman, B.K., & Lower, R.R. (2007). Six-minute walk test and health status assessment in sarcoidosis. *Chest, 132*, 207–213.

Belardinelli, R., Paolini, I., Cianci, G., Piva, R., Georgiou, D., & Purcaro, A. (2001). Exercise training intervention after coronary angioplasty: The ETICA trial. *Journal of the American College of Cardiology, 37*, 1891–1900.

Belza, B., Steele, B.G., Hunziker, J., Lakshminaryan, S., Holt, L., & Buchner, D.M. (2001). Correlates of physical activity in chronic obstructive pulmonary disease. *Nursing Research, 50*, 195–202.

Bocalini, D., dos Santos, L., & Serra, A. (2008). Physical exercise improves the functional capacity and quality of life in patients with heart failure. *Clinics, 64*, 437–442.

Bourbonnais, J.M., & Samavati, L. (2010). Effects of gender on health related quality of life in sarcoidosis. *Sarcoidosis Vasculitis and Diffuse Lung Disease, 27*(2), 96–102.

Brubaker, P., Moore, B., Stewart, K., Wesley, D., & Kitzman, D. (2009). Endurance exercise training in older patients with heart failure: Results from a randomized, controlled, single-blind trial. *Journal of the American Geriatrics Society, 57*, 1982–1989.

Carod-Artal, J., Egido, J., Gonzalez, J., & de Seijas, E. (2000). Quality of life among stroke survivors evaluated 1 year after stroke: Experience of a stroke unit. *Stroke, 31*, 2995–3000.

Chang, J.A., Curtis, J.R., Patrick, D.L., & Raghu, G. (1999). Assessment of health-related quality of life in patients with interstitial lung disease. *Chest, 116*, 1175–1182.

Chen, M., & Rimmer, J. (2011). Effects of exercise on quality of life in stroke survivors: A meta-analysis. *Stroke, 42*, 832–837.

Cheng, B., Huang, Y., Shu, C., Lou, X., Fu, Z., & Zhao, J. (2010). A cross-sectional survey of participation of asthmatic children in physical activity. *World Journal of Pediatrics, 6*(3), 238–243.

Chien, C., Lee, C., Wu, Y., Chen, T., & Wu, Y. (2006). Home-based exercise increases exercise capacity but not quality of life in people with chronic heart failure: A systematic review. *Australian Journal of Physiotherapy, 54*, 87–93.

Combs, S., Dugan, E., Passmore, M., Riesner, C., Whipker, D., Yingling, E., & Curtis, A.B. (2010). Balance, balance confidence, and health-related quality of life in persons with chronic stroke after body weight-supported treadmill training. *Archives of Physical Medicine Rehabilitation, 91*, 1914–1919.

De Weerd, L., Rutgers, W., Groenier, K., & van der Meer, K. (2011). Perceived wellbeing of patients one year post stroke in general practice-recommendations for quality aftercare. *BMC Neurology, 11*, 42.

Dogra, S., Kuk, J.L., Baker, J., & Jamnik, V. (2011). Exercise is associated with improved asthma control in adults. *The European Respiratory Journal: Official Journal of the European Society for Clinical Respiratory Physiology, 37*(2), 318–323.

Dugmore, L., Tipson, R., Phillips, M., Flint, E., Stentiford, N., Bone, M., & Littler, W.A. (1999). Changes in cardiorespiratory fitness, psychological wellbeing, quality of life, and vocational status following a 12-month cardiac exercise rehabilitation programme. *Heart, 81*, 359–366.

Elley, C., Kerse, N., Arroll, B., & Robinson, E. (2003). Effectiveness of counseling patients on physical activity in general practice: Cluster randomized controlled trial. *British Medical Journal, 326*, 1–6.

Emery, C., Frid, D., Engebretson, T., Alonzo, A., Fish, A., Ferketich, A., . . . Stern, S.L. (2004). Gender differences in quality of life among cardiac patients. *Psychosomatic Medicine, 66*, 190–197.

Emery, C.F., Schein, R.L., Hauck, E.R., & MacIntyre, N.R. (1998). Psychological and cognitive outcomes of a randomized trial of exercise among patients with chronic obstructive pulmonary disease. *Health Psychology, 17*(3), 232–240.

Fanelli, A., Cabral, A.L.B., Neder, J.A., Martins, M.A., & Carvalho, C.R.F. (2007). Exercise training on disease control and quality of life is asthmatic children. *Medicine and Science in Sports and Exercise, 39*, 1474–1480.

Fernandez, F., Garcia, M., Alvarez, C., Giron, M., & Aguirre-Jaime, A. (2007). Is there an association between physical exercise and the quality of life of hypertensive patients? *Scandinavian Journal of Medicine & Science in Sports, 17*, 348–355.

Flynn, K., Pina, I., Whellan, D., Lin, L., Blumenthal, J., Ellis, S., . . . Weinfurt, K.P.; HF-ACTION Investigators (2009). Effects of exercise training on health status in patients with chronic heart failure: Findings from the HF-ACTION randomized controlled trial. *Journal of the American Medical Association, 301*, 1451–1459.

Ford, E.S., Mannino, D.M., Redd, S.C., Moriarty, D.G., & Mokdad, A.H. (2004). Determinants of quality of life among people with asthma: Findings from the behavioral risk factor surveillance system. *Journal of Asthma, 41*(3), 327–336.

Gary, R., Sueta, C., Dougherty, M., Rosenberg, B., Cheek, D., Preisser, J., . . . McMurray, R. (2004). Home-based exercise improves functional performance and quality of life in women with diastolic heart failure. *Heart and Lung, 33*, 210–218.

Greenlund, K., Giles, W., Keenan, N., Croft, J., Mensah, G., & Huston, S. (2002). Physician advice, patient actions, and health-related quality of life in secondary prevention of stroke through diet and exercise: The physician's role in helping patients to increase physical activity and improve eating habits. *Stroke, 33*, 565–571.

Gulmans, V.A.M., de Meer, K., Brackel, H.J.L., Faber, J.A.J., Berger, R., & Helders, P.J.M. (1999). Outpatient exercise training in children with cystic fibrosis: Physiological effects, perceived competence, and acceptability. *Pediatric Pulmonology, 28*, 39–46.

Hebestreit, H., Kieser, S., Junge, S., Ballmann, M., Hebestreit, A., Schindler, C., . . . Kriemler, S. (2010). Long-term effects of a partially supervised conditioning programme in cystic fibrosis. *European Respiratory Journal, 35*(3), 578–583.

Holland, A.E., Hill, C.J., Conron, M., Munro, P., & McDonald, C.F. (2008). Short-term improvement in exercise capacity and symptoms following exercise training in interstitial lung disease. *Thorax, 63*, 549–554.

Hung, C., Daub, B., Black, B., Welsh, R., Quinney, A., & Haykowsky, M. (2004). Exercise training improves overall physical fitness and quality of life in older women with coronary artery disease. *Chest, 126*, 1026–1031.

Janz, N., Janevic, M., Dodge, J., Fingerlin, T., Schork, A., Mosca, L., & Clark, N.M. (2001). Factors influencing quality of life in older women with heart disease. *Medical Care, 39*, 588–598.

Jastrzębski , D., Gumola, A., Gawlik, R., & Kozielski, J. (2006). Dyspnea and quality of life in patients with pulmonary fibrosis after six weeks of respiratory rehabilitation. *Journal of Physiology and Pharmacology, 57*(Supp 4), 139–149.

Jette, D., & Downing, J. (1996). The relationship of cardiovascular and psychological impairments to the health status of patients enrolled in cardiac rehabilitation programs. *Physical Therapy, 76*, 130–139.

Juenger, J., Schellberg, D., Kraemer, S., Haunstetter, A., Zugck, C., Herzog, W., & Haass, M. (2002). Health related quality of life in patients with congestive heart failure: Comparison with other chronic diseases and relation to functional variables. *Heart, 87*, 235–241.

Katsura, H., Yamada, K., Wakabayashi, R., & Kida, K. (2005). The impact of dyspnoea and leg fatigue during exercise on healh-related quality of life in patients with COPD. *Respirology, 10*, 485–490.

Klijn, P.H.C., Oudshoorn, A., van der Ent, C.K., van der Net, J., Kimpen, J.L., & Helders, P.J.M. (2004). Effects of anaerobic training in children with cystic fibrosis. *Chest, 125*, 1299–1305.

Lacasse, Y., Goldstein, R., Lasseron, T.J., & Martin, S. (2006). Pulmonary rehabilitation for chronic obstructive pulmonary disease. *Cochrane Database of Systematic Reviews*, Issue 4. Art. No.: CD003793. doi:10.1002/14651858.CD003793.pub2

Langhammer, B., Stanghelle, J., & Lindmark, B. (2008). Exercise and health-related quality of life during the first year following acute stroke. A randomized controlled trial. *Brain Injury, 22*, 135–145.

Lloyd-Jones, D., Adams, R., Brown, T., Carnethon, M., Dai, S., De Simone, G., . . . Wylie-Rosett, J.; American Heart Association Statistics Committee and Stroke Statistics Subcommittee (2010). Heart disease and stroke statistics—2010 update: A report from the American Heart Association. *Circulation, 121*, e46–e215.

Lloyd-Williams, F., Mair, F., & Leitner, M. (2002). Exercise training and heart failure: A systematic review of current evidence. *British Journal of General Practice, 52*, 47–55.

Mandic, S., Tymchak, W., Kim, D., Daub, B., Quinney, H., Taylor, D., . . . Haykowsky, M.J. (2008). Effects of aerobic or aerobic and resistance training on cardiorespiratory and skeletal muscle function in heart failure: A randomized controlled pilot trial. *Clinical Rehabilitation, 23*, 207–216.

Mannino, D., & Buist, A.S. (2007). Global burden of COPD: Risk factors, prevalence, and future trends. *Lancet, 370*, 765–773.

Marchionni, N., Fattirolli, F., Fumagalli, S., Oldridge, N., Del Lungo, F., Morosi, L., . . . Masotti, G. (2003). Improved exercise tolerance and quality of life with cardiac rehabilitation of older patients after myocardial infarction: Results of a randomized, controlled trial. *Circulation, 107*, 2201–2206.

Mendes, F.A.R., Gonçalves, R.C., Nunes, M.P.T., Saraiva-Romanholo, B.M., Cukier, A., Stelmach, R., . . . Carvalho, C.R.F. (2010). Effects of aerobic training on psychosocial morbidity and symptoms in patients with asthma: A randomized clinical trial. *Chest, 138*, 331–337.

Mereles, D., Ehlken, N., Kreuscher, S., Ghofrani, S., Hoeper, M.M., Halank, M., . . . Grünig, E. (2006). Exercise and respiratory training improve exercise capacity and quality of life in patients with severe chronic pulmonary hypertension. *Circulation, 114*(14), 1482–1489.

Miche, E., Roelleke, E., Zoller, B., Wirtz, U., Schneider, M., Huerst, M., . . . Radzewitz, A. (2009). A longitudinal study of quality of life in patients with chronic heart failure following an exercise program. *European Journal of Cardiovascular Nursing, 8*, 281–287.

Nieuwland, W., Berkhuysen, M., van Veldhuisen, D., Brugemann, J., Landsman, M., van Sonderen, E., . . . Rispens, P. (2000). Differential effects of high-frequency versus low-frequency exercise training in rehabilitation of patients with coronary artery disease. *Journal of the American College of Cardiology, 36*, 202–207.

Nishiyama, O., Kondoh, Y., Kimura, T., Kato, K., Kataoka, K., Ogawa, T., . . . Taniguchi, H. (2008). Effects of pulmonary rehabilitation in patients with idiopathic pulmonary fibrosis. *Respirology, 13*, 394–399.

Okano, Y., Hirawa, N., Tochikubo, O., Mizushima, S., Fukubara, S., Kihara, M., . . . Umemura, S. (2004). Relationships between diurnal blood pressure variation, physical activity, and health-related quality of life. *Clinical and Experimental Hypertension, 26*, 145–155.

Park, Y., Song, M., Cho, B., Lim, J., Song, W., & Kim, S. (2010). The effects of an integrated health education and exercise program in community-dwelling older adults with hypertension: A randomized controlled trial. *Patient Education and Counselling, 82*, 133–137.

Patwala, A., Woods, P., Sharp, L., Goldspink, D., Tan, L., & Wright, D. (2009). Maximizing patient benefit from cardiac resynchonization therapy with the addition of structure exercise training. *Journal of the American College of Cardiology, 53*, 2332–2339.

Pihl, E., Cider, A., Stromberg, A., Fridlund, B., & Martensson, J. (2011). Exercise in elderly patients with chronic heart failure in primary care: Effects on physical capacity and health-related quality of life. *European Journal of Cardiovascular Nursing, 10*, 150–158.

Povoa, T., Jardim, P., Lima, A., Salgado, C., Souza, C., Pachecho, I., . . . Jardim, L. (2010). Effects of aerobic and resistance training on quality of life and functional capacity in hypertensive women. *Journal of Hypertension, 28*, e374.

Raghu, G., Weycker, D., Edelsberg, J., Bradford, W.Z., & Oster, G. (2006). Incidence and prevalence of idiopathic pulmonary fibrosis. *American Journal of Respiratory Critical Care Medicine, 174*, 810–816.

Rand, D., Eng, J., Tang, P., Hung, C., & Jeng, J. (2010). Daily physical activity and its contribution to the health-related quality of life of ambulatory individuals with chronic stroke. *Health and Quality of Life Outcomes, 8*, 1–8.

Ries, A.L., Kaplan, R.M., Myers, R., & Prewitt, L.M. (2003). Maintenance after pulmonary rehabilitation in chronic lung disease: A randomized trial. *American Journal of Respiratory and Critical Care Medicine, 167*, 880–888.

Ringbaek, T., Brøndum, E., Martinez, G., Thøgersen, J., & Lange, P. (2010). Long-term effects of 1-year maintenance training on physical functioning and health status in patients with COPD: A randomized controlled study. *Journal of Cardiopulmonary Rehabilitation and Prevention, 30*, 47–52.

Ruo, B., Rumsfeld, J., Hlatsky, M., Liu, H., Browner, W., & Whooley, M. (2003). Depressive symptoms and health-related quality of life: The heart and soul study. *Journal of the American Medical Association, 290*, 215–221.

Santos, J., & Brofman, P. (2008). Six-minute walk test and quality of life in heart failure: A correlative study with a Brazilian sample. *Insuficiencia Cardiaca, 3,* 72–75.

Saunders, D., Greig, C., Mead, G., & Young, A. (2009). Physical fitness training for stroke patients. *Cochrane Database of Systematic Reviews.* Issue 4. Art. No.: CD003316. doi:10.1002/14651858.CD003316.pub3

Schmid, A., Duncan, P., Studenski, S., Lai, S., Richards, L., Perera, S., . . . Wu, S.S. (2007). Improvements in speed-based gait classification are meaningful. *Stroke, 38,* 2096–2100.

Seki, E., Watanabe, Y., Sunayama, S., Iwama, Y., Shimada, K., Kawakami, K., . . . Daida, H. (2003). Effects of phase III cardiac rehabilitation programs on health-related quality of life in elderly patients with coronary artery disease. *Circulation Journal, 67,* 73–77.

Selvadurai, H.C., Blimkie, C.J., Cooper, P.J., Mellis, C.M., & Van Asperen, P.P. (2004). Gender differences in habitual activity in children with cystic fibrosis. *Archives of Disease in Childhood, 89,* 928–933.

Selvadurai, H.C., Blimkie, C.J., Meyers, N., Mellis, C.M., Cooper, P.J., & Van Asperen, P.P. (2002). Randomized controlled study of in-hospital exercise training programs in children with cystic fibrosis. *Pediatric Pulmonology, 33*(3), 194–200.

Smart, N., & Marwick, T. (2005). Risks and benefits of exercise in cardiac disease. *Heart and Metabolism, 26,* 10–14.

Spruit, M.A., Thomeer, M.J., Gosselink, R., Troosters, T., Karsan, A., Debrock, A.J.T., . . . Decramer, M. (2005). Skeletal muscle weakness in patients with sarcoidosis and its relationship with exercise intolerance and reduced health status. *Thorax, 60,* 32–38.

Taichman, D.B., Shin, J., Hud, L., Archer-Chicko, C., Kaplan, S., Sager, J.S., . . . Palevsky, H. (2005). Health-related quality of life in patients with pulmonary arterial hypertension. *Respiratory Research, 6*(1), 92.

Taylor, R., Brown, A., Ebrahim, S., Jolliffe, J., Noorani, H., Rees, K., . . . Oldridge, N. (2004). Exercise-based rehabilitation for patients with coronary heart disease: Systematic review and meta-analysis of randomized controlled trials. *American Journal of Medicine, 116,* 682–692.

Tomioka, H., Imanaka, K., Hashimoto, K., & Iwasaki, H. (2007). Health-related quality of life in patients with idiopathic pulmonary fibrosis: Cross-sectional and longitudinal study. *Internal Medicine, 46,* 1533–1542.

Tsai, J., Yang, H., Wang, W., Hsieh, M., Chen, P., Kao, C., . . . Chan, P. (2004). The beneficial effect of regular endurance exercise training on blood pressure and quality of life in patients with hypertension. *Clinical and Experimental Hypertension, 26,* 255–265.

Turner, S., Eastwood, P., Cook, A., & Jenkins, S. (2011). Improvements in symptoms and quality of life following exercise training in older adults with moderate/severe persistent asthma. *Respiration; International Review of Thoracic Diseases, 81*(4), 302–310.

Van de Port, I., Wood-Dauphinee, S., Lindeman, E., & Kwakkel, G. (2007). Effects of exercise training programs on walking competency after stroke: A systematic review. *American Journal of Physical Medicine & Rehabilitation, 86,* 935–951.

Van den Berg-Emmons, R., Bussmann, J., Balk, A., & Stam, H. (2005). Factors associated with the level of movement-related everyday activity and quality of life in people with chronic heart failure. *Physical Therapy, 85,* 1340–1348.

Van Tol, B., Huijsmans, R., Kroon, D., Schothorst, M., & Kwakkel, G. (2006). Effects of exercise training on cardiac performance, exercise capacity and quality of life in patients with heart failure: A meta-analysis. *European Journal of Heart Failure, 8,* 841–850.

Verrill, D. Barton, C., Beasley, W., & Lippard, W.M. (2005). The effects of short-term and long-term pulmonary rehabilitation on functional capacity, perceived dyspnea, and quality of life. *Chest, 128*(2), 673–683.

Ware, J.E., & Sherbourne, C.D. (1992). The MOS 36-item short-form health survey (SF-36), I: Conceptual framework and item selection. *Medical Care, 30,* 473–483.

36

PHYSICAL ACTIVITY AND PSYCHOSOCIAL HEALTH AMONG CANCER SURVIVORS

Jeffrey Vallance, S. Nicole Culos-Reed, Michael Mackenzie, and Kerry S. Courneya

In the United States alone, approximately 1.6 million new cases of cancer (excluding skin cancer) are expected to be diagnosed in 2012 and close to 577,000 Americans are expected to die from cancer, making it the second most common cause of death in the United States after heart disease (American Cancer Society, 2012). The four most common cancers – prostate, breast, colorectal, and lung – are expected to account for approximately 50% of all new cancer cases and 50% of all new cancer deaths in 2010 (2012). The 5-year relative survival rate in the United States across all cancers and disease stages is 67% (2012). The high incidence coupled with good survival rates have resulted in nearly 12 million cancer survivors currently living in the United States (2012). Consequently, there is a growing population of cancer survivors.

Cancer and cancer treatments

Cancer consists of over 100 forms of diseases that grow at different rates and respond to different treatments. Cancer presents as either a malignant (i.e., invasive) or benign (i.e., non-invasive, encapsulated) solid tumor, or a nonsolid leukemia in the body's circulatory system (Ecsedy & Hunter, 2002). Individuals require cancer treatment that is aimed at their specific kind of cancer (e.g., breast, lung, colorectal). The most common treatment modalities for cancer are surgery, systemic therapy (i.e., chemotherapy, hormone replacement therapy), and radiation therapy. While these treatments have been shown to improve survival rates, cancer survivors are also at increased risk for many acute, chronic, and late effects of their disease and treatments, including cancer recurrence, second cancers, cardiac dysfunction, weight gain, bone loss, lymphedema, arthralgias, cognitive dysfunction, and menopausal symptoms (Shaprio & Recht, 2001).

A more immediate and often overlooked adverse consequence of cancer and its treatments is the impaired psychosocial health of survivors often experienced throughout the cancer trajectory. Data strongly suggest that survivors undergoing cancer treatment(s) often report poorer psychosocial health (Gao, Bennett, Stark, Murray, & Higginson, 2010). The adverse side-effects of cancer treatments have spurred a major research effort into strategies to alleviate and minimize treatment effects, both physical and psychosocial.

Psychosocial health and cancer

A cancer diagnosis and related treatments are often associated with increased emotional distress and reduced psychosocial health (Patrick et al., 2004). This process often leaves survivors overwhelmed, worried, depressed, and anxious, causing clinically significant and persistent psychosocial morbidity (i.e., impaired psychosocial health). These responses may arise from pain, a fear of recurrence, or treatment side-effects (e.g., nausea, fatigue) (Reddick, Nanda, Campbell, Ryman, & Gaston-Johansson, 2005). For some survivors, poor psychosocial health indicators, such as depression and anxiety, may be acute. However, for many survivors this depression and anxiety often is sustained well into survivorship (Carlson, Waller, Groff, Giese-Davis, & Bultz, 2011). Recent evidence also appears to suggest that depression may predict mortality, with recent meta-analytic data indicating a statistically significant associated risk (Satin, Linden, & Phillips, 2009).

Non-pharmacological modes by which to facilitate optimal psychosocial health profiles among cancer survivors are varied and can include group psychotherapy, educational resources, art therapy, music therapy, and individual one-on-one counseling. While data suggest that these intervention modalities have small effects on psychosocial health outcomes, they are unlikely to also address the physical and functional concerns experienced by cancer survivors. One intervention that has been found to enhance both the physical and psychosocial health of cancer survivors is physical activity. Clinically relevant and exciting evidence continues to emerge that supports the role of physical activity as a safe and effective intervention to facilitate favorable psychosocial health outcomes across various cancer survivor groups. This chapter will examine recent research on the associations between physical activity and psychosocial health among cancer survivors. Practical implications from this research will also be presented.

Physical activity and psychosocial health among cancer survivors

Among the general population, physical activity is a useful tool in both the prevention and treatment of anxiety (Conn, 2010a; Herring, O'Connor, & Dishman, 2010) and depression (Conn, 2010b), and improved positive affect (Reed & Buck, 2009). Given elevated levels of anxiety, depression, and distress among cancer survivors, researchers have attempted to understand the associations and effects of physical activity on psychosocial health outcomes across the cancer trajectory. Systematic reviews, as well as both cross-sectional and experimental studies in the cancer context, have demonstrated significant associations and effects between physical activity and several psychosocial health outcomes such as anxiety, stress, depression, self-esteem, and mood.

Conn and colleagues' recent meta-analysis of physical activity interventions for cancer survivors is one of the few to include a well-being component other than health-related quality of life – mood (Conn, Hafdahl, Porock, McDaniel, & Nielsen, 2006). Dependent on the instrument used to measure mood, indices of psychosocial health including stress, anxiety, and depression can be assumed. The results indicated small positive effects on well-being outcomes. For two-group comparisons there was a modest positive effect size for mood (0.19), although effect sizes were larger for single-group pre-post design studies. This meta-analysis clearly highlights the heterogeneity across the literature. The analyses also found that there were more favorable mood outcomes for interventions delivered after treatment compared to during, and improvement in mood was only found in the physical activity trials done after treatment completion. This is an important consideration when looking for potential benefits of physical activity on the psychosocial health outcomes in cancer survivors.

Research in the field of physical activity and cancer is now starting to examine the effects of exercise on specific psychosocial indicators. For example (and most recently) Craft and colleagues (Craft, Vaniterson, Helenowski, Rademaker, & Courneya, 2012) conducted a systematic review and meta-analysis to determine the antidepressant effects of exercise among cancer survivors. Studies included (N=15) were randomized controlled trials comparing exercise interventions to usual care using a self-report inventory or clinician rating to assess depressive symptoms. There was a significant overall effect size (-0.22) suggesting that exercise may have modest positive effects on depression symptoms.

Future well-designed studies are required to further our understanding of the role of physical activity for the psychosocial health of cancer survivors, on or off treatment. Clearly, a number of limitations are highlighted by the physical activity and cancer reviews, including most specifically the relatively sparse focus on the psychosocial health in relation to physical activity. Additional limitations include the heterogeneity across studies [intervention characteristics – duration, type and intensity, cancer type, treatment status (on/off)] and small sample size. The discord between the qualitative and quantitative findings regarding potential benefits from a physical activity intervention reflects the need to interpret the findings with caution until additional interventions confirm the findings. Finally, there has also been a lack of intervention work in cancer based on a needs-based approach (i.e., targeting individuals based on their need for improvement on a desired psychosocial health outcome).

Cross-sectional evidence

A more in-depth look at some specific studies may help to explain or elucidate the inconsistencies noted in the above reviews. In the cross-sectional literature, studies across several tumor groups have reported significant and beneficial relationships between physical activity, depression, anxiety, and self-esteem (Belanger, Plotnikoff, Clark, & Courneya, 2011; Faul et al., 2011; Jones et al., 2004; Penttinen et al., 2011; Rogers, Markwell, Courneya, McAuley, & Verhulst, 2011). For example, in a recent study of 192 mixed cancer survivors beginning chemotherapy (Faul et al., 2011), weekly metabolic equivalents (METs) were significantly associated with lower levels of anxiety and depression. Weekly METs were also associated with lower psychosocial composite scores on the SF-36. In a second study of 483 rural cancer survivors who were post-treatment, Rogers et al. found that those survivors who reported no leisure time physical activity had significantly higher depression scores compared to those survivors who were accruing at least 500 METs per week, the equivalent of 150 minutes per week of at least moderate-intensity physical activity (Rogers et al., 2011). This study also explored the associations between sitting time and depression. While a positive trend between sitting time and depression symptoms was apparent, there were no statistically significant relationships. It is important to note that this finding is not unique to cancer, as numerous cross-sectional studies in the general population have also reported no significant associations of physical activity with psychosocial health, depression, and self-esteem (Mosher et al., 2009; Taylor, Nicholls, et al., 2010).

Several cross-sectional studies demonstrate that these associations between physical activity and depression appear to be influenced by demographic and cancer treatment variables. For example, in a sample of 588 young adult cancer survivors, women demonstrated a clear dose-response relationship between different physical activity levels and depression, with only the two most active groups showing evidence of a physical activity and depression relationship (Belanger et al., 2011). These physical activity levels included (a) completely sedentary, (b) insufficiently active, (c) active within public health guidelines, and (d) exceeding public health activity guidelines. The same study also found that chemotherapy status (i.e., received chemotherapy vs.

no chemotherapy) moderated the relationships of physical activity level with depression, stress, and self-esteem. That is, for young adult survivors who received chemotherapy, it is likely that even smaller amounts of physical activity may be beneficial, where for survivors that did not receive chemotherapy, it appears that achieving physical activity guidelines may be required for benefits related to depression, self-esteem, and stress. In another study of cancer survivors beginning chemotherapy (Faul et al., 2011), weekly METs accounted for a significant portion of the variance in both anxiety and depression after controlling for BMI and age. In other words, physical activity was independently associated with lower anxiety and depression scores.

Experimental evidence

Several randomized controlled trials with cancer survivors have demonstrated significant and positive effects on depression, anxiety, overall psychological distress, self-esteem, and happiness outcomes (Courneya et al., 2003, 2007, 2009; Midtgaard et al., 2011; Morey et al., 2009; Noble, Russell, Kraemer, & Sharratt, 2012; Ream, Richardson, & Alexander-Dann, 2006; Sprod, Hsieh, Hayward, & Schneider, 2010). In one randomized controlled trial examining aerobic activity in 122 lymphoma survivors (Courneya et al., 2009), survivors in the aerobic group reported significantly higher ratings of happiness and significantly lower depression symptoms compared to those in a usual care control group. Courneya and colleagues have also published two randomized controlled trials in the breast cancer context (Courneya et al., 2003, 2007). In the START trial (Supervised Trial of Aerobic and Resistance Training During Chemotherapy) (Courneya et al., 2007), data suggested that those in the resistance-training group reported significantly higher self-esteem compared to those in the usual care control group. Among a sample of post-treatment (post-menopausal) breast cancer survivors, Courneya and colleagues (Courneya et al., 2003) reported significant changes in both happiness and self-esteem ratings compared to the control group. In one of the largest studies to date, Morey and colleagues randomized 641 older, overweight, long-term cancer survivors to either a home-based physical activity program or a wait-list control group (Morey et al., 2009). Data indicated that survivors in the intervention group reported significantly higher scores on the psychosocial health composite component of the SF-36 compared to the control group.

While these aforementioned studies are all positive, the evidence from other randomized controlled trials reports conflicting results. For example, a trial by Midtgaard and colleagues found significant effects on depression, but not anxiety, in a sample of 209 patients undergoing chemotherapy (Midtgaard et al., 2011). Further, Basen-Engquist reported no significant effects on psychosocial composite scores from the SF-36 after a 6-month lifestyle intervention (Basen-Engquist et al., 2006). Given the conflicting evidence, much remains to be understood. Future randomized trials need to continue to explore and elucidate the association between physical activity and psychosocial health outcomes.

Yoga, psychosocial health, and cancer

While research has primarily examined aerobic exercise, and to a lesser extent resistance training, recent research is exploring the role of other less traditional modes of physical activity. Given the permutations of developing interventions specifically designed to address psychosocial outcomes, yoga stands out as a field of interest as it consists of a low-intensity form of physical activity that may directly access mechanisms that improve patients' psychosocial health (Lin, Hu, Chang, Lin, & Tsauo, 2011; Smith & Pukall, 2009). Potential mechanisms for yoga's benefits to cancer survivors have included increased positive affect (Danhauer et al., 2009), improvements in measures of mindfulness, best understood as a special form of non-discursive attentional regulation (Salmon, Lush, Jablonski, & Sephton, 2009), and improved regulation of the autonomic nervous system (Jerath, Edry, Barnes, & Jerath, 2006; Khattab, Khattab, Ortak, Richardt, & Bonnemeier, 2007; Sarang & Telles, 2006). Further research will elucidate the role of yoga as a means of enhancing the mental health of cancer survivors.

Mechanisms of action

Mechanisms behind physical activity-related improvements in psychosocial health are unclear, given the complexity of these relationships. Purported mechanisms are numerous and have largely been divided into psychological and physiological models. Described here are two psychological models that include the role of self-efficacy and positive affect, while two such physiological models include stress adaptation and neurobiological explanations.

Self-efficacy

Within the context of physical activity, self-efficacy refers to a person's confidence in their ability to engage in physical activity under a variety of circumstances (Pinto, Rabin, & Dunsiger, 2009). Self-efficacy influences physical activity behavior such that the stronger an individual's sense of self-efficacy, the more likely they will both respond favorably and adhere to physical activity, which subsequently further bolsters self-efficacy (Blacklock, Rhodes, Blanchard, & Gaul, 2010). Interestingly, the appraisal of physiological sensations as either positive or negative will respectively increase or decrease self-efficacy, which, in turn, also predicts adherence to physical activity (Perkins, Baum, Taylor, & Basen-Engquist, 2009).

Positive affect

A current area of clinical research interest is the study of positive affect as an independent, adaptive pathway in the cancer experience (Hou, Law, & Fu, 2010). This emerging field of research suggests both baseline positive affect and the enhancement of positive affect are important components of symptom management and cancer recovery (Lyubomirsky, King, & Diener, 2005). In general, positive affect tends to increase pre- to post-physical activity following non-exhaustive physical activity intensities and may also predict improved program adherence, further solidifying the benefits obtained through regular physical activity (Ekkekakis, Parfitt, & Petruzzello, 2011; Garber et al., 2011). This engagement in behaviors that result in greater state positive affect may, over time, result in dispositional trait-like changes and enhancement of both quality of life and psychosocial health indices (Hirsch, Floyd, & Duberstein, 2012).

Stress adaptation

In general, cancer and its treatment have far-reaching effects on the totality of physiological functioning, leading to inappropriate and sustained stress responses (Fagundes et al., 2011). While physical activity may initially further intensify these stress responses, the subsequent recovery may more appropriately down-regulate these responses (Ekkekakis et al., 2011). For example, aerobic fitness may confer stress-buffering effects to psychosocial stressors via a smaller overall stress response and more rapid recovery from stressors (Forcier et al., 2006). This shorter-duration stress response could have the effect of reducing overall wear and tear on the body (Spalding, Lyon, Steel, & Hatfield, 2004).

Neurobiology

Current research in the area of neuroscience also suggests that physical activity is responsible for a number of neurobiological changes that may impact psychosocial health (Harvey, Hotopf, Overland, & Mykletun, 2010). Ernst and colleagues suggest physical activity decreases depressive symptoms by increasing brain neurogenesis. They suggest four molecular mechanisms that could play a role in mediating the effects of physical activity on increased neurogenesis: increased levels of beta-endorphins, vascular endothelial growth factor, brain derived neurotrophic growth factor, and serotonin (Ernst, Olson, Pinel, Lam, & Christie, 2006).

An argument must be made that psychology and physiology are not discrete entities and that a psycho-physiological model may be the one that accounts for the most variance (Netz, 2009). Future research must explore the complementary psycho-physiological mechanisms by which these relationships occur and develop parsimonious explanations to better explore and describe the mediating role of physical activity in improving cancer survivor psychosocial health outcomes in general, and the antidepressive and anxiolytic effects of physical activity (Strohle, 2009). More importantly, therapies directed toward addressing the functional links between mind and body may be particularly effective in treating symptoms associated with chronic illness (Taylor, Goehler, Galper, Innes, & Bourguignon, 2010).

Mediators of change

Unfortunately, relatively few interventions have examined mediating variables that may be responsible for observed changes in psychosocial health outcomes. For example, Courneya and colleagues have reported that while physical fitness parameters (i.e., peak oxygen consumption and peak power output) may mediate changes in health-related quality of life and fatigue, no such mediation was found for self-esteem, happiness, or depression (Courneya et al., 2003, 2009). While these findings suggest that improving physical fitness outcomes may be the most effective way to realize improvements in the physical and functional aspects of health-related quality of life, these studies suggest that other aspects of physical activity programs and interventions (e.g., social support, group interaction) may be responsible for changes in psychosocial health outcomes.

Limitations and future directions

Despite the aforementioned studies demonstrating several characteristics that are indicative of well-conducted, high-quality research (e.g., large sample sizes, targeted samples, randomized controlled trial methodology), several limitations remain that should be mentioned. First, while several studies have reported physical function as a primary outcome, no studies have developed a physical activity intervention specifically for alleviating psychosocial outcomes such as depression and anxiety symptoms, or improving self-esteem. Psychosocial health outcomes are most often included within a secondary analysis and are largely exploratory. Thus, the randomized controlled trials published to date are not statistically powered to detect specific changes in psychosocial health outcomes. Future studies should be designed with specific psychosocial health outcomes as the targeted outcome, and thus be appropriately powered to detect such changes.

Issues also remain with the assessment of physical activity. In all of the (associative) studies in the cancer context, physical activity was assessed via self-report. Across these studies, the self-report tools used varied considerably. While the limitations of self-reported physical activity are well documented (e.g., over-reporting, difficulty with recall), future research should make use of the recent technological advances in physical activity measurement. For example, step pedometers and accelerometers are two methods that provide a more objective index of physical activity behavior. While pedometers primarily capture walking activities, accelerometers (considered the gold standard of physical activity measurement) provide information relating to the intensity of the movement/activity being performed and may be particularly useful within the cancer context (Rogers, 2010). Accelerometers are able to provide information not just related to light, moderate, and vigorous physical activity, but also information related to time spent being sedentary. Using more objective indicators of physical activity may provide more detailed insight into the physical activity (and the emerging science of sedentary behavior), and psychosocial health relationship.

Across the studies, psychosocial health outcomes were also assessed in a variety of ways. While depression is the most commonly reported outcome across the studies, several assessments of depression symptom frequency are used (e.g., Center for Epidemiological Studies – Depression Scale, Hospital Anxiety and Depression Scale). The most common depression assessment used is the Center for Epidemiological Studies – Depression Scale (CES-D) (Kohout, Berkman, Evans, & Cornoni-Huntley, 1993; Radloff, 1977). The CES-D is a measure of depressive symptom frequency. Across studies, data suggest that the mean depression symptom frequency is actually quite low. For example, CES-D baseline mean are typically <10 on a 0–30-point scale (Belanger et al., 2011; Courneya et al., 2009). Therefore, it seems reasonable to suggest that physical activity interventions are simply able to reduce already somewhat low frequencies of depression symptoms. Future large-scale trials should determine whether physical activity interventions are able to reduce the actual clinical occurrence of depression, rather than simply mean symptom frequency, which is documented to be relatively low. To do so, future research must utilize more appropriate and clinically relevant assessments of depression. For example, the Patient Health Questionnaire – 9 (Kroenke, Spitzer, & Williams, 2001) asks individuals, "Over the last 2 weeks, how often have you been bothered by any of the following problems?" for each of the 9 DSM-IV criteria, which included such items as "Feeling tired or having little energy" and "Feeling down, depressed, or hopeless." Response options are "not at all," "several days," "more than half the days," and "nearly every day." Major depression is diagnosed if five or more symptoms are present, including depressed mood or anhedonia (i.e., inability to experience pleasurable emotions). Other depression is diagnosed if two to four depressive symptoms are present, including depressed mood or anhedonia (Kroenke et al., 2001).

Implementation

This chapter has highlighted the largely positive associations and effects observed in studies examining physical activity and psychosocial health outcomes. The evidence supports the role of physical activity across the cancer context and across tumor groups for facilitating some psychosocial health outcomes such as depression and self-esteem. Given the low rates of physical activity among a variety of tumor groups, clearly the challenge of facilitating physical activity behavior in this population remains. Several currently ongoing randomized controlled trials are exploring the effects of physical activity on a range of psychosocial health outcomes across a variety of tumor groups (Jones et al., 2010; Kampshoff et al., 2010; Persoon et al., 2010). These studies will add to the literature by providing critical information about the effects of physical activity on psychosocial health by examining different tumor groups and exploring different doses of physical activity. Research into factors that help cancer survivors engage in lifelong physical activity may not only result in more optimal psychosocial health profiles, but also reduce the risk of recurrence and facilitate longer survival for millions of cancer survivors. Staging these efforts within a theoretical framework appears to be one effective way to encourage and facilitate the adoption and maintenance of physical activity behavior in various cancer survivor groups

(Vallance, Courneya, Plotnikoff, & Mackey, 2008). While new trials continue to explore the physical activity and psychosocial health relationship among cancer survivors, resulting data should be used to develop physical activity behavior change trials and population health campaigns designed to facilitate the psychosocial health of this population.

The recent ACSM roundtable on "Exercise guidelines for cancer survivors" (Schmitz et al., 2010) concluded physical activity is safe both during and after cancer treatments, resulting in improvements in physiological, physical, and psychosocial health outcomes across several cancer survivor groups. Current recommendations suggest an overall volume of weekly activity of 150 minutes of moderate-intensity physical activity, or 75 minutes of vigorous-intensity physical activity, or an equivalent combination (Schmitz et al., 2010). Suggested strength training recommendations are to perform two to three weekly sessions including physical activities for all major muscle groups. Flexibility guidelines suggest stretching on days other physical activities are performed. These guidelines are embedded within the proviso that physical activity programs must be adapted for the individual on the basis of their health status, treatments, and anticipated disease trajectory.

Research indicates the timing of these interventions may also be important. It is suggested that although regular physical activity may improve outcomes during treatment, it may provide greater benefits during the survivorship phase (Courneya & Friedenreich, 2007; Doyle et al., 2006). However, this reported enhanced physical activity benefit post-treatment may be a reflection of survivors' treatment completion and lessening of medical demands, creating additional time and energy for cancer survivors to devote to and benefit from physical activity. ACSM roundtable guidelines suggest that cancer survivors, regardless of where they are in the treatment continuum, should avoid inactivity and that any level of physical activity carries with it some benefit (Schmitz et al., 2010).

The goals of the physical activity program and unique psychosocial health needs of cancer survivors should guide the development of tailored physical activity prescription. Research has strongly encouraged these programs to be as prescriptive as possible to meet survivors not only where they are in the cancer trajectory but also based on a host of other concerns, which may well include psychosocial health (Hacker, 2009). Deciding on the best approach for people with cancer requires detailed knowledge of the individual's current abilities, past physical activity experience, specific cancer, cancer treatment and recovery, and co-morbid conditions to best tailor the physical activity intervention program. It has been further suggested interventions should include multiple options based on preferences of targeted cancer-specific subgroups (Rogers, Markwell, Verhulst, McAuley, & Courneya, 2009).

To be prescriptive, survivors are best served by highly knowledgeable health and fitness professionals who have not only cancer-specific training but also understand the intricacies of prescribing physical activity for psychosocial health and wellness. To this end, the recent Cancer Exercise Specialist (CES) initiative by ACSM is a critical addition to cancer-specific physical activity testing and prescription. The potential for this professional designation, along with more established designations of Clinical Physical Activity Specialist and Clinical Physical Activity Physiologist, to serve as a springboard for better prescribing physical activity to cancer survivors for a variety of health concerns, not least for the express aim of mitigating symptoms and improving health in general with an eye toward psychosocial health, is highly warranted. In addition, as oncology in and of itself is a highly interdisciplinary endeavor, physical activity clinicians should be prepared to work with other treatment team members including physicians, nurses, and psychosocial health professionals.

Reaching this level of complexity in physical activity prescription will be contingent on state-of-science knowledge of cancer etiology and treatment as well as clinical physical activity physiology and behavioral health interventions. This requires a health professional well versed in all three areas. In the meantime, ACSM recommendations serve as a strong starting point for most individuals that can be further broken down into activities they enjoy, feel good doing, and derive benefit from. In maintaining such a regime, the by-product appears to be enhanced psychosocial health profiles, regardless of intervention specifics.

Summary

Unfortunately, the majority of cancer survivors will not realize these aforementioned psychosocial health benefits due to overwhelmingly low physical activity participation rates (Blanchard, Courneya, & Stein, 2008). Despite the accumulating evidence documenting the associated benefits of physical activity after a cancer diagnosis, most cancer survivors are not meeting the minimal amounts of physical activity required for the accrual of health benefits (Blanchard et al., 2008; Coups & Ostroff, 2005; Courneya, Katzmarzyk, & Bacon, 2008). Cancer care professionals can expect that less than 10% of cancer survivors will engage in physical activity during treatments and between 20% and 30% will engage in regular physical activity after their treatments. Developing and evaluating strategies to assist cancer survivors in adopting and maintaining physical activity so that psychosocial health benefits can be realized are critical. These initiatives need to be developed based on current knowledge of the determinants of physical activity in this population.

Acknowledgments

Jeffrey Vallance is supported by a Population Health Investigator Award from Alberta Innovates–Health Solutions and a New Investigator Award from the Canadian Institutes of Health Research. Michael Mackenzie is supported by a Social Sciences and Humanities Research Council Graduate Student Award and an Alberta Innovates–Health Solutions Health Research Studentship. Kerry Courneya is supported by the Canada Research Chairs Program.

References

American Cancer Society. (2012). *Cancer facts & figures 2012*. Atlanta, GA: American Cancer Society.

Basen-Engquist, K., Taylor, C. L., Rosenblum, C., Smith, M. A., Shinn, E. H., Greisinger, A., . . . Rivera, E. (2006). Randomized pilot test of a lifestyle physical activity intervention for breast cancer survivors. *Patient Education and Counselling, 64*(1–3), 225–234.

Belanger, L. J., Plotnikoff, R. C., Clark, A., & Courneya, K. S. (2011). Physical activity and health-related quality of life in young adult cancer survivors: A Canadian provincial survey. *Journal of Cancer Survivorship, 5*(1), 44–53.

Blacklock, R., Rhodes, R., Blanchard, C., & Gaul, C. (2010). Effects of exercise intensity and self-efficacy on state anxiety with breast cancer survivors. *Oncology Nursing Forum, 37*(2), 206–212.

Blanchard, C. M., Courneya, K. S., & Stein, K. (2008). Cancer survivors' adherence to lifestyle behavior recommendations and associations with health-related quality of life: Results from the American Cancer Society's SCS-II. *Journal of Clinical Oncology, 26*(13), 2198–2204.

Carlson, L. E., Waller, A., Groff, S. L., Giese-Davis, J., & Bultz, B. D. (2013). What goes up does not always come down: Patterns of distress, physical and psychosocial morbidity in people with cancer over a one year period. *Psychooncology, 22*(1), 168–176.

Conn, V. S. (2010a). Anxiety outcomes after physical activity interventions: Meta-analysis findings. *Nursing Research, 59*(3), 224–231.

Conn, V. S. (2010b). Depressive symptom outcomes of physical activity interventions: Meta-analysis findings. *Annals of Behavioral Medicine, 39*(2), 128–138.

Conn, V. S., Hafdahl, A. R., Porock, D. C., McDaniel, R., & Nielsen, P. J. (2006). A meta-analysis of exercise interventions among people treated for cancer. *Supportive Care in Cancer, 14*(7), 699–712.

Coups, E. J., & Ostroff, J. S. (2005). A population-based estimate of the prevalence of behavioral risk factors among adult cancer survivors and noncancer controls. *Preventive Medicine, 40*(6), 702–711.

Courneya, K. S., & Friedenreich, C. M. (2007). Physical activity and cancer control. *Seminars in Oncology Nursing, 23*(4), 242–252.

Courneya, K. S., Katzmarzyk, P. T., & Bacon, E. (2008). Physical activity and obesity in Canadian cancer survivors: Population-based estimates from the 2005 Canadian Community Health Survey. *Cancer, 112*(11), 2475–2482.

Courneya, K. S., Mackey, J. R., Bell, G. J., Jones, L. W., Field, C. J., & Fairey, A. S. (2003). Randomized controlled trial of exercise training in postmenopausal breast cancer survivors: Cardiopulmonary and quality of life outcomes. *Journal of Clinical Oncology, 21*(9), 1660–1668.

Courneya, K. S., Segal, R. J., Mackey, J. R., Gelmon, K., Reid, R. D., Friedenreich, C. M., . . . McKenzie, D. C. (2007). Effects of aerobic and resistance exercise in breast cancer patients receiving adjuvant chemotherapy: A multicenter randomized controlled trial. *Journal of Clinical Oncology, 25*(28), 4396–4404.

Courneya, K. S., Sellar, C. M., Stevinson, C., McNeely, M. L., Peddle, C. J., Friedenreich, C. M., . . . Reiman, T. (2009). Randomized controlled trial of the effects of aerobic exercise on physical functioning and quality of life in lymphoma patients. *Journal of Clinical Oncology, 27*(27), 4605–4612.

Craft, L. L., Vaniterson, E. H., Helenowski, I. B., Rademaker, A. W., & Courneya, K. S. (2012). Exercise effects on depressive symptoms in cancer survivors: A systematic review. *Cancer Epidemiology, Biomarkers & Prevention, 21*(1), 3–19.

Danhauer, S. C., Mihalko, S. L., Russell, G. B., Campbell, C. R., Felder, L., Daley, K., & Levine, E. A. (2009). Restorative yoga for women with breast cancer: Findings from a randomized pilot study. *Psychooncology, 18*(4), 360–368.

Doyle, C., Kushi, L. H., Byers, T., Courneya, K. S., Demark-Wahnefried, W., Grant, B., . . . Andrews, K. S.; 2006 Nutrition, Physical Activity and Cancer Survivorship Advisory Committee; American Cancer Society. (2006). Nutrition and physical activity during and after cancer treatment: An American Cancer Society guide for informed choices. *CA: A Cancer Journal for Clinicians, 56*(6), 323–353.

Ecsedy, J., & Hunter, D. (2002). The origin of cancer. In H. Adami, D. Hunter, & D. Trichopoulos (Eds.), *Textbook of cancer epidemiology* (pp. 29–53). New York: Oxford University Press.

Ekkekakis, P., Parfitt, G., & Petruzzello, S. J. (2011). The pleasure and displeasure people feel when they exercise at different intensities: Decennial update and progress towards a tripartite rationale for exercise intensity prescription. *Sports Medicine, 41*(8), 641–671.

Ernst, C., Olson, A. K., Pinel, J. P., Lam, R. W., & Christie, B. R. (2006). Antidepressant effects of exercise: Evidence for an adult-neurogenesis hypothesis? *Journal of Psychiatry & Neurosciences, 31*(2), 84–92.

Fagundes, C. P., Murray, D. M., Hwang, B. S., Gouin, J. P., Thayer, J. F., Sollers, J. J., 3rd, . . . Kiecolt-Glaser, J. K. (2011). Sympathetic and parasympathetic activity in cancer-related fatigue: More evidence for a physiological substrate in cancer survivors. *Psychoneuroendocrinology, 36*(8), 1137–1147.

Faul, L. A., Jim, H. S., Minton, S., Fishman, M., Tanvetyanon, T., & Jacobsen, P. B. (2011). Relationship of exercise to quality of life in cancer patients beginning chemotherapy. *Journal of Pain & Symptom Management, 41*(5), 859–869.

Forcier, K., Stroud, L. R., Papandonatos, G. D., Hitsman, B., Reiches, M., Krishnamoorthy, J., & Niaura, R. (2006). Links between physical fitness and cardiovascular reactivity and recovery to psychological stressors: A meta-analysis. *Health Psychology, 25*(6), 723–739.

Gao, W., Bennett, M. I., Stark, D., Murray, S., & Higginson, I. J. (2010). Psychological distress in cancer from survivorship to end of life care: Prevalence, associated factors and clinical implications. *European Journal of Cancer, 46*(11), 2036–2044.

Garber, C. E., Blissmer, B., Deschenes, M. R., Franklin, B. A., Lamonte, M. J., Lee, I. M., . . . Swain, D. P.; American College of Sports Medicine. (2011). American College of Sports Medicine position stand. Quantity and quality of exercise for developing and maintaining cardiorespiratory, musculoskeletal, and neuromotor fitness in apparently healthy adults: Guidance for prescribing exercise. *Medicine & Science in Sports & Exercise, 43*(7), 1334–1359.

Hacker, E. (2009). Exercise and quality of life: Strengthening the connections. *Clinical Journal of Oncology Nursing, 13*(1), 31–39.

Harvey, S. B., Hotopf, M., Overland, S., & Mykletun, A. (2010). Physical activity and common mental disorders. *British Journal of Psychiatry, 197*(5), 357–364.

Herring, M. P., O'Connor, P. J., & Dishman, R. K. (2010). The effect of exercise training on anxiety symptoms among patients: A systematic review. *Archives of Internal Medicine, 170*(4), 321–331.

Hirsch, J. K., Floyd, A. R., & Duberstein, P. R. (2012). Perceived health in lung cancer patients: The role of positive and negative affect. *Quality of Life Research, 21*(2), 187–194.

Hou, W. K., Law, C. C., & Fu, Y. T. (2010). Does change in positive affect mediate and/or moderate the impact of symptom distress on psychological adjustment after cancer diagnosis? A prospective analysis. *Psychology & Health, 25*(4), 417–431.

Jerath, R., Edry, J. W., Barnes, V. A., & Jerath, V. (2006). Physiology of long pranayamic breathing: Neural respiratory elements may provide a mechanism that explains how slow deep breathing shifts the autonomic nervous system. *Medical Hypotheses, 67*(3), 566–571.

Jones, L. W., Courneya, K. S., Vallance, J. K., Ladha, A. B., Mant, M. J., Belch, A. R., . . . Reiman, T. (2004). Association between exercise and quality of life in multiple myeloma cancer survivors. *Supportive Care in Cancer, 12*(11), 780–788.

Jones, L. W., Douglas, P. S., Eves, N. D., Marcom, P. K., Kraus, W. E., Herndon, J. E., 2nd, . . . Peppercorn, J. (2010). Rationale and design of the Exercise Intensity Trial (EXCITE): A randomized trial comparing the effects of moderate versus moderate to high-intensity aerobic training in women with operable breast cancer. *BMC Cancer, 10,* 531.

Kampshoff, C. S., Buffart, L. M., Schep, G., van Mechelen, W., Brug, J., & Chinapaw, M. J. (2010). Design of the Resistance and Endurance exercise After ChemoTherapy (REACT) study: A randomized controlled trial to evaluate the effectiveness and cost-effectiveness of exercise interventions after chemotherapy on physical fitness and fatigue. *BMC Cancer, 10,* 658.

Khattab, K., Khattab, A. A., Ortak, J., Richardt, G., & Bonnemeier, H. (2007). Iyengar yoga increases cardiac parasympathetic nervous modulation among healthy yoga practitioners. *Evidence Based Complementary & Alternative Medicine, 4*(4), 511–517.

Kohout, F. J., Berkman, L. F., Evans, D. A., & Cornoni-Huntley, J. (1993). Two shorter forms of the CES-D (Center for Epidemiological Studies Depression) depression symptoms index. *Journal of Aging & Health, 5*(2), 179–193.

Kroenke, K., Spitzer, R. L., & Williams, J. B. (2001). The PHQ-9: Validity of a brief depression severity measure. *Journal of General Internal Medicine, 16*(9), 606–613.

Lin, K. Y., Hu, Y. T., Chang, K. J., Lin, H. F., & Tsauo, J. Y. (2011). Effects of yoga on psychological health, quality of life, and physical health of patients with cancer: A meta-analysis. *Evidence Based Complementary & Alternative Medicine, 2011,* 659876.

Lyubomirsky, S., King, L., & Diener, E. (2005). The benefits of frequent positive affect: Does happiness lead to success? *Psychological Bulletin, 131*(6), 803–855.

Midtgaard, J., Stage, M., Moller, T., Andersen, C., Quist, M., Rorth, M., . . . Adamsen, L. (2011). Exercise may reduce depression but not anxiety in self-referred cancer patients undergoing chemotherapy. Post-hoc analysis of data from the "Body & Cancer" trial. *Acta Oncologica, 50*(5), 660–669.

Morey, M. C., Snyder, D. C., Sloane, R., Cohen, H. J., Peterson, B., Hartman, T. J., . . . Demark-Wahnefried, W. (2009). Effects of home-based diet and exercise on functional outcomes among older, overweight long-term cancer survivors: RENEW: A randomized controlled trial. *Journal of the American Medical Association, 301*(18), 1883–1891.

Mosher, C. E., Sloane, R., Morey, M. C., Snyder, D. C., Cohen, H. J., Miller, P. E., & Demark-Wahnefried, W. (2009). Associations between lifestyle factors and quality of life among older long-term breast, prostate, and colorectal cancer survivors. *Cancer, 115*(17), 4001–4009.

Netz, Y. (2009). Type of activity and fitness benefits as moderators of the effect of physical activity on affect in advanced age: A review. *European Reviews of Aging & Physical Activity, 6*(1), 19–27.

Noble, M., Russell, C., Kraemer, L., & Sharratt, M. (2012). UW WELL-FIT: The impact of supervised exercise programs on physical capacity and quality of life in individuals receiving treatment for cancer. *Supportive Care in Cancer, 20*(4), 865–873.

Patrick, D. L., Ferketich, S. L., Frame, P. S., Harris, J. J., Hendricks, C. B., Levin, B., . . . Vernon, S.W.; National Institutes of Health State-of-the-Science Panel. (2004). National Institutes of Health State-of-the-Science Conference Statement: Symptom management in cancer: pain, depression, and fatigue, July 15–17, 2002. *Journal of the National Cancer Institute Monographs* (32), 9–16.

Penttinen, H. M., Saarto, T., Kellokumpu-Lehtinen, P., Blomqvist, C., Huovinen, R., Kautiainen, H., . . . Hakamies-Blomqvist, L. (2011). Quality of life and physical performance and activity of breast cancer patients after adjuvant treatments. *Psychooncology, 20*(11), 1211–1220.

Perkins, H. Y., Baum, G. P., Taylor, C. L., & Basen-Engquist, K. M. (2009). Effects of treatment factors, comorbidities and health-related quality of life on self-efficacy for physical activity in cancer survivors. *Psychooncology, 18*(4), 405–411.

Persoon, S., Kersten, M. J., Chinapaw, M. J., Buffart, L. M., Burghout, H., Schep, G., . . . Nollet, F. (2010). Design of the EXercise Intervention after Stem cell Transplantation (EXIST) study: A randomized controlled trial to evaluate the effectiveness and cost-effectiveness of an individualized high intensity physical exercise program on fitness and fatigue in patients with multiple myeloma or (non-) Hodgkin's lymphoma treated with high dose chemotherapy and autologous stem cell transplantation. *BMC Cancer*, *10*, 671.

Pinto, B. M., Rabin, C., & Dunsiger, S. (2009). Home-based exercise among cancer survivors: Adherence and its predictors. *Psychooncology*, *18*(4), 369–376.

Radloff, L. (1977). The CES-D scale: A self report depression scale for research in the general population. *Applied Psychological Measurement*, *1*, 385–401.

Ream, E., Richardson, A., & Alexander-Dann, C. (2006). Supportive intervention for fatigue in patients undergoing chemotherapy: A randomized controlled trial. *Journal of Pain & Symptom Management*, *31*(2), 148–161.

Reddick, B. K., Nanda, J. P., Campbell, L., Ryman, D. G., & Gaston-Johansson, F. (2005). Examining the influence of coping with pain on depression, anxiety, and fatigue among women with breast cancer. *Journal of Psychosocial Oncology*, *23*(2–3), 137–157.

Reed, J., & Buck, S. (2009). The effect of regular aerobic exercise on positive-activated affect: A meta-analysis. *Psychology of Sport & Exercise*, *10*(6), 581–594.

Rogers, L. Q. (2010). Objective monitoring of physical activity after a cancer diagnosis: Challenges and opportunities for enhancing cancer control. *Physical Therapy Reviews*, *15*(3), 224–237.

Rogers, L. Q., Markwell, S. J., Courneya, K. S., McAuley, E., & Verhulst, S. (2011). Physical activity type and intensity among rural breast cancer survivors: Patterns and associations with fatigue and depressive symptoms. *Journal of Cancer Survivorship*, *5*(1), 54–61.

Rogers, L. Q., Markwell, S. J., Verhulst, S., McAuley, E., & Courneya, K. S. (2009). Rural breast cancer survivors: Exercise preferences and their determinants. *Psychooncology*, *18*(4), 412–421.

Salmon, P., Lush, E., Jablonski, M., & Sephton, S. E. (2009). Yoga and mindfulness: Clinical aspects of an ancient mind/body practice. *Cognitive & Behavioral Practice*, *16*(1), 59–72.

Sarang, P., & Telles, S. (2006). Effects of two yoga based relaxation techniques on heart rate variability (HRV). *International Journal of Stress Management*, *13*(4), 460–475.

Satin, J. R., Linden, W., & Phillips, M. J. (2009). Depression as a predictor of disease progression and mortality in cancer patients: A meta-analysis. *Cancer*, *115*(22), 5349–5361.

Schmitz, K. H., Courneya, K. S., Matthews, C., Demark-Wahnefried, W., Galvao, D. A., Pinto, B. M., . . . Schwartz. A. L.; American College of Sports Medicine. (2010). American College of Sports Medicine roundtable on exercise guidelines for cancer survivors. *Medicine & Science in Sports & Exercise*, *42*(7), 1409–1426.

Shaprio, C. L., & Recht, A. (2001). Side effects of adjuvant treatment of breast cancer. *New England Journal of Medicine*, *344*, 1977–2008.

Smith, K. B., & Pukall, C. F. (2009). An evidence-based review of yoga as a complementary intervention for patients with cancer. *Psychooncology*, *18*(5), 465–475.

Spalding, T. W., Lyon, L. A., Steel, D. H., & Hatfield, B. D. (2004). Aerobic exercise training and cardiovascular reactivity to psychological stress in sedentary young normotensive men and women. *Psychophysiology*, *41*(4), 552–562.

Sprod, L. K., Hsieh, C. C., Hayward, R., & Schneider, C. M. (2010). Three versus six months of exercise training in breast cancer survivors. *Breast Cancer Research & Treatment*, *121*(2), 413–419.

Strohle, A. (2009). Physical activity, exercise, depression and anxiety disorders. *Journal of Neural Transmission*, *116*(6), 777–784.

Taylor, A. G., Goehler, L. E., Galper, D. I., Innes, K. E., & Bourguignon, C. (2010). Top-down and bottom-up mechanisms in mind-body medicine: Development of an integrative framework for psychophysiological research. *Explore (NY)*, *6*(1), 29–41.

Taylor, D. L., Nichols, J. F., Pakiz, B., Bardwell, W. A., Flatt, S. W., & Rock, C. L. (2010). Relationships between cardiorespiratory fitness, physical activity, and psychosocial variables in overweight and obese breast cancer survivors. *International Journal of Behavioral Medicine*, *17*(4), 264–270.

Vallance, J. K., Courneya, K. S., Plotnikoff, R. C., & Mackey, J. R. (2008). Analyzing theoretical mechanisms of physical activity behavior change in breast cancer survivors: Results from the activity promotion (ACTION) trial. *Annals of Behavioral Medicine*, *35*(2), 150–158.

37

PHYSICAL ACTIVITY AND QUALITY OF LIFE IN MULTIPLE SCLEROSIS

Robert W. Motl

Multiple sclerosis (MS) is a prevalent, non-traumatic, and chronic disabling neurological disease among adults in the United States and worldwide. The National Multiple Sclerosis Society (NMSS) estimates that there are approximately 400,000 cases of MS in the United States with an incidence of nearly 200 new cases each week (NMSS, 2005). Others have indicated that MS affects an estimated 1 per 1,000 persons in the United States (Mayr et al., 2003). There are an estimated 2.5 million cases of MS worldwide (NMSS, 2005). The majority of people with MS are diagnosed between 20 and 50 years of age, and women are affected between two and three times more often than men (NMSS, 2005). MS is more common among people with northern European ancestry than people of African, Asian, and Hispanic descent (NMSS, 2005).

MS itself is typically characterized by intermittent and unpredictable, but recurrent, episodes of focal inflammation in the central nervous system (CNS; Hemmer, Nessler, Zhou, Kieseier, & Hartung, 2006) that eventually result in the demyelination and transection of axons in the brain, optic nerve, and spinal cord (Trapp & Nave, 2008). The axonal damage interferes with the smooth and rapid propagation of electrical potentials along neuronal pathways in the CNS (Bjartmar & Trapp, 2001). Over the course of the disease, there are further neurodegenerative processes that presumably are characterized by insufficient neurotrophic support rather than inflammation within the CNS, although this latter process is not completely understood (Bjartmar & Trapp, 2001; Trapp & Nave, 2008). The inflammatory and neurodegenerative processes are associated with the accumulation of symptoms, neurological impairment, and disability over time in persons with MS. Symptoms of MS commonly include walking and cognitive impairments, visual and bowel/bladder disturbances, and depression, fatigue, and pain (NMSS, 2005; Riazi et al., 2003). Ultimately, the disease process and its manifestations compromise quality of life (QOL) in persons with MS.

Multiple sclerosis and quality of life

There has been an increased interest by researchers and clinicians in the study of QOL among persons with MS (Benito-León, Morales, Rivera-Navarro, & Mitchell, 2003; Mitchell, Benito-León, Gonzalez, & Rivera-Navarro, 2005). QOL can be described as an umbrella term that consists of a number of outcomes that are considered important within a person's life (Rejeski & Mihalko, 2001). These outcomes can include physical, social, psychological, and spiritual

530

dimensions of one's well-being (Benito-León et al., 2003). Overall, QOL represents a judgment from the respondent's perspective that reflects how well they are living based on consideration of those dimensions of well-being.

There is a wealth of evidence indicating that persons with MS have lower QOL than other populations, including persons with or without a chronic disease condition (Benito-León et al., 2003; Mitchell et al., 2005). For example, persons with MS had significantly lower overall and domain-specific QOL than controls without a chronic disease in one cross-sectional study (Lobentanz et al., 2004). Other descriptive studies have reported that QOL in persons with MS is reduced even when compared with those who have inflammatory bowel disease, ischemic stroke, and rheumatoid arthritis (Lankhorst et al., 1996; Naess, Beiske, & Myhr, 2008; Rudick, Miller, Clough, Gragg, & Farmer, 1992). Several features of MS likely contribute to compromised QOL, including (1) onset of MS during the most productive years of one's life, (2) uncertain and unstable course of MS, (3) diffuse effects of MS on the CNS and mental processes, and (4) absence of convincing disease-modifying treatment (Benito-León et al., 2003). Obviously, mitigating reductions or even improving QOL is an important objective of clinical research and care of persons with MS. Such goals might be accomplished by understanding the factors that influence QOL in those with MS.

Factors influencing quality of life in multiple sclerosis

There are many modifiable factors that are associated with QOL in persons with MS and such factors represent possible targets or approaches for improving QOL in this population. Disability is one of the primary factors associated with reduced QOL in persons with MS (Amato et al., 2001; Lobentanz et al., 2004; Merkelbach, Sittinger, & Koenig, 2002) and in the context of MS is typically characterized by a restriction or inability to perform ambulatory activities in the manner considered normal. By extension, disability is often measured among persons who have MS by using the Expanded Disability Status Scale (EDSS; Kurtzke, 1983). In previous cross-sectional studies, EDSS scores were negatively correlated with overall QOL and physical aspects of health-related QOL in persons with MS (Amato et al., 2001; Lobentanz et al., 2004). Importantly, the effect of disability on QOL remained statistically significant even when controlling for other factors such as fatigue, cognitive impairment, anxiety, depression, and social support (Henriksson, Fredrikson, Masterman, & Jonsson, 2001; Stuifbergen, Seraphine, & Roberts, 2000).

Based on a prominent literature review, there are other factors such as the mood states of anxiety and depression, self-efficacy, social support, pain, and fatigue that are associated with QOL in those with MS (Mitchell et al., 2005). Mood states, namely anxiety and depression, as measured by the Hospital Anxiety and Depression Scale, have been significantly and negatively correlated with physical and mental aspects of health-related QOL in a cross-sectional study of patients with MS, even after controlling for EDSS scores (Janssens et al., 2003). Another study reported that personal beliefs regarding confidence in coping with challenging situations (i.e., self-efficacy), as measured by the MS Self-Efficacy Scale, were positively associated with physical and psychological aspects of QOL in a cross-sectional study of MS patients (Riazi, Thompson, & Hobart, 2004). Both social support (i.e., a person's perception of support and assistance from family, friends, and acquaintances) and self-efficacy were positively associated with overall QOL in a cross-sectional sample of 786 persons with MS, even after controlling for disability (Stuifbergen et al., 2000). Pain, as assessed by the McGill Pain Questionnaire, was inversely correlated with aspects of QOL in two recent cross-sectional studies of persons with MS (Kalia & O'Connor, 2005; Svendsen, Jensen, Hansen, & Bach, 2005). Fatigue assessed by the Fatigue

Severity Scale has been negatively correlated with aspects of QOL in cross-sectional studies of MS patients (Benedict et al., 2005; Lobentanz et al., 2004). Collectively, these findings are consistent with the notion that anxiety, depression, self-efficacy, social support, pain, and fatigue are additional modifiable factors that are associated with QOL in persons with MS (Benito-León et al., 2003; Stuifbergen & Roberts, 1997).

There is a wealth of evidence on factors associated with QOL in persons with MS, but until recently researchers had not examined the possible association between co-occurring or symptom clusters and QOL in this population. Symptom clusters have been defined as "three or more concurrent symptoms (e.g., pain, fatigue, sleep insufficiency) that are related to each other" (Dodd, Miaskowski, & Paul, 2001, p. 465). Symptom clusters consist of multiple symptoms that are interrelated through a common etiology or statistically as a cluster or latent variable (Miaskowski, Dodd, & Lee, 2004). Conceptually, the study of symptom clusters recognizes that co-occurring symptoms likely provide a better understanding of consequences (e.g., behavior, function, or QOL) compared with a single symptom. To that end, one study examined the symptom cluster of fatigue, pain, and depression as a correlate of reduced QOL in persons with MS (Motl & McAuley, 2010). The sample included 291 persons with a definite diagnosis of MS who were enrolled in a 6-month longitudinal study of physical activity and QOL. The participants completed baseline measures of fatigue, depression, and pain and follow-up measures of QOL. Cluster analysis initially identified three subgroups differing in experiences of fatigue, depression, and pain. Analysis of variance then indicated that the subgroup with the lowest scores on all three symptoms had the highest QOL, whereas the subgroup with the highest scores on the symptoms had the worst QOL. Such findings provide preliminary support for fatigue, pain, and depression as a symptom cluster that predicts reduced QOL in persons with MS.

Another study subsequently replicated those findings with a slightly broader symptom cluster of fatigue, pain, depression, and perceived cognitive complaints, and examined its association with QOL in 133 persons with a definite diagnosis of MS (Motl, Suh, & Weikert, 2010). Results indicated that (1) there were moderate bivariate correlations between fatigue, depression, pain, and perceived cognitive complaint scores; (2) the correlations between scores from the pairs of symptoms were attenuated when expressed as partial correlations controlling for the covariance of the remaining pair of symptoms; (3) exploratory and confirmatory factor analyses supported a single-factor model for the associations among fatigue, depression, pain, and perceived cognitive complaint scores; (4) cluster analysis identified three subgroups differing in experiences of fatigue, depression, pain, and perceived cognitive complaints; and (5) analysis of variance indicated a possible dose-response relationship between worsening symptoms and decreases in the psychological and physical domains of QOL. Such findings provide initial support for a possible dose-response relationship between worsening symptoms of fatigue, pain, depression, and perceived cognitive complaints with QOL in persons with MS.

Lifestyle factors such as physical activity, spiritual growth, health responsibility, interpersonal relations, nutrition, and stress management have been associated with QOL in persons with MS (Stuifbergen, 1995; Stuifbergen et al., 2000). For example, participation in lifestyle activities to improve overall health and well-being, as measured by overall scores on the Health Promotion Lifestyle Profile II, was positively and weakly to moderately associated with increased QOL in small (Stuifbergen, 1995) and large (Stuifbergen et al., 2000) samples of persons with MS, even after controlling for disability, perceived barriers, self-efficacy, and social support. One particular lifestyle factor that has been identified as important for QOL in MS is physical activity.

Physical activity and quality of life

Physical activity is a lifestyle factor that has been associated with many benefits among persons living with MS. The benefits of physical activity for persons with MS have been summarized in a general literature review (Garrett & Coote, 2009), a systematic Cochrane review (Rietberg, Brooks, Uitdehaag, & Kwakkel, 2005), and meta-analyses (Motl & Gosney, 2008; Snook & Motl, 2009). Some of the benefits of physical activity in persons with MS include improved strength, body composition, and cardiorespiratory fitness as well as management of fatigue, depression, anxiety, and cognitive impairment. One meta-analysis indicated that physical activity, in the form of exercise training, was associated with improved walking mobility in persons with MS (Snook & Motl, 2009). This body of literature is important as it identifies that physical activity is associated with important disease-specific benefits among those with MS.

Physical activity may have additional benefits relative to QOL. This is noteworthy as MS is associated with a reduction in QOL (Benito-León et al., 2003) and an improvement in QOL through an active lifestyle might be an even more meaningful outcome than general health benefits for those with MS (Benito-León, 2011). Descriptive, cross-sectional, and experimental evidence links physical activity, exercise training, and QOL among persons with MS. Stuifbergen (1997) conducted a descriptive study that focused on physical activity and QOL in those with MS. This descriptive study ($N = 37$) reported a positive relationship between physical activity and QOL as measured by the general health and physical functioning components of the SF-36 and weaker correlations with the vitality and social functioning components of the same scale. The effect of physical activity on QOL in this study was not limited to structured exercise programs, but generalized to forms of physical activity such as gardening and housework. However, these findings should be interpreted with caution given the small sample size, descriptive research design, and use of a self-report physical activity measure. Self-report physical activity measures have been criticized for issues of poor reliability and validity, whereas objective measures presumably have fewer psychometric issues (Dishman, Washburn, & Schoeller, 2001).

Recent cross-sectional studies have provided additional evidence of an association between physical activity and QOL in MS. One study examined the association between self-reported and objectively measured physical activity and QOL, using generic and disease-targeted instruments, in persons with MS (Motl, McAuley, Snook, & Gliottoni, 2008). The results from this cross-sectional analysis indicated that physical activity was positively associated with QOL, and this did not differ based on type of physical activity measure or QOL instrument. Another cross-sectional study reported that physical activity was favorably associated with QOL in a sample of 121 patients with MS (Stroud & Minahan, 2009). Such findings are stronger than descriptive studies, but should be interpreted with caution given the cross-sectional nature of the research designs and lack of evidence on the temporal nature of the association among variables.

Multiple intervention studies have examined the effect of exercise training programs on various indices of QOL in MS. Petajan et al. (1996) examined the effects of a 15-week aerobic training intervention versus a non-exercise control condition on mood, daily activities, and fatigue among 54 persons with MS. The exercise intervention was associated with transient improvements in depression and anger mood scores, prolonged improvements in daily activity scores on variables such as social interaction, emotional behavior, and home management, and no effect on fatigue severity scores. This study provided evidence that exercise training influenced factors related to QOL, although the study did not actually measure QOL and did not account for social interaction among participants (Sutherland, Andersen, & Stoove, 2001).

Sutherland et al. (2001) demonstrated that a 10-week aerobic exercise intervention resulted in improvements in physical, social, and mental components of QOL as measured by the Multiple

Sclerosis Quality of Life-54 scale. Mostert and Kesselring (2002) reported that a 4-week aerobic training intervention resulted in improvements on only two dimensions of the SF-36, vitality and social function, among MS patients. Similar improvements in vitality were reported after a 6-month program of yoga and aerobic exercise among individuals with MS (Oken et al., 2004). One final study reported positive effects of an 8-week aerobic training intervention on QOL as measured by the Hamburg Quality of Life Questionnaire for Multiple Sclerosis (HAQUAMS) (Schulz et al., 2004). There were relatively modest, though statistically significant, improvements in social function, mood, and total scores on the HAQUAMS in the exercise-training group. We note, however, that these intervention studies generally focused on aerobic exercise programs instead of lifestyle physical activity and included small samples of persons with MS. The intervention studies generally focused on QOL as a subsidiary, rather than primary, study outcome.

Using meta-analytic procedures, one study examined the overall effect of exercise training interventions on QOL among persons with MS (Motl & Gosney, 2008). To do this, the researchers searched MEDLINE, PsychINFO, and Current Contents Plus for the period of 1960 to November 2006 using the keywords exercise, physical activity, and physical fitness in conjunction with QOL and MS. The researchers further conducted a manual search of bibliographies of retrieved papers and literature reviews, and contacted study authors about additional studies. Twenty-five journal articles were located and reviewed, of which only 13 provided enough data to compute effect sizes expressed as Cohen's d. The 13 studies with 484 MS participants yielded 109 effect sizes with a weighted mean effect size of $g = 0.23$ (95% CI = 0.15, 0.31). There were larger effects associated with MS-specific measures of QOL when compared with general measures of QOL. The nature of the exercise stimulus further influenced the magnitude of the mean effect size, with aerobic exercise yielding the largest effects on QOL. The cumulative evidence from the meta-analysis supports that exercise training is associated with a small improvement in QOL among persons with MS; there currently is not evidence from interventions on lifestyle physical activity and improvements in QOL among those with MS.

Factors accounting for the positive association between physical activity and QOL

Previously identified factors such as disability, mood, self-efficacy, social support, and pain might account for the association between physical activity and QOL in persons with MS. This proposition was initially based on conceptual arguments and supported by empirical research involving older adults. For example, disability might account for the relationship between physical activity and QOL among those with MS. This possibility is best conceptualized within Nagi's (1965) disablement model. The disablement model and its operational definitions (Verbrugge & Jette, 1994) describe the pathway from disease to disability. The pathway involves the transition from (1) pathology (i.e., disease) to impairment (i.e., dysfunction in specific body systems), (2) impairment to functional limitation (i.e., restrictions in basic physical and mental actions), and (3) functional limitation to disability (i.e., difficulty with activities of daily life). Physical activity influences this process through effects on transitions from impairment to functional limitation and functional limitation to disability (Guralnik & Ferrucci, 2003; Stewart, 2003). The stunting of the disability process might enhance QOL and provide a basis for examining the indirect effect of physical activity on QOL through disability. Physical activity, disability, and QOL have been related among those with MS (NMSS, 2005; Pearson, Busse, van Deursen, & Wiles, 2003, 2004; Stuifbergen, 1997), and support an examination of the indirect effect of physical activity on QOL through disability in this population.

Psychological factors such as self-efficacy and self-esteem might account for the effect of physical activity on QOL in those with MS. Such a position has been proposed by Stewart and King (1991) and supported empirically in research by Elavsky et al. (2005) and McAuley et al. (2006). Indeed, Stewart and King (1991) conceptualized a comprehensive framework of QOL outcomes of relevance for physical activity research with older adults. This framework views function and well-being as two broad QOL categories with several underlying elements (e.g., physical, cognitive, emotional). This conceptualization has its basis in the Medical Outcomes Study and its seminal measure the Short-Form 36 or SF-36. As noted by Rejeski and Mihalko (2001), QOL in such a framework represents an umbrella term for multiple positive outcomes. These multiple positive outcomes allow for an inference or judgment of QOL. The underlying elements of such a model are specific, proximal outcomes of physical activity and may be viewed as intermediate factors in a broader model that includes global, distal QOL constructs. Such proximal effects of physical activity influence more distal QOL constructs (Rejeski & Mihalko, 2001).

This proposition was recently examined in two studies of mediators of the association between physical activity and QOL among older adults (Elavsky et al., 2005; McAuley et al., 2006). Participants in one study completed psychosocial and QOL measures at 1 and 5 years following enrollment in a 6-month randomized controlled exercise trial. The analyses indicated that (1) physical activity was cross-sectionally associated with self-efficacy, self-esteem, and positive affect, and, in turn, self-efficacy and positive affect were associated with QOL, and (2) changes in physical activity were associated with changes in self-esteem and positive affect, but only change in positive affect was associated with change in QOL. The other study examined the associations among physical activity, health status, self-efficacy, and QOL in older Black and White women as part of the baseline assessment of a 24-month prospective study (McAuley et al., 2006). The analyses indicated that physical activity was indirectly associated with QOL through a pathway that included self-efficacy and health status. Such findings support the position that physical activity effects on QOL are indirect and provided seminal support for a social-cognitive perspective on the association between physical activity and QOL in older adults.

Based on conceptual arguments and the empirical research with older adults, one study examined variables that might account for the relationship between physical activity and QOL in a sample ($N = 292$) of persons with a definite diagnosis of MS (Motl, McAuley, Snook, & Gliottoni, 2009). The participants wore an accelerometer for 7 days and then completed self-report measures of physical activity, QOL, disability, fatigue, mood, pain, self-efficacy, and social support. Covariance modeling indicated that those who were more physically active reported lower levels of disability ($\gamma = -.50$), depression ($\gamma = -.31$), fatigue ($\gamma = -.46$), and pain ($\gamma = -.19$), and higher levels of social support ($\gamma = .20$), self-efficacy for managing MS ($\gamma = .41$), and self-efficacy for regular physical activity ($\gamma = .49$). Those who reported lower levels of depression ($\beta = -.37$), anxiety ($\beta = -.15$), fatigue ($\beta = -.16$), and pain ($\beta = -.08$) and higher levels of social support ($\beta = .26$) and self-efficacy for controlling MS ($\beta = .17$) reported higher levels of QOL. The observed pattern of relationships supports the possibility that physical activity is indirectly associated with improved QOL in persons with MS via depression, fatigue, pain, social support, and self-efficacy for managing MS.

Those findings were then replicated in a prospective examination of depression, fatigue, pain, self-efficacy, and social support as possible intermediaries in the pathway between changes in physical activity and QOL over a 6-month period of time in persons with MS (Motl & McAuley, 2009). Adults with a definite diagnosis of MS wore an accelerometer for 7 days and then completed a battery of questionnaires at baseline ($N = 292$) and 6-months' follow-up ($N = 276$). The initial data analysis indicated that change in physical activity was associated with a statistically significant and small residual change in QOL ($\beta = .07$). The subsequent data analysis indicated that change in physical activity was associated with residual changes in fatigue ($\gamma = -.17$), pain ($\gamma = -.13$), social support ($\gamma = .07$), and self-efficacy ($\gamma = .11$), and, in turn, changes in fatigue ($\beta = -.13$), pain ($\beta = -.09$), social support ($\beta = .18$), and self-efficacy ($\beta = .10$) were associated with a residual change in QOL. The observed pattern of associations supports the possibility that physical activity is indirectly associated with improved QOL through pathways that include fatigue, pain, social support, and self-efficacy in persons with MS.

One other study focused specifically on the role of self-efficacy in the association between physical activity and QOL in MS (Motl & Snook, 2008). This was based on evidence that self-efficacy and physical activity have been positively associated with QOL in persons with MS, and using a social-cognitive perspective (McAuley et al., 2006), the association between physical activity and QOL might be indirect and accounted for by self-efficacy. The study tested the hypothesis that physical activity would be indirectly associated with QOL through a pathway that included self-efficacy. Participants were 133 persons with a definite diagnosis of MS who completed the Godin Leisure-Time Exercise Questionnaire, Multiple Sclerosis Self-Efficacy Scale, and Multiple Sclerosis Impact Scale. Path analysis indicated that those with MS who were more physically active had greater self-efficacy for function and control, and self-efficacy for function and control were associated with greater physical and psychological components of QOL. Such findings further support physical activity as a possible modifiable behavior for mitigating reductions of QOL by improving self-efficacy in persons with MS.

Limitations of existing research

There is an emerging body of research on physical activity and QOL in MS, but not all researchers have considered the evidence compelling based on methodological challenges (Mayo & Asano, 2009). Indeed, this area of exercise in MS has been plagued by challenges including choosing and prioritizing the outcomes, designing and dosing the intervention to target the focal outcome, monitoring and ensuring compliance with the intervention, and recruiting an appropriate sample based on a power analysis (Mayo & Asano, 2009). This is countered by other recommendations that promotion of physical activity represents a critical part of the clinical armamentarium of clinicians who manage the consequences of MS (Benito-León, 2011). Collectively, there is not yet universal agreement, but continued investigation, perhaps within the context of a large multi-centered randomized controlled trial, will highlight the value of exercise and physical activity in the lives of persons with MS.

Next steps

Previous studies have provided evidence for the range of factors influencing QOL in persons with MS. Physical activity is one modifiable behavior that has been consistently associated with QOL in descriptive, cross-sectional, and longitudinal studies, and intervention studies have further demonstrated favorable effects of exercise training on QOL in persons with MS. Despite the beneficial effects of exercise training on QOL, this type of physical activity may present many barriers for persons with MS including accessibility, cost, and the need for specialized staff and equipment. The focus on exercise training might explain the high rate of sedentary behavior among persons with MS (Motl, McAuley, & Snook, 2005). By comparison, lifestyle physical activity that occurs in the context of the daily lives of persons with MS might represent a more accessible and reasonable interventional target for improving QOL and achieving other benefits in persons with MS. To date, there is a lack of intervention studies that targeted an increase in lifestyle physical activity as an approach for improving QOL or other outcomes among persons with MS. We are aware of two studies that have demonstrated an increase in self-reported (Motl, Dlugonski, Wójcicki, McAuley, & Mohr, 2011) and objective physical activity (Dlugonski, Motl, & McAuley, 2011) after participation in a 12-week Internet-based behavioral intervention among persons with MS. Perhaps future studies should adopt a similar behavioral approach for increasing physical activity and examining its influence on QOL and other meaningful outcomes in persons with MS. QOL is a putative meaningful benefit associated with living an active lifestyle that researchers should continue exploring in order to improve the overall health and well-being of persons with MS.

Summary

MS is associated with a substantial reduction in QOL (Miltenburger & Kobelt, 2002). This is likely caused by (1) onset of MS during the most productive years of life, (2) uncertain and unstable course of MS, (3) diffuse effects of MS on the CNS and mental processes, and (4) absence of a convincing disease-modifying treatment (Benito-León et al., 2003). QOL has been identified as a key outcome variable in clinical research and practice of those living with MS. Physical activity is a modifiable lifestyle factor that is favorably associated with QOL in those with MS. The significance of this observation is that physical activity has a potentially strong role to play in improving the QOL of those with MS. Encouraging physical activity among those with MS, although challenging, is potentially crucial for improvements in QOL. There is further benefit in that physical activity is an inexpensive option for limiting disability and improving QOL with potential economic and personal payoffs for those with MS. This is significant as there is a link between the costs of MS and QOL (Henriksson et al., 2001; McCabe & De Judicibus, 2005; Miltenburger & Kobelt, 2002).

By further examining the physical activity and QOL relationship, we might be in a better position for designing activity programs that maximize QOL benefits. In particular, future research should seek to better understand the effects of lifestyle physical activity, not solely exercise behavior, on QOL in persons with MS. Physical activity is a modifiable lifestyle factor, and provides researchers and clinicians with an effective, non-pharmacological approach for increasing QOL in those with MS. Researchers and clinicians might be able to identify and then manipulate environmental, social, or personal variables in an effort to increase physical activity and induce QOL benefits. This translational component obviously requires studies that examine correlates of physical activity in those with MS and, ultimately, the design of interventions to promote factors associated with the improvement of QOL in persons with MS. Researchers have made great strides in identifying correlates and designing behavioral interventions, and continued research will highlight the efficacy of such approaches for increasing physical activity and improving the QOL of persons living with MS.

Acknowledgments

I would like to thank Deirdre Dlugonski for assistance with writing this chapter and recognize financial support from the National Multiple Sclerosis Society (RG 3926A2/1).

References

Amato, M. P., Ponziani, G., Rossi, F., Liedl, C. L., Stefanile, C., & Rossi, L. (2001). Quality of life in multiple sclerosis: The impact of depression, fatigue and disability. *Multiple Sclerosis*, 7(5), 340–344.

Benedict, R. H., Wahlig, E., Bakshi, R., Fishman, I., Munschauer, F., & Zivadinov, R. (2005). Predicting quality of life in multiple sclerosis: Accounting for physical disability, fatigue, cognition, mood disorder, personality, and behavior change. *Journal of Neurological Sciences, 231*(1–2), 29–34.

Benito-León, J. (2011). Physical activity in multiple sclerosis: The missing prescription. *Neuroepidemiology, 36*, 192–193.

Benito-León, J., Morales, J. M., Rivera-Navarro, J., & Mitchell, A. J. (2003). A review about the impact of multiple sclerosis on health-related quality of life. *Disability and Rehabilitation, 25*(23), 1291–1303.

Bjartmar, C., & Trapp, B. D. (2001). Axonal and neuronal degeneration in multiple sclerosis: Mechanisms and functional consequences. *Current Opinions Neurology, 14*(3), 271–278.

Dishman, R. K., Washburn, R. A., & Schoeller, D. A. (2001). Measurement of physical activity. *Quest, 53*(3), 295–309.

Dlugonski, D., Motl, R. W., & McAuley, E. M. (2011). Increasing physical activity in multiple sclerosis: Replicating internet intervention effects using objective and self-report outcomes. *Journal of Rehabilitation Research, 48*(9), 1129–1136.

Dodd, M. J., Miaskowski, C., & Paul, S. M. (2001). Symptom clusters and their effect on the functional status of patients with cancer. *Oncology Nursing Forum, 28*(3), 465–470.

Elavsky, S., McAuley, E., Motl, R. W., Konopack, J. F., Marquez, D. X., & Hu, L. (2005). Physical activity enhances long-term quality of life in older adults: Efficacy, esteem, and affective influences. *Annals of Behavioral Medicine, 30*(2), 138–145.

Garrett, M., & Coote, S. (2009). Multiple sclerosis and exercise in people with minimal gait impairment: A review. *Physical Therapy Reviews, 14*(3), 169–180.

Guralnik, J. M., & Ferrucci, L. (2003). Assessing the building blocks of function: Utilizing measures of functional limitation. *American Journal of Preventive Medicine, 25*(3 Suppl 2), 112–121.

Hemmer, B., Nessler, S., Zhou, D., Kieseier, B., & Hartung, H. P. (2006). Immunopathogenesis and immunotherapy of multiple sclerosis. *Nature Clinical Practice Neurology, 2*(4), 201–211.

Henriksson, F., Fredrikson, S., Masterman, T., & Jonsson, B. (2001). Costs, quality of life and disease severity in multiple sclerosis: A cross-sectional study in Sweden. *European Journal of Neurology, 8*(1), 27–35.

Janssens, A. C., van Doorn, P. A., de Boer, J. B., Kalkers, N. F., van der Meche, F. G., & Passchier, J. (2003). Anxiety and depression influence the relation between disability status and quality of life in multiple sclerosis. *Multiple Sclerosis, 9*(4), 397–403.

Kalia, L. V., & O'Connor, P. W. (2005). Severity of chronic pain and its relationship to quality of life in multiple sclerosis. *Multiple Sclerosis, 11*(3), 322–327.

Kurtzke, J. F. (1983). Rating neurologic impairment in multiple sclerosis: An expanded disability status scale (EDSS). *Neurology, 33*(11), 1444–1452.

Lankhorst, G. J., Jelles, F., Smits, R. C. F., Polman, C. H., Kuik, D. J., & Pfennings, L. E. M. A. (1996). Quality of life in multiple sclerosis: The disability and impact profile (DIP). *Journal of Neurology, 243*(6), 469–474.

Lobentanz, I. S., Asenbaum, S., Vass, K., Sauter, C., Klosch, G., & Kollegger, H. (2004). Factors influencing quality of life in multiple sclerosis patients: Disability, depressive mood, fatigue and sleep quality. *Acta Neurologica Scandinavica, 110*(1), 6–13.

Mayo, N. E., & Asano, M. (2009). Not another meta-analysis! *Multiple Sclerosis, 15*, 409–411.

Mayr, W. T., Pittock, S. J., McClelland, R. L., Jorgensen, N. W., Noseworthy, J. H., & Rodriguez, M. (2003). Incidence and prevalence of multiple sclerosis in Olmsted County, Minnesota, 1985–2000. *Neurology, 61*(10), 1373–1377.

McAuley, E., Konopack, J. F., Motl, R. W., Morris, K. S., Doerksen, S. E., & Rosengren, K. R. (2006). Physical activity and quality of life in older adults: Influence of health status and self-efficacy. *Annals of Behavioral Medicine, 31*(1), 99–103.

McCabe, M. P., & De Judicibus, M. (2005). The effects of economic disadvantage on psychological well-being and quality of life among people with multiple sclerosis. *Journal of Health Psychology, 10*(1), 163–173.

Merkelbach, S., Sittinger, H., & Koenig, J. (2002). Is there a differential impact of fatigue and physical disability on quality of life in multiple sclerosis? *Journal of Nervous and Mental Disease, 190*(6), 388–393.

Miaskowski, C., Dodd, M., & Lee, K. (2004). Symptom clusters: The new frontier in symptom management research. *Journal of the National Cancer Institute Monographs* (32), 17–21.

Miltenburger, C., & Kobelt, G. (2002). Quality of life and cost of multiple sclerosis. *Clinical Neurology and Neurosurgery, 104*(3), 272–275.

Mitchell, A. J., Benito-León, J., Gonzalez, J. M. M., & Rivera-Navarro, J. (2005). Quality of life and its assessment in multiple sclerosis: Integrating physical and psychological components of wellbeing. *Lancet Neurology, 4*(9), 556–566.

Mostert, S., & Kesselring, J. (2002). Effects of a short-term exercise training program on aerobic fitness, fatigue, health perception and activity level of subjects with multiple sclerosis. *Multiple Sclerosis, 8*(2), 161–168.

Motl, R. W., Dlugonski, D., Wójcicki, T. R., McAuley, E. M., & Mohr, D. C. (2011). Internet intervention for increasing physical activity in persons with multiple sclerosis. *Multiple Sclerosis, 17*(1), 116–128.

Motl, R. W., & Gosney, J. L. (2008). Effect of exercise training on quality of life in multiple sclerosis: A meta-analysis. *Multiple Sclerosis, 14*(1), 129–135.

Motl, R. W., & McAuley, E. (2009). Pathways between physical activity and quality of life in adults with multiple sclerosis. *Health Psychology, 28*(6), 682–689.

Motl, R. W., & McAuley, E. (2010). Symptom cluster and quality of life: Preliminary evidence in multiple sclerosis. *Journal of Neuroscience Nursing, 42*(4), 212–216.

Motl, R. W., McAuley, E., & Snook, E. M. (2005). Physical activity and multiple sclerosis: A meta-analysis. *Multiple Sclerosis, 11*(4), 459–463.

Motl, R. W., McAuley, E., Snook, E. M., & Gliottoni, R. C. (2008). Does the relationship between physical activity and quality of life differ based on generic versus disease-targeted instruments? *Annals of Behavioral Medicine, 36*(1), 93–99.

Motl, R. W., McAuley, E., Snook, E. M., & Gliottoni, R. C. (2009). Physical activity and quality of life in multiple sclerosis: Intermediary roles of disability, fatigue, mood, pain, self-efficacy, and social support. *Psychology, Health, & Medicine, 14*(1), 111–124.

Motl, R. W., & Snook, E. M. (2008). Physical activity, self-efficacy, and quality of life in multiple sclerosis. *Annals of Behavioral Medicine, 35*(1), 111–115.

Motl, R. W., Suh, Y., & Weikert, M. (2010). Symptom cluster and quality of life in multiple sclerosis. *Journal of Pain and Symptom Management, 39*(6), 1025–1032.

Naess, H., Beiske, A. G., & Myhr, K. M. (2008). Quality of life among young patients with ischaemic stroke compared with patients with multiple sclerosis. *Acta Neurologica Scandinavica, 117*(3), 181–185.

Nagi, S. (1965). Some conceptual issues in disability and rehabilitation. In M. B. Sussman (Ed.), *Sociology and rehabilitation* (p. 100–113). Washington, DC: American Sociological Association.

National Multiple Sclerosis Society (NMSS) (2005). *Multiple sclerosis information sourcebook.* Information Resource Center and Library of the National Multiple Sclerosis Society, New York, NY.

Oken, B. S., Kishiyama, S., Zajdel, D., Bourdette, D., Carlsen, J., & Haas, M. (2004). Randomized controlled trial of yoga and exercise in multiple sclerosis. *Neurology, 62*(11), 2058–2064.

Pearson, O. R., Busse, M. E., van Deursen, R. W., & Wiles, C. M. (2003). Monitored ambulatory activity monitoring: Relation with observed or perceived walking assessments in multiple sclerosis. *Multiple Sclerosis, 9,* S149.

Pearson, O. R., Busse, M. E., van Deursen, R. W., & Wiles, C. M. (2004). Quantification of walking mobility in neurological disorders. *Quarterly Journal of Medicine, 97*(8), 463–475.

Petajan, J. H., Gappmaier, E., White, A. T., Spencer, M. K., Mino, L., & Hicks, R. W. (1996). Impact of aerobic training on fitness and quality of life in multiple sclerosis. *Annals of Neurology, 39*(4), 432–441.

Rejeski, W. J., & Mihalko, S. L. (2001). Physical activity and quality of life in older adults. *The Journals of Gerontology, Series A: Biological Sciences, 56*(2), 23–35.

Riazi, A., Hobart, J. C., Lamping, D. L., Fitzpatrick, R., Freeman, J. A., & Jenkinson, C. (2003). Using the SF-36 measure to compare the health impact of multiple sclerosis and Parkinson's disease with normal population health profiles. *Journal of Neurology, Neurosurgery, & Psychiatry, 74*(6), 710–714.

Riazi, A., Thompson, A. J., & Hobart, J. C. (2004). Self-efficacy predicts self-reported health status in multiple sclerosis. *Multiple Sclerosis, 10*(1), 61–66.

Rietberg, M. B., Brooks, D., Uitdehaag, B. M. J., & Kwakkel, G. (2005). Exercise therapy for multiple sclerosis. *Cochrane Database Systematic Reviews* (1), CD003980.

Rudick, R. A., Miller, D., Clough, J. D., Gragg, L. A., & Farmer, R. G. (1992). Quality-of-life in multiple-sclerosis – Comparison with inflammatory bowel-disease and rheumatoid-arthritis. *Archives of Neurology, 49*(12), 1237–1242.

Schulz, K. H., Gold, S. M., Witte, J., Bartsch, K., Lang, U. E., & Hellweg, R. (2004). Impact of aerobic training on immune-endocrine parameters, neurotrophic factors, quality of life and coordinative function in multiple sclerosis. *Journal of the Neurological Sciences, 225*(1–2), 11–18.

Snook, E. M., & Motl, R. W. (2009). Effect of exercise training on walking mobility in multiple sclerosis: A meta-analysis. *Neurorehabilitation and Neural Repair, 23*(2), 108–116.

Stewart, A. L. (2003). Conceptual challenges in linking physical activity and disability research. *American Journal of Preventive Medicine, 25*(3 Suppl 2), 137–140.

Stewart, A. L., & King, A. C. (1991). Evaluating the efficacy of physical activity for influencing quality-of-life outcomes in older adults. *Annals of Behavioral Medicine, 13*(3), 108–116.

Stroud, N. M., & Minahan, C. L. (2009). The impact of regular physical activity on fatigue, depression and quality of life in persons with multiple sclerosis. *Health and Quality of Life Outcomes, 7*, 68.

Stuifbergen, A. K. (1995). Health-promoting behaviors and quality of life among individuals with multiple sclerosis. *Scholarly Inquiry for Nursing Practice, 9*(1), 31–50.

Stuifbergen, A. K. (1997). Physical activity and perceived health status in persons with multiple sclerosis. *Journal of Neuroscience Nursing, 29*(4), 238–243.

Stuifbergen, A. K., & Roberts, G. J. (1997). Health promotion practices of women with multiple sclerosis. *Archives of Physical Medicine and Rehabilitation, 78*(12 Suppl 5), S3–S9.

Stuifbergen, A. K., Seraphine, A., & Roberts, G. (2000). An explanatory model of health promotion and quality of life in chronic disabling conditions. *Nursing Research, 49*(3), 122–129.

Sutherland, G., Andersen, M. B., & Stoove, M. A. (2001). Can aerobic exercise training affect health-related quality of life for people with multiple sclerosis? *Journal of Sport and Exercise Psychology, 23*(2), 122–135.

Svendsen, K. B., Jensen, T. S., Hansen, H. J., & Bach, F. W. (2005). Sensory function and quality of life in patients with multiple sclerosis and pain. *Pain, 114*(3), 473–481.

Trapp, B. D., & Nave, K. A. (2008). Multiple sclerosis: An immune or neurodegenerative disorder? *Annual Review of Neuroscience, 31*, 247–269.

Verbrugge, L. M., & Jette, A. M. (1994). The disablement process. *Social Science & Medicine, 38*(1), 1–14.

38

EXERCISE AS AN ADJUNCT TREATMENT FOR SCHIZOPHRENIA

Guy Faulkner, Paul Gorczynski, and Kelly Arbour-Nicitopoulos

Schizophrenia is the most disabling and persistent form of severe mental illness. It is generally considered a disease related to brain abnormalities caused by a range of specific genetic and/or environmental factors (Tandon, Keshavan, & Nasrallah, 2008a). Its annual incidence averages 15 per 100,000, and the risk of developing the illness over one's lifetime is approximately 0.7% (Tandon, Keshavan, & Nasrallah, 2008b). The usual presentation in late adolescence/early adulthood places incredible demands on individuals, their families, and society itself. The symptoms of schizophrenia can be divided into positive and negative symptoms because of their impact on diagnosis and treatment, although it is important to highlight that the range and nature of symptoms vary widely between individuals (USDHHS, 1999). Positive symptoms are those that appear to reflect an excess or distortion of normal functions and are manifested in symptoms such as delusions, hallucinations, and thought disorder. Negative symptoms are those that appear to reflect a reduction or loss of normal functions and reflect symptoms such as affective flattening, apathy, social withdrawal, and cognitive impairments.

Unfortunately, schizophrenia is considered as a chronic and relapsing disorder with incomplete remissions (Tandon, Nasrallah, & Keshavan, 2009). Antipsychotic medication is the front-line treatment for schizophrenia. While such medication can be efficacious for controlling the positive symptoms, it is typically less so in alleviating negative symptoms and cognitive deficits (Tandon, Moller, et al., 2008). Notably, some researchers have suggested that motivational deficits are the central link between negative symptoms and functional impairment in schizophrenia (Foussias, Mann, Zakzanis, van Reekum, & Remington, 2009) – an obvious challenge for developing and implementing psychosocial interventions in this population.

Recovery from schizophrenia and reintegration into the community is fundamentally threatened by ignoring the physical health needs of these patients. Excess mortality is at least twice that observed in the general population and this differential mortality gap has worsened in recent decades (Saha, Chant, & McGrath, 2007). Life expectancy is shorter by 15 years, primarily because of coronary artery disease (Hennekens, Hennekens, Hollar, & Casey, 2005; McGrath, Saha, Chant, & Welham, 2008). Individuals with schizophrenia also do not receive the same level of medical services as the general population. For example, despite the development of numerous guidelines, psychiatrists have not translated these recommendations for medical monitoring into clinical practice (Druss, 2007). In sum, schizophrenia is a lifelong, often debilitating illness that strikes individuals in their prime. Successful recovery is considered multi-factorial and extends beyond symptomatic remission – quality of life for those with schizophrenia also includes physical and mental health (Ramon, Healy, & Renouf, 2007).

The case for physical activity/exercise

Physical benefits

A greater awareness of the scope and magnitude of obesity in schizophrenia has turned focus to developing strategies in managing this weight gain and assessing the impact of pharmacological and non-pharmacological interventions. While it is difficult to identify the relative contributions of disease-specific factors such as genetics, medication side-effects, or lifestyle factors such as diet, smoking, and inactivity, it is clear that helping individuals with schizophrenia become more physically active must be one component of such interventions for a number of reasons. First, current best practice guidelines in the management of obesity dictate that pharmacological interventions (e.g., sibutramine, orlistat) be used in conjunction with non-pharmacological strategies (Padwai, Li, & Lau, 2004). Second, such non-pharmacological therapy should involve physical activity and dietary counselling within a behavioural modification programme (Faulkner, Cohn, & Remington, 2007). Third, regardless of weight loss, physical inactivity is itself a major cause of morbidity and mortality, and merits the same level of concern as other cardiovascular disease risk factors (e.g., Wei et al., 1999). The majority of individuals with schizophrenia have lower cardiorespiratory fitness and physical functional capacity than population standards (Strassnig, Brar, & Ganguli, 2011).

Psychological benefits

The physical benefits alone from regular physical activity in reducing morbidity and mortality in this population are sufficient justification for the inclusion of exercise in programmes of rehabilitation (Faulkner & Biddle, 1999). However, irrespective of weight and fitness outcomes, reviews have concluded that increased physical activity improves psychological health and social well-being in this population (Faulkner & Biddle, 1999; Faulkner, 2005). The aim of this chapter is to update these earlier systematic reviews of the research base (quasi-experimental and experimental designs) concerning the mental health benefits of physical activity for individuals with schizophrenia, and identify key research gaps that must be addressed in the future.

Methods

A recent review of the effects of physical activity or exercise on the mental health of individuals with schizophrenia (Faulkner, 2005) included four quasi-experimental studies and two experimental studies. The review identified studies using Social Science Citation Index and Embase via BIDS, PsychLit, Medline, and Sport Discus. Keywords included exercise, physical activity, fitness, and schizophrenia. Three decades of literature, from 1974 to 2004, were searched with only English language studies selected. Using the same search strategy, an update to the review was conducted, searching the literature from 2004 to 2011 using Medline, PsychINFO, and Sport Discus. The search was supplemented by examining the references of the retrieved papers. Only quasi-experimental or experimental studies were included in this update, although we acknowledge the value of qualitative designs in highlighting the role of physical activity in the lives of people with serious mental illness (Faulkner & Sparkes, 1999). Studies were excluded if exercise/physical activity was not the specific intervention examined, if mental health outcomes were not reported, and/or the sample used did not specifically consist of individuals with a diagnosis of schizophrenia. Overall, seven studies were added to the current review (Acil et al., 2008; Beebe et al., 2005; Behere et al., 2011; Dodd et al., 2011; Duraiswamy et al., 2007; Marzolini et al., 2009; Warren et al., 2010).

The results are presented in two sections and classified by means of Campbell and Stanley's (1963) quasi-experimental and experimental categories. Additionally, a number of other categories are included. "Participants" describes the general nature of participants involved; "Design" expands on the research design that was used; "Treatment" describes the content of the exercise programme offered; "Psychological instruments" refers to the dependent measures assessed at pre and post treatment; and "Outcome" describes the effects of exercise participation for the participants. Statistical significance criteria are presented where available.

Results

Quasi-experimental research

Six studies (n = 230) in this category were located that used control group comparisons, repeated measures, or cross-over designs. A summary can be found in Table 38.1. The participants were predominantly adult males representing both inpatient and outpatient populations. All had diagnoses of chronic schizophrenia. Standardised psychological instruments used included the Brief Symptom Inventory (BSI; Derogatis & Melisaratos, 1983), the Brief Psychiatric Rating Scale (BPRS; Overall & Gorham, 1962), the Clinical Global Impression severity of illness item (CGI; Guy, 1976), the Nurses' Observation Scale for In-Patient Evaluation (NOSIE; Honigfeld, Gillis, & Klett, 1965), the Profile of Mood States (POMS; McNair, Lorr, & Droppleman, 1971), the Physical Estimation and Attraction Scales (PEAS; Sonstroem, 1978), the Physical Self-Efficacy (PSE; Ryckman, Robbins, Thorton, & Cantrell, 1982) and Perceived Competence Scales (PCS; Harter, 1982), the Positive and Negative Symptom Scale (PANSS; Kay, Fiszbein & Opler, 1987), the Scale for the Assessment of Negative Symptoms (SANS; Derogatis, 1993), the Scale for the Assessment of Positive Symptoms (SAPS; Andreasen, 1990), the State-Trait Anxiety Inventory (STAI; Spielberger, Gorsuch, Lushene, Vagg, & Jacobs, 1983), the Symptoms Check List-90 (SCL-90; Derogatis, Lipman, Rickels, Uhlenhuth, & Covi, 1974), and the Visual Analogue Scale (VAS; Carlsson, 1983).

Exercise programmes lasted from 3 weeks to 24 weeks and consisted of 40-minute aerobic sessions three times a week, 30 minutes of aerobic exercises and 30 minutes of walking twice a week, 20-minute walking/jogging sessions three times a week, 45 minutes of moderate skills-based physical activity five times a week, or 30 to 50 minutes of light or moderate activity twice a week.

Outcome results indicated that most studies reported some improvement on the inventory measures used (components of BPRS, BSI, NOSIE, POMS, PSE, SCL-90, SANS, SAPS, and STAI) except for the PEAS scale, where no change was reported on perceived self-image scores. In contrast, Bergman and colleagues (1993) found no improvement in psychopathological characteristics among their adolescent sample.

Experimental research

Seven further studies (n = 198) were identified that incorporated randomisation into their research design (Acil et al., 2008; Beebe et al., 2005; Behere et al., 2011; Duraiswamy et al., 2007; Lukoff, Wallace, Liberman, & Burke, 1986; Marzolini et al., 2009; Pelham et al., 1993) (see Table 38.2 for a summary).

Table 38.1 Quasi-experimental research examining psychological effects of exercise for individuals with schizophrenia

Study	Participants	Design	Treatment	Psychological instruments	Outcome
Bergman et al. (1993)	15 adolescent inpatients (9 m; 6 f; M =19.13 yrs)	Quasi-experimental (cross-over)	3 weeks, 5 days/wk, 45 mins' low-intensity activity. Alternative educational group activity	BSI, VAS; PSE, PCS	Significant improvements in physical self-efficacy only.
Chamove (1986)	40 outpatients (21 m; 19 f; M = 51 yrs)	Quasi-experimental	Normal variations in participation in one of the following: swimming, gardening, keep fit, occupational therapy. Rated blindly by nurses on days of in/activity for ≥2 days of each	NOSIE	All patients rated better on all NOSIE measures on active days. Greatest benefits for less severely disturbed, sedentary, overweight & female subjects.
Dodd et al. (2011)	8 inpatients (6 m, 2 f; M = 45.8 yrs +/- 10.1)	Single-group, pre-post pilot study; baseline familiarisation phase followed by a 24-week exercise and walking programme.	Small-group aerobic exercise programme for up to 30 min each session, twice/week and a 30-min weekly walking session	PANSS	No significant improvement in PANSS, cardio-respiratory fitness ($\dot{V}O_2$max) or walking endurance (6-min walk test).
Gimino & Levin (1984)	80 inpatients	Quasi-experimental 40 in treatment 40 in wait-list control matched for sex, age, diagnosis	10 weeks of 40 mins' jogging, 3/week	POMS, SCL-90, STAI, PEAS	Significant decrease on depression (p<.05) & tension (p<.02) of POMS for exercise group only; no difference in self-image scores.
Hatlova & Basny sen (1995)	70 inpatients (45m; 25 f)	Quasi-experimental 3 groups: 1. warmup/ stretching exercises; 2. more active; sport games for men, aerobics for women; 3. no exercise	Groups 1 and 2, 6 months, 2/wk, 30–50 min	BPRS	Group 1 improved by 12.3% on BPRS, Group 2 by 8.8% with group 3 improving by 1.3%. Greater acceptance of programme by participants in Group 2.

Warren et al. (2010) | 17 outpatients and inpatients (11 m, 6 f; M = 39.9 yrs +/- 10.1) | Single-group, quasi-experimental | 10-week programme of 3 supervised walking/jogging sessions per week progressing to completing a 5 km course | BPRS, SANS, CGI | No significant changes in any mental health measure.

Table 38.2 Experimental research examining psychological effects of exercise for individuals with schizophrenia

Study	Participants	Design	Treatment	Psychological instruments	Outcome
Acil et al. (2008)	30 outpatients (18 m; 12 f; M = 32.4 yrs)	RCT: Treatment (n =15) or control (n = 15) group	10-week group-based aerobic exercise programme consisting of 40 min/day sessions, 3 days/wk	SANS; SAPS; BSI; WHOQOL–BREF-TR	Significant improvements (p < .05) on SANS, SAPS and BSI in exercise group. Significant improvements in physical and mental domains (p<.05) of the WHOQOL in the exercise group.
Beebe et al. (2005)	10 outpatients (8 m, 2 f; M = 52 yrs)	RCT: Exercise (n = 4) or waitlist control (n = 6) group	16-week, group-based treadmill exercise programme 3 days/wk (building to 30 min/session)	PANSS	Non-significant improvements on the PANSS and 6-Min Walking Distance (6MWD) in the exercise group.
Behere et al. (2011)	66 outpatients (47 m, 19 f; M = 31.8 yrs)	RCT: Yoga (n = 27), exercise (n = 17) or waitlist control (n = 22) group	One month of instruction followed by 2 months of home-based practice of yoga or exercises (brisk walking, jogging, and aerobic and stretching exercises)	PANSS, SOFS, TRENDS, TRACS	Significant improvement in positive and negative symptoms, socio–occupational functioning and performance on TRENDS (p<0.05) in the yoga group only.

Table 38.2 Continued

Study	Participants	Design	Treatment	Psychological instruments	Outcome
Duraiswamy et al. (2007)	41 outpatients (28 m, 13 f; M = 30.4 yrs +/- 7.9)	RCT: Yoga (n = 21) or physical training (i.e., brisk walking, jogging, and stretching) (n = 10) group	Participants in both groups received 3 weeks of instruction and then asked to participate in a 3-month programme (5 days/wk for 1 hr/day)	PANSS, SOFS, SAS, AIMS, WHOQOL-BREF	Yoga group had significantly less psychopathology, and significantly greater social and occupational functioning and quality of life than those in the training group at the end of 4 months.
Lukoff et al. (1986)	28 male inpatients	RCT: Social skills (n =14) or holistic treatment (n=14) intervention (including exercise and education in stress management)	Holistic intervention included 30 min of walking/running each weekday for 9 weeks	Symptom Checklist-90, PAS, NGI, TSC	Significant increase in fitness in holistic group. Significant improvement in both groups on psychopathology measures at the end of the 9-week intervention. No change for either group in self-concept.
Marzolini et al. (2009)	13 outpatients (8 m, 5 f; M = 44.6 yrs +/- 2.6)	RCT: Exercise (n = 7) or standard care (n = 6) group	Supervised exercise group met for 90 mins 2/wk for 12 weeks. Each session included 20 minutes of resistance training and 60 minutes of walking and flexibility exercises	MHI	Significant improvement in total MHI score (p < 0.03) for the exercise group only. Non-significant increase on the 6-minute walk test among the exercise group only.
Pelham et al. (1993)	10 outpatients (18–45 yrs)	RCT: Aerobic (n = 5) or non-aerobic (n = 5) condition	Aerobic: 30 minutes of bike ergometry, 65–75% HR reserve, 4 times/wk for 8 weeks. Non-aerobic: muscle tone/strengthening exercises, 30 min, 4 times/wk for 8 weeks	Predicted $\dot{V}O_2$ max, BDI	Significant increase in $\dot{V}O_2$max and reduction in BDI (ps<.05) from baseline to the end of week 12 for the aerobic condition only.

As with the quasi-experimental studies, participants were predominantly adult males and recruited from outpatient settings. Common psychological instruments used included the Brief Symptom Inventory (BSI; Derogatis & Melisaratos, 1983), the Positive and Negative Symptom Scale (PANSS; Kay et al., 1987), the Scale for the Assessment of Negative Symptoms (SANS; Derogatis, 1993), the Scale for the Assessment of Positive Symptoms (SAPS; Andreasen, 1990), the World Health Organization Quality of Life Scale – Turkish Version (WHOQOL-BREF-TR; Fidaner, Elbi, & Fidaner, 1999), and the Mental Health Inventory (MHI; Veit & Ware, 1983).

Exercise programmes lasted from 8 weeks to 16 weeks with a frequency ranging from 2 to 5 sessions per week and session duration of 30 minutes to 1 hour. After a 16-week group-based treadmill walking programme, PANSS scores decreased in the experimental group, but changes were not significant (Beebe et al., 2005). The 10-week study by Acil, Dogan, and Dogan (2008) demonstrated significant reductions in negative and positive symptoms as measured by the SANS, SAPS, and BSI. Additionally, self-reported ratings of physical and mental health quality of life improved significantly, but social and environmental ratings did not change.

After 2 months of home-based yoga and aerobic and stretching exercises, Behere et al. (2011) found ratings of PANSS and SOFS (Saraswat, Rao, Subbakrishna, & Gangadhar, 2006) decreased in both the yoga and aerobic and stretching exercise groups from baseline, but only in the yoga group were changes significant. Additionally, TRENDS (Behere et al., 2008) scores increased in both groups, but again, only in the yoga group were changes significant. This study was based on the work of Duraiswamy et al. (2007), which found similar positive effects of yoga after 3 months. In their study, PANSS scores and SOFS scores decreased significantly in the yoga and physical training groups, with greater decreases found in the yoga group. Results from the other psychological instruments varied, with two measures, the Simpson Angus Scale (Simpson & Angus, 1970) and the AIMS, indicating a decrease in symptom scores for both groups, with no significant difference between the two groups. Findings for the WHOQOL-BREF (Skevington, Lotfy, & O'Connell, 2004) were more favourable for the yoga group than the exercise group, with increases in the yoga group being significantly different than baseline measures.

In Pelham and colleagues' (1993) study, a time-series analysis showed that five chronic outpatients randomly assigned to a 12-week aerobic exercise group had significant reductions in depression scores (BDI), along with increases in aerobic fitness. Conversely, five clients assigned to a 12-week non-aerobic training group did not improve in aerobic fitness or BDI scores. No explanation was offered for the difference in BDI scores across the two conditions.

In Marzolini et al.'s (2009) study, the MHI showed improvements in ratings for depression, positive affect, behaviour, and anxiety for the combined aerobic and strength-training group, but changes were not significantly different from the control group. Similarly, there were fitness improvements for the exercise participants but no significant differences were found between the treatment and control conditions.

Lukoff and colleagues (1986) found that both a social skills group and an aerobic exercise group (which included education) showed similar but substantial and significant reductions in overall psychopathology over the course of their 9-week programme. There were no dropouts in the exercise group and an increase in fitness, as measured by the Cooper 12-minute aerobic fitness test, was reported. However, there was a high rate of relapse (79%) in the exercise group during the 2-year follow-up. The authors suggest that participants had difficulty transferring the skills obtained during the highly structured inpatient programme to the community. Given the multiple components within this intervention, it would be impossible to attribute any outcomes specifically to exercise.

Discussion

Reaching firm conclusions regarding the role of exercise in improving the mental health of individuals with schizophrenia is difficult given the wide range of outcome measures used, the heterogeneous nature of exercise interventions and samples, and generally small sample sizes. At the very least, the existing research clearly demonstrates that physical activity interventions are possible with this population group. Adherence to supervised exercise programmes among individuals with schizophrenia appears comparable to that of the general population when it is reported. Furthermore, existing evidence also suggests that physical activity participation is associated with modest improvements in some measures of mental health – typically those associated with the negative symptoms of schizophrenia. Such findings are more consistent with studies reporting stronger research designs (i.e., RCTs). These improvements appear largely independent of changes in physical measures, including fitness or body weight.

No research has directly investigated the potential mechanisms underpinning the positive benefits reported. Qualitative case studies tend to infer that any benefit is largely related to hypothesised psycho-social mechanisms such as increased social interaction, physical self-esteem, and competence (Faulkner & Sparkes, 1999). Further research will be needed comparing different types of activity in order to identify which programme works best for this population and in what way. In the absence of a single generic mechanism, a range of exercise modes and intensities should be recommended based on the participants' previous exercise experiences, preferences, and goals. Current guidelines for lifestyle activity and exercise appear just as acceptable to individuals with schizophrenia in terms of potential mental health benefit. That is, accumulating at least 150 minutes of moderate- to heavy-intensity physical activity during the week should apply equally to this population, although modest short-term goals will be most appropriate for sedentary individuals. Richardson and colleagues (2005) have described examples of structured, supervised, facility-based exercise programmes as well as lifestyle physical activity interventions that encourage participants to incorporate walking into their everyday life, and discuss a range of practical issues related to physical activity promotion with this population.

Implications for researchers

There is a range of limitations in the existing research that need to be tackled. Some of these limitations can be addressed by better reporting of study design and outcomes. The exact nature of the exercise programme must be clearly defined with the duration, frequency, and intensity of exercise reported. Adherence must also be clearly reported. Changes in fitness levels should also be documented, as well as the incorporation of follow-up measures in research designs. The participants should be clearly described in terms of their age, sex, diagnosis, duration of illness, and medication regimen. Outcome measures should include measures relevant to schizophrenia-related symptomatology, particularly the negative symptoms, and consider broader clinical outcomes such as use of health services, medication compliance, and rate of relapse (Faulkner, 2005).

Other limitations are related to the samples typically used and the nature of the exercise intervention. These do present some interesting opportunities. In terms of sample, efforts should be made to increase the representation of women in research studies. It may be that exercise programmes need to be specifically tailored to be more attractive and enjoyable for women. Increasing female participation is critical as the prevalence of metabolic syndrome is even higher in women than in men (McEvoy et al., 2005). Comparison of lifestyle and structured interventions to increase physical activity should also be conducted, as we do not know whether less structured interventions can work with this population. Their flexibility, lower cost, and easy integration into daily schedules might be particularly appealing to individuals with schizophrenia.

The most notable absence in reviewing these studies is any explicit theoretical framework being used to guide the intervention in helping participants initiate and maintain physical activity. That is, it is not known how best to get this population engaged in exercise programmes in order to derive mental health benefits. Although adherence is not always reported, this lack of theory may contribute to the relatively modest changes in mental health and certainly the generally insignificant changes in physical fitness reported. Accordingly, future studies should describe how their intervention is theoretically informed and measure changes in the theoretically proposed mediators of behaviour change. Recent work has started to address this gap. Although mental health outcomes are not reported, Beebe and colleagues (2010a, b) describe the development of an intervention informed by self-efficacy theory. Modest increases in walking and exercise self-efficacy were reported in the intervention group. We have also completed a pilot study of a behavioural intervention for women with schizophrenia (see case study; Arbour-Nicitopoulos et al., 2010).

A 6-week weight management programme for women with schizophrenia: the need for women-centred, theory-based interventions

An example of a theory-based programme implemented among women with schizophrenia is the HEalthy Lifestyle Promotion Program (HELPP). This programme is a 6-week group-based weight management educational programme that was designed by an interdisciplinary team of health care professionals in the areas of psychiatry, exercise psychology, recreation therapy, and nutrition. A total of 23 women (5 inpatients, 18 outpatients; M_{age} = 41.7 yrs; M_{BMI} = 38.8 kg/m2) diagnosed with schizophrenia or schizoaffective disorder successfully completed the programme, and 10 participants returned for a 6-week follow-up session. Below is a description of the theoretical framework used to develop HELPP, as well as the implementation and evaluation of the programme.

Theoretical framework

The underlining theoretical framework was Social Cognitive Theory (SCT; Bandura, 1977, 1997). The primary objective of the programme was to increase self-managed behaviour. The programme targeted the four sources of self-efficacy: mastery experience (i.e., engaging in group-based physical activity), vicarious experiences (e.g., discussing how to be physically active at home), verbal persuasion (e.g., positive reinforcement of healthy behaviours from interventionists), and physiological feedback (e.g., educating participants on normal heart rate response during physical activity). Participants were taught how to use self-regulatory skills (e.g., self-monitoring, planning) to facilitate self-managed physical activity and healthy eating. As per group dynamics theory (Cartwright, 1972), the group functioned as an agent of change to facilitate participants' learning and practising of these self-regulatory skills.

Programme implementation

HELPP was offered twice per week for 90 minutes per session, and was facilitated by a recreation therapist and registered dietician. The focus of the programme was on individuals developing the self-regulatory skills necessary for participating in physical activity and maintaining healthy eating habits (e.g., self-monitoring, relapse prevention). Each session consisted of two components: 60-minute education and skill-development and 30-minute lifestyle physical activity participation.

Programme evaluation

Pre- to post-programme changes

Primary outcomes: Overall, 19 of the 23 women (83%) completed the programme, and 10 (44%) returned for a follow-up booster session. Mean attendance was 64% (see Figure 38.1a). Improvements in daily servings of fruits and vegetables and fat, and weekly minutes of moderate physical activity were also found (Figure 38.1b).

Secondary outcomes: Improvements were also shown for body image and self-efficacy *(ps* < .05), as well as the quality of life domains pertaining to perceived general health (*p* < .05), and social and physical functioning (*ps* < .10). No changes in BMI or waist circumference were found.

6-week follow-up

Ten women completed a 6-week follow-up session. Among these women, we found:

- Post-programme improvements in physical activity, self-efficacy, body image, and quality of life were maintained at follow-up
- A significant decrease in physical functioning from post- to 6-week follow-up
- No change in BMI and waist circumference from post- to 6-week follow-up.

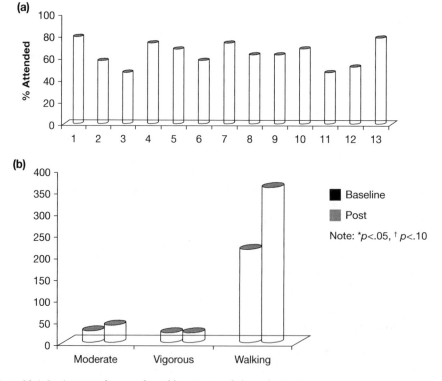

Figure 38.1 Session attendance and weekly minutes of physical activity

---

Lessons learned

Overall, HELPP was a feasible programme that was associated with short-term changes in physical and psychological health. While this was a pilot programme, the results suggest certain constructs (i.e., self-efficacy, body image, and quality of life) to target in future theory-informed intervention work within the schizophrenia population. This work also speaks to the potential of using a group-based format as an agent of change within the schizophrenia population, and the need for inter-disciplinary collaboration to deal with the increasing complexity of care in this population.

Research quality has improved if the increasing number of RCTs (n = 6) is taken as an overall indicator of quality. It is encouraging to see that since the first systematic review (Faulkner & Biddle, 1999), the number of RCTs has increased from one to seven. Clearly, exercise research with populations characterised by serious mental illness such as schizophrenia is relatively scarce in comparison to clinical depression. When conducted, sample sizes are small. This may not be helped. The overall burden of schizophrenia far outweighs the low prevalence of this condition. Researchers may be able to draw from only a relatively small pool of potential participants. Recruiting patients with schizophrenia can be time-consuming as many may be unable or unwilling to comply with study and intervention requirements. Multi-site trials will probably be required to run adequately powered randomised controlled trials examining the efficacy of exercise.

Speculatively, the small number of studies may be related to difficulties in accessing funding or institutional commitment to support such work. First, relative to the motivational and cognitive deficits characteristic of schizophrenia, health behaviour change among this population might be considered as too difficult. Describing this as therapeutic nihilism, Le Fevre (2001) suggests that this is a result of physical health in schizophrenia being largely ignored by the medical profession. Increasing obesity and diabetes prevalence among individuals with schizophrenia, particularly associated with atypical antipsychotic medication, is now recognised as a clinical concern (Allison et al., 2009). A focus on physical activity may be getting lost within broader intervention considerations targeting weight management either through medication switching, pharmacological adjuncts, or behavioural interventions that tend to largely target diet (Faulkner et al., 2007).

This might be changed by the investigation of therapeutic mechanisms that link the outcomes of physical activity with symptom reduction in schizophrenia. A novel and exciting line of research provides an example of such an approach. There are a range of neurobiological alterations in the domains of brain structure, physiology, and neurochemistry among individuals with schizophrenia (see Keshavan, Tandon, Boutros, & Nasrallah, 2008). The chronic and relapsing nature of schizophrenia might be explained by these deficits. For example, the hippocampus has been considered central to the neuropathology and pathophysiology of schizophrenia (Harrison, 2004). Meta-analysis findings demonstrate that whole-brain and hippocampal volume are reduced and that ventricular volume is increased relative to healthy controls (Steen, Mull, McClure, Hamer, & Lieberman, 2006). These deficits likely contribute to the neuropsychological impairments of schizophrenia rather than the positive symptoms (Harrison, 2004).

Given that adult neurogenesis in the hippocampus can be stimulated through exercise, Pajonk and colleagues (2010) investigated the effects of exercise on hipppocampal volume and vascularisation in chronic schizophrenia patients. Patients and healthy controls were randomised to either aerobic exercise (cycling ergometry) three times per week (30-minute sessions) for 12 weeks or a comparison condition where participants played table football matched for a similar frequency and duration. Following training, relative hippocampal volume increased significantly in both patients and healthy controls, with no change in the non-exercise patients. Patients in the exercise group had a 34% increase in a short-term memory measure while control subjects had a 17% lower score. Overall, this study suggests that hippocampal volume in individuals with schizophrenia is plastic in response to exercise. Future research replicating this finding, and linking exercise-associated improvements in hippocampal volume with meaningful clinical changes, is clearly warranted. This line of research may further legitimise exercise as an important component of treatment planning for individuals with schizophrenia.

Conclusion

Good physical health is a realistic goal for people with mental illness (Le Fevre, 2001). It is a challenging population to work with, yet this review demonstrates that physical activity intervention is possible and qualitative research consistently suggests that patients want support in leading healthier lives (e.g., Soundy, Faulkner, & Taylor, 2007). Theoretically driven research is required to examine how to reliably assist individuals with schizophrenia adopt and maintain physical activity in the face of significant motivational and cognitive deficits that are inherent to schizophrenia. Such work will be needed if the potential mental health benefits of exercise are to be maximised for this population.

Acknowledgements

The writing of this review was supported in part by an operating grant from the Canadian Institutes of Health Research (CIHR).

References

Acil, A. A., Dogan, S., & Dogan, O. (2008). The effects of physical exercises to mental state and quality of life in patients with schizophrenia. *Journal of Psychiatric and Mental Health Nursing, 15*, 808–815.

Allison, D. B., Newcomer, J. W., Dunn, A. L., Blumenthal, J. A., Fabricatore, A. N., Daumit, G. L., . . . Alpert, J. E. (2009). Obesity among those with mental disorders: A National Institute of Mental Health meeting report. *American Journal of Preventive Medicine, 36*, 341–350.

Andreasen, N. C. (1990). Methods for assessing positive and negative symptoms. *Modern Problems of Pharmacopsychiatry, 24*, 73–88.

Arbour-Nicitopoulos, K. P., Faulkner, G. E., Shyu, V., Cohn, T. A., Golding, N., & Hsueh, R. (2010). A 6-week weight management program for women with schizophrenia: The need for women-centred interventions. *Journal of Sport & Exercise Psychology, 32*, S140.

Bandura, A. (1977). Self-efficacy: Toward a unifying theory of behavioural change. *Psychological Review, 84*, 191–215.

Bandura, A. (1997). *Self-efficacy: The exercise of control.* New York: W.H. Freeman & Co.

Beebe, L. H., Tian, L., Morris, N., Goodwin, A., Swant Allen, S., & Kuldau, J. (2005). Effects of exercise on mental and physical health parameters of persons with schizophrenia. *Issues in Mental Health Nursing, 26*, 661–676.

Beebe, L. H., Smith, K., Burk, R., McIntyre, K., Dessieux, O., Tavakoli, A., . . . Velligan, D. (2011). Effect of a motivational intervention on exercise behaviour in persons with schizophrenia spectrum disorders. *Community Mental Health Journal, 47*(6), 628–636. doi:10.1007/s10597-010-9363-8

Beebe, L. H., Smith, K., Burk, R., Dessieux, O., Velligan, D., Tavakoli, A., & Tennison, C. (2010). Effect of a motivational group intervention on exercise self-efficacy and outcome expectations for exercise in schizophrenia spectrum disorders. *Journal of the American Psychiatric Nurses Association, 16*, 105–113.

Behere, R. V., Arasappa, R., Jagannathan, A., Varambally, S., Venkatasubramanian, G., Thirthalli, J., . . . Gangadhar, B. N. (2011). Effect of yoga therapy on facial emotion recognition deficits, symptoms and functioning in patients with schizophrenia. *Acta Psychiatricia Scandinavica, 123*, 147–153.

Behere, R. V., Raghunandan, V. N., Venkatasubramanian, G., Subbakrishna, D. K., Jayakumar, P. N., & Gangadhar, B. N. (2008). TRENDS: A Tool for Recogniton of Emotions in Neuropsychiatric Disorders. *Indian Journal of Psychological Medicine, 30*, 32–38.

Bergman, U., Hutzler, Y., Stein, D., Avidan, G., & Wozner, Y. (1993). Therapeutic physical activity for adolescents in a closed psychiatric ward. *Issues in Special Education and Rehabilitation, 8*, 41–54.

Campbell, D., & Stanley, J. (1963). *Experimental and quasi-experimental designs for research.* Chicago: Rand McNally.

Carlsson, A. M. (1983). Assessment of chronic pain: Aspects of reliability and validity of the visual analogue scale. *Pain, 16*, 87–101.

Cartwright, D. (1972). Achieving change in people: Some applications of group dynamics theory. In: E. P. Hollander & R. G. Hunt (Eds.), *Classic contributions to social psychology* (pp. 352–361). New York: Oxford University Press.

Chamove, A. S. (1986). Positive short-term effects of activity on behavior in chronic schizophrenic patients. *British Journal of Clinical Psychology, 25*, 125–133.

Derogatis, L. R. (1993). *BSI Brief Symptom Inventory. Administration, scoring, and procedures manual.* Minneapolis, MN: National Computer Systems.

Derogatis, L. R., Lipman, R. S., Rickels, K., Uhlenhuth, E. H., & Covi, L. (1974). The Hopkins Symptom Checklist (HSLC): A self report symptom inventory. *Behavioral Science, 19*, 1–15.

Derogatis, L. R., & Melisaratos, N. (1983). The brief symptom inventory: An introduction report. *Psychological Medicine, 13*, 595–605.

Dodd, K. J., Duffy, S., Stewart, J. A., Impey, J., & Taylor, N. (2011). A small group aerobic exercise programme that reduces body weight is feasible in adults with severe chronic schizophrenia: A pilot study. *Disability and Rehabilitation, 33*, 1222–1229.

Druss, B. G. (2007). Improving medical care for persons with serious mental illness: Challenges and solutions. *Journal of Clinical Psychiatry, 68*(Suppl. 4), 40–44.

Duraiswamy, G., Thirthalli, J., Nagendra, H. R., & Gangadhar, B. N. (2007). Yoga therapy as an add-on treatment in the management of patients with schizophrenia – A randomized controlled trial. *Acta Psychiatrica Scandinavica, 116*, 226–232.

Faulkner, G. (2005). Exercise as an adjunct treatment for schizophrenia. In G. Faulkner & A. Taylor (Eds.), *Exercise, health and mental health: Emerging relationships* (pp. 27–47). London: Routledge.

Faulkner, G., & Biddle, S. (1999). Exercise and schizophrenia: A review. *Journal of Mental Health, 8*, 441–457.

Faulkner, G., Cohn, T., & Remington, G. (2007). Interventions to reduce weight gain in schizophrenia. *Cochrane Database of Systemic Reviews, 24*, CD005148.

Faulkner, G., & Sparkes, A. (1999). Exercise as therapy for schizophrenia: An ethnographic study. *Journal of Sport and Exercise Psychology, 21*, 52–69.

Fidaner, H., Elbi, H., Fidaner, C., et al. (1999). The measurement of quality of life, WHOQOL-100 and WHOQOL-TR-BREF (in Turkish). *3P Dergisi, 7*(Suppl. 2), 5–13.

Foussias, G., Mann, S., Zakzanis, K. K., van Reekum, R., & Remington, G. (2009). Motivational deficits as the central link to functioning in schizophrenia: A pilot study. *Schizophrenia Research, 115*, 333–337.

Gimino, F. A., & Levin, S. J. (1984). The effects of aerobic exercise on perceived self-image in post-hospitalized schizophrenic patients. *Medicine and Science in Sports and Exercise, 16*, 139.

Guy, W. (1976). *ECDEU assessment manual for psychopharmacology: Nurses' Global Impressions Scale.* Washington, DC: U.S. Government Printing Office.

Harrison, P. J. (2004). The hippocampus in schizophrenia: A review of the neuropathological evidence and its pathophysiological implications. *Psychopharmacology, 174*, 151–162.

Harter, S. (1982). The perceived competence scale for children. *Child Development, 53*, 87–97.

Hatlova, B., & Basny sen, Z. (1995). Kinesiotherapy – Therapy using two different types of exercises in curing schizophrenic patients. *Physical activity for life: East and west, south and north* (pp. 426–429). International Society for Comparative PE and Sport. Proceedings of the 9th Biennial Conference, July 2–7, 1994, Prague. Aachen, Germany: Meyer & Meyer Verlag.

Hennekens, C. H., Hennekens, A. R., Hollar, D., & Casey, D. E. (2005). Schizophrenia and increased risks of cardiovascular disease. *American Heart Journal, 150*, 1115–1121.

Honigfeld, G., Gillis, R. D., & Klett, C. J. (1965). Nurses' observation scale for inpatient evaluation: A new scale for measuring improvement in chronic schizophrenia. *Journal of Clinical Psychology, 21*, 65–71.

Kay, S. R., Fiszbein, A., & Opler, L. A. (1987). The positive and negative syndrome scale (PANSS) for schizophrenia. *Schizophrenia Bulletin, 13*, 261–276.

Keshavan, M. S., Tandon, R., Boutros, N. N., & Nasrallah, H. A. (2008). Schizophrenia, "Just the Facts": What we know in 2008. Part 3: Neurobiology. *Schizophrenia Research, 106*, 89–107.

Le Fevre, P. D. (2001). Improving the physical health of patients with schizophrenia: Therapeutic nihilism or realism? *Scottish Medical Journal, 46*, 11–31.

Lukoff, D., Wallace, C. J., Liberman, R. P., & Burke, K. (1986). A holistic program for chronic schizophrenic patients. *Schizophrenia Bulletin, 12*, 274–282.

Marzolini, S., Jensen, B., & Melville, P. (2009). Feasibility and effects of a group-based resistance and aerobic exercise programme for individuals with severe schizophrenia: A multidisciplinary approach. *Mental Health and Physical Activity, 2*, 29–36.

McEvoy, J. P., Meyer, J. M., Goff, D. C., Nasrallah, H. A., Davis, S. M., Sullivan, L., . . . Lieberman, J. A. (2005). Prevalence of the metabolic syndrome in patients with schizophrenia: Baseline results from the Clinical Antipsychotic Trials of Intervention Effectiveness (CATIE) schizophrenia trial and comparison with national estimates from NHANES III. *Schizophrenia Research, 80*(1), 19–32.

McGrath, J., Saha, S., Chant, D., & Welham, J. (2008). Schizophrenia: A concise overview of incidence, prevalence, and mortality. *Epidemiologic Reviews, 30*, 67–76.

McNair, D. M., Lorr, M., & Droppleman, L. F. (1971). *Manual for the profile of mood states.* San Diego, CA: Educational and Industrial Testing Service.

Overall, J. E., & Gorham, D. R. (1962). The Brief Psychotic Rating Scale. *Psychological Reports, 10*, 799–812.

Padwai, R., Li, S. K., & Lau, D. C. W. (2004). Long-term pharmacotherapy for obesity and overweight. *Cochrane Database of Systematic Reviews, 3*, CD004094.

Pajonk, F. G., Wobrock, T., Gruber, O., . . . Falkai, P. (2010). Hippocampal plasticity in response to exercise in schizophrenia. *Archives of General Psychiatry, 67*, 133–143.

Pelham, T. W., Campagna, P. D., Ritvo, P. G., & Birnie, W. A. (1993). The effects of exercise therapy on clients in a psychiatric rehabilitation program. *Psychosocial Rehabilitation Journal, 16*, 75–84.

Ramon, S., Healy, B., & Renouf, N. (2007). Recovery from mental illness as an emergent concept and practice in Australia and the UK. *International Journal of Social Psychiatry, 53*, 108–122.

Richardson, C., Faulkner, G., McDevitt, J., Skrinar, G. S., Hutchison, D. S., & Piette, J. D. (2005). Integrating physical activity into mental health services for individuals with serious mental illness. *Psychiatric Services, 56*, 324–331.

Ryckman, R. M., Robbins, M. A., Thornton, B., & Cantrell, P. (1982). Development and validation of a physical self-efficacy scale. *Journal of Personality and Social Psychology, 42*, 891–900.

Saha, S., Chant, D., & McGrath, J. (2007). A systematic review of mortality in schizophrenia: Is the differential mortality gap worsening over time. *Archives of General Psychiatry, 64*, 1123–1131.

Saraswat, N., Rao, K., Subbakrishna, D. K., & Gangadhar, B. N. (2006). The Social Occupational Functioning Scale (SOFS): A brief measure of functional status in persons with schizophrenia. *Schizophrenia Research, 81*, 301–309.

Simpson, G. M., & Angus, J. W. S. (1970). A rating scale for extrapyramidal side effects. *Acta Psychiatrica Scandinavica, 212*, 11–19.

Skevington, S. M., Lotfy, M., & O'Connell, K. A. (2004). The World Health Organization's WHOQOL-BREF quality of life assessment: Psychometric properties and results of the international field trial. A report from the WHOQOL group. *Quality of Life Research, 13*, 299–310.

Sonstroem, R. J. (1978). Physical estimation and attraction scales: Rationale and research. *Medicine and Science in Sports, 10*, 97–102.

Soundy, A., Faulkner, G., & Taylor, A. (2007). Exploring variability and perceptions of lifestyle physical activity among individuals with severe and enduring mental health problems: A qualitative study. *Journal of Mental Health, 16*, 1–11.

Spielberger, C. D., Gorsuch, R. L., Lushene, R., Vagg, P. R., & Jacobs, G. A. (1983). *Manual for the State-Trait Anxiety Inventory (Form Y1).* Palo Alto, CA: Consulting Psychologists Press.

Steen, R. G., Mull, C., McClure, R., Hamer, R. M., & Lieberman, J. A. (2006). Brain volume in first-episode schizophrenia: Systematic review and meta-analysis of magnetic resonance imaging studies. *British Journal of Psychiatry, 188*, 510–518.

Strassnig, M., Brar, J. S., & Ganguli, R. (2011). Low cardiorespiratory fitness and physical functional capacity in obese patients with schizophrenia. *Schizophrenia Research, 126*(1–3), 103–109.

Tandon, R., Keshavan, M. S., & Nasrallah, H. A. (2008a). Schizophrenia, "Just the Facts" What we know in 2008. Part 1: Overview. *Schizophrenia Research, 100*, 4–19.

Tandon, R., Keshavan, M. S., & Nasrallah, H. A. (2008b). Schizophrenia, "Just the Facts" What we know in 2008. Part 2: Epidemiology and etiology. *Schizophrenia Research, 102,* 1–18.

Tandon, R., Moller, H-J., Belmaker, R. H., . . . Moeller, H. J.; Section of Pharmacopsychiatry, World Psychiatric Association. (2008). World Psychiatry Association Pharmacopsychiatry Section statement on comparative effectiveness of antipsychotics in the treatment of schizophrenia. *Schizophrenia Research, 100,* 20–38.

Tandon, R., Nasrallah, H. A., & Keshavan, M. S. (2009). Schizophrenia, "Just the Facts" 4. Clinical features and conceptualization. *Schizophrenia Research, 110,* 1–23.

United States Department of Health and Human Services. (1999). Mental health: A report of the Surgeon General. Atlanta, GA: U.S. Department of Health and Human Services, Centers for Disease Control and Prevention, National Center for Chronic Disease Prevention and Health Promotion.

Veit, C. T., & Ware, J. E. (1983). The structure of psychological distress and well-being in general populations. *Journal of Consulting and Clinical Psychology, 51,* 730–742.

Warren, K. R., Ball, M. P., Feldman, S., Liu, F., McMahon, R. P., & Kelly, D. L. (2010). Exercise program adherence using a 5-kilometer (5K) event as an achievable goal in people with schizophrenia. *Biological Research in Nursing, 13*(4), 383–390. doi:10.1177/1099800410393272

Wei, M., Kampert, J. B., Barlow, C. E., Nichaman, M. Z., Gibbons, L. W., Paffenbarger, R. S. Jr., & Blair, S. N. (1999). Relationship between low cardiorespiratory fitness and mortality in normal weight, overweight and obese men. *Journal of American Medical Association, 282,* 1547–1553.

POSTSCRIPT

Panteleimon Ekkekakis

The ambitious goal of this handbook is to provide a comprehensive, state-of-the-science, balanced, and accessible overview of the evidence on physical activity and mental health. As discussed in the introductory chapter, evaluating this literature has become immensely challenging due to numerous contradictory statements, the technical complexity of the methods involved, and, by several indications, the growing influence of bias, both in favor of and against physical activity. The combination of these factors has resulted in confusion and a large number of clinical professionals reporting limited awareness of the evidence linking physical activity to mental health outcomes. The chapters in this landmark volume will hopefully help alleviate most of the confusion and usher in a new era of intensified research efforts and more evidence-based clinical application. On the basis of the data summarized herein, the following proposals for facilitating future progress can be made.

Promote the standardization and transparency of systematic reviews. As noted in the introductory chapter, the discrepant conclusions reached in systematic reviews and meta-analyses on the effects of physical activity on the various aspects of mental health indicate a systemic dysfunction. Of course, subjectivity will always be an inextricable part of any review process that includes evaluation of evidence. However, for readers to be able to make sense of the evidence, it is important to ensure that the reasons for any discrepancies are fully transparent. If certain types of evidence are excluded (e.g., from observational, smaller-scale experimental, or neuroscientific and neuroimaging studies), the reasons should be stated. If individual studies are dismissed due to methodological weaknesses, these should be specified on a study-by-study basis; condemning an entire literature because some studies are weak seems arbitrary. Finally, it should be clear that the evaluation of methodological quality cannot be reduced to simply checking for allocation concealment, intention-to-treat, and assessor blinding; bias comes in many forms and detecting it requires considerably more scrutiny, critical thought, experience, and expertise. For these reasons, moving toward the standardization of the methodology of systematic reviews and adhering to established reporting standards seems to hold promise.

Prominent examples of standardized systems include the Preferred Reporting Items for Systematic Reviews and Meta-Analyses (PRISMA; Moher, Liberati, Tetzlaff, & Altman, 2009) and the Grading of Recommendations Assessment, Development, and Evaluation (GRADE; Guyatt, Oxman, Schünemann, Tugwell, & Knottnerus, 2011; Guyatt et al., 2008). According to PRISMA, for example, "authors should specify the methodological components that they assessed" and "if authors exclude studies from the review, or any subsequent analyses on the basis of the risk of bias, they should tell readers which studies they excluded and explain the reasons for those exclusions" (Liberati et al., 2009, p. W76). Similarly, according to GRADE, "including a risk of bias table that summarizes key criteria used to assess study limitations for each outcome for each study helps ensure transparency" (Guyatt, Oxman, Vist, et al., 2011, p. 414).

Raise visibility and adhere to reporting standards. Researchers investigating the relationship between physical activity and mental health should be encouraged to adopt a more extraverted attitude, actively raising the visibility of their work in fields like psychiatry, clinical psychology, primary care, and public health. The publication of studies solely in "specialty" journals in the field of exercise science may be one of the factors that have contributed to the low level of awareness of the evidence among many mental health researchers and clinicians. Furthermore, even when this is not mandated by journal policies, authors are encouraged to adhere closely to reporting guidelines such as the Strengthening the Reporting of Observational Studies in Epidemiology (STROBE; von Elm et al., 2007) and the Consolidated Standards of Reporting Trials (CONSORT; Boutron, Moher, Altman, Schulz, & Ravaud, 2008).

Focus on methodological rigor and establishing causation. There are still indications of inadequate efforts to eliminate sources of bias, particularly in observational and small-scale experimental trials. It should be clear that, at this stage of knowledge development, the continued accumulation of data from studies with serious methodological weaknesses is likely to be appraised as weakening, rather than strengthening, the evidence base. While both internal and external validity should be considered, establishing cause and effect must remain a top priority. In recent years, the first empirical evidence of genetic pleiotropy has emerged, suggesting that, at the population level, observed associations between physical activity and positive mental health might be explained by common genetic variation (de Geus & de Moor, 2008, 2011; de Moor, Boomsma, Stubbe, Willemsen, & de Geus, 2008):

> [W]e should consider the alternative possibility that the association between exercise behavior and mental health reflects the effects of genes that influence the propensity to exercise as well as a disposition for well-being or, framed inversely, that genes preventing people [from exercising] are also involved in the risk for anxious and depressive symptoms.
>
> *(de Geus & de Moor, 2008, pp. 55–56)*

Intensify efforts to understand motivational processes. The transition from research evidence to effective clinical practice will be impossible unless dramatic progress is made in understanding the psychological and psychobiological processes underlying the motivation for physical activity participation. Unfortunately, on this issue there has been very little substantive progress, despite the investment of considerable research funds and the accumulation of a voluminous literature. Whether physical activity can benefit mental health or not can become a purely academic exercise unless research can answer the two "most vexing questions in the field of exercise intervention: why exercisers exercise, and why non-exercisers do not" (de Geus & de Moor, 2008, p. 57). The development of physical activity interventions that maximize adherence and minimize dropout, especially among individuals facing mental health challenges, should be considered an absolute prerequisite for the successful application of physical activity in clinical practice.

References

Boutron, I., Moher, D., Altman, D.G., Schulz, K.F., & Ravaud, P. (2008). Extending the CONSORT statement to randomized trials of nonpharmacologic treatment: Explanation and elaboration. *Annals of Internal Medicine, 148*, 295–309.

de Geus, E.J.C., & de Moor, M.H.M. (2008). A genetic perspective on the association between exercise and mental health. *Mental Health and Physical Activity, 1*, 53–61.

de Geus, E.J.C., & de Moor, M.H.M. (2011). Genes, exercise, and psychological factors. In C. Bouchard & E.P. Hoffman (Eds.), *Genetic and molecular aspects of sport performance* (pp. 294–305). Chichester, UK: Blackwell.

de Moor, M.H.M., Boomsma, D.I., Stubbe, J.H., Willemsen, G., & de Geus, E.J.C. (2008). Testing causality in the association between regular exercise and symptoms of anxiety and depression. *Archives of General Psychiatry, 65*, 897–905.

Guyatt, G.H., Oxman, A.D., Schünemann, H.J., Tugwell, P., & Knottnerus, A. (2011). GRADE guidelines: A new series of articles in the *Journal of Clinical Epidemiology*. *Journal of Clinical Epidemiology, 64*, 380–382.

Guyatt, G.H., Oxman, A.D., Vist, G.E., Kunz, R., Falck-Ytter, Y., Alonso-Coello, P., & Schünemann, H.J. (2008). GRADE: An emerging consensus on rating quality of evidence and strength of recommendations. *British Medical Journal, 336*, 924–926.

Guyatt, G.H., Oxman, A.D., Vist, G., Kunz, R., Brozek, J., Alonso-Coello, P., . . . Schünemann, H.J. (2011). GRADE guidelines: Rating the quality of evidence – study limitations (risk of bias). *Journal of Clinical Epidemiology, 64*, 407–415.

Liberati, A., Altman, D.G., Tetzlaff, J., Mulrow, C., Gøtzsche, P.C., Ioannidis, J.P.A., . . . Moher, D. (2009). The PRISMA statement for reporting systematic reviews and meta-analyses of studies that evaluate health care interventions: Explanation and elaboration. *Annals of Internal Medicine, 151*, W65–W94.

Moher, D., Liberati, A., Tetzlaff, J., & Altman, D.G. (2009). Preferred Reporting Items for Systematic Reviews and Meta-Analyses: The PRISMA statement. *Annals of Internal Medicine, 151*, 264–269.

von Elm, E., Altman, D.G., Egger, M., Pocock, S.J., Gøtzsche, P.C., & Vandenbroucke, J.P. (2007). The Strengthening the Reporting of Observational Studies in Epidemiology (STROBE) statement: Guidelines for reporting observational studies. *Annals of Internal Medicine, 147*, 573–577.

INDEX

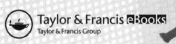